Amplification for Children with Auditory Deficits

edited by

Fred H. Bess
Judith S. Gravel
and
Anne Marie Tharpe

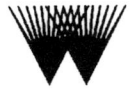

Bill Wilkerson Center Press
Nashville, Tennessee

AMPLIFICATION FOR CHILDREN WITH AUDITORY DEFICITS

Copyright © 1996 by Bill Wilkerson Center Press

All rights reserved.
No part of this book may be reproduced in any form except as may be expressly permitted by the publisher. All inquiries should be addressed to Bill Wilkerson Center Press, 1114 19th Avenue South, Nashville, Tennessee 37212.

Proceedings of the International Symposium on Amplification for Children with Auditory Deficits held October 12-16, 1994, in Palm Springs, California, cosponsored by the Bill Wilkerson Center, the Division of Hearing and Speech Sciences Vanderbilt University School of Medicine, and the Academy of Dispensing Audiologists with funding support from Oticon, Inc. Supported in part by Project #MCJ-TN 217 from the Maternal and Child Health Resources and Services Administration, Department of Health and Human Services.

Library of Congress Catalog Card Number: 95-078697
ISBN 0-9631439-3-X

This book was manufactured in the United States of America.

Contents

Preface vii
Contributors ix

PART I. Auditory Capabilities of Children with Hearing Impairment

Freeman E. McConnell Memorial Lecture
Chapter 1 1
    Amplification for Children: The Process Begins
    Mark Ross

Chapter 2 29
    Audition and the Development of Oral Communication Competency
    Arlene Earley Carney

Chapter 3 55
    Speech Perception and Production in Children with Hearing Impairment
    Arthur Boothroyd, Orna Eran, and Laurie Hanin

Chapter 4 75
    Binaural Auditory Processing and the Effects of Hearing Loss
    Wayne O. Olsen

PART II. Issues in Pediatric Amplification

Chapter 5 107
    Fitting Hearing Aids in the Pediatric Population: A Survey of Practice Procedures
    Andrea Hedley-Williams, Anne Marie Tharpe, and Fred H. Bess

Chapter 6 123
    Initiating Early Amplification: *TIPS* for Success
    Allan O. Diefendorf, Patricia S. Reitz, Michelle W. Escobar, and Michael K. Wynne

Chapter 7 145
    Amplification Selection Considerations in the Pediatric Population
    Kathryn Laudin Beauchaine and Kris Frisbie Donaghy

Chapter 8 161
    Traditional and Theoretical Approaches to Selecting Amplification for
    Infants and Young Children
    *Richard C. Seewald, K. Shane Moodie, Sheila T. Sinclair, and
    Leonard E. Cornelisse*

Chapter 9 193
    Situational Hearing Aid Response Profile (SHARP)
    Patricia G. Stelmachowicz, Ann Kalberer, and Dawna E. Lewis

Chapter 10 215
    Monitoring and Management of Amplification Systems for Children
    Jackson Roush

Chapter 11 229
    Sound-Field Amplification in the Classroom: Applied and
    Theoretical Issues
    Carl C. Crandell and Joseph J. Smaldino

PART III. New Technologies

Chapter 12 253
    Transposition Hearing Aids for Children
    Judith S. Gravel and Patricia M. Chute

Chapter 13 273
    Behind-the-Ear FM Systems: New Technology for Children
    Patricia A. Chase and Fred H. Bess

Chapter 14 283
    Cochlear Implants and Tactile Aids for Children with Profound
    Hearing Impairment
    *Mary Joe Osberger, Amy M. Robbins, Susan L. Todd, Allyson Riley,
    Karen Iler Kirk, and Arlene Earley Carney*

PART IV. Amplification and Special Populations

Chapter 15 311
    The Potential Benefits of Amplification for Young Children with
    Normal Hearing
    Noel D. Matkin

Chapter 16 321
    Amplification for Children with Minimal Hearing Loss
    Carol Flexer

Chapter 17 339
    Special Considerations for Children with Fluctuating/Progressive
    Hearing Loss
    Anne Marie Tharpe

PART V. Management of Children with Auditory Deficits

Chapter 18 369
    Developing Auditory Capabilities in Children with Severe and
    Profound Hearing Loss
    Diane Brackett

Chapter 19 383
    Auditory Intervention for Children with Mild Auditory Deficits
    Carolyn Edwards

Appendix 1 399
    Position Statement: Amplification for Infants and Children
    with Hearing Loss

Appendix 2 431
    Case Study: Amplification in Children
    Sheila T. Sinclair, K. Shane Moodie, and Richard C. Seewald

Appendix 3 441
    Clinical Grand Rounds

Author Index 455

Subject Index 469

Preface

In September 1979, Vanderbilt University School of Medicine and the Bill Wilkerson Center sponsored a meeting designed to offer an update on the status of amplification in education. Although it was recognized at that time that a properly fitted and functioning hearing aid was critical to successful habilitation/rehabilitation, many unanswered questions remained about amplification and its proper use with infants and young children. More than 300 participants from the United States and Canada attended the conference. Papers from that symposium culminated in the book *Amplification in Education* (Bess, Freeman, and Sinclair 1981).

In the intervening years, we have seen our knowledge in the area of amplification and its application for young children increase significantly. Indeed, we have witnessed numerous changes in hearing aid technology, we have learned more about early identification, assessment, and management of young children with hearing impairment, and we have developed innovative procedures to select and fit amplification. Despite these developments, we are struck by the many challenges that remain in the area of amplification for young children.

The chapters contained within this book represent the proceedings of the conference Amplification for Children with Auditory Deficits held in Palm Springs, California, October 1994. This symposium was sponsored by the Bill Wilkerson Center, the Division of Hearing and Speech Sciences Vanderbilt University School of Medicine, and the Academy of Dispensing Audiologists, and we extend our appreciation to Oticon, Inc., for their funding support of the conference. More than 200 scholars, investigators, and clinicians assembled for the purpose of generating, challenging, and promoting innovative ideas in pediatric amplification.

The purpose of this text is to provide a current review of amplification in children and to promote an appreciation for the importance and complexity of providing amplification for infants and children. Reflecting this purpose, the book is organized into six sections: Part I deals with the auditory capabilities of children with hearing impairment; Part II covers issues in pediatric amplification; Part III discusses new technologies in amplification; Part IV addresses special problems/considerations; Part V covers the issues of management; and the appendixes offer a position statement and grand rounds/case presentations on amplification in children. It is our sincere hope that the contents of this book will provide guidance for audiologists who shoulder the responsibility of providing amplification to infants and children with hearing loss.

Numerous individuals contributed to the success of the symposium and this book. In particular, the authors and editors recognize Kathy Hollis and Shelia Lewis, who assisted with many of the details throughout the conference, including the local arrangements, and who typed all the correspondence concerned with the symposium. Georgia Walker typed and formatted the chapters for this book. Mary Sue Fino-Szumski coordinated manuscript preparation and oversaw the entire publication process. We also acknowledge Carol Davis and Ken Smith, representing the Academy of Dispensing Audiologists, which served as the cosponsor of the International Symposium. We thank a number of our colleagues who generously reviewed the chapters in this book including Martha Anne Ellis, Raymond M. Hurley, Bronya Keats, and Tad Zelski. John Bamford, Ruth Bentler, Arthur Boothroyd, Allan Diefendorf, David Hawkins, Judy Kopun, Noel Matkin, and Gus Mueller served as reviewers and made helpful comments on the position statement on Amplification for Infants and Children with Hearing Loss, which appears in Appendix 1. We are especially grateful to Arthur Boothroyd, whose comprehensive and critical review strongly influenced the final version of the position statement. In addition, we are grateful to the Maternal and Child Health Bureau, which recognized the need for such a meeting.

Finally, we wish to thank our spouses, Susie, Bruce, and Jim, and our children, Amy and Danny, Jay and Julie, Roy and Julia, who never complained about our time or attention away from them while working on this book. Their contributions have not gone unnoticed.

Fred H. Bess, Judith S. Gravel, and Anne Marie Tharpe, editors

REFERENCE

Bess, F.H., Freeman, B.A., and Sinclair, J.S. 1981. *Amplification in education.* Washington, D.C.: Alexander Graham Bell Association for the Deaf.

Contributors

Kathryn Laudin Beauchaine, M.A.
Department of Audiology
Boys Town National Research
 Hospital
Omaha, Nebraska

Fred H. Bess, Ph.D.
Division of Hearing and Speech
 Sciences
Vanderbilt University School of
 Medicine and
Bill Wilkerson Center
Nashville, Tennessee

Arthur Boothroyd, Ph.D.
Graduate School
City University of New York
New York, New York

Diane Brackett, Ph.D.
CHIP Hearing Services
University of Connecticut
Storrs, Connecticut

Arlene Earley Carney, Ph.D.
Department of Communication
 Disorders
University of Minnesota
Minneapolis, Minnesota

Patricia A. Chase, M.S.
Division of Hearing and Speech
 Sciences
Vanderbilt University School of
 Medicine
Nashville, Tennessee

Patricia M. Chute, Ed.D.
Children's Cochlear Implant Center
Manhattan Eye, Ear, and Throat
 Hospital
New York, New York

Leonard E. Cornelisse, M.S.
Hearing Health Care Research Unit
Department of Communicative
 Disorders
The University of Western Ontario
London, Ontario, Canada

Carl C. Crandell, Ph.D.
Department of Communication
 Processes and Disorders
University of Florida
Gainesville, Florida

Allan O. Diefendorf, Ph.D.
Department of Otolaryngology-Head
 and Neck Surgery
Indiana University School of Medicine
Indianapolis, Indiana

Kris Frisbie Donaghy
Department of Audiology
Omaha Public Schools
Omaha, Nebraska

Carolyn Edwards, M.Cl.Sc., M.B.A.
Auditory Management Services
Toronto, Ontario, Canada

Orna Eran, M.Phil.
Graduate School
City University of New York
New York, New York

Michelle W. Escobar, M.A.
Department of Otolaryngology-Head
  and Neck Surgery
Indiana University School of Medicine
Indianapolis, Indiana

Carol Flexer, Ph.D.
School of Communicative Disorders
The University of Akron
Akron, Ohio

Judith S. Gravel, Ph.D.
Albert Einstein College of Medicine
Bronx, New York

Laurie Hanin, Ph.D.
New York League for the Hard of
  Hearing
New York, New York

Andrea Hedley-Williams, M.S.
Bill Wilkerson Center
Nashville, Tennessee

Ann Kalberer, M.S.
Boys Town National Research
  Hospital
Omaha, Nebraska

Karen Iler Kirk, Ph.D.
Department of Otolaryngology
Indiana University School of Medicine
Indianapolis, Indiana

Dawna E. Lewis, M.A.
Boys Town National Research
  Hospital
Omaha, Nebraska

Noel D. Matkin, Ph.D.
Hearing and Speech Sciences
University of Arizona
Tucson, Arizona

K. Shane Moodie, M.Cl.Sc.
Department of Communicative
  Disorders
The University of Western Ontario
London, Ontario, Canada

Wayne O. Olsen, Ph.D.
Section of Audiology
Department of Otorhinolaryngology
Mayo Clinic
Rochester, Minnesota

Mary Joe Osberger, Ph.D.
Advanced Bionics Corporation
Sylmar, California

Patricia S. Reitz, M.A.
Department of Otolaryngology-Head
  and Neck Surgery
Indiana University School of Medicine
Indianapolis, Indiana

Allyson Riley, M.S.
Department of Otolaryngology
Indiana University School of Medicine
Indianapolis, Indiana

Amy M. Robbins, M.S.
Department of Otolaryngology
Indiana University School of Medicine
Indianapolis, Indiana

Mark Ross, Ph.D.
University of Connecticut
Storrs, Connecticut

Jackson Roush, Ph.D.
Division of Speech and Hearing
  Sciences, School of Medicine
University of North Carolina
Chapel Hill, North Carolina

Richard C. Seewald, Ph.D.
Hearing Health Care Research Unit
Department of Communicative
 Disorders
The University of Western Ontario
London, Ontario, Canada

Sheila T. Sinclair, M.Cl.Sc.
Hearing Health Care Research Unit
Department of Communicative
 Disorders
The University of Western Ontario
London, Ontario, Canada

Joseph J. Smaldino, Ph.D.
Department of Communicative
 Disorders
University of Northern Iowa
Cedar Falls, Iowa

Patricia G. Stelmachowicz, Ph.D.
Boys Town National Research
 Hospital
Omaha, Nebraska

Anne Marie Tharpe, Ph.D.
Department of Communication
 Disorders
Louisiana State University Medical
 Center
New Orleans, Louisiana

Susan L. Todd, M.A.
Department of Otolaryngology
Indiana University School of Medicine
Indianapolis, Indiana

Michael K. Wynne, Ph.D.
Department of Otolaryngology-Head
 and Neck Surgery
Indiana University School of Medicine
Indianapolis, Indiana

DEDICATED TO MARK ROSS

Pioneer in pediatric audiology; steadfast leader in advocating the early and appropriate selection and use of amplification for young children with hearing impairment; consummate clinician and educator. His monumental contributions to children with hearing impairment and their families have strongly inspired and influenced all of us in the profession.

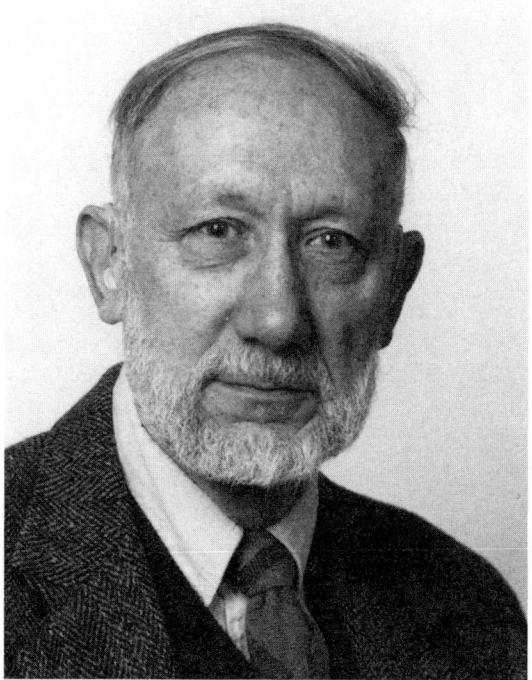

"Whatever we do, it is necessary to keep in mind that when we test and treat a young child with hearing impairment, we are also dealing with the parents—their dreams for their child—and, further, that what we do has an impact that transcends time and place. It is the children and their families who must live with the consequences of our early actions."

Mark Ross 1992

PART I.

Auditory Capabilities of Children with Hearing Impairment

Freeman E. McConnell Memorial Lecture

Amplification for Children:
The Process Begins

Mark Ross

PREAMBLE

As an undergraduate and master's student, I was fortunate to have Dr. Robert West, one of the founders of the American Speech-Language-Hearing Association (ASHA), as a major professor. I still remember two examples he gave to illustrate the clinical and scientific learning process, both of which are relevant in this context. In one, he drew a small circle on the blackboard. The area within the circle represented our current knowledge in any area, while the periphery defined the unknown. Since the border of a periphery is much greater than the area within a circle, it demonstrated that the unknown is always greater than the known. Furthermore, as the circle representing knowledge increases, the periphery increases correspondingly and so does the unknown. In other words, the more we know, the more there is to know. I would not take this literally in all areas of knowledge, but the example illustrates the continuing challenge we face as professionals: When we learn or do something new, we often seem to be opening up more questions than answers.

In the second example, Dr. West likened much of clinical progress to a spiral spring. Oftentimes, while we may appear to be circling back to where we were, we are actually at a higher level but at the same azimuth point. As we figuratively look down, our perspective is enriched by the knowledge of what did and did not work in the past—or it should be but sometimes is not, which is one of the themes of this chapter.

As I survey the literature and consider my own experiences in the field, it is clear that we have an abundant body of knowledge regarding amplification for children. We now possess an enormous quantity of information on this topic—our circle has grown to what appears to be monstrous proportions—yet the periphery remains as a challenge and a goad for continuing investigations. The path leading to the current state of the art is the spiral of which Dr. West spoke. Current developments, concepts, technology, and so on are often foreshadowed by previous events; that is, to truly appreciate where we are, we should know where we have been. And this is another theme of the chapter.

In my time in the field, I have often observed that for many of our colleagues, their professional history begins when they enter the field. Perhaps their professors exposed them to the older literature, but amidst the stresses of entering a new profession, much of the historical background they did get was probably relegated to the "not now relevant" category. This is understandable when one is faced with the immediacy of meeting the needs of a waiting client. Still, to be a member of a profession, one has to place oneself in a historical context; we build on the contributions of our predecessors, as we hope that those who follow us will stand on our shoulders. Of course, the older one gets, the more history one will have lived through; what for me is simply a recapitulation of my professional activities may be ancient history for some of you. In the following pages, I shall review some of the highlights of amplification for children from a truly ancient history perspective (that is, from before I entered the field) and from the time I began working with children with hearing impairment. Since I know my own work best, I shall probably devote an inordinate amount of time to my opinions and practices as they have evolved over the years while acknowledging the contributions made by others toward my own thinking.

My review of "the beginning of the process," that is, the historical approach, will acknowledge the work of some of our early colleagues on the topic. More often than not, what we herald as a new development is simply a refinement of previous technology and applications, accompanied by a relabeling process that obscures the debt owed to previous generations.

The subtitle of this chapter, "the process begins," was selected to convey the reason we engage in this activity in the first place, and that is to give children with hearing losses the best auditory access we can to their language. Really, this is what we are all about. The ultimate goal of amplification for children is a reduction of the auditory consequences of a hearing loss. This does not automatically follow when even the best of amplification systems are provided. A crucial step has been taken; concurrently and continually, all the other ingredients of a comprehensive habilitation program have to be applied to invest this step with its true significance (Luterman 1979, 1991; Ross, Brackett, and Maxon 1991; Roush and Matkin 1994). Notwithstanding the existence of a high degree of technological sophistication and the availability of comprehensive habilitation programs, there is no guarantee that these will be used for a *particular child. Social forces and attitudes influence their application. Because something can be done does not mean that it will be done or even that it should be done. And this will be the final theme of this chapter.*

THE BEGINNING OF THE PROCESS

THE PREELECTRONICS AGE

In its earliest manifestations, amplification for children was inextricably associated with their education. Scattered through the history of Deaf education were reports of children who were deaf being able to hear if one spoke loudly enough directly into their ears or used an ear trumpet (Bender 1981). The realization that some of these children could hear was formally recognized in the middle 18th century, with public demonstrations of miraculous cures (reported by Goldstein 1933, 1939). By their own classification, educators in the 19th century reported that more than 30% of the children in schools for the Deaf were semi-deaf, partial hearing, or hard of hearing. These children had significant degrees of residual hearing that could be stimulated by *ad concham* presentations (which Wedenberg [1951] did with his son some years later) or with a speaking tube of some kind.

The observations that *some* children who were deaf and attended special schools could hear undoubtedly stimulated the development of modern amplification systems. In the preamplification age, at a time when there was a higher incidence of untreatable and untreated conductive hearing losses than at the present time, there also were a greater number of children who were partially deaf (or partially hearing, depending upon whether one views a cup as half empty or full) but could potentially respond to high-level auditory inputs. The fact that Deaf children are not always deaf has been a source of confusion, simplification, misdiagnosis, and mismanagement from that time to the present day (Ross and Calvert 1967).

In the United States, Max Goldstein, founder of the Central Institute for the Deaf (CID) in 1914, based his theory and work on his previous training with Urbantschitsch in Vienna in the late 1800s. His book *The Acoustic Method* (1939) and many other of his published articles, plus his work at CID, clearly nominate him as the founder of the auditory method for training children with hearing impairment in the U.S. (However, E.M. Gallaudet in 1884, as well as others at that time, recognized that children who were semi-deaf could benefit from a program that stimulated their residual hearing.) Goldstein began his work at the St. Joseph School in St. Louis and later carried on his work at CID. As one reads through his book, his disappointment in the way that other schools practiced the acoustic method is clearly evident: "The pedagogic technique . . . has not been applied with sufficient care, detail and persistency . . . and with sufficient regard for the

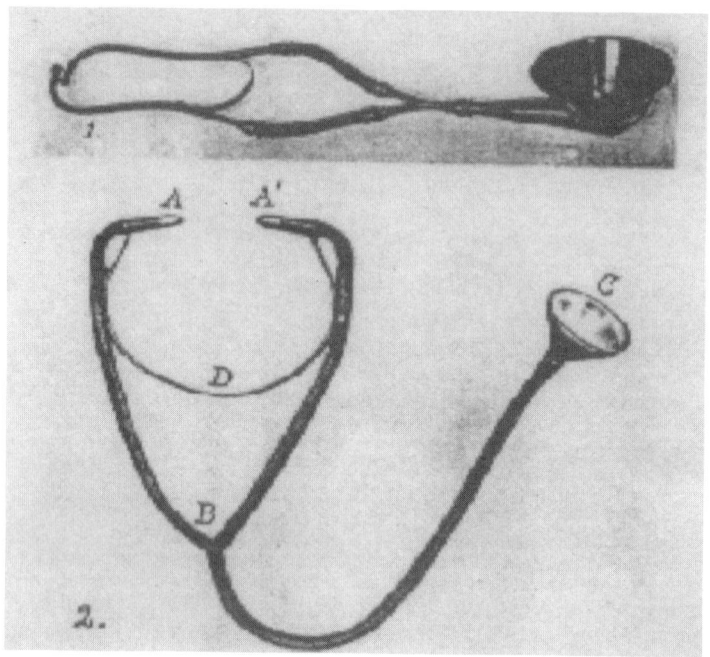

Figure 1. Two speaking tubes. From Goldstein 1939. Reprinted with the permission of the *Laryngoscope*.

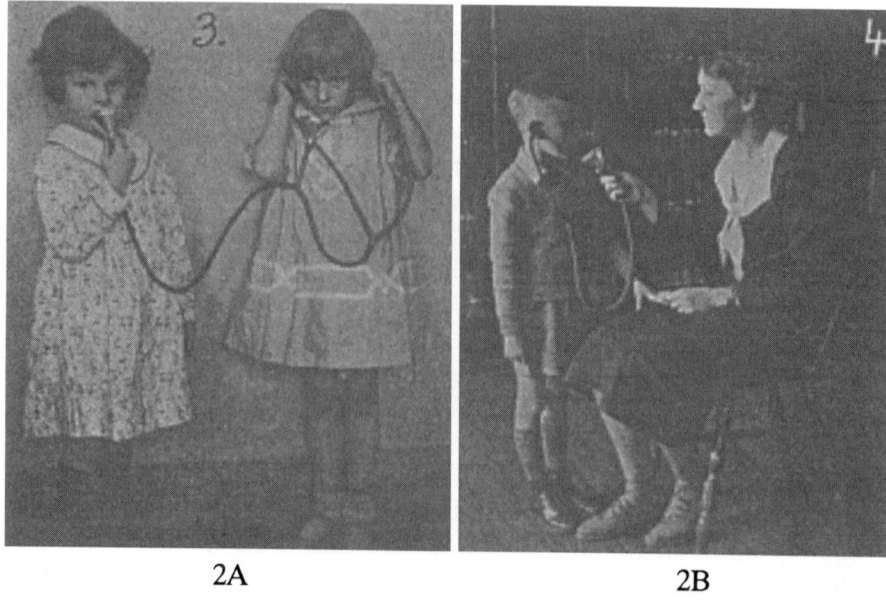

Figure 2A. Child-to-child communication with speaking tube. **2B.** Example of self-monitoring with speaking tube. From Goldstein 1939. Reprinted with the permission of the *Laryngoscope*.

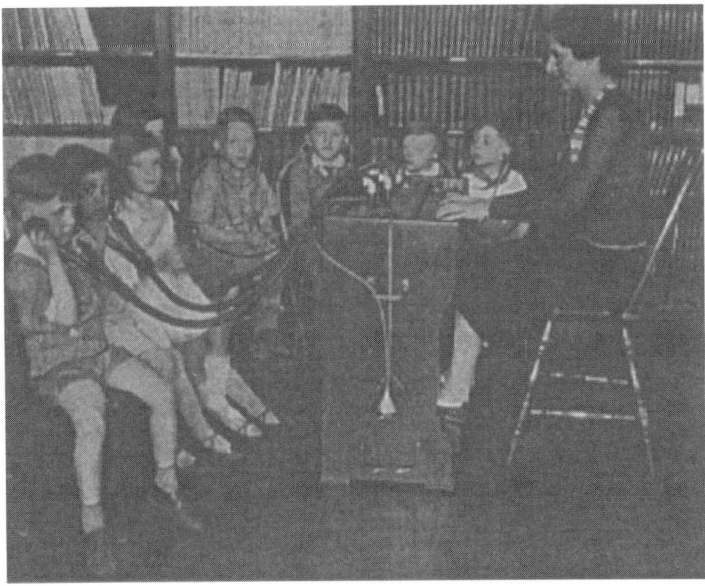

Figure 3. Auditory stimulation with organ. From Goldstein 1939. Reprinted with the permission of the *Laryngoscope*.

fundamental principles" (Goldstein 1939, p. 17). (In passing, we can note that this complaint and observation also apply today in respect to our much greater potential, and our relative failure, to fully stimulate residual hearing in many more children.) Often described as a complete proponent of an analytic method of training, Goldstein does incorporate synthetic exercises designed for the auditory comprehension of speech and language. Sound exercises were conducted first with various musical instruments, speaking tubes (figure 1) used for individual instruction (figures 2A and 2B), and a specially constructed organ for group instruction (figure 3).

DEVELOPMENT OF GROUP AUDITORY TRAINING SYSTEMS

It was apparent to the early teachers who used the speaking tube that the device was not sufficiently powerful for many children. Something else was needed. The first electrical auditory training system specifically designed for sound stimulation in an educational setting was used at CID (figure 4). This rather massive device has to be considered the forerunner of group auditory training systems as well as personal hearing aids. From that time onward, the goal was to design better and smaller amplification devices (although I doubt that any teacher or clinician could have conceived of the present generation of miniature hearing aids).

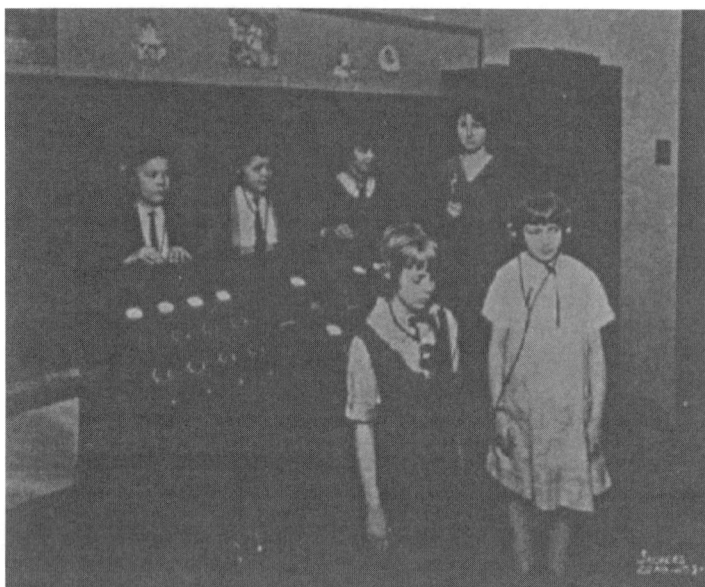

Figure 4. First electrical group hearing aid. Note "auditory only" listening task. From Goldstein 1939. Reprinted with the permission of the *Laryngoscope*.

Coupled to the realization that many children who were deaf could hear, the increased acceptance, or at least prominence, of the acoustic method appears to have stimulated the continued development of electrical group auditory training systems. In the *Volta Review* alone, 39 articles were published prior to World War II (WWII) devoted to stimulating residual hearing with various auditory training procedures, beginning with a 1904 article by Urbantschitsch (Goldstein's mentor). Eight more were published during this period in the *Annals of the Deaf* on the same topic. Educators began expanding the use of amplification beyond its application with children who were clearly hard of hearing to those classified as deaf. Reports published in the 1920s and the 1930s indicated various degrees of success in stimulating residual hearing among children who were deaf and not just children who were partially deaf. Undoubtedly, many of these students who were considered deaf had significant degrees of residual hearing, which could not be tested with the audiometric tools available at that time (Urbantschitsch used a lack of response to tuning fork stimulation to define total deafness).

Beginning with just one installation in 1926, the number of schools possessing group auditory training systems increased until by 1936, the majority of schools (day, residential, and private) reported using them (Watson and Watson 1937). This came out of a professional association committee report that recommended an increased focus on using the residual hearing of children in schools. This same report expresses concerns that have a modern ring to them, covering such topics as the effectiveness of selective amplification, the negative impact of poor classroom acoustics, the necessity of providing soundproof-testing facilities, and the need to improve the quality of the amplified sound produced by group hearing aids. All of these concerns were expressed *before* audiology existed as a separate profession. An immersion into this older literature is a healthy antidote to the misconception that audiologists were the first to discover and exploit the residual hearing of children in schools.

In going through this literature, I found particularly interesting the changes in terminology that took place during this time. *Auricular training* was initially the "in" term describing the stimulation and use of residual hearing, later overlapping and superseded by *acoustic method*, *acoustic training*, and *auditory training*. As best as I can determine, they were basically describing the same phenomenon. Most used *unisensory* acoustic inputs at some stage but reverted to multisensory stimulation for the major part of the training process. As a matter of fact, Goldstein (1939, p. 18) did try to bring order to the terminological chaos by insisting on the term the *acoustic method*. Unfortunately, he sadly underestimated the need to own a procedure by employing a new label to describe more or less minute variations on an existing concept, a propensity that is evidently still among us *(aurilism, auditory-oral, aural-oral, acoupedic, unisensory, auditory-verbal*—did I miss any?).

Whatever the differences or similarities between the methods (mostly regarding varying degrees of dependency on the visual channel) and whatever the term used to describe them, they all had in common the necessity of an amplification system that could present an audible amplified speech signal to the children. Group auditory training systems were limited in furthering the goals of these early teachers since they could be employed only in classrooms. The typical procedure was to provide auditory training exercises for some period during the school day. More often than not, the exercises were purely listening and, possibly, speaking activities, and not incorporated as part of the usual academic program. That is, subject matter was not necessarily taught during auditory training. Although the group trainer may have been used during subject matter teaching, the nature of auditory sensations remained basically irrelevant (when it could be perceived at all). The children depended on speechreading or the amalgamation of signs used by teachers with normal hearing for message comprehension.

The message this sent was that hearing is a structured classroom activity with little or no relevance in real life. The fallacy in this mode of operation was apparent early in the 1950s, with the research results of Hudgins (1953) and Clarke (1957), among others. They pointed out that to be effective, amplified sound not only had to be employed in all classrooms throughout the school day but also had to be stressed as an avenue for language comprehension and development. Their research supported the advantages of amplified sound, with the children who were systematically amplified doing better in speech, speech perception, and academic attainments than children who were not amplified (Clarke 1957) or who were exposed to an inferior auditory training system (Hudgins 1953).

Some of the auditory training systems developed during the 1950s would still be considered acceptable today in terms of their electroacoustic characteristics, if not their size and convenience. One developed in Germany at that time included a wide-frequency band, undistorted high output, a microphone mounted on the earphones with an on-off switch, and individual ear volume (but not tone) controls (Schmael 1960). The one used at CID and at the Clarke School for the Deaf at that time also included a wide-frequency band (100 to 8000 Hz) and high output (up to 140 dB), with a teacher microphone and four additional microphones suspended by wires over the children, ensuring improved self-monitoring and child-to-child communication. However, there were no individual tone or volume control provisions (Hudgins 1953). In terms of the lack of tone controls, it was not until the early 1970s that our "modern" FM auditory training systems included this feature.

In the description of the auditory training system given above by Hudgins (1953), as well as by a number of other early educators of children with hearing impairment, the importance of ensuring adequate auditory self-monitoring of speech and child-to-child communication is explicitly emphasized. These people were very well aware of the significance of the teacher's and children's microphone position. While writing this section, I was reminded that this attitude was hardly universal by an experience I had in the early 1960s (we are beginning to move up to the modern era, as I define it). I was visiting a school for the Deaf and noticed that only one microphone was connected to the group auditory training system, located next to the teacher. When I commented to the principal who was accompanying me that it would not enable the children to monitor their voices, she said, and I quote, "It is against the school policy for the children to hear themselves when they talk"! At hearing that, I also became speechless.

DEVELOPMENT OF PERSONAL HEARING AIDS

A number of early writers noted that to be truly effective, residual hearing had to be stimulated all the time, not just during classroom activities. Beginning approximately in the late 1920s and early 1930s, advances in electronics made possible the development of wearable hearing aids (Watson and Tolan 1949). They were wearable, I should note, only by the standards of that day (figures 5 and 6). (Although if the advantages of hearing are

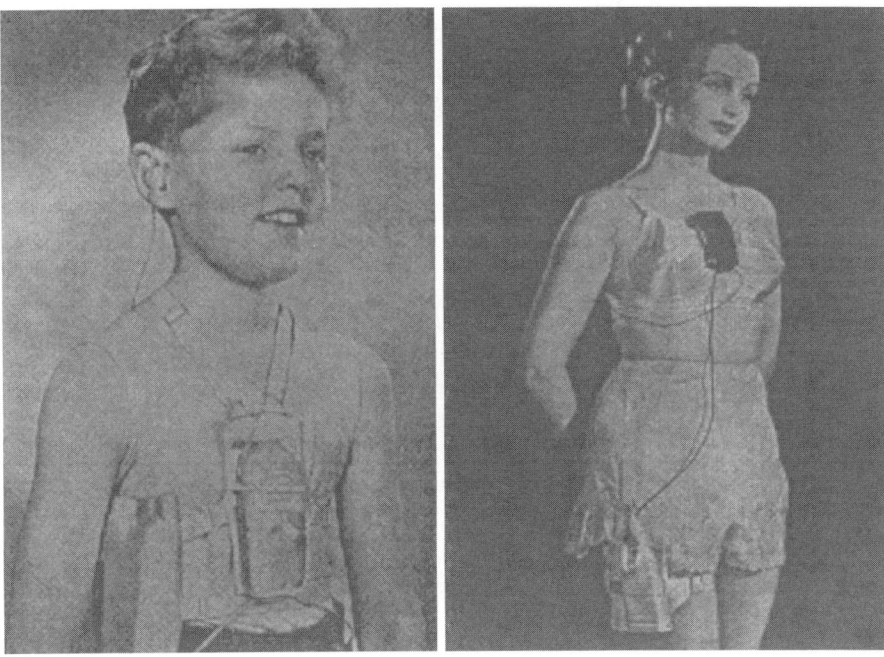

Figures 5 and 6. Duopack body-worn aid on young boy and on young woman. From Davis 1951. Reprinted with the permission of Holt, Rinehart and Winston, Inc.

sufficiently salient, any size device will be accepted—cochlear implants being a case in point.) That educators—not audiologists who did not exist at the time—were seriously considering using personal aids in their schools can be seen by the 12 articles devoted to personal hearing aids published in the *Volta Review* and the *American Annals of the Deaf* prior to WWII.

Actually, judging from the appearance and limitations of these early instruments, it is a wonder that they were used as often as these articles imply (O'Connor 1938). Perhaps that was due to the relatively greater occurrence of milder and conductive hearing losses among the children in schools for the Deaf in those days, since children with these hearing losses were more likely to benefit from amplification. Approximately one-third of the children used bone-conduction vibrators with their individual and group hearing aids, which gives us some insight into the relative ineffectiveness of medical intervention for middle ear disorders at that time (Watson and Watson 1937). For the vast majority of the children, during the period prior to WWII, when amplified sound was provided at all, it was through group auditory training systems, and then in only a relatively few schools.

By today's standards, these hearing aids were large, and they performed very poorly (Watson and Tolan 1949). Their bandwidth was

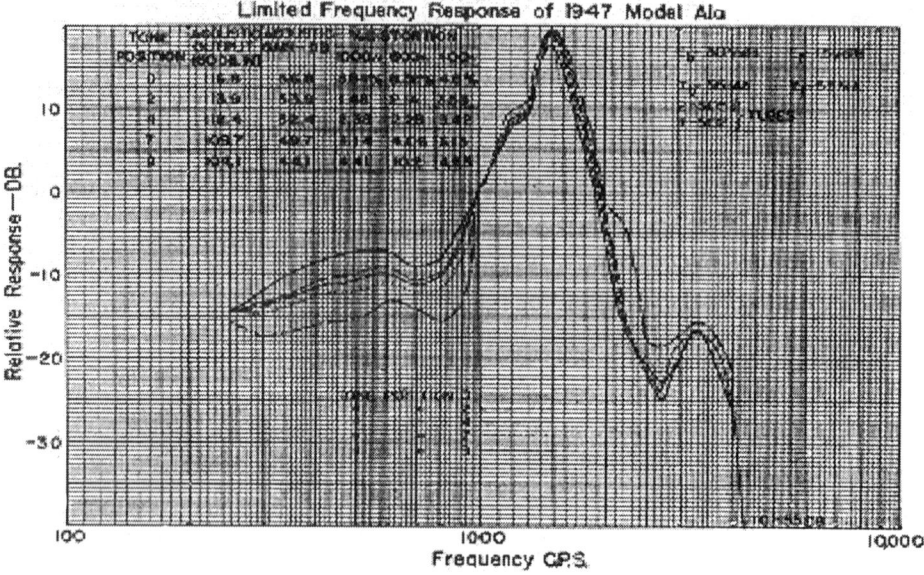

Figure 7. Frequency response of a 1947 hearing aid. From Watson and Tolan 1949. Reprinted with the permission of Williams and Wilkins.

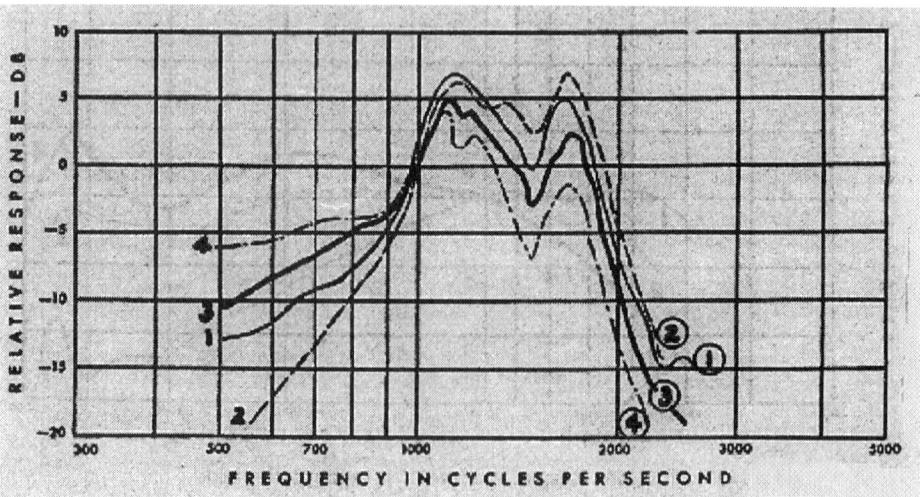

Figure 8. Frequency response of widely available hearing aid. From Watson and Tolan 1949. Reprinted with the permission of Williams and Wilkins.

limited, the response was peaked, and they displayed excessive distortion (figures 7 and 8). Their imposing physical dimensions essentially precluded a binaural fitting, particularly for younger children. That they accessed and improved auditory capabilities for some children cannot be doubted, particularly children with conductive hearing losses; that these hearing aids could provide significant benefit for any child with a sensorineural hearing loss or one with a greater than a moderate hearing loss was doubtful.

Complicating hearing aid fittings at that time was the necessity to take ear impressions using a plaster of Paris mixture (high quality to be sure). In taking such an impression on a squirming child, one had to be very certain that the cotton block was in place, that the child remained perfectly still during the period the impression material set, and that all of the material could be removed (Watson and Tolan 1949). Although not specifically mentioned in the older literature, the difficulty of doing all this must have influenced the provision of hearing aids for young children. Plaster of Paris was used in the first number of ear impressions made on me, and I can still remember how the technician (no audiologist) stressed the necessity to remain perfectly still while the impression set, and how uncomfortable the heat it generated in my ear became.

In the post-WWII era, rapid and continuing advances in electronics led to significant improvement in hearing aid performance. During this period, audiologists entered the scene, bringing their special skills and research orientation with them. Hearing aids became smaller and more convenient to wear. In early 1952, the size and performance characteristics of the first body hearing aid I wore seemed quite adequate. In spite of being a vacuum tube hearing aid, and requiring two rather large batteries, it was only a little larger than a pack of cigarettes—about the same size as current body aids (the few that are still around). Its frequency extended from about 300 Hz to about 3 kHz. The response was evidently based on the bandwidth of telephones (Watson and Tolan 1949, p. 327), which permitted adequate speech comprehension for adults with sophisticated preexisting language competencies.

Children, however, are another matter. Unfortunately, wearable hearing aids designed for adults had to be used with children as well. Because a hearing aid response may be sufficient to permit adults to *recognize* a known language does not mean that it is optimal for children with congenital hearing impairment to *develop* auditory-verbal competency in the same language. The linguistic information carried by frequencies above 3 kHz is considerable. The *lowest* spectral peak of the phoneme /s/, for example, is in the vicinity of 5 to 6 kHz in different vowel contexts (Boothroyd and Medwetsky 1992). These authors suggest that the upper frequency range of wearable hearing aids should be in the vicinity of 10 kHz. As it happens, at relatively high-output levels the upper frequency range of modern hearing aids, necessary for children with severe and profound hearing losses, rarely exceeds 4 kHz. In this area, at least, there is much room for improvement.

Sam Lybarger, a pioneer in this field if there ever was one, recognized the need for a wider bandwidth in wearable hearing aids more than 60 years ago when he and a colleague recommended a frequency range of 100 to 6000 kHz (Haller and Lybarger 1933).

THE PROCESS BEGINS

In organizing this section, I am going to proceed more or less chronologically, from the initial fitting process to the use of amplification as an educational tool, reviewing and commenting on the evolution of some of the practices and issues that particularly interest me. Since much of the following material is based on my own experiences and memories, not every assertion will be buttressed by a citation from the literature.

THE FIRST VISITS

The process begins when the child is diagnosed as having a hearing loss (McConnell 1968; McConnell and Liff 1975). I would hope to have hearing aids selected for children by their first birthday, a goal that has been expressed for at least the last 40 years (Pickles 1957) but is still far from a reality (Benoit 1994; Ross and Green 1990; see figure 9). My reasoning for this recommendation is simple and has been expressed in detail elsewhere (Ross 1986; Ross et al. 1991).

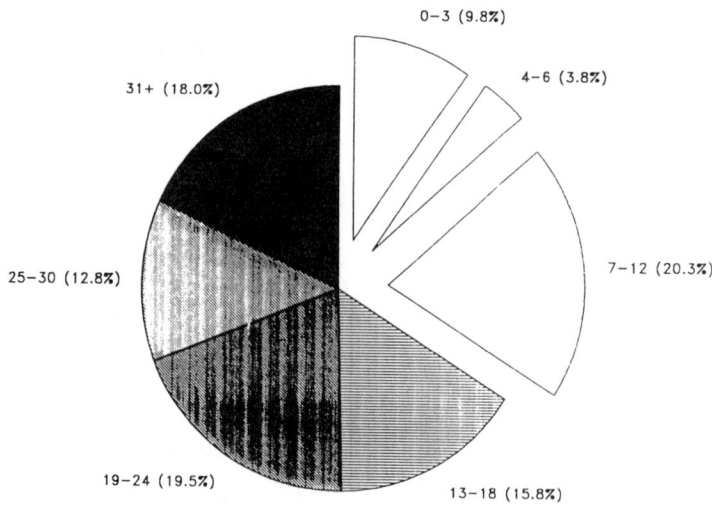

Figure 9. Age (in months) of initial identification of congenital hearing loss. From Benoit 1994. Reprinted with permission.

By starting earlier, we have an opportunity to employ a *developmental* rather than a *remedial* approach to training. In adopting this clinical approach, I was heavily influenced by the work of Whetnall and Fry (1964), Tervoort (1964), McNeill (1966), and Lennenberg (1967), among others. The implication of these authors' work was that children have an innate and biologically based capacity to develop speech and language, *provided that they receive an appropriate sample of the language*. The language exposure has to be early in a child's life—how early has never really been defined other than the earlier the better—and has to take place in a conversational context. Although this capacity is not tied exclusively to the auditory channel, as an audiologist I felt it my obligation, and I still do, to try to ensure that the auditory channel was fully stimulated before considering a purely visual approach.

Insofar as the use of residual hearing for children was concerned, it was soon apparent to me that this endeavor was not a very high priority among clinical audiologists. The significant literature was not being published in the U.S. To understand the application and priority placed on residual hearing, it was necessary to examine the work done by our colleagues in England and elsewhere in Europe (Ewing 1957, 1960; Ewing and Ewing 1961; Watson 1961). These authors stressed the efficacy and the many variables affecting the use of residual hearing (i.e., early intervention, modifications of the electroacoustic response, monaural/binaural, effect of room acoustics, and auditory training/learning procedures). Coming to this continent from England in the early 1960s, Dan Ling brought much of this information with him, and he has added his own creative contributions to the prerequisite conditions for fostering the auditory-verbal learning process (Ling 1976).

Early amplification is also necessary to try to preclude or limit the auditory sensory deprivation effects. The evidence on this topic seemed sufficiently salient more than 20 years ago to warrant review in a small monograph (Ross 1972a). Since then the phenomenon has received increasing attention. The initial research with animals convincingly demonstrated that early sound deprivations were associated with anatomic and physiologic sequelae. It could be argued that children are not animals (though there are times that some parents would disagree with this assertion) and therefore that this research was not applicable to them. I have always felt that the presumption should always be in the children's favor, and that we should act as if auditory sensory deprivation also affects children unless proven otherwise. Recent research supports the wisdom of this orientation, in that deprivation effects were evident in only one twin with episodes of recurrent otitis media (Brown 1994), and in the nonaided ear of children fit with monaural hearing aids (Gelfand and Silman 1993). The convincing evidence supporting the concept of "adult-onset auditory deprivation" (reviewed in the *Journal of the American Academy of Audiology*, Sept. 1993) adds additional weight to this orientation. As with the developmental approach, we really do not know how early is early—three months, six months, one year, two years, later? Again, lacking concrete evidence with children, we have to operate with the presumption that earlier *is* better, that the longer children with hearing impairment are deprived of an amplified speech signal, the more possible auditory deprivation effects will limit their potential auditory accomplishments.

Some of the ardent exponents of early amplification were not audiologists at all, but dedicated teachers tremendously devoted to children who were deaf (Beebe 1953; Griffiths 1964; Pollack 1964). They were teachers and therapists, and their results were reported in case history rather than "scientific" formats. They had in common their belief in the efficacy of amplified sound for the overwhelming majority of children with hearing impairment. I think they made an immense contribution to our current clinical practices with young children. They would fit hearing aids on children at an age much younger than any audiologist would feel comfortable doing it while stressing the potency of even the tiniest bit of residual hearing. My recollection is that they made many audiologists uncomfortable. We were measuring hearing thresholds, and we knew that some children really were deaf. Then, too, they were too zealous, too much believers to communicate effectively with a young profession that felt "truth" lay somewhere between an analysis of variance and a matched control group. Their basic approach is recycled now as the auditory-verbal approach, and its merits have become clinically respectable.

Early detection will also help us assist parents to deal with the reality of children's hearing loss before possible secondary problems emerge. I do not know of any evidence suggesting that our intervention with parents can be more effective if we begin to assist them while the children are younger, but again, I would make a presumption in the parents' favor. We should also recognize that there is a reciprocal relationship between parents and children; if we work with the children earlier, and they show clearly defined auditory-verbal progress, the parents are going to feel better. Their attitude will in turn influence how they interact with their children, which should foster further progress in the children, and so on. This should not be interpreted to mean that parents are responsible if their child fails to demonstrate adequate auditory-verbal progress. Too many other variables are involved. Success, too, has many dimensions, not the least of which is a happy child. Fostering a sense of guilt among caring parents is just too easy to do and helps no one.

The professional community is increasingly recognizing the centrality of the parental role (Luterman 1979, 1991). It was not always so. Parents were often viewed, at best, as chauffeurs responsible for bringing a child to the clinic or, at worst, as obstacles to our "ideal" clinical interventions. More often than not, they were tolerated rather than embraced as people with a major stake in the outcome. Counseling often consisted of some words in the waiting room as the child was brought back from the test or therapy room. Often, parents were given a role to assist the clinician in getting the child ready for a hearing test by engaging in preliminary play audiometry games at home, which included getting a child used to wearing headphones (thank goodness for the present generation of insert earphones).

Since it was a common practice to delay hearing aid fitting until accurate bilateral thresholds were obtained, the process of fitting an aid could take many months. If one were fortunate enough to detect and diagnose a hearing loss in a child by age 2 or 3—and this has not gotten a lot better in recent years (Benoit 1994)—it would still take lots of preparation time before the hearing aid (monaural, usually, at that time) could be fit. First, it was necessary to schedule hearing testing training sessions. These would consist of a therapist playing with the child, trying to get the child to associate a sound with some action—that is, preliminary play audiometry. My memory of this is that of a wailing child being torn from the mother's breast and carried down to the therapy room, where the first 15 or 20 minutes would be spent trying to gain rapport. Sometimes this distress went on for months, at weekly intervals, until the child was "conditioned" to take a hearing test. The same separation trauma occurred even after accurate air conduction thresholds were obtained, since hearing aids were not generally fit without an introductory program of auditory training (Carhart 1947; Newby 1958; Streng, Fitch, Hedgecock, Phillips, and Carrell 1958), carried out in a therapy room without the parents (although in "modern" clinics they could see and hear their child's distress through a one-way mirror).

Such an auditory training program could last many months. One goal was to have children enjoy listening to the sound; if they objected, one point of view was that amplification should not be forced on them. A child should not be "burdened" with wearing a hearing aid unless he could understand the purpose of the hearing aid, learn how to manipulate it, and "make known his responses to amplification" (Streng et al. 1958, p. 144). That was not an unusual attitude at that time. Considering that monopack hearing aids had just been recently developed, and that hearing aids were truly a physical burden to be worn, the feeling becomes more understandable. The problem is that this attitude is still with us to some extent. Instead of viewing hearing aids as a technical miracle, as a way a growing child can access more of the communication code of his or her culture, there is a feeling that we are inflicting children with a burden by requiring them to use hearing aids. The devices become visible signs of the children's impairment rather than tools for reducing its impact (I will, below, address the attitude that children with severe and profound hearing losses should not be amplified because they are members, potentially at any rate, of a visually oriented culture, in which case the entire idea of hearing aids becomes irrelevant).

Since we learn from our mentors, that was the way I practiced audiology when I first became an audiologist. But I soon changed. It was much easier to test a child with the mother (few clinics saw fathers in those days) holding or in the same room with the child. We did not have auditory brainstem response (ABR) or visual reinforcement audiometry (VRA) tests at that time; mainly, we depended on behavioral observations and history (McConnell 1968; Ross and Lerman 1966). Yet some of us began fitting aids on children when we were pretty sure they had a hearing loss without requiring precise thresholds. Every once in a while, and I shudder to think of those times, we tested some children using a Galvanic Skin Response (GSR) Audiometer in an attempt to establish accurate thresholds (Knox 1972). Basically, this test measures the changes in skin resistance produced by an electrical shock, weak to be sure. A tone is associated with the shock, and after a few pairings, the idea is that the tone by itself would soon elicit the change in skin resistance. It was a required test in the Veterans Administration audiology clinic I worked in before I entered academia. The adults feared and disliked it, but being adults they could, and did, voice their displeasure.

There was also a great deal of interest in using the test for measuring the hearing of young, "difficult" children with multiple disabilities. The kids hated it, the parents hated it, and I hated it. Pretty soon, I began thinking for myself and decided that in spite of all the "authority" associated with the test, the disadvantages more than outweighed the advantages. This lesson is still germane. Learning from one's mentors and predecessors does not mean abrogating one's own intelligence, experience, and instincts. As I recall commenting to my students on more than one occasion: "If five years from now you are still practicing what we taught you here, then you haven't learned very much."

FITTING THE FIRST HEARING AID

But how does one fit a child with a hearing aid when the audiometric information is so sparse? Carefully, of course, and in a way that potential benefits clearly outweigh possible problems. Even without the current armamentarium of tests, it was usually possible to get some idea about the degree of hearing loss, if not the configuration and possible disparities between the ears. So only general recommendations were made, with scheduled and frequent follow-ups part of the procedure. We required a sturdy aid (since kids have not changed, this requirement is still valid!), minimal distortion, adjustable output controls (from about 120 to 135 dB), and a wide-frequency range (Ross 1975; Ross and Lerman 1966). When we did not have information about the relative hearing status of the two ears—the usual case—we used a Y cord to ensure that each ear received some auditory stimulation. As more precise audiometric information was obtained, electroacoustic changes were made accordingly. When individual ear thresholds were obtained, the child was fit with binaural body aids. As soon as we could, we used aided audiograms to determine possible changes in the tone control settings, testing each ear separately.

Functional gain measurements are, of course, quite common now, but we should not forget that for a long time they were in disrepute because of possible standing wave effects generated by using pure tones in a sound field. Because of the complex phase relationships between the direct and reflected sounds, the sound field could demonstrate rapid changes in intensity with minor positional changes. The validity of functional gain measures was the topic of my 1958 master's thesis at Brooklyn College under the direction of John Duffy, who had been using aided audiograms since WWII. The availability of warble tones and narrow band stimuli rather than pure tones soon dissipated some of the validity concerns. It was, and is, however, such a simple technique that it soon became overused and misinterpreted. For example, clinicians were measuring what they thought were aided thresholds, but in reality they were measuring masked thresholds, from either low-frequency noise in the test booth or internal noise in the hearing aid.

What really concerned me (and still does) was the frequent use of aided thresholds in counseling parents to demonstrate how "normal" the amplification system had made their child's hearing loss. It should be clear that *aided* thresholds of 15 or 20 dB HL do not produce equivalent suprathreshold sensations as those of *unaided* 15 or 20 dB HL thresholds.

Another problem was the goal of some clinicians in aiming to achieve the lowest aided thresholds possible. Some would note with pride that they were able to obtain aided thresholds of 5 or 10 dB HL in the presence of unaided thresholds of 60 or 70 dB HL or more. (And I am assuming that I do not have to explain why this is not a desirable practice, or why the same aided and unaided thresholds do not produce equivalent suprathreshold sensations.)

Before there were dedicated hearing aid test boxes, and long before probe-tube microphone measures, there was the Bruel & Kjaer (B & K) electroacoustic measuring system. It became an important part of our hearing aid fitting procedure. We knew that the response in a real ear, particularly a child's ear, was going to be different from that displayed in the 2cc coupler (the real-ear-to-coupler difference, or RECD), but we did not know how much or how to document this difference, so we used the B & K to make *relative* changes in the hearing aid performance. We knew that when we added more high frequencies, extended the frequency range, or modified the output, this dimension would be similarly changed in the real ear. The goal was to provide an amplified speech sensation level across frequency that would give a child maximum access to the raw acoustic material of the speech signal. With the advent of real-ear measures, and the development of the desired sensation level (DSL) method (see chapter 8), we are finally in a position to ensure that this goal can be reached and validly observed.

WEARING THE FIRST HEARING AID

Recommending a hearing aid is relatively easy compared to getting a young child to wear it. Clinicians seem to have their own way of doing it, based on what seems logical and what they are comfortable with (Ross 1995). I have always felt that recipes of incrementally increasing wear time were counterproductive. These formulations usually required a child to put the aid on for a few minutes a day the first week, then gradually increase the time over a several week period. If a child objected, the clinician would point to a clock and try to cajole the child into a few minutes more. If there ever was a procedure that set up a power struggle between the child and the adults, that was it, and it was one in which the child held the high cards. I would not suggest that hearing aids be casually fit on youngsters, but we should not explicitly call attention to them either. If we are dealing with a very young child, as I hope we are, he or she is probably not aware that something all that unusual is going on. Why then call attention to it? The point is, we cannot give young children a choice when it comes to amplification, any more than we can give them a choice in eating, sleeping, or playing with matches.

Certainly, the clinician has to carefully observe the child, and of course, the earmolds have to fit properly, and yes, the real-ear aided output has to be below discomfort levels, but once these precautions are taken, the child should be expected to wear the aid(s) all day every day. (Although it does seem to make sense in a new fitting to gradually increase the gain over several days while observing the child.) The last thing in the world we want to do is to approach a child with a pitying, sorrowful expression on our faces, conveying this attitude: "You may not like it, but it's good for you"!

I think a gradualist attitude really reflected discomfort with fitting hearing aids on young children. Without the aids, the children looked like other children; with the aids, they appeared disabled. The public attitude toward hearing aids was, and to a great extent still is, that they are devices that stigmatize the wearer. It was and still is very hard for parents to accept the reality of a child's hearing loss. By insisting that the child needed to wear hearing aids, clinicians were bringing the parental pain to the surface and making it worse. And none of us entered this field to inflict pain. Beyond that, because we are members of the same public and influenced by the same feelings that hearing aids stigmatize children, I think some of this outlook influenced our comfort level in selecting hearing aids for children. Some clinicians were not really convinced of the therapeutic potency of properly used amplified sounds (based, perhaps, by their own unsuccessful clinical experiences and by the relative paucity of hard scientific evidence). Thus, if aids had to be worn, they should be as inconspicuous as possible and in only one ear. A binaural fitting gave the impression of a greater impairment, and many clinicians apparently recommended one aid to soften the impact of the child's hearing loss for parents. Monaural recommendations were being made long after the general superiority of binaural aids became evident (Ross 1980).

In my opinion, a modern equivalent of this attitude is the reluctance of many audiologists to recommend an FM system as the first and primary amplification device for a young child. In this day and age, one should not have to extol the auditory virtues of an increased speech-to-noise (S/N) ratio. Every person with hearing impairment can benefit from increasing the S/N ratio, but of all of them, children with hearing losses can benefit the most. But because an FM system requires that a parent use a clearly visible microphone and transmitter, and because the child has to wear a body-worn FM receiver or two rather large behind-the-ear (BTE) FM receivers, many audiologists apparently feel (no research, just my impressions) that such a fitting would unduly burden the parents and the children or feel that the parents are not ready for such a dramatic fitting.

THE LISTENING ENVIRONMENT

The most appropriate electroacoustic system and the most carefully designed therapy program will not do children any good if the primary signal—speech—is buried in the background of noise. The sine qua non of any auditory approach, however it is defined, is the necessity that children detect as much of the acoustic elements of speech as their hearing losses permit. Very little literature on the effect of environmental acoustics on the speech perception of people with hearing impairment appeared in U.S. journals in the 1950s and early 1960s. One article in the *Volta Review* (Watson 1961) briefly mentioned the negative impact of classroom acoustics, but as a lecturer at the University of Manchester in England, he was reviewing the work done there.

Perhaps because of my own hearing loss, I have long been sensitized to the effect that noise could have on the language development of children with hearing impairment. If I, as an adventitiously hard of hearing adult, had difficulty *understanding* speech in a noisy classroom, how in the world could we expect that children with congenital hearing impairment *develop* their auditory language skills in those same conditions? This question and this concern were virtually absent from our post-WWII literature, although comments about the effect of acoustic conditions could be found before that period (Haller and Lybarger 1933; O'Connor 1938; Watson and Watson 1937). It was only when I discovered the European literature on the topic

(Ewing 1960; Ewing and Ewing 1961; John 1957; John and Thomas 1957; Tolk 1961; Watson 1962) that I was able to teach and write on the topic (Ross 1972b).

There is still, in my opinion, insufficient emphasis on the effect of environmental acoustics on children's use of residual hearing. I take the fact of its omission from this volume as an indication that the phenomenon has already been established and not that it is irrelevant. We know that most people with hearing losses will experience a disproportionate impact on speech perception in poor, or even average, acoustic conditions (Nabelek and Nabelek 1994), and that children with uncertain language skills will likely show an even greater effect (Ross 1992a). The significant challenge is not to refine our current insights on environmental acoustics but to apply what we already know. Although some features in modern (and not-so-modern) hearing aids can improve speech perception in noisy places—such as directional microphones, multiband amplification, wide-frequency range, and low distortion instruments—none of them will deliver the same positive S/N ratio as can an FM system. As anybody with ears (or hearing aids) can attest, the world is not getting any quieter; and as the cacophony grows, so does the need for an improved S/N ratio.

There really is a need for more creativity in developing new features in FM systems that can further improve speech perception in noise. Several of the newer generation of FM systems include a muting circuit that decreases the gain of the environmental microphones when an FM signal is received, a feature that was available—albeit imperfectly—almost 20 years ago (Ross 1977a). A good muting circuit should help negate the effect of open environmental microphones on the perception of the teacher's speech (Hawkins and Yacullo 1984). At least 15 years ago, Siemens Hearing Instruments manufactured an FM system for classroom use (not marketed in the U.S. as far as I know) that incorporated a built-in spring-loaded FM microphone on each child's receiver (Ross 1981). The child would press the microphone to talk. The signal would be picked up by the teacher's FM receiver and retransmitted to the other children. This is the only system I know of that permits excellent child-to-child communication, but it can work only in a classroom with other students with hearing impairment. It is not, however, currently available.

What we really need is a small handheld FM microphone/transmitter, perhaps the size of a ballpoint pen, that can be laser aimed at a talker some distance away, judge the distance and adjust microphone sensitivity accordingly, reject or mute all sounds off the aiming point, and transmit the detected signal to BTE FM receivers. An additional "third" ear if you will, as a partial compensation for the two existing ones with poor hearing. Before this gets dismissed as a wild-eyed dream, I would like to quote a comment made just 40 years ago. In a section on the gullibility of people to "Quack

Hearing Devices," these authors wrote, "Even a thoroughly rational person is likely to wonder why a hearing aid can't fit entirely within the ear and provide satisfactory amplification" (Streng et al. 1958). In other words, the authors dismissed this possibility as sheer fantasy. I think the technological distance between the hearing aids of 1955 and a completely-in-the-canal (CIC) aid of 1996 is greater than existing FM microphones and my wild-eyed dream.

At any rate, clinicians who work with children with hearing impairment should fantasize, and should challenge the manufacturers to develop amplification systems that will help children access more of the auditory code of our language. We are not concerned with reality, research and development costs, market share, and so on. Not that these concerns are irrelevant—of course, they are relevant—but they are not ours. As a case in point, I offer the example of the current availability of BTE FM systems. Their need was apparent for years; as a matter of fact, I wrote about the desirability of this feature nearly 20 years ago (discussion in Rubin 1976; Ross 1977a). Several years ago, one was introduced on the market, now there are two, and soon a third one will be available. With the technological possibilities being what they are now, I hope the gestation period of future "fantasies" will not take quite so long.

IMPLEMENTING OUR GOOD INTENTIONS

If we take a developmental view of the history of amplification with children, it is clear that we are infinitely better off than our predecessors were in the preelectronic and the early electronic age. They could not even dream of the technical capacities we now possess, or the laws that mandate educational opportunities for children with hearing impairments. Though we too seldom use all our available resources for specific children, we pretty much know the components of an optimal auditory management program for a young child with hearing impairment. Moreover, we have the technical capacity to deliver such a program. I find it ironic that the acoustic method, begun in schools for the Deaf more than a hundred years ago, is now meeting its greatest contemporary opposition among the staff and personnel in other schools for the Deaf.

It would not be accurate to assume that this current opposition to amplification in some schools and among some members of the Deaf community is reversing successful programs of auditory management in schools for the Deaf. At least until the last few years, all such schools possessed classroom amplification systems, and most of the children owned hearing aids, but the presence of these devices rarely guaranteed that they were being employed properly. The attempts to stimulate residual hearing that took place in schools shortly before and after WWII seldom seemed to take root and get translated into an informed, enthusiastic, and long-term commitment. In the hundreds of classrooms and schools that I visited over the years, even a superficial examination revealed that audition was rarely used effectively in most of them. I always saw something that could be improved, which became distressingly apparent after I actually listened through the classroom system. The output was much too low or distorted, the teacher's voice was buried in the classroom noise, it was impossible to hear myself or the other children, or individual ear adjustments could not be made. In the oral schools, the teachers seemed to talk with exaggerated lip movements, but with little voice, while in the total communication schools, the input speech was too soft and grammatically fragmented (Ross and Calvert 1984). It seemed that in most such settings, these devices were purchased and displayed in response to social pressures rather than a belief in their efficacy. Even so, approximately 25% of the children in schools for the Deaf rarely or never used either a personal or a group hearing aid in their classrooms, while 45% never or rarely used hearing aids at home or in the dormitories. Furthermore, this percentage increased as the students got older (Karchmer and Kirwin 1977).

These statistics do not imply that the other children, the ones using some sort of amplification system, were deriving acceptable benefit from it. Since the landmark article by Gaeth and Lounsbury (1966), the evidence has consistently revealed that a high percentage of children in schools use non- or malfunctioning amplification devices (Ross 1977b). Moreover, this research was not concerned with such factors as provisions for self-monitoring, the effect of classroom acoustics, whether monaural or binaural aids were used, and the characteristics of the amplified speech output in a child's ear. In view of all these confounding factors, it is highly unlikely that most of the children received an adequate, much less optimal, amplified speech signal for any portion of the day. Twenty-four years ago I wrote, "We do not know how far we can go with the use of amplified sound because, generally speaking, we have not used it appropriately" (Ross 1972b). I wish I could be convinced that, on a national scale, the situation is very different today. My optimistic view, when I see what *has* been accomplished with some children, is that clearly discernible progress has been made. My pessimistic view is that in relation to what *can* be done, given the possibilities inherent in modern technology and current law, we have simply been treading water.

A case in point is the observation by Rose (1994) that 73% of the children in schools for the Deaf who had received cochlear implants were no longer using them. He uses this finding—rightfully, in my opinion—to question the implant selection and habilitation process for these children. The fact that they rejected the implants, either for social reasons or for their insufficient benefits, is not surprising. Their rejection or failure to benefit from the implants is, in my view, an extension of how residual hearing is being underused or neglected in these same settings. One can hardly expect reasonable auditory-verbal progress subsequent to being implanted, given the informed, sustained, and dedicated commitment necessary to realize significant progress with a cochlear implant, if children with moderate and severe hearing losses were not being helped to use, and benefit from, conventional amplification systems.

To go back to the opening statement in this section, the greatest future challenge we face regarding amplification for children is not new technical developments, impressive as they are, but changes in social attitudes. If residual hearing is thought to be, at best, irrelevant and, at worst, an imposition by the hearing world on one's personal identity, then there would be no chance to demonstrate what modern hearing technology and habilitation procedures can offer.

It seems that the advent of cochlear implants with children has stirred the worst fears of the Deaf community and rekindled an attitude regarding acoustic amplification that has been extant, but relatively quiescent. They see cochlear implants as a development that holds the possibility of threatening the future existence of the Deaf community and as an unjustifiable intrusion on the natural identity of children born deaf. Some of their more outspoken advocates reject the concept that their hearing is impaired; rather, they view themselves as members of a visually oriented cultural and linguistic subgroup (Tucker 1993). These attitudes have percolated throughout the Deaf community and have strongly influenced the view and acceptance of amplification in special education settings. Three major schools for the Deaf that I know of have completely abolished classroom amplification systems and any encouragement of personal hearing aids by the children. The prevailing value system appears to be giving them a choice: Be a proud Deaf person and a member of this community, or by using an amplification system, be a misfit, neither here nor there. And it is having an effect. I have recently talked to dozens of educators and audiologists, from both total communication (TC) and oral schools, and they all agreed that a student's acceptance of amplification is being increasingly seen as a betrayal of one's own natural identity. Certainly, this outlook has not affected all the students or staff, deaf or hearing, in all schools, but it does seem to be an increasingly prevailing outlook.

The effect of this attitude can be seen in the results of the student questionnaire administered by the audiology department at the National Technical Institute for the Deaf (NTID) to entering students (1994). In 1994, only 36% wanted to have their hearing tested, 33% were willing to learn about their hearing loss, hearing aids, or hearing test results, 39% wanted to have their hearing aids rechecked, and practically none (15 out of 187 students) wanted to use an FM system. I doubt that these figures indicate perfect satisfaction with their hearing aid, or recent knowledge regarding the nature of their hearing status. These figures do suggest the students' disinterest in exploring the possibilities inherent in using their residual hearing. I cannot help feeling, however, that these students would have been less influenced by this attitude had their experiences with amplification been long-term, positive, and rewarding. Because NTID has a history of encouraging students to use their residual hearing, it is likely that the use and interest in amplification would be even less prevalent in other postsecondary programs.

The Deaf community does have a point: The effective use of residual hearing can very well threaten the long-term viability of the community. Most of the children who are the beneficiaries of an optimal auditory management program will function as hard of hearing and not deaf. They may well be lost to the Deaf community. As audiologists, however, we are primarily concerned not with the viability of the Deaf community—though by no means should we consider ourselves their adversaries either—but with the well-being of the children with hearing impairments we see in our clinics. *They* are our primary professional responsibility. We select and supervise amplification for children, and no other group can fulfill this role. In the beginning, before we know the precise dimensions of a child's hearing loss or the functional capabilities of the residual hearing, we must ensure the best amplification selections we can. Depending on how we view the world, the sense of hearing is a gift given to us by our biological forebears, an evolutionary inheritance, or a God-given attribute. I see it as our ethical obligation to use whatever hearing remains to the maximum extent possible (Ross 1992b). Certainly, we have to be sensitive to the wishes of the parents and to the developing situation with a child, but our initial stance has to be proamplification.

In the history of education for persons who are deaf, the pendulum always seems to be located at one extreme or another, never finding a resting place in the middle (oral *or* manual, day *or* residential, mainstreaming *or* segregated, natural *or* structured language, deaf *or* hearing, etc.). Now we see this same extremist tendency being applied in regard to providing amplification for children with hearing impairment: hearing *or* silence. As I understand the position being advocated by most forceful spokepersons for the Deaf community, the acceptance of amplification implies a rejection of their community. They point out that a full and fruitful life can be achieved without sound, as indeed it can, and that therefore whatever aesthetic and communicative advantages accrue to the use of amplified sound are irrelevant and unnecessary. The implication is that group solidarity and identity are threatened by people who are able to derive some benefit from amplified sound, that they are not fully accepting of themselves and their own natural group. I find this a sad formulation, the notion that the ticket for admission to a supportive and often very necessary group is the foreclosing of whatever benefit the world of sound can offer.

Adults can make up their own minds regarding the choice they want to make, after experiencing (I hope) an optimal auditory management program as a child. Children, however, are another matter. Some 90% of children with hearing impairment are born to parents with normal hearing, and more than 90% of all children with hearing impairment have some residual hearing. At the time of detection, we usually do not know precisely how much of a hearing loss they have or how well they will be able to use their residual hearing. It seems that we must give these children the opportunity to enter the world of sound, to realize its potential value, to the degree that their hearing loss permits. The time will come when the children we work with will be all grown up, and they will be responsible and capable of making their own decisions. And that is how it should be. We will have fulfilled our role when they make their own decisions, when they have the capabilities and experiences to choose between options, one of which should be feeling at home in both the Deaf and the hearing worlds.

REFERENCES

Beebe, H.H. 1953. *A guide to help the severely hard of hearing child.* Basel, Switzerland: S. Karger.
Bender, R.E. 1981. *The conquest of deafness.* 3d ed. Danville, Ill.: Interstate Printers and Publishers.
Benoit, R. 1994. Infant hearing screening task force work paper, Newington Children's Hospital, Newington, Connecticut.
Boothroyd, A., and Medwetsky, L. 1992. Spectral distribution of /s/ and the frequency response of hearing aids. *Ear and Hearing* 13:150-157.
Brown, D.P. 1994. Speech recognition in recurrent otitis media: Results in a set of identical twins. *Journal of the American Academy of Audiology* 5:1-6.
Carhart, R. 1947. Auditory training. In H. Davis (ed.), *Hearing and deafness.* New York: Rinehart Books.
Clarke, B.R. 1957. Use of a group hearing aid by profoundly deaf children. In A.W.G. Ewing (ed.), *Educational guidance and the deaf child.* Manchester, England: Manchester University Press.
Davis, H. (ed.). 1951. *Hearing and deafness.* New York: Rinehart Books.
Ewing, A.W.G. (ed.). 1957. *Educational guidance and the deaf child.* Manchester, England: Manchester University Press.
Ewing, A. 1960. *The modern educational treatment for deafness.* Manchester, England: Manchester University Press.
Ewing, I.R., and Ewing, A.W.G. 1961. *New opportunities for deaf children.* 2d ed. London, England: University of London Press.
Gaeth, J.H., and Lounsbury, E. 1966. Hearing aids and children in elementary schools. *Journal of Speech and Hearing Disorders* 31:282-289.
Gelfand, S.A., and Silman, S. 1993. Apparent auditory deprivation in children: Implications of monaural versus binaural amplification. *Journal of the American Academy of Audiology* 44:313-318.

Goldstein, M. 1933. *Problems of the deaf*. St. Louis, Mo.: Laryngoscope.
Goldstein, M. 1939. *The acoustic method*. St. Louis, Mo.: Laryngoscope.
Griffiths, C. 1964. The auditory approach for pre-school deaf children. *Volta Review* 66:387-397.
Haller, G.L., and Lybarger, S.F. 1933. Selection of electrical apparatus for auricular training. *Volta Review* 35:295-298.
Hawkins, D.B., and Yacullo, W.S. 1984. Signal-to-noise advantage of binaural hearing aids and directional microphones under different levels of reverberation. *Journal of Speech and Hearing Disorders* 49:278-286.
Hudgins, C.V. 1953. The response of profoundly deaf children to auditory training. *Journal of Speech and Hearing Disorders* 18:273-288.
John, J.E.J. 1957. Acoustics and efficiency in the use of hearing aids. In A.W.G. Ewing (ed.), *Educational guidance and the deaf child*. Manchester, England: Manchester University Press.
John, J.E.J., and Thomas, H. 1957. Design and construction of schools for the deaf. In A.W.G. Ewing (ed.), *Educational guidance and the deaf child*. Manchester, England: Manchester University Press.
Karchmer, M.A., and Kirwin, L.A. 1977. The use of hearing aids by hearing impaired students in the United States. Series S, no. 2. Washington, D.C.: Office of Demographic Studies, Gallaudet University.
Knox, A.W. 1972. Electrodermal audiometry. In J. Katz (ed.), *Handbook of clinical audiology*. Baltimore: Williams and Wilkins.
Lennenberg, E.H. 1967. *Biological foundations of language*. New York: John Wiley and Sons.
Ling, D. 1976. *Speech and the hearing-impaired child: Theory and practice*. Washington, D.C.: Alexander Graham Bell Association for the Deaf.
Luterman, D. 1979. *Counselling parents of hearing-impaired children*. Boston: Little, Brown.
Luterman, D. 1991. *When your child is deaf*. Baltimore: York Press.
McConnell, F. 1968. *Proceedings of the conference on current practices in the management of deaf infants (1-3 years)*. Nashville, Tenn.: Bill Wilkerson Hearing and Speech Center.
McConnell, F., and Liff, S. 1975. The rationale for early identification and intervention. *Otolaryngological Clinics of North America* 8:77-87.
McNeill, D. 1966. Developmental psycholinguistics. In F. Smith and G.A. Miller (eds.), *The genesis of language*. Cambridge: MIT Press.
Nabelek, A., and Nabelek, I. 1994. Room acoustics and speech perception. In J. Katz (ed.), *Handbook of clinical audiology*. 4th ed. Baltimore: Williams and Wilkins.
National Technical Institute for the Deaf. 1994. Audiology Department Entrance Questionnaire. Rochester, New York.
Newby, H.A. 1958. *Audiology: Principles and practices*. New York: Appleton-Century Crofts.
O'Connor, C.D. 1938. What every superintendent of a school for the deaf should know about hearing aids and their use. *Volta Review* 40:710-717.
Pickles, A.M. 1957. Home training with hearing aids. In A.W.G. Ewing (ed.), *Educational guidance and the deaf child*. Manchester, England: Manchester University Press.
Pollack, D. 1964. Acoupedics: A uni-sensory approach to auditory training. *Volta Review* 66:400-409.
Rose, D.E. 1994. Cochlear implants in children with prelingual deafness: Another side of the coin. *American Journal of Audiology* 3:6.

Ross, M. 1972a. *Principles of aural rehabilitation*. The Bobbs-Merrill Studies in Communication Disorders. New York: Bobbs-Merrill.
Ross, M. 1972b. Classroom acoustics and speech intelligibility. In J. Katz (ed.), *Handbook of clinical audiology* (p. 769). Baltimore: Williams and Wilkins.
Ross, M. 1975. Hearing aid selection for pre-verbal hearing impaired children. In M.C. Pollack (ed.), *Amplification for the hearing impaired*. New York: Grune and Stratton.
Ross, M. 1977a. Classroom amplification. In W.R. Hodgson and P.D. Skinner (eds.), *Hearing aid assessment and use in audiologic habilitation*. Baltimore: Williams and Wilkins.
Ross, M. 1977b. A review of studies on the incidence of hearing aid malfunctions. In *The condition of hearing aids worn by children in a public school program*. Stock No. 017-080-91724-5, Washington, D.C.: U.S. Government Printing Office.
Ross, M. 1980. Binaural vs. monaural amplification. In E.R. Libby (ed.), *Binaural hearing*. Chicago, Ill.: Zentron.
Ross, M. 1981. Classroom amplification. In W.R. Hodgson and P.H. Skinner (eds.), *Hearing aid assessment and use in aural rehabilitation*. Baltimore: Williams and Wilkins.
Ross, M. 1986. *Principles of aural habilitation*. Austin: Pro-Ed.
Ross, M. 1992a. Room acoustics and speech perception. In M. Ross (ed.), *FM auditory training systems: Characteristics, selection and use*. Baltimore: York Press.
Ross, M. 1992b. Implications of audiological success. *Journal of the American Academy of Audiology* 1:4.
Ross, M. 1995. Post-selection considerations. In F. Martin and J. Clark (eds.), *Children with hearing disorders*. Boston: Allyn and Bacon.
Ross, M., and Calvert, D.R. 1967. The semantics of deafness. *Volta Review* 69:644-649.
Ross, M., and Calvert, D.R. 1984. Semantics of deafness revisited: Total communication and the use and misuse of residual hearing. *Audiology: A Journal of Continuing Education* 9:127-148.
Ross, M., and Green, R.R. 1990. Detection and management of hearing-impaired children: A follow-up questionnaire study. *Hearing Rehabilitation Quarterly* 15(2):4-5, 14-15.
Ross, M., and Lerman, J.W. 1966. Hearing aid selection and usage in young hearing-impaired children. *Connecticut Medicine* 30(11):793-795.
Ross, M., Brackett, D., and Maxon, A.B. 1991. *Assessment and management of mainstreamed hearing-impaired children: Principles and practices*. Austin: Pro-Ed.
Roush, J., and Matkin, N.D. 1994. *Infants and toddlers with hearing loss*. Baltimore: York Press.
Rubin, M. 1976. *Hearing aids: Current developments and concepts*. Discussion comment by Ross, p. 196. Baltimore: University Park Press.
Schmael, O. 1960. The use and benefits of hearing aids in German schools for the deaf. In A.W.G. Ewing (ed.), *The modern educational treatment for deafness*. Manchester, England: Manchester University Press.
Streng, A., Fitch, W.J., Hedgecock, L.D., Phillips, J.W., and Carrell, J.A. 1958. *Hearing therapy in children*. 2d ed. New York: Grune and Stratton.
Tervoort, B. 1964. Development of language and the "critical period." *Acta Otolaryngologica* (Suppl.) 206:247-251.
Tolk, J. 1961. Acoustics, intelligibility of speech and electro-acoustics systems in classrooms. *Proceedings of the 2nd International Course in Paedo-Audiology* (pp. 103-109). The Netherlands: Groningen University.

Tucker, B. 1993. Deafness: 1993-2013—The dilemma. *Volta Review* 95:105-108.
Watson, L.A., and Tolan, T. 1949. *Hearing tests and hearing instruments*. Baltimore: Williams and Wilkins.
Watson, T.J. 1961. The use of residual hearing in the education of deaf children: Part III. *Volta Review* 63:435-440.
Watson, R.B., and Watson, N.A. 1937. Hearing aids in schools for the deaf. *Volta Review* 39:261-266.
Watson, T.J. 1962. The use of residual hearing in the education of deaf children. Washington, D.C.: The Volta Bureau.
Wedenberg, E. 1951. Auditory training of deaf and hard of hearing children. *Acta Otolaryngologica* (Stockholm) Suppl. 94:1-130.
Whetnall, E., and Fry, D.B. 1964. *The deaf child*. Springfield, Ill.: Charles C. Thomas.

2

Audition and the Development of Oral Communication Competency

Arlene Earley Carney

INTRODUCTION

In the field of early intervention for infants and children with hearing losses, few topics are as controversial or as debated as the importance of audition in the development of long-term oral communication competency. The discussion focuses not on whether audition *is* important in the development of oral skills (that much, at least, would be conceded by all concerned) but on *how much* audition is needed, *how best* are auditory skills developed, and *when* are auditory skills manifested in oral communication competency. The debate is further complicated by the paucity of data in this area, despite the long history of specialists in the field who have stressed the importance of early intervention for providing the auditory input necessary for the development of oral communication (Boothroyd 1988; Fry 1978; Geers and Moog 1987; Matkin 1984; Northern and Downs 1991).

The lack of closure in this ongoing debate suggests that we take a newer and different approach to this old problem to seek a fresher solution. The purpose of this chapter is to examine ways in which we might begin to study and quantify the problems in the development of oral communication competency in infants and children with hearing losses and thus arrive at more effective solutions. Four general areas will be discussed: (1) how speech perception and production develop in parallel in young children with normal hearing; (2) what changes in speech perception and production might be expected as a result of hearing loss; (3) how oral communication competency was affected in selected children with differing degrees of hearing loss; and

(4) what further research is indicated from the examination of models of speech perception and production and from the case studies presented.

DEVELOPMENT OF SPEECH PRODUCTION AND PERCEPTION IN CHILDREN WITH NORMAL HEARING

Aslin and Smith (1988) described an interesting and comprehensive model of perceptual development in children for all the perceptual systems. However, it has particular applicability to the auditory perceptual system and its development in children with hearing losses. Aslin and Smith described three levels of perceptual development: the sensory primitive level, the perceptual representation level, and the cognitive/linguistic representation level.

At the level of the sensory primitive, the focus is on the basic sensory input to the child—in our case, an auditory stimulus. This is the most peripheral level of auditory development. We ask, What stimulus is the child receiving, and how is this stimulus processed initially? A behavioral, perceptual response at the sensory primitive level is that of detection: Is sound present or absent? The sensory primitive level can be discussed physiologically as well, with such techniques as auditory brainstem response testing or the measurement of otoacoustic emissions. For such testing, our question becomes: Is sound being processed by the auditory brainstem and cochlea of an infant or child? This level does not extend beyond simple reception of the incoming auditory stimulus. Audiologically, our efforts to implement early identification are all focused at this sensory primitive level.

At the next, intermediary level of perceptual representation in the Aslin and Smith (1988) model, the focus is on understanding what type of complex encoding of the stimulus occurs at some higher, or more neural, level, but before auditory stimuli would be processed as real words. In the area of auditory perceptual development, the large literature on infant speech perception addresses this level. Researchers have asked infants to discriminate between speech tokens that differ phonetically but to ignore nonimportant acoustic differences, such as within phonetic category variations, gender of the speaker, or to listen for differences that are important or unimportant for their language-learning environment (Eilers, Gavin, and Wilson 1979; Jusczyk 1986; Kuhl 1979, 1983, 1988; Kuhl, Williams, Lacerda, Stevens, and Lindblom 1992; Werker 1991; Werker, Gilbert, Humphrey, and Tees 1981; Werker and Lalonde 1988). This is clearly a level of more complex perception, but it does not involve the recognition or comprehension of some message, only the categorization or discrimination of stimuli based on complex acoustic features. Even for adult listeners, audiologists have not routinely examined this level of auditory perception.

For children with hearing losses, some investigators are beginning to develop procedures that are independent of word recognition and tap this general area of auditory perceptual representation more directly (Boothroyd 1991; Carney, Osberger, Carney, Robbins, Renshaw, and Miyamoto 1993; Osberger, Miyamoto, Zimmerman-Phillips, Kemink, Stroer, Firszt, and Novak 1991). The procedures used by these investigators involve the discrimination of nonsense syllables in three-stimuli forced choice procedures (Boothroyd 1991) or in strings of syllables that change or remain the same (Carney et al. 1993; Osberger et al. 1991).

The third level of perceptual development is that of cognitive/linguistic representation. Here, the complex neural/acoustic code of the perceptual representation level is transformed into meaningful words. Individual speech sounds become part of meaningful whole units. Listeners may still be able to break down the words into component speech sounds, but the processing is more of the whole word than of the phonemes of speech. Audiologically, we have a long history of assessing auditory skill at this level of word recognition, both for children and for adults. This is evident in the lists of tests used by pediatric audiologists for assessing word recognition in children with hearing loss, such as the Word Intelligibility by Picture Identification Test (Ross and Lerman 1970), the Northwestern University Children's Perception of Speech (Elliott and Katz 1980), the Minimal Pairs Test (Robbins, Renshaw, Miyamoto, Osberger, and Pope 1988), or the Hoosier Auditory Visual Enhancement Test (Renshaw, Robbins, Miyamoto, Osberger, and Pope 1988).

A parallel model of speech production development was developed by Carney (1993a) and described briefly in Moeller and Carney (1993). This model of speech production development follows the perceptual model of Aslin and Smith (1988). Once again, there are three levels of development: the production primitive level, the production representation level, and the cognitive/linguistic production level. Like its perceptual counterpart of the sensory primitive level, the production primitive level is the most basic level of speech output. Infants cry, make vegetative sounds, or have undifferentiated vocalizations, made with a generally closed vocal tract (Oller 1980; Stark 1980). This is typical of infants through the first few months of life.

Very quickly, infants move to the production representation level in which they begin to produce more complex vocal sequences that more closely resemble adult speech patterns in timing, syllabic structure, and phonetic content. Some of these syllables have very distinct consonantlike and vowel-like portions and have been called canonical syllables (Oller 1980). Between 5 and 8 months of age, infants with normal hearing begin to produce canonical syllables that are recognizable reliably to their parents (Eilers and Oller 1994; Oller and Eilers 1988). These infant utterances with their adultlike timing and phonetic patterns are recognized as the necessary precursors for the first oral words produced by children in the earliest stages of language development (Oller, Wieman, Doyle, and Ross 1975).

The third level of production development is cognitive/linguistic representation. At this stage, listeners begin to identify clear phonemes and syllabic patterns from the parent language in the vocal repertoire of infants and toddlers. By 12 to 15 months of age, the average toddler may have broad phonetic and phonemic inventories and is producing a few recognizable words (Bauer 1988; Kent and Bauer 1985; Stoel-Gammon 1985; Vihman, Ferguson, and Elbert 1986). Phonemes in speech strings begin to be used meaningfully in real words.

DEVELOPMENT OF SPEECH PRODUCTION AND PERCEPTION IN CHILDREN WITH HEARING LOSSES

Hearing loss of any degree interrupts this parallel development of speech perception and production. In the perceptual mode, hearing loss immediately reduces or even eliminates the sensory primitive, depending on the degree and extent of auditory damage. As a result, the level of perceptual representation, at best, is distorted or, at worst, is absent, again depending on the extent of auditory damage. The final result is a delayed cognitive/linguistic representation for oral language. In contrast, infants with hearing losses who are presented with very early sign input may have a well-developed cognitive/linguistic representation through the visual modality with no auditory sensory primitive or auditory perceptual representation. Despite one's view of the importance, or even the necessity, of oral communication competency for children with hearing losses, it is critical to recognize that high levels of cognitive/linguistic representation can be achieved through either the auditory or the visual modality (through the acquisition of sign language).

When we add amplification to this developing system, we are attempting to increase the intensity and to broaden the spectrum of the input to the damaged sensory primitive level. Our hearing aid selection procedures are based on the premise that we can overcome a damaged sensory primitive with appropriate adjustments to the incoming signal even if we cannot alter the sensory primitive itself. Our goal is to restore the sensory primitive to what we think is a normal state through manipulation of the incoming stimuli. When we monitor the effects of amplification during infancy, we are most often evaluating and adjusting the input to the sensory primitive through instrumental procedures, such as using real-ear probe microphone techniques, or through perceptual procedures, such as assessing the aided detection of speech or nonspeech sounds. It is rare to address any perceptual process beyond detection. We make a variety of assumptions that the input we provide via this adjusted sensory primitive will be adequate to develop the appropriate perceptual representation and cognitive/linguistic representations necessary for the recognition of words or the comprehension of discourse. Throughout childhood, we continue to monitor amplification with the types of procedures we use with infants, those directed at the sensory primitive level, and we expand our assessments to the cognitive/linguistic representation level, with more or less success. In our interpretation of the results of word recognition tests, we may conclude that the poor performance of children with hearing losses is due to language or vocabulary effects, despite the fact that these may be familiar words that we believe are audible. We may not consider that we simply do not know what intermediate perceptual steps may have been missing for a child.

Hearing loss affects the development of speech production as well. This has been well documented by the work of Oller, Eilers, and associates (Eilers and Oller 1994; Oller and Eilers 1988; Oller, Eilers, Bull, and Carney 1985), as well as others (Kent, Osberger, Netsell, and Hustedde 1987; Stoel-Gammon 1988; Stoel-Gammon and Otomo 1986). In the current model, the production primitive may be quite prolonged. The production representation stage may be seriously delayed by profound hearing loss. The absence of canonical babbling by age 12 months is now becoming recognized as an indicator of severe-to-profound hearing loss (Eilers and Oller 1994; Oller and Eilers 1988). Cognitive/linguistic representation may be delayed by even mild or moderate hearing loss and certainly by severe-to-profound hearing losses (Abraham 1989; Carney 1986, 1993b; Dodd 1976; Geffner 1980; Ling 1976; Monsen 1978, 1983; Oller, Jensen, and Lafayette 1978; Oller and Kelly 1974; Osberger and McGarr 1982). Without the orderly progression of these stages of speech production development, the ability to use oral communication functionally is greatly at risk.

CASE STUDIES OF SPEECH PRODUCTION DEVELOPMENT IN INFANTS WITH HEARING LOSSES

In this section, speech production data are presented from four infants with different degrees of hearing, characterized according to a sensory primitive level. That is, each infant's hearing is described in terms of his or her detection ability, as we do in standard clinical practice. The first infant, a male, had hearing thresholds within normal limits bilaterally. The second infant, a female, had a moderate sensorineural hearing loss with a pure-tone average of 53 dB HL (ANSI 1989) in her better ear. The third infant, a male, had a progressive sensorineural hearing loss that changed from moderate to severe levels (pure-tone average of 73 dB HL [ANSI 1989] in his better ear) by the time the vocalization data were collected. The second and third infants with hearing losses were younger siblings of older children with profound hearing losses and were identified as being hearing impaired in the first three months of life. The fourth infant, a female, had a profound hearing loss with essentially no residual hearing (responses were obtained only at 250 and 500 Hz at the output limits of 90 and 110 dB HL, respectively). In addition, this fourth infant was identified relatively late, around 12 months of age. All three infants with hearing losses were fitted with appropriate amplification at Boys Town National Research Hospital. They wore their hearing aids regularly and were being followed in an ongoing parent-infant program when these data were collected.

These four infants were participants in a larger study of the development of infant vocalization in children with normal hearing and with hearing losses ranging from moderate to profound. Each infant was videotaped and audiotaped in one of two environments every two weeks beginning at 8 months of age through approximately 24 months of age. The first environment was a large sound-treated room designed as an informal play setting. The second environment was a room in the infant's home. In both environments, vocalizations were recorded with pressure zone microphones (PZM) placed on a wall or table that were directed to the super VHS camcorder and audiocassette recorder. The infant's mother and/or father were present in the session along with one tester. The infant was permitted to move around the room freely and to play with any toys available. The tester and parents did not attempt to elicit any vocalizations directly but engaged in conversation until the infant began vocalizing when adult talking ceased. Recording was carried out for approximately an hour each time.

Two examiners in consensus analyzed and transcribed the videotaped samples. Both examiners had to agree on a coding category for each part of the vocalization sample. Vocalizations that could not be agreed upon were marked, and a third examiner broke the tie between the original two transcribers. For all the analyses that are described below, each sample of vocalizations was initially separated into syllables and utterances. For all measures in this current investigation, a syllable is considered to be a production with some vocalic nucleus. The syllable may contain a consonantal margin in either prevocalic or postvocalic position, but the consonant portion is not necessary for the production to be called a syllable. Thus, a single vocalic nucleus produced would be considered a single syllable. An utterance is composed of any number of syllables produced in a single breath group (Lynch, Oller, and Steffens 1989; Oller and Lynch 1992).

Syllables and utterances were broken down further into a hierarchy based on syllabic complexity: canonical syllables, marginal syllables, fully resonant vocalic nuclei, and quasi-resonant nuclei. The characteristics of each of these were described in Oller (1983). A canonical syllable has a clear vocalic portion and a clear consonantal margin with timing characteristics like those of adult speech, that is, the transition from vocalic to consonantal portion should not exceed 120 ms and should be continuous, and there should be a considerable amplitude difference between the vocalic and consonantal portions of the syllable. In contrast, a marginal syllable is one with both consonantal and vocalic portions that are less distinct, with much longer transitions between the two portions of this protosyllable and with little amplitude difference between the vocalic and consonantal portions. A fully resonant vocalic nucleus has clear areas of resonance and is produced with an open vocal tract. Finally, a quasi-resonant nucleus, generally produced at a very early stage of development, is a phonated production without the full resonances observed. The vocal tract is in a semiclosed state with no observable movement of the articulators.

All four infants were observed to produce a number of vocalizations beyond the production primitive level for at least parts of the sessions observed. That is, all four infants produced vocalizations beyond the early, vegetative stage. Consequently, the analysis of speech production development focused on the production representation level and the use of the syllable and nucleus types described above.

Four measures of production representation were made: canonical babbling ratios, marginal babbling ratios, vocalic ratios, and quasi-resonant nuclei ratios. All four ratios show the relationship between a particular type of speech production relative to the number of syllables or utterances produced by the infant. Two calculations were made for the canonical babbling ratio (CBR). The first has been described by Oller and Eilers (1988). CBR (Oller) is the ratio of the number of canonical syllables divided by the number of utterances in a sample. In general, infants produce reduplicated or repeated syllable strings (e.g., *da da da*) or variegated syllable strings (e.g., *na da na da*) once they produce canonical syllables (Mitchell and Kent 1990; Oller 1983). Consequently, the numerator of this CBR can be very large relative to the denominator, the number of utterances. The CBR (Oller) has no natural upper limit. The second CBR was described by Carney (1991). The CBR (Carney) is the ratio of the number of utterances with at least one canonical syllable divided by the number of utterances. This CBR (Carney) varies between 0 and 1; a CBR of 1 would indicate that all utterances contain at least one canonical syllable.

The marginal babbling ratios (MBR) are calculated the same way. The MBR (Oller) is the ratio of the number of marginal syllables divided by the number of utterances. Once again, this ratio has no upper limit. The MBR (Carney) is the ratio of the number of utterances with a marginal syllable as its most complex syllable type divided by the number of utterances. That is, if an utterance has both canonical and marginal syllables, it would be coded as a canonical utterance for the CBR (Carney) and the MBR (Carney).

Carney (1991) added two additional ratios to this type of analysis: the vocalic ratio and the quasi-resonant nucleus (QRN) ratio. A vocalic utterance has only vowel-like portions with no recognizable consonantlike portion. The vocalic ratio is the number of vocalic utterances divided by the number of utterances. Similarly, the QRN ratio is the ratio of utterances with QRN divided by the number of utterances. For both ratios, the vocalic nucleus and the QRN are the most sophisticated syllable types in each utterance.

The analysis of vocalization types for each of the four infants is shown in figures 1 through 4. The upper portion of each figure shows the results for canonical and marginal babbling ratios, whereas the lower portion shows the results for the vocalic and quasi-resonant nuclei ratios. The results for the infant with normal hearing are shown in figure 1 at three points in time—8,

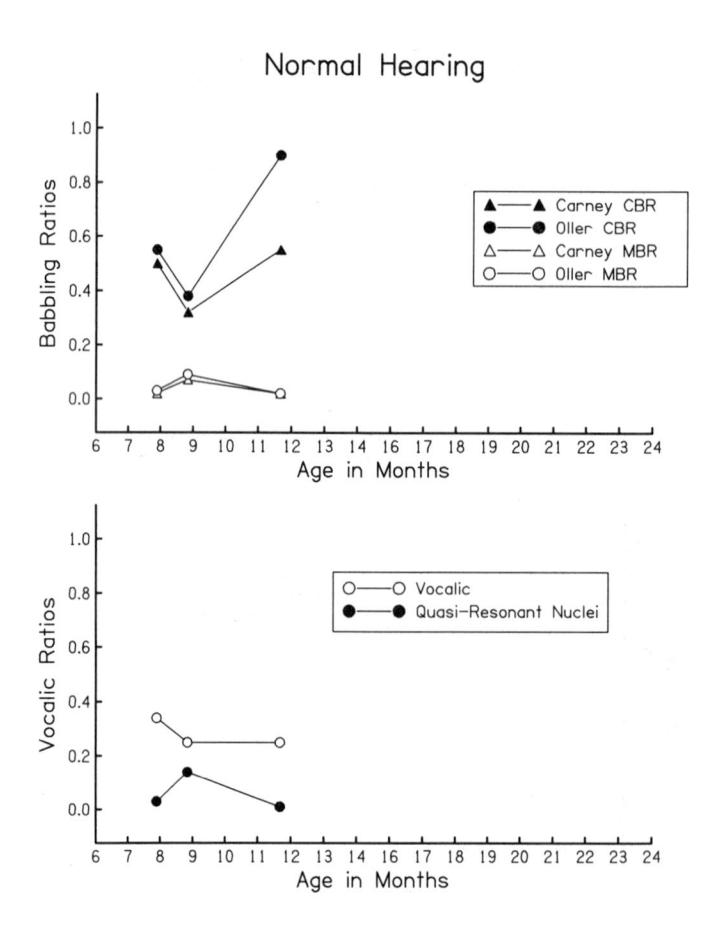

Figure 1. Babbling and vocalic ratios for one infant with normal hearing over time. Two different canonical babbling ratios (CBR) and two different marginal babbling ratios (MBR) are shown, one described by Oller and Eilers (1988) and the other by Carney (1991).

9, and 12 months of age. For this infant, both MBRs (Oller and Carney) are close to 0 for all three points in time. This infant clearly shows a high proportion of canonical syllable production, according to either CBR. According to Oller and Eilers (1988), a CBR of .2 suggests that the infant is in a canonical stage (that is, some consistent production of canonical syllables is observed). This infant has some variation in the CBRs (Carney) between 8 and 12 months, with an upper limit of approximately .55. The higher value of the CBR (Oller), particularly at 12 months, shows simply that this infant is producing a number of multisyllabic utterances that contain many canonical syllables. This infant also shows a decrease in the proportion of vocalic

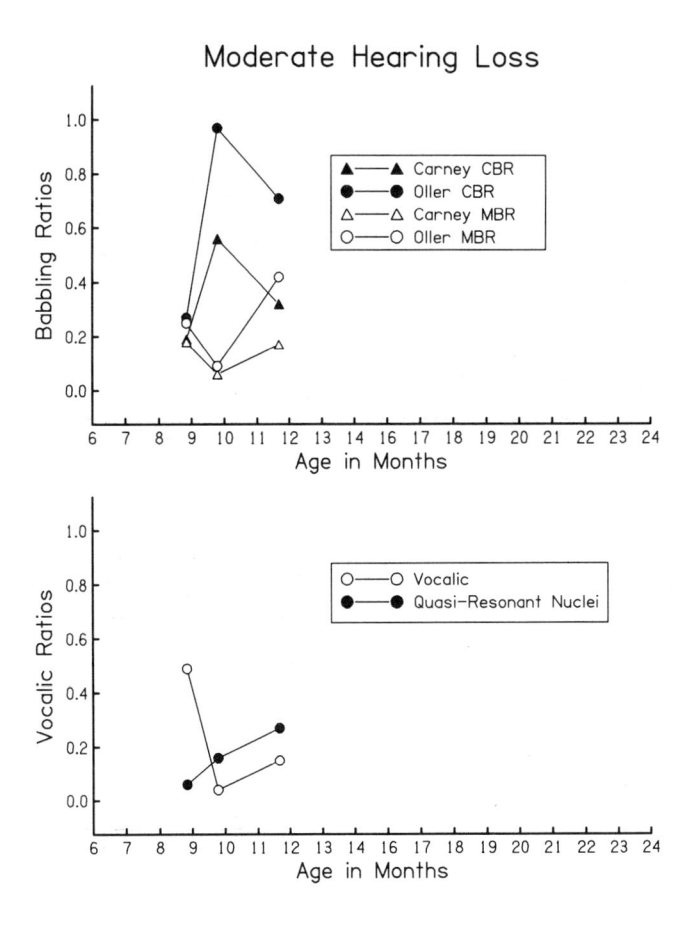

Figure 2. Babbling and vocalic ratios for one infant with a moderate hearing loss over time. Two different canonical babbling ratios (CBR) and two different marginal babbling ratios (MBR) are shown, one described by Oller and Eilers (1988) and the other by Carney (1991).

utterances over time, holding at about .3. For each point in time, the four ratios (CBR [Carney], MBR [Carney], vocalic ratio, QRN ratio) add up to 1. For this infant with normal hearing, the 9-month recording showed some decrease in canonical activity and increase in QRN and marginal syllable activity. However, by 12 months, the proportion of canonical syllables is again the greatest of all four types.

The results of the analysis for the infant with a moderate hearing loss (53 dB HL PTA) are shown in figure 2 for three points in time—9, 10, and 12 months. This infant shows a different picture of timing characteristics compared to the infant with normal hearing. At 9 months of age (1 month

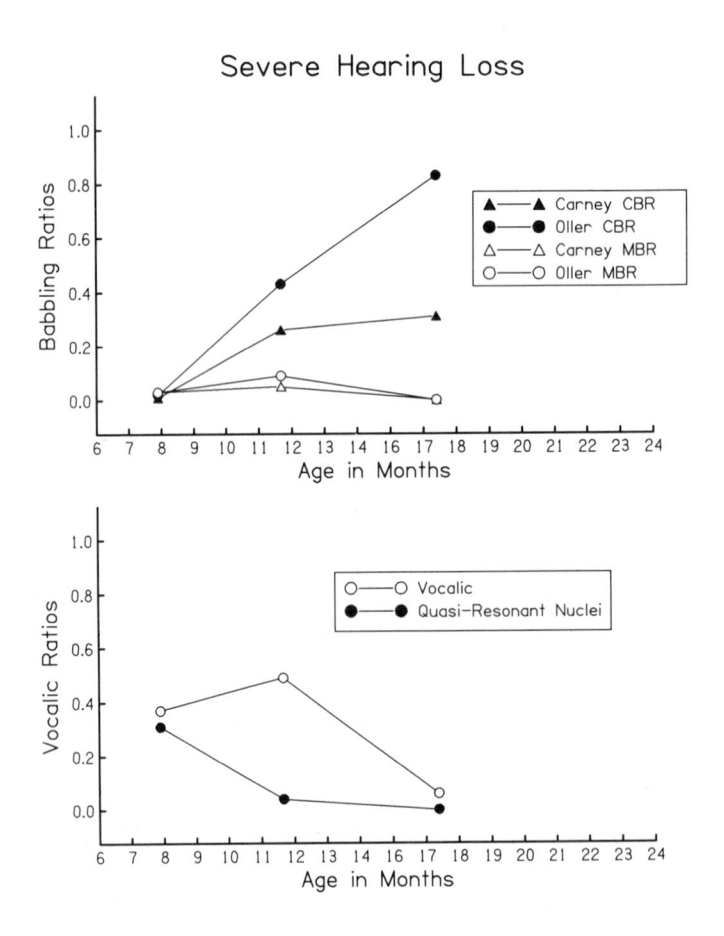

Figure 3. Babbling and vocalic ratios for one infant with a severe hearing loss over time. Two different canonical babbling ratios (CBR) and two different marginal babbling ratios (MBR) are shown, one described by Oller and Eilers (1988) and the other by Carney (1991).

Profound Hearing Loss

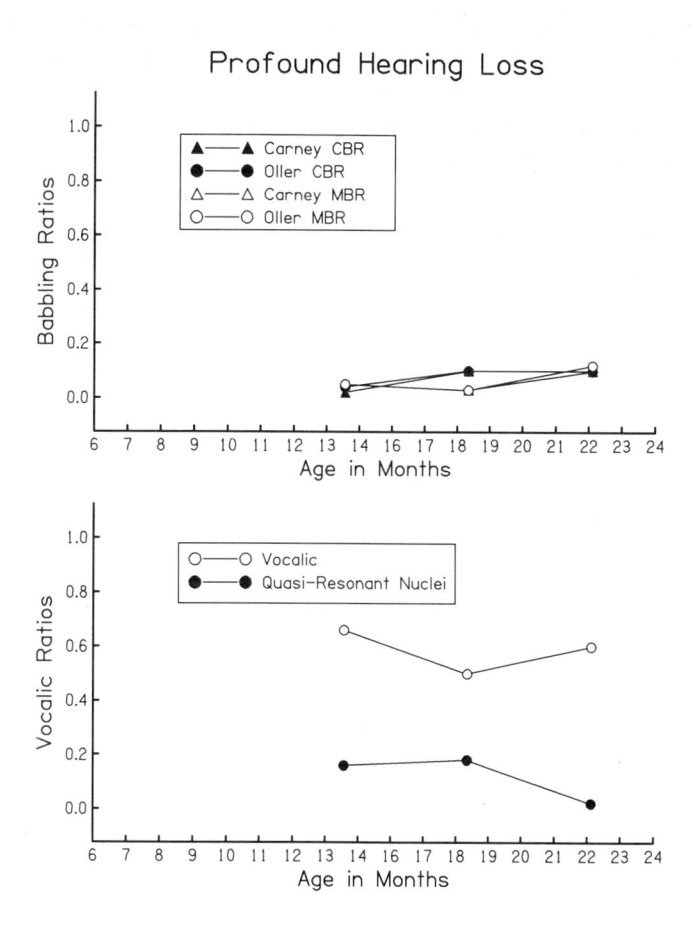

Figure 4. Babbling and vocalic ratios for one infant with a profound hearing loss over time. Two different canonical babbling ratios (CBR) and two different marginal babbling ratios (MBR) are shown, one described by Oller and Eilers (1988) and the other by Carney (1991).

older than the infant with normal hearing), this infant with moderate hearing loss has CBRs close to .2 (both Oller and Carney), indicating that the infant is in the canonical stage. For this same session, the infant has a very high proportion of vocalic utterances (.5) with few QRNs. By 10 months of age, there is a dramatic increase in both CBRs, as well as a drop-off in both MBRs and vocalic nuclei, with a small increase in QRNs. CBR production decreases at 12 months to levels just above that at 8 months for the CBR (Carney) but with a higher value of CBR (Oller) than at 9 months. Once again, the results of the CBR (Oller) show an increase in the number of syllables produced per utterance. Both of these infants show a session-to-session variability, even over a three- or four-month period.

The results of this timing analysis are shown in figure 3 for the infant with the severe loss (73 dB HL PTA) at three points in time—8, 12, and 17 months. At 8 months of age, this infant has CBRs (both Carney and Oller) considerably less than .2, a different pattern from either the infant with normal hearing or the infant with a moderate hearing loss. At 8 months of age, this infant produces predominantly vocalic and QRN utterances. Again, in contrast to the other two infants, the infant with severe hearing loss continues to increase both CBRs by 17 months of age. His CBR (Oller) is quite high, approaching 1, which suggests a high proportion of multisyllabic strings. His CBR (Carney) hovers around .3, a level similar to that of the infant with moderate loss but lower than the infant with normal hearing at only 12 months of age. By 17 months of age, canonical syllables predominate for this child with very marginal syllables, vocalic nuclei, and QRN.

In figure 4 are shown the results from the infant with profound hearing loss at three later points in time—14, 18, and 22 months of age. These points were selected due to her late identification of hearing loss, relative to the other two infants. The pattern is strikingly different for this infant. She never reaches the criterion level of .2 CBR for either the Oller or Carney metric. There is a very small, gradual increase in both canonical and marginal activity. The predominant type of vocalization is vocalic across all three points in time.

The results from these four infants are consistent with the results reported by Oller and Eilers (1988) and Eilers and Oller (1994). Even by 22 months of age, the infant with profound hearing loss does not demonstrate a pattern of canonical babbling. Her utterances are of the more primitive vocalic type. In contrast, the two infants with moderate and severe hearing losses do reach the criterion level of a CBR (Oller) of .2 by 12 months of age, the date suggested as a cutoff by Eilers and Oller. In addition, the infant with a moderate hearing loss shows a pattern of babbling that is more similar to the infant with normal hearing than does the infant with the severe hearing loss. These case studies suggest that degree of hearing loss (or impact of damage on the sensory primitive) appears to have some predictable effects on the development of timing characteristics in the vocalizations of infants. Specifically, it appears that there is a delay in the onset and use of canonical babbling that increases as hearing loss increases.

To examine another area of production representation, a different type of analysis was performed. In addition to coding utterances by syllable type, each utterance was transcribed with a system called Reduced Aspect Feature Transcription (RAFT), described by Carney (1990). In this system, global features of consonantlike or vowel-like productions are coded rather than providing each with a phonetic label from the International Phonetic Alphabet (IPA). In RAFT, the two most important considerations are the speaker's use of vocal tract space and vocal tract manipulation. That is, focus would be on the production of a vowel-like sound that would be made with the tongue up high and in the front of the vocal tract rather than on the production of the vowel /i/. The analysis in this chapter will focus only on vowel-like productions in the samples coded for timing characteristics for the four infants already discussed.

In coding with RAFT, the height of each vocalic portion of each syllable in each utterance is first determined—high, mid, or low. Then the place of each vowel-like production is coded—front, mid, or back. No attempt is made to give the vowel-like portions phonetic labels. Instead, each vowel-like portion would be labeled with one height parameter and one place parameter. Thus, vowel-like productions might be coded as "high-back" or "mid-mid." As with the coding of timing characteristics, transcription was done by consensus. Two transcribers had to agree on the coding of each vowel-like token.

The results of this analysis are shown in the figures 5 through 8. These figures demonstrate the distribution of the use of vocal tract space for vowel-like productions. Three parameters per figure are shown, one for each

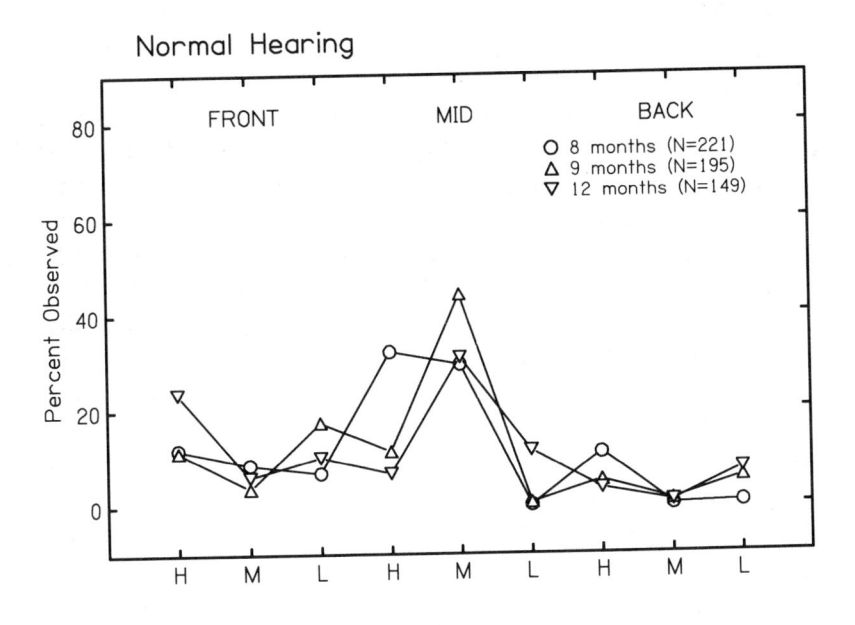

Figure 5. Results of RAFT analysis of the use of vocal tract space for vowel-like tokens for one infant with normal hearing over time. (H = high, M = mid, and L = low. Each point represents a combination of the high, mid, or low parameter with the front, mid, or back parameter. N = the number of vowel-like tokens produced at each recording time.)

point in time at which a recording was made. Each figure is arranged so that the first three data points from left to right represent vocalizations that were coded as vowel-like productions made in the front of the vocal tract; the next three points were made in the middle of the vocal tract (from front to back); and the last three points were made in the back of the vocal tract. Under each of the place categories are three letters representing the height categories—high (H), mid (M), and low (L). For each point in time, each figure has a data point that shows the percentages of productions observed that are high and front, mid and front, low and front; high and mid, mid and mid, low and mid; high and back, mid and back, low and back. The values of the percentage observed should sum to 1 for each point in time at which a recording was done. In addition, the number of total utterances coded at each recording time is shown next to the recording time.

Four points will be discussed per figure for each infant's vocalizations. Three are the locations of the point vowels—high-front, high-back, and low-back. The fourth is the mid-mid location. The latter is of particular interest for children with hearing losses because a number of investigators have reported on the predominance of central or neutralized vowels in the speech of children who are deaf (Monsen 1978, 1983; Smith 1975). Results from the infant with normal hearing are shown in figure 5. At each of the three recording times—8, 9, and 12 months—the infant has the highest proportion of mid-mid vowels, ranging from 30% to 45% observed. By 12 months, this infant was producing approximately 25% of his vowels as high-front tokens, with much smaller percentages (5% to 10%) observed for high- and low-back vowel-like tokens. The infant with normal hearing appears to have a tendency to favor a neutralized vowel position but to continue to expand his use of vocal tract space somewhat over time.

The results of this analysis for the infant with moderate hearing loss are shown in figure 6. For this infant, the proportion of mid-mid vowel-like tokens *increases* over time, a pattern opposite to that of the infant with normal hearing. At 12 months, this infant has fewer tokens in the high-front and high-back areas, with the same very low proportion of low-back vowels as before. In contrast to the infant with normal hearing, there is less expansion of vocal tract space over time, despite the similarity in timing characteristics observed in the first analysis.

The results for the infant with the severe hearing loss are shown in figure 7. Overall, at all three recording times, this infant has an exceptionally high proportion of mid-mid vowels, with an increase to over 75% of the vowel-like tokens observed by 17 months. There are no high-front vowel-like tokens observed at any of the three recording times. In addition, the proportion of high-back vowels decreased steadily from 8 to 17 months. Only the low-back vowels continue to increase up to 20% of the vowel-like tokens observed.

AUDITION AND ORAL COMMUNICATION • 43

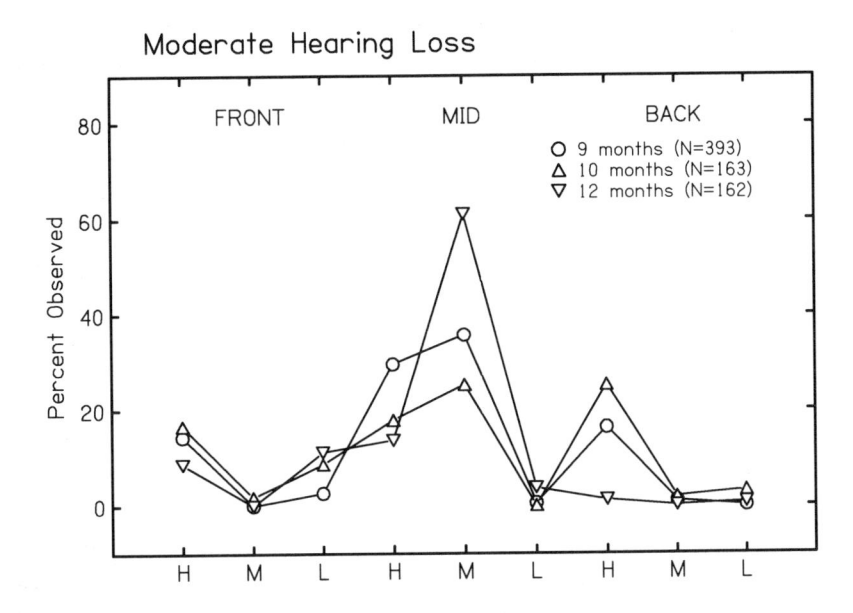

Figure 6. Results of RAFT analysis of the use of vocal tract space for vowel-like tokens for one infant with a moderate hearing loss over time. (H = high, M = mid, and L = low. Each point represents a combination of the high, mid, or low parameter with the front, mid, or back parameter. N = the number of vowel-like tokens produced at each recording time.)

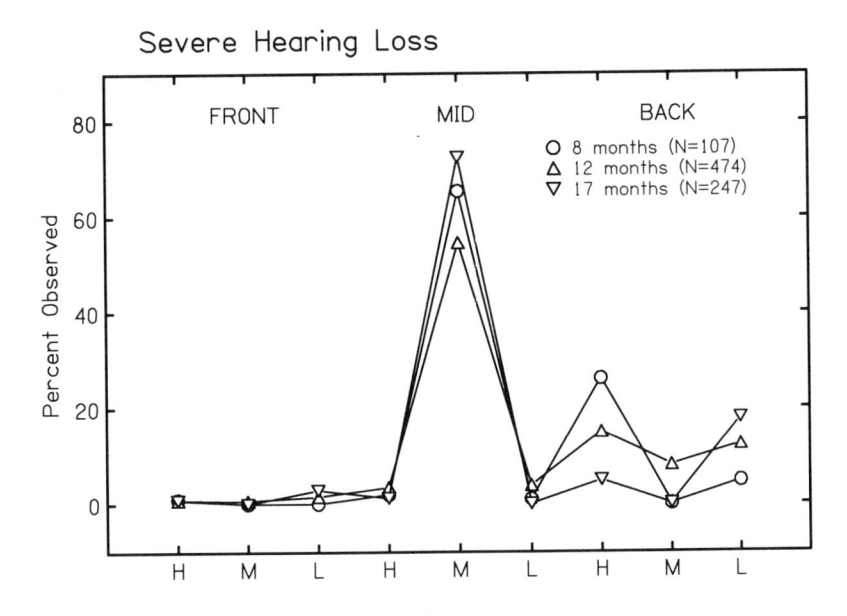

Figure 7. Results of RAFT analysis of the use of vocal tract space for vowel-like tokens for one infant with a severe hearing loss over time. (H = high, M = mid, and L = low. Each point represents a combination of the high, mid, or low parameter with the front, mid, or back parameter. N = the number of vowel-like tokens produced at each recording time.)

Profound Hearing Loss

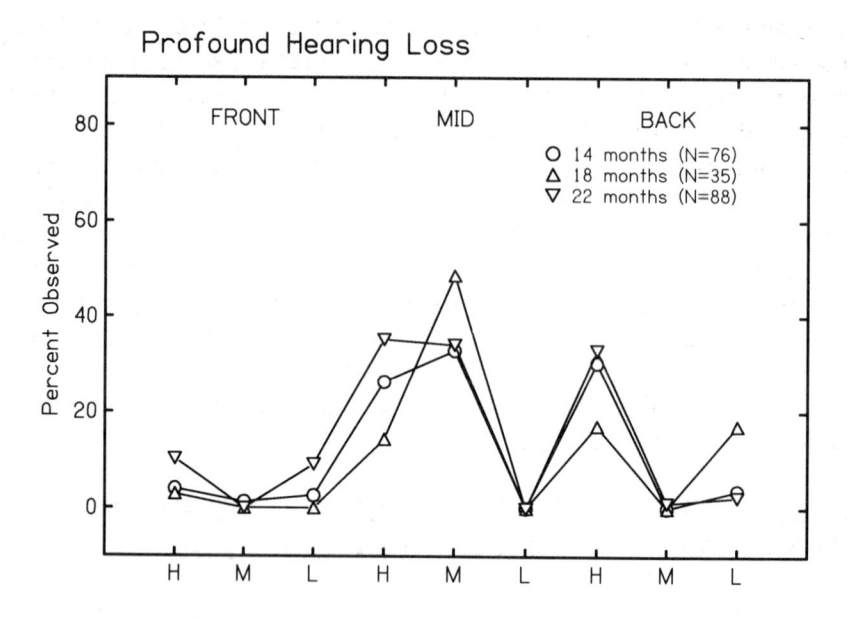

Figure 8. Results of RAFT analysis of the use of vocal tract space for vowel-like tokens for one infant with a profound hearing loss over time. (H = high, M = mid, and L = low. Each point represents a combination of the high, mid, or low parameter with the front, mid, or back parameter. N = the number of vowel-like tokens produced at each recording time.)

Finally, the results for the infant with profound hearing loss are shown in figure 8. This pattern departs from the one observed for the infant with the severe hearing loss. The infant with a profound hearing loss has two peaks in her function—one for mid-mid and high-mid vowel-like tokens and a second for high-back vowel-like tokens. Each accounts for a little less than one-third of the vowel-like tokens observed. In addition, about 10% of the tokens are coded as high-front vowel-like productions. The move to a predominance of neutralized vowels is not as apparent for this infant. However, there is one striking difference in vocalizations for this infant in comparison to the other three. This infant produced many fewer vocalizations overall than the other infants. For example, the infant with a severe hearing loss produced 107, 474, and 247 vowel-like tokens at 8, 12, and 17 months, respectively, whereas the infant with a profound hearing loss produced 76, 35, and 88 vowel-like tokens at 14, 18, and 22 months, respectively. These tokens were also produced in vocalic nuclei and QRN only because the canonical and marginal syllable output was so low.

The results of the RAFT analysis suggest that even infants with normal hearing use a neutralized vowel space in the early stages of vocal development. As vocalizations mature in timing characteristics and more canonical syllables are produced, more of the vocal tract space begins to be used as well. For the two infants with moderate and severe hearing losses, the pattern was reversed; over time, more vowel-like tokens became neutralized, despite the fact that they produced canonical syllables with appropriate timing characteristics. This was particularly dramatic for the infant with the severe hearing loss. One interpretation of these data is that infants with hearing losses even in the moderate range fail to expand their vocal tract space use rather than to collapse their vocal tract space, as described earlier for older children (Monsen 1978). The data for the infant with profound loss are puzzling because they do not follow the pattern set by the other two infants. However, the small set of vocalizations to be coded as well as the absence of appropriate timing characteristics distinguishes the data from those of any infant with normal hearing.

CASE STUDIES OF SPEECH PRODUCTION DEVELOPMENT IN PRESCHOOL-AGE CHILDREN WITH HEARING LOSSES

The question of oral communication competency clearly becomes more important as a child leaves infancy and reaches the preschool years. In these years clinicians and teachers begin to look for evidence of phoneme production, exemplars of the cognitive/linguistic representation level. For children with normal hearing, speech production skills are highly developed at this level. We wanted to demonstrate that the types of analysis used for infants can be expanded to accommodate the more complex productions of children above the age of 3 years. In this section of the chapter, we apply the analysis procedures of RAFT to a corpus of utterances from four children between the ages of 3 and 5 years with profound sensorineural hearing losses, whose pure-tone averages range from 92 to greater than 115 dB HL (ANSI 1989; Carney, Carotta, Dettman, and Karasek 1991). Again, the children were characterized by a severely damaged sensory primitive level. All four children were fitted with appropriate amplification at Boys Town National Research Hospital. They wore their hearing aids regularly, in addition to using FM systems in their self-contained preschool classrooms. All four children were enrolled in preschool classes at Boys Town National Research Hospital. Classroom teachers used a total communication approach, with Signing Exact English (SEEII) as the form of manually coded English used. In addition, each child received daily speech intervention in a combination of group and individual activities.

The four children were asked to name pictures after a tester in an interactive repetition task. The pictures prompted a wide range of vowel, diphthong, and consonant stimuli produced in both open and closed syllables. This task, which was called the Diagnostic Speech Inventory, was developed by Carotta and described by Carotta, Carney, and Dettman (1990).

As with the infant data, transcribers in consensus coded the vocalic portions of the syllables with RAFT according to vowel height and place parameters. In addition, they used a strict criterion for determining whether a real English vowel was produced as well for each vocalic token; that is, after a determination that a token was a high-back vowel, transcribers would then determine if the vowel was sufficiently well formed to be considered a /u/. This analysis revealed the way in which the use of vocal tract space translated into the production of actual recognizable phonemes (Carney et al. 1991).

These data are shown in figures 9 through 12 in a different format from that used for the infant data. Each figure has nine boxes, representing the nine possible vowel areas by height and place. The boxes are oriented so that height and place correspond roughly to the traditional vowel quadrilateral. Vowel height is shown along the ordinate and vowel place along the abscissa. In each of the nine squares, the number represents how many tokens were coded as being produced in the vowel space. Within some of the spaces is a second number, next to an IPA symbol for a vowel. This indicates how many of those actual vowels the child produced.

RAFT analysis results are shown in figure 9 for Subject 1, the child with the poorest hearing. Her pure-tone average is in excess of 115 dB HL

Vowel Inventory Subject 1

Vowel Height	Front	Mid	Back
High	10	2	47 u–2 ʊ–11
Mid	43 ɛ–8	273 ʌ–93	49 o–5
Low	13	1	77 ɑ–27

Vowel Place

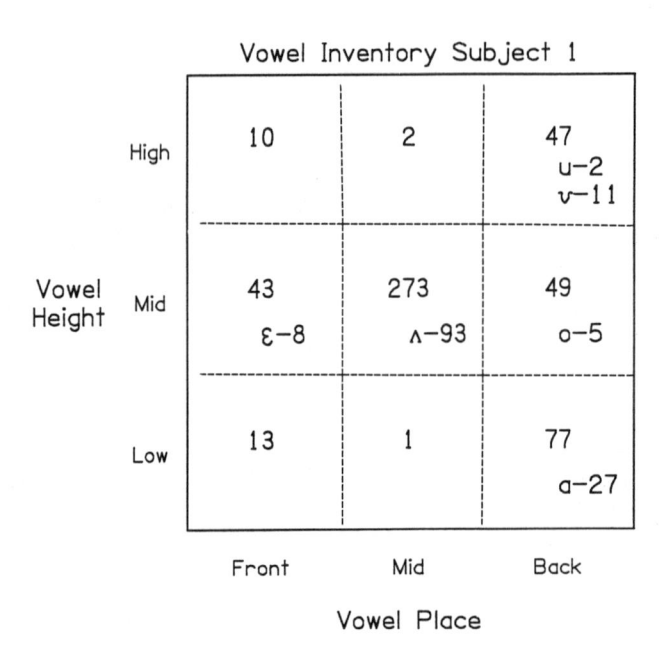

Figure 9. Results of RAFT analysis of the use of vocal tract space for vowel-like tokens for Subject 1, a child with a profound hearing loss (PTA > 115 dB HL). Numbers in each box represent the number of vowel-like tokens coded with that vowel height and vowel place parameter. IPA symbols and numbers indicate how many of the vowel-like tokens were also coded as real vowels within each vowel height and place category.

Vowel Inventory Subject 2

	Front	Mid	Back
High	72 I–4	8	49 u–2
Mid	38 e–1	208 ʌ–12	36
Low	18	11	29

Vowel Height (y-axis) / Vowel Place (x-axis)

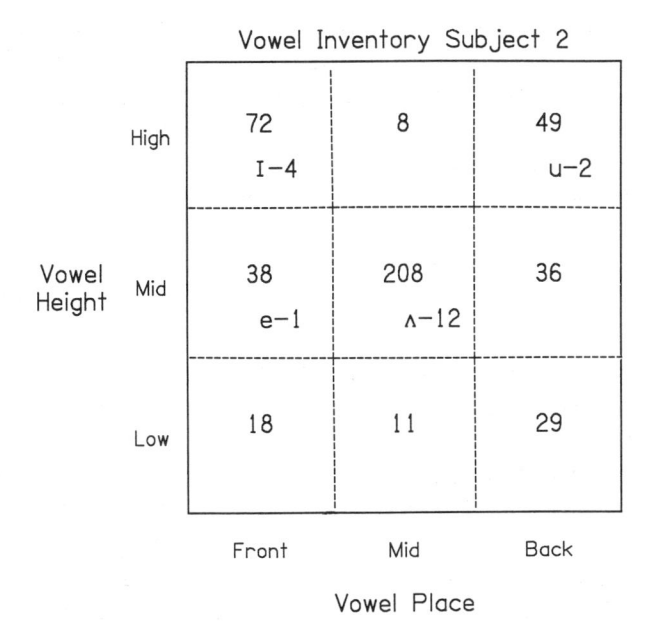

Figure 10. Results of RAFT analysis of the use of vocal tract space for vowel-like tokens for Subject 2, a child with a profound hearing loss (PTA of 105 dB HL). Numbers in each box represent the number of vowel-like tokens coded with that vowel height and vowel place parameter. IPA symbols and numbers indicate how many of the vowel-like tokens were also coded as real vowels within each vowel height and place category.

in her better ear. By far, most of her vowel tokens (N= 273) were produced in the mid-mid space, clearly indicating vowel neutralization. Of these 273 tokens, only 93 were coded as the vowel /ʌ/; the rest did not meet the strict transcription criteria. This child has a vowel inventory of six vowels. About 28% of her total utterances were coded as real vowels, most of them as /ʌ/.

The results of this analysis for Subject 2 are shown in figure 10. This child has a better-ear pure-tone average of 105 dB HL (ANSI 1989). Once again, the predominant vowel space used is that of the mid-mid portion, with 208 tokens coded with that label. In contrast to Subject 1, who has somewhat poorer hearing, only 12 of these mid-mid vowels were coded as the actual vowel /ʌ/. For this subject, only 4% of her productions are transcribed as real vowels. Her vowel inventory is smaller, consisting of only four vowels. This child shows somewhat less use of vocal tract space and manipulation ability than does Subject 1, who has poorer hearing thresholds.

The results of the RAFT analysis for Subject 3 are shown in figure 11. This child has a better-ear pure-tone average of 103 dB HL. This child has a more expanded vowel space and a greater vowel inventory of eight vowels. Fewer of her vocalic tokens are produced in the mid-mid space (N = 142). Thirteen percent of her utterances contain real vowels. All three of these

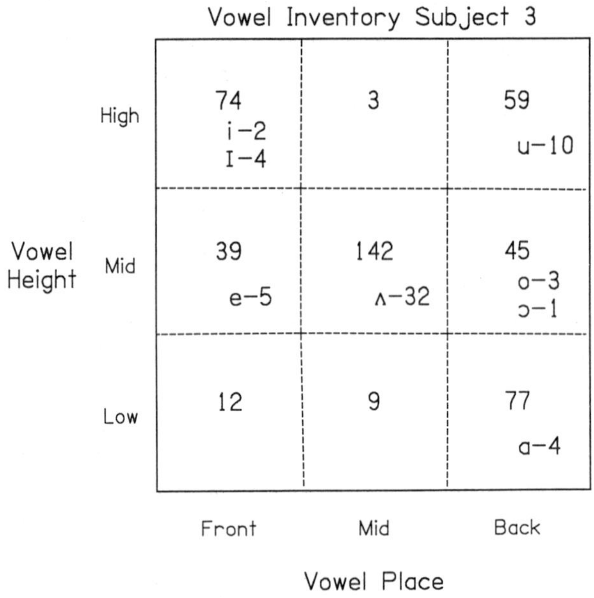

Vowel Inventory Subject 3

Vowel Height	Front	Mid	Back
High	74 i–2 I–4	3	59 u–10
Mid	39 e–5	142 ʌ–32	45 o–3 ɔ–1
Low	12	9	77 ɑ–4

Vowel Place

Figure 11. Results of RAFT analysis of the use of vocal tract space for vowel-like tokens for Subject 3, a child with a profound hearing loss (PTA of 103 dB HL). Numbers in each box represent the number of vowel-like tokens coded with that vowel height and vowel place parameter. IPA symbols and numbers indicate how many of the vowel-like tokens were also coded as real vowels within each vowel height and place category.

children are quite similar in their speech production skills. They all appear to be in various stages of the production representation level, with some limited productions at the cognitive/linguistic representation level.

Finally, RAFT results from Subject 4 are shown in figure 12. This subject has the best pure-tone average (92 dB HL; ANSI 1989) of the four children. In comparison to the other three children, he has the greatest use of vocal tract space and the largest vowel inventory. For this subject, 86% of his tokens are coded as real vowels. In addition, his vowel inventory has 12 vowels. In contrast to the other three preschool children, this child is well into the cognitive/linguistic representation stage and is much readier for functional oral communication.

From these case study data, we can see that profound hearing loss has a great effect on children's speech production ability at the earlier stages of the speech production model, at the subphonemic level. That is, there is substantial impact of hearing loss on the production representation level. This, in turn, has a direct effect on the cognitive/linguistic representation level of speech production.

Vowel Inventory Subject 4

Vowel Height	Front	Mid	Back
High	115 i–36 I–68	1	88 u–29 ʊ–49
Mid	49 e–23 ɛ–19	60 ɝ–1 ʌ–44	63 o–30 ɔ–28
Low	28 æ–27	0	112 ɑ–96

Vowel Place

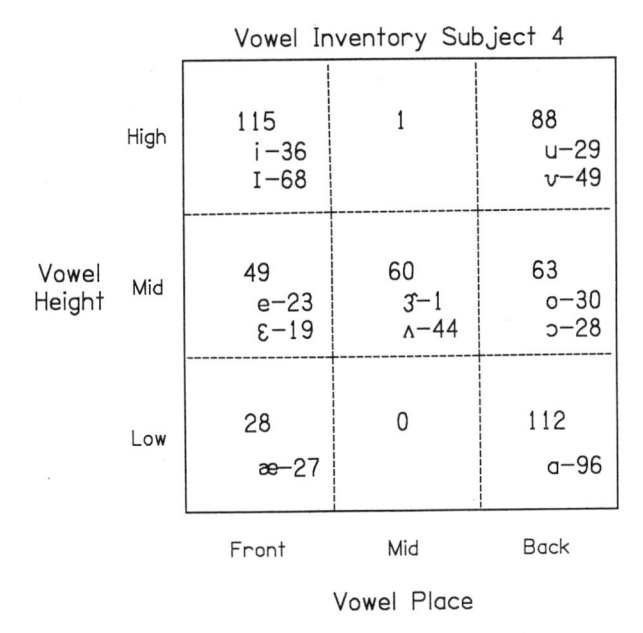

Figure 12. Results of RAFT analysis of the use of vocal tract space for vowel-like tokens for Subject 4, a child with a profound hearing loss (PTA of 92 dB HL). Numbers in each box represent the number of vowel-like tokens coded with that vowel height and vowel place parameter. IPA symbols and numbers indicate how many of the vowel-like tokens were also coded as real vowels within each vowel height and place category.

FUTURE DIRECTIONS

The clear direction of this work is to determine how changes in auditory skill and development can change oral communication competency. Today, the largest change in auditory skill development is likely to come from the receipt of a cochlear implant by a child with a very damaged sensory primitive level and poorly developed speech production skills, particularly if that child is very young. The addition of a cochlear implant leads to immediate changes in the sensory primitive and reorganization of the perceptual representation level. How the cochlear implant affects the production primitive and the production representation level will be a particularly interesting focus of future research. Such studies are currently being conducted in the laboratory at Boys Town National Research Hospital and the University of Minnesota. These data further suggest that the study of children who are hard of hearing is also valuable at all stages of speech production development and not just at the cognitive/linguistic level.

The approaches described in this chapter, in the areas of both perception and production, address newer ways to examine oral communication competency. Although these data are preliminary, they show us that we may be ignoring important information about speech perceptual and production development. Through analyses such as those described, we may be able to select communication modalities in a more informed and evenhanded manner, make prognoses for development, and monitor progress in smaller but quantified steps. Through the implementation of parallel models of perceptual and production development, we may be able to determine the perception-production link for an individual child in order to design more appropriate intervention strategies and to understand better how sensory aids and prostheses affect all aspects of receptive and expressive behavior.

ACKNOWLEDGMENTS

The research reported in this chapter was completed while the author was affiliated with Boys Town National Research Hospital in Omaha, Nebraska. This work was supported in part by grants to Boys Town National Research Hospital from the National Institutes of Health-National Institute on Deafness and Other Communication Disorders #P60DC00982 and #P50DC00215. I would like to thank Ann Kalberer, Renee Zakia, Denise Dettman, Catherine Carotta, and Jeffrey Hicks for assistance with data collection and analysis and Edward Carney for technical assistance in this project. In particular, I would like to thank the parents and children for their faithful participation in these longitudinal studies.

REFERENCES

Abraham, S. 1989. Using a phonological framework to describe speech errors of orally trained, hearing-impaired school-agers. *Journal of Speech and Hearing Disorders* 54:600-649.

American National Standards Institute. 1989. Specifications for audiometers. ANSI S3.6-1989. New York: American National Standards Institute.

Aslin, R.N., and Smith, L.B. 1988. Perceptual development. *Annual Review of Psychology* 39:435-473.

Bauer, H. 1988. The ethologic model of phonetic development: I. Phonetic contrast estimators. *Clinical Linguistics and Phonetics* 2:347-380.

Boothroyd, A. 1988. *Hearing impairments in young children.* Washington, D.C.: Alexander Graham Bell Association for the Deaf.

Boothroyd, A. 1991. Speech perception measures and their role in the evaluation of hearing aid performance in a pediatric population. In J.A. Feigin and P.G. Stelmachowicz (eds.), *Proceedings of the 1991 national conference on pediatric amplification.* Omaha, Nebr.: Boys Town National Research Hospital.

Carney, A.E. 1986. Understanding speech intelligibility in the hearing impaired. *Topics in Language Disorders* 6:47-59.

Carney, A.E. 1990. Reduced Aspect Feature Transcription (RAFT) as an index of speech intelligibility. *Journal of the Acoustical Society of America* 87:S89(A).

Carney, A.E. 1991. Vocal development in hearing-impaired infants. *Journal of the Acoustical Society of America* 90:2298(A).

Carney, A.E. 1993a. Speech production assessment. Presentation at the conference Intervention for Children with Cochlear Implants: Auditory, Speech, and Educational Aspects, June, Boys Town National Research Hospital, Omaha, Nebraska.

Carney, A.E. 1993b. Research on home use of FM systems: Impact on speech production-phonological analysis. Presentation at the 1993 Conference on Development in Pediatric Audiology: Assessment and Amplification, September, Boys Towns National Research Hospital, Omaha, Nebraska.

Carney, A.E., Carotta, C., Dettman, D., and Karasek, A. 1991. Estimating phonetic inventories for young hearing-impaired children. *Asha* 33:149(A).

Carney, A.E., Osberger, M.J., Carney, E., Robbins, A.M., Renshaw, J.J., and Miyamoto, R.T. 1993. A comparison of speech discrimination with cochlear implants and tactile aids. *Journal of the Acoustical Society of America* 94:2036-2049.

Carotta, C., Carney, A.E., and Dettman, D. 1990. Assessment and analysis of speech production in hearing-impaired children. *Asha* 32:59(A).

Dodd, B.J. 1976. The phonological systems of deaf children. *Journal of Speech and Hearing Disorders* 41:185-198.

Eilers, R.E., Gavin, W., and Wilson, W.R. 1979. Linguistic experience and phonemic experience in infancy: A cross-linguistic study. *Child Development* 50:14-18.

Eilers, R.E., and Oller, D.K. 1994. Infant vocalizations and the early diagnosis of severe hearing impairment. *Journal of Pediatrics* 12:199-203.

Elliott, L., and Katz, D. 1980. *Development of a new children's test of speech discrimination.* St. Louis: Auditec.

Fry, D.B. 1978. The role and primacy of the auditory channel in speech and language development. In M. Ross and T.G. Giolas (eds.), *Auditory management of hearing-impaired children: Principles and prerequisites for intervention.* Baltimore: University Park Press.

Geers, A., and Moog, J. 1987. Predicting spoken language acquisition in profoundly deaf children. *Journal of Speech and Hearing Disorders* 52:84-94.

Geffner, D. 1980. Feature characteristics of spontaneous speech production in young deaf children. *Journal of Communication Disorders* 13:443-454.

Jusczyk, P.W. 1986. Toward a model of the development of speech perception. In J. Perkell and D. Klatt (eds.), *Invariance and variability in speech processes.* Hillsdale, N.J.: Lawrence Erlbaum Associates.

Kent, R.D., and Bauer, H. 1985. Vocalizations of one-year olds. *Journal of Child Language* 12:491-526.

Kent, R.D., Osberger, M.J., Netsell, R., and Hustedde, C. 1987. Phonetic development in identical twins who differ in auditory function. *Journal of Speech and Hearing Disorders* 52:64-75.

Kuhl, P.K. 1979. Speech perception in early infancy: Perceptual constancy for spectrally dissimilar vowel categories. *Journal of the Acoustical Society of America* 66:1668-1679.

Kuhl, P.K. 1983. Perception of auditory equivalence classes for speech in early infancy. *Infant Behavior and Development* 6:263-285.

Kuhl, P.K. 1988. Auditory perception and the evolution of speech. *Human Evolution* 3:19-43.

Kuhl, P.K., Williams, K.A., Lacerda, F., Stevens, K.N., and Lindblom, B. 1992. Linguistic experience alters phonetic perception in infants by six months of age. *Science* 255:606-608.

Ling, D. 1976. *Speech and the hearing-impaired child: Theory and practice.* Washington, D.C.: Alexander Graham Bell Association for the Deaf.

Lynch, M., Oller, D.K., and Steffens, M. 1989. Development of speech-like vocalizations in a child with congenital absence of cochleas: The case of total deafness. *Journal of Applied Psycholinguistics* 10:315-333.

Matkin, N.D. 1984. Early recognition and referral for hearing-impaired children. *Pediatrics in Review* 6:151-156.

Mitchell, P.R., and Kent, R.D. 1990. Phonetic variation in multisyllabic babbling. *Journal of Child Language* 17:247-265.

Moeller, M.P., and Carney, A.E. 1993. Assessment and intervention with preschool hearing-impaired children. In J. Alpiner and P. McCarthy (eds.), *Rehabilitative audiology: Children and adults.* 2d ed. Baltimore: Williams and Wilkins.

Monsen, R.B. 1978. Toward measuring how well hearing-impaired children speak. *Journal of Speech and Hearing Research* 21:197-219.

Monsen, R.B. 1983. The oral speech intelligibility of hearing-impaired talkers. *Journal of Speech and Hearing Disorders* 48:286-296.

Northern, J.L., and Downs, M.P. 1991. *Hearing in children.* 4th ed. Baltimore: Williams and Wilkins.

Oller, D.K. 1980. The emergence of the sounds of speech in infancy. In G.H. Yeni-Komshian, J.F. Kavanagh, and C.A. Ferguson (eds.), *Child phonology,* vol. 1: *Production.* New York: Academic Press.

Oller, D.K. 1983. Infant babbling as a manifestation of capacity for speech. In S.E. Gerber and G.T. Mencher (eds.), *The development of auditory behavior.* New York: Grune and Stratton.

Oller, D.K., and Eilers, R.E. 1988. The role of audition in infant babbling. *Child Development* 59:441-449.

Oller, D.K., Eilers, R.E., Bull, D.H., and Carney, A.E. 1985. Pre-speech vocalizations of a deaf infant: A comparison with normal metaphonological development. *Journal of Speech and Hearing Research* 28:47-63.

Oller, D.K., Jensen, H., and Lafayette, R. 1978. The relatedness of phonological processes of a hearing-impaired child. *Journal of Communication Disorders* 11:97-105.

Oller, D.K., and Kelly, C. 1974. Phonological substitution processes of a hard-of-hearing child. *Journal of Speech and Hearing Disorders* 39:65-74.

Oller, D.K., and Lynch, M. 1992. Infant vocalization and innovations in infraphonology. In C.A. Ferguson, L. Menn, and C. Stoel-Gammon (eds.), *Phonological development: Models, research, implications.* Timonium, Md.: York Press.

Oller, D.K., Wieman, L.A., Doyle, W., and Ross, C. 1975. Infant babbling and speech. *Journal of Child Language* 3:1-11.

Osberger, M.J., and McGarr, N.S. 1982. Speech production characteristics of the hearing impaired. In N. Lass (ed.), *Speech and language: Advances in basic research and practice,* vol. 8. New York: Academic Press.

Osberger, M.J., Miyamoto, R.T., Zimmerman-Phillips, S., Kemink, J., Stroer, B.S., Firszt, J., and Novak, M. 1991. Independent evaluation of the speech perception abilities of children with the Nucleus 22-channel cochlear implant system. *Ear and Hearing* 12 (Suppl.):105-115.

Renshaw, J.J., Robbins, A.M., Miyamoto, R.T., Osberger, M.J., and Pope, M.L. 1988. *Hoosier Auditory Visual Enhancement Test.* Indianapolis: Indiana University School of Medicine.

Robbins, A.M., Renshaw, J.J., Miyamoto, R.T., Osberger, M.J. and, Pope, M.L. 1988. *Minimal Pairs Test.* Indianapolis: Indiana University School of Medicine.

Ross, M., and Lerman, J. 1970. A picture identification test for hearing-impaired children. *Journal of Speech and Hearing Research* 13:44-53.

Smith, C.R. 1975. Residual hearing and speech production in deaf children. *Journal of Speech and Hearing Research* 18:795-811.

Stark, R.E. 1980. Stages of speech development in the first year of life. In G.H. Yeni-Komshian, J.F. Kavanagh, and C.A. Ferguson (eds.), *Child phonology*, vol. 1: *Production.* New York: Academic Press.

Stoel-Gammon, C. 1985. Phonetic inventories: 15 to 24 months: A longitudinal study. *Journal of Speech and Hearing Research* 28:505-512.

Stoel-Gammon, C. 1988. Prelinguistic vocalizations of hearing-impaired and normally hearing subjects: A comparison of consonantal inventories. *Journal of Speech and Hearing Disorders* 53:302-315.

Stoel-Gammon, C., and Otomo, K. 1986. Babbling development of hearing-impaired and normally hearing subjects. *Journal of Speech and Hearing Disorders* 51:33-41.

Vihman, M., Ferguson, C.A., and Elbert, M. 1986. Phonological development from babbling to speech: Common tendencies and individual differences. *Applied Psycholinguistics* 7:3-40.

Werker, J.F. 1991. The ontogeny of speech perception. In G. Mattingly and M. Studdert-Kennedy (eds.), *Modularity and the motor theory of speech perception.* Hillsdale, N.J.: Lawrence Erlbaum Associates.

Werker, J.F., Gilbert, J.H.V., Humphrey, K., and Tees, R.C. 1981. Developmental aspects of cross-language speech perception. *Child Development* 52:349-355.

Werker, J.F., and Lalonde, C.E. 1988. Cross-language speech perception: Initial capabilities and developmental change. *Developmental Psychology* 24:672-683.

3

Speech Perception and Production in Children with Hearing Impairment

Arthur Boothroyd, Orna Eran, and Laurie Hanin

INTRODUCTION

Speech perception and production are, to say the least, complex processes. They involve capacities, skills, and knowledge at many levels, including sensorimotor, phonetic, phonologic, lexical, syntactic, semantic, pragmatic, cognitive, and sociocognitive. Childhood deafness can affect all of these levels. The effects can be direct, as in the effect of sensorineural damage on the capacity for perceiving details in the acoustic signal, or they can be indirect, as in the effects of an impoverished acoustic input on speech and language development. The complexity of the processes and the many ways in which they are affected by deafness make the meaningful assessment of speech perception and production in children who are deaf very difficult. In part, the difficulties arise because the many possible perception and production tasks that can be used for assessment place differing demands on the various components of the processes, and on the various capacities, skills, and knowledge bases of the child (Boothroyd 1983, 1984, 1985a, b, 1991; Erber and Alencewicz 1976; Hudgins 1949; Monsen 1978; Risberg 1976; Subtelny 1977; Tyler 1993).

The present chapter deals with two of the more basic aspects of these complex processes. The first is the capacity to perceive phonologically significant contrasts in the utterances of others. The second is the ability to produce utterances that convey phonologically significant contrasts to others. Information about these two aspects by no means represents a complete description. Nevertheless, they are essential to the higher level components of speech perception and production. That is, the perception and production of phonologically significant contrasts among speech sounds are necessary for the development of effective speech production and perception, though admittedly, not sufficient. A second reason for choosing these basic aspects for study is that it should be possible to evaluate them in relatively young children without having to wait many years for the combined effects of maturation and instruction.

Much is already known about the effects of hearing impairment on speech perception at a phonetic level (Bilger and Wang 1976; Erber 1972, 1974, 1981; Hack and Erber 1982; Hudgins and Numbers 1942; Pickett et al. 1972; Risberg 1976; Ross and Giolas 1978; Walden and Montgomery 1975). We know, for example, that performance, on average, decreases with increasing hearing loss. We also know, however, that pure-tone threshold is not a perfect predictor of auditory speech perception at the phonetic level. Two children with identical thresholds may perform very differently on basic speech perception tasks. We also know that, for a given degree of hearing loss, some aspects of speech tend to be perceived auditorily better than others. Suprasegmental patterns, for example, are perceived better than segments, vowels better than consonants, vowel height better than vowel place, consonant voicing better than consonant manner, and consonant place the least accurately (Boothroyd 1984). In visual perception, or speechreading, the pattern is different. Segments are seen better than suprasegmental patterns, vowels better than consonants, and place of articulation better than voicing or manner. To a certain extent, the phonetic-level information available from residual hearing and vision is complementary (Erber 1969, 1972). The aspects of speech that cannot be heard are likely to be seen, and the ones that cannot be seen are likely to be heard.

Despite several years of research on phonetic-level perception in children who are deaf, however, many questions remain unanswered. To what extent, for example, have the published data been influenced by the electroacoustic characteristics of the equipment used to amplify sound? Do the data represent the physical limitations of the damaged auditory system, or are they telling us more about the effects of auditory training, acclimatization, and/or phonologic development? Is there a level of hearing loss at which auditory speech perception capacity is effectively zero? What are the psychoacoustic correlates of decreased auditory speech perception capacity in damaged ears? And are speech production skills a significant factor in determining how the subjects perform on perception tasks?

Similarly, in the area of speech production at the phonetic level there is much that is known, and many questions are unanswered (Boothroyd 1986; Ling 1976; McGarr 1983; McGarr and Harris 1980; Nickerson 1975; Osberger and McGarr 1982; Rubin 1984; Smith 1975; Stark and Levitt 1974). We know, again, that production performance tends to deteriorate, on average, with increasing hearing loss but that children with the same hearing loss may have different abilities. We know that when a child with hearing impairment can use amplified sound as a primary avenue for speech acquisition, he or she tends to produce best the aspects of speech that he or she can perceive best. We also know that, when speech must be learned without benefit of audition, the production problems can be many and serious. Errors have been documented in breathing, laryngeal control, velar control, valving, articulation, coarticulation, and interarticulator timing. At the acoustic/phonetic level, these errors produce abnormal voice quality, rhythm, average pitch, intonation contours, and vowels, and they result in consonant distortions, omissions, additions, and substitutions. Children who are deaf and acquire production skills through a combination of individual aptitude and excellent teaching, but without the benefit of residual hearing, tend to produce vowels and consonants quite well but often have serious difficulties with rhythm, pitch, intonation, and voice quality.

Among the unknowns are the relative contributions of inherent capacity and educational opportunity. Does the research literature on speech production by children who are deaf really tell us something about hearing impairment, or is it, as Ling has suggested, more of a commentary on quality of instruction (Ling 1976)? Along the same lines, the adequacy of the amplification equipment used to provide children with hearing impairment with speech input and feedback is an unknown factor in terms of the production data. And what exactly is the relationship between auditory speech perception capacity and speech production performance in children with hearing impairment?

ASSESSING SPEECH PERCEPTION AND PRODUCTION

The remainder of this chapter is devoted to reviewing some of the relevant findings of ongoing research at the City University of New York. Specifically, the relationships and dependencies among phonetic-level speech perception, phonetic-level speech production, pure-tone threshold, sensation level, age, and primary communication mode are examined. The general goal of this research has been to establish a database of auditory speech perception capacity in aided children with various degrees of hearing loss that can be used as a frame of reference against which to assess the efficacy of cochlear implants. The results will be reported in full elsewhere. The present chapter reviews a sample of the findings.

IMSPAC

The data to be reported were obtained with an *IM*itative test of the perception of *S*peech *PA*ttern *C*ontrasts known as IMSPAC. The basic

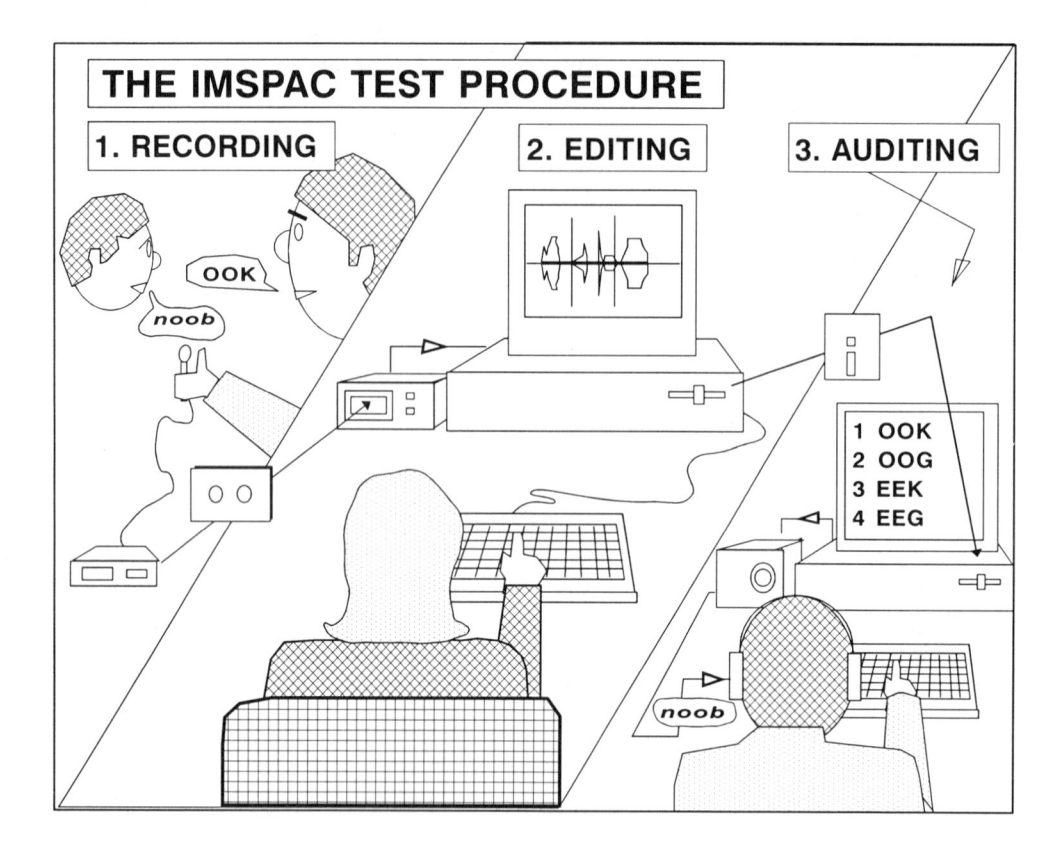

Figure 1. The IMSPAC test procedure has three stages: first, recording of the child's imitations; second, digitization and editing of the recordings to generate files containing only the child's imitations; and third, presentation of the child's utterances to a team of auditors in a forced-choice paradigm. The complete test involves 40 imitations of auditory-visual models and 40 of auditory-only models.

concept is straightforward. The child is asked to imitate a syllable, for example, *ook*. The child's imitation is then heard by a hearing adult who is asked to decide whether the child was imitating, for example, *ook, oog, eek,* or *eeg,* as shown in figure 1. The response of *ook* or *oog* is scored correct for vowel place. The response of *ook* or *eek* is scored correct for final consonant voicing. Each pair of contrasts is represented in a single subtest by eight syllables. There are five subtests, representing ten contrasts:

syllable number (e.g., *oo* versus *oo-oo*)
intonation (e.g., *aw!* versus *aw?*)
vowel height (e.g., *boo* versus *baw*)
vowel place (e.g., *koo* versus *kee*)
initial consonant voicing (e.g., *gaw* versus *kaw*)

final consonant voicing (e.g., *awt* versus *awd*)
initial consonant continuance (e.g., *zoo* versus *doo*)
final consonant continuance (e.g., *eech* versus *eesh*)
initial consonant place (e.g., *seh* versus *feh*)
final consonant place (e.g., *awg* versus *awk*)

To increase face validity as a measure of capacity for development of speech perception and production skills at the sentence level, the phonetic context of the test contrast changes from trial to trial within a test.

A single administration of the test involves two presentations of 40 syllables each. In the first presentation, the child is given every possible input (hearing, speechreading and, if appropriate, print). The results are intended to provide information on the child's best production performance. In the second presentation, using a different form of the test, the child must imitate using only an auditory input. The results are intended to provide information on auditory capacity, at least up to any ceiling determined by production ability. Thus, if the scores by audition alone are significantly poorer than those obtained with all possible inputs, we may assume that the auditory-only score reflects auditory capacity. If the two scores are equal, we may assume that the auditory capacity is at least as good as that reflected by production performance (though possibly better). If the auditory-visual score approaches zero, however, this test is ineffective as a test of auditory capacity.

The data reported here were obtained from tape-recorded imitations collected at several collaborating centers. Auditory input was provided by linear amplification, without compression or limiting, at the highest comfortable listening level, up to a maximum of 136 dB SPL (sound pressure level). Recordings of the imitations were digitized and edited at the City University of New York, to remove all but the child's utterances, and audited by teams of four hearing adults, using the four-alternative forced-choice response format. The hardware, software, and procedures were developed in-house for this and related work.

The results of this procedure are composite scores, for each child under the auditory-only and auditory-visual input conditions. Each score is averaged across ten contrasts, each involving eight utterances judged by four auditors. In addition, separate scores are obtained for the ten contrasts.

The subjects for whom data are to be reported were 97 children who were severely and profoundly deaf in various educational settings around the United States. There were 49 boys and 48 girls. Twenty-one were of minority status (African American, Latin American, or Asian). All were users of hearing aids. Ages at onset of hearing loss ranged from zero to 4 years, but only six subjects became deaf after age 2. Hearing losses ranged from 70 to 117 dB with a mean of 97 dB. Ages ranged from 3 to 15 years with a mean of 9 years. Sixty-two were in schools for the Deaf. Twenty-four were in a day program for children who are hearing impaired. The remainder were mainstreamed. The primary mode of communication was reported to be oral for 61 of the subjects and total communication (TC) for 36.

PREDICTORS OF PERFORMANCE

In multiple regression analyses, the only significant predictor of performance, under the auditory-only condition, was degree of hearing loss. As shown in the left panel of figure 2, hearing loss accounted for 50% of the variance in the auditory-only score. In other studies, test-retest variability has been found to account for approximately 10% of the variance, leaving approximately 40% unexplained. Note that age accounted for only a nonsignificant 1.5%, while communication mode, age at onset, and minority status were unrelated to performance.

Under the auditory-visual condition, hearing loss was still the primary predictor of performance, but it accounted for only 30% of the variance, as

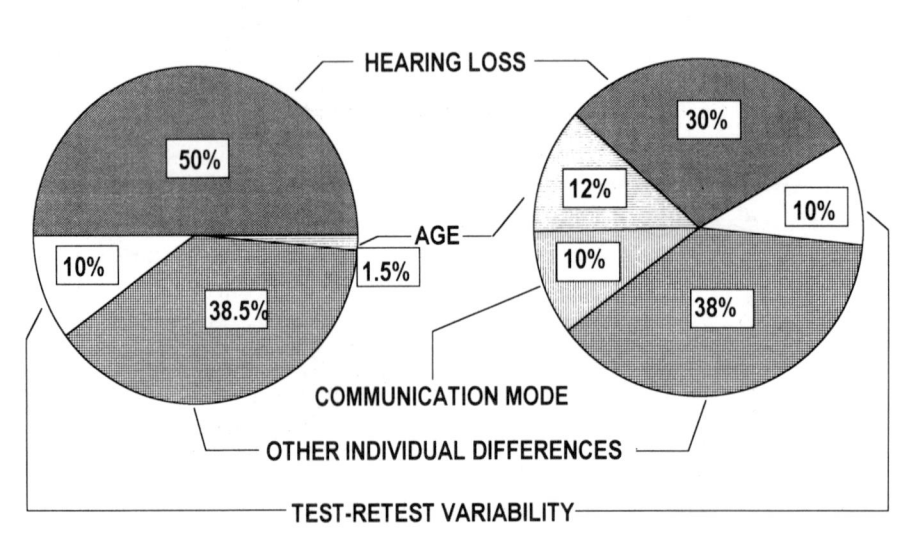

Figure 2. The IMSPAC test was administered to 97 children who were severely and profoundly deaf, ages 3 through 15 years, at the highest comfortable listening level. Composite scores were examined using stepwise multiple linear regression analysis. This figure shows the resulting attribution of variance. The auditory-only scores depended mainly on degree of hearing loss. The auditory-visual scores were somewhat less dependent on hearing loss but were significantly dependent on age and communication mode. In both cases, about 40% of the variance was unaccounted for and may be attributed to individual factors other than degree of loss, age, and communication mode.

shown in the right panel of figure 2. Both age and communication mode accounted for significant proportions of the variance (12% and 10%, respectively). As with the auditory-only scores, approximately 40% of the variance was unexplained by the variables examined here.

These data are in keeping with the conclusion that the auditory-only score is, indeed, a measure of auditory capacity that is set by the inherent physical characteristics of the auditory system and is not amenable to change through maturation and/or instruction. The auditory-visual score, on the other hand, although strongly reflecting degree of hearing loss, does appear also to be responsive to the effects of maturation and instruction.

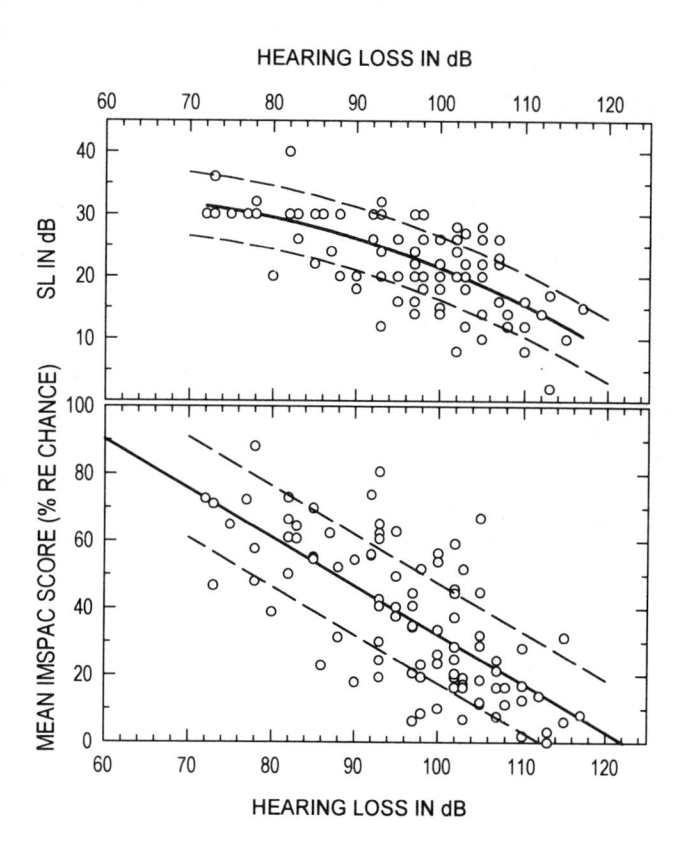

Figure 3. The upper panel shows the sensation levels at which stimuli were presented to 97 children who were severely and profoundly deaf during IMSPAC testing, as a function of three-frequency average hearing loss. The lower panel shows the resulting composite scores under the auditory-only condition. The lines show regression functions (quadratic in the upper panel and linear in the lower) plus and minus 1 standard error or prediction. These data emphasize that a significant contributor to the poor IMSPAC performance of the subjects who were more profoundly deaf is the fact that their reduced dynamic range of hearing mandates sensation levels below the nominal 30 dB needed for full audibility of the speech signal.

HEARING LOSS, SENSATION LEVEL, AND AUDITORY CAPACITY

In the lower panel of figure 3, the mean IMSPAC score of each child, for the auditory-only condition, is plotted as a function of three-frequency average threshold in the better ear (which was also the ear tested). Note that the scores have been corrected for guessing, using the transform:

$$y = (x-g)(100-g)*100 \qquad (1)$$

where: y = corrected score in %
x = raw score in %
and   g = score expected from guessing (50% in this case). Using this transform, the range from 50% to 100% is expanded to become 0% to 100%.

The solid line in the lower panel of figure 3 shows the linear regression function for score on loss. It is the expected score of the average subject. The broken lines show the standard error of prediction. Roughly two-thirds of the scores fall between these lines. It will be seen that the score of the average subject is 0% for a loss of 120 dB. It rises at the rate of 1.4 percentage points per dB for losses below 120 dB. The upper panel of figure 3 shows the sensation levels at which the auditory models were presented to the subjects. (The lines show the quadratic regression function +/-1 standard error of prediction.) These data emphasize that one of the reasons for the poorer performance of children who are deafer is that they simply do not have access to the full acoustic signal. The useful information in the speech signal is usually estimated to cover a range of about 30 dB (from the loudest vowel to the weakest consonant). Full audibility of speech, therefore, requires a sensation level of approximately 30 dB. It will be seen from figure 3 that this criterion was met for the average subject with a hearing loss of 80 dB, but not for those with greater losses. Indeed, for a loss around 115 dB, the typical sensation level was only 10 dB. At such a sensation level, even subjects with normal hearing score only about 30% on this type of test (Boothroyd and Martin-Evans 1990).

These data are in keeping with the conclusion that limited audibility of the amplified signal is a significant contributor to the reduced speech perception capacity of people who are profoundly deaf. The extent to which this problem might be addressed by amplitude compression and/or speech coding has still to be determined (Boothroyd, Springer, Smith, and Shulman 1988; Braida, Durlach, DeGennaro, Peterson, and Bustamante 1982; Braida, Durlach, Lippmann, Hicks, Rabinowitz, and Reed 1980). In the meantime, it is sobering to realize that our efforts to use amplification to provide basic audibility of the speech signal may be inadequate for children who are profoundly deaf despite the technological advances of recent decades.

PERCEPTION, PRODUCTION, AND HEARING LOSS

In figure 4, the data have been grouped according to hearing loss in 10 dB intervals. The benefit of this approach is that, unlike linear regression analysis, it makes no assumptions about the form of the underlying relationships. Group size is shown at the top of the figure. Group means for the auditory-only and auditory-visual conditions are shown; plus and minus standard errors derived from the pooled error variance in an analysis of variance. These data show that both scores fall with increasing hearing loss, but the mean audiovisual score is about 25 percentage points higher than the auditory-only score. The difference is relatively independent of degree of hearing loss. Note that the group with the most profound hearing loss appears to obtain very little information by hearing alone but, given the visual input, can produce imitations in which 40% of the contrasts are identifiable by the auditors.

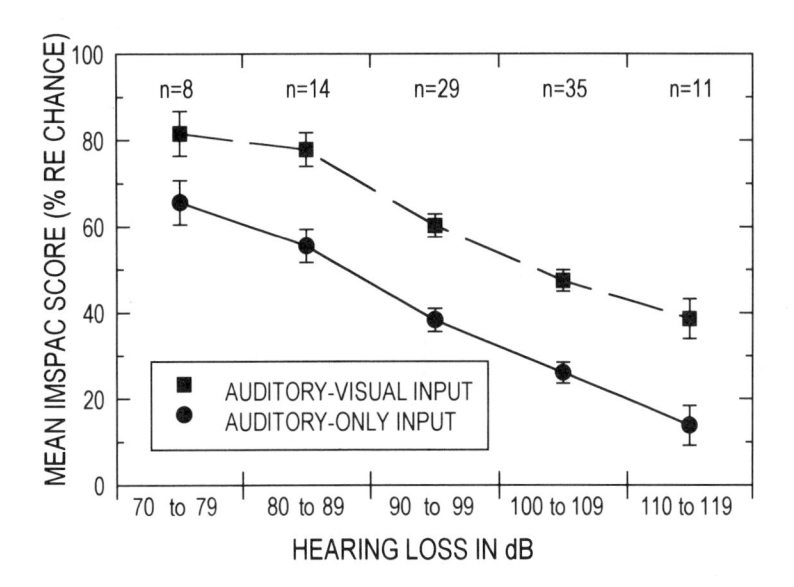

Figure 4. Auditory-visual and auditory-only IMSPAC scores of subjects grouped according to hearing loss in 10 dB intervals. Data points are group means plus and minus 1 standard error (derived from the error term in a repeated-measures analysis of variance). It is clear from these data that the auditory-only scores are not being limited by production ability. It seems probable that they are, therefore, revealing limits set by auditory perceptual capacity.

These data add further support to the conclusion that the imitations produced under the auditory-only condition are an index of auditory capacity. If their quality was being limited by the speech production capabilities of the children, then the auditory-visual scores would be no better than the auditory-only scores. The data also support the conclusion that the absence of auditory capacity need not exclude the possibility of acquiring motor speech skills. At the same time, they illustrate that good hearing is an enormous asset in the acquisition of those skills.

PERCEPTION, PRODUCTION, LOSS, AND COMMUNICATION MODE

In figure 5, the loss by modality data of the previous figure are shown separately for the oral and TC subjects. The overall pattern is similar for the two groups. However, the auditory-visual scores for the oral subjects are some 35 to 40 percentage points higher than the auditory-only scores. The difference is only about 15 percentage points (but still significant) for the TC subjects. Note that the conclusion that motor speech skills can be acquired in the absence of significant auditory capacity is less strongly supported for the TC group. These data support the conclusion that the development of phonetic level speech production skills, beyond the limits set by auditory capacity, is strongly influenced by learning opportunity.

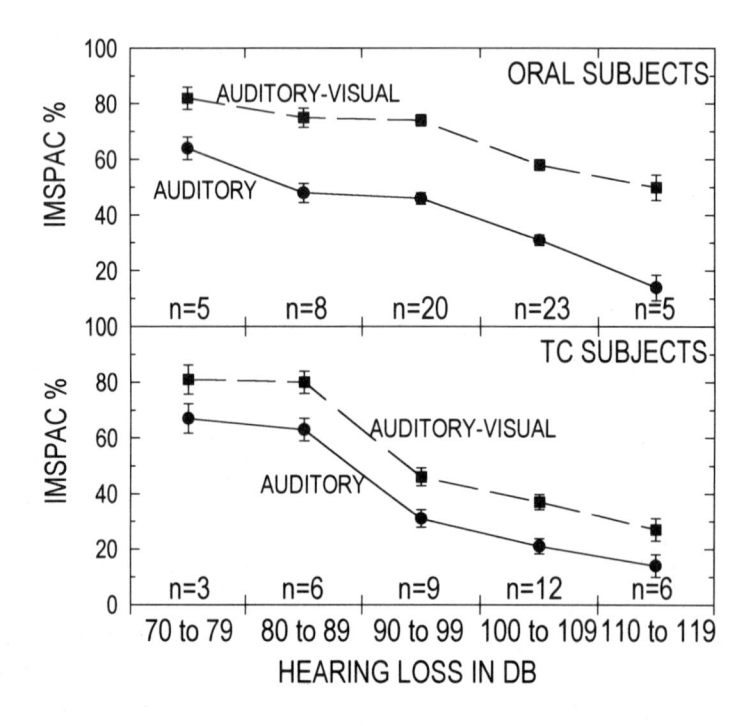

Figure 5. The comparison between auditory-visual and auditory-only IMSPAC scores, as a function of hearing loss, is shown separately in the figure for the oral and total communication (TC) subjects. The modality effect is much greater for the oral groups. It is still significant, however, for the TC groups.

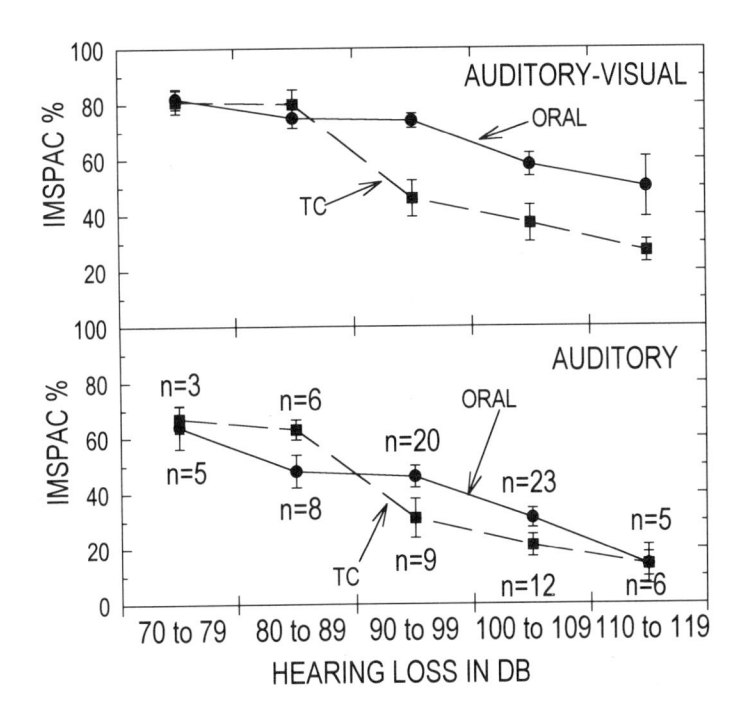

Figure 6. In this figure, the data of figure 5 have been rearranged to show the oral/TC effect separately for the auditory-visual and auditory-only presentations of IMSPAC. In analyses of variance, it was found that the oral/TC difference was present only for the auditory-visual condition and then only for subjects with losses of 90 dB or more. The absence of a significant oral/TC effect for the auditory-only condition lends further support to the conclusion that these scores reveal limits set by auditory capacity rather than by production abilities. Note that the error bars in this figure are standard errors based on the pooled within-group variance.

Figure 6 shows the same data as figure 5 but rearranged to emphasize several points. In the upper panel are the auditory-visual scores for the oral and TC subjects. The better scores for the oral subjects are present only for hearing losses of 90 dB or more. This observation is in keeping with the conclusion that, given enough auditory capacity, specific instruction in speech production does not necessarily influence performance. For people who are profoundly deaf, however, optimal speech production skills cannot be expected to follow spontaneously from hearing.

In the lower panel are the auditory-only scores for the two groups. In an analysis of variance, the main effect of modality was nonsignificant, and there was no significant interaction between modality and hearing loss group. In other words, the auditory-only scores for the oral and TC subjects were, to all intents and purposes, identical. This finding further supports the conclusion that the auditory-only score provides a measure of inherent auditory capacity, without confounding by maturation and learning.

PERCEPTION, PRODUCTION, AND AGE

In figure 7, the auditory-visual and auditory-only scores are shown as a function of age group in four-year intervals. Significant differences between the two measures are shown by asterisks, and significant differences between adjacent age groups are shown by heavy lines. The youngest and oldest groups had lower mean hearing losses than the other two groups. In figure 7, therefore, the confounding of age and hearing loss has been corrected by adjusting each mean to its predicted value for a loss of 100 dB, using the regression functions for IMSPAC score on loss. The auditory-only scores are relatively unaffected by age. There is a significant rise for the oldest group, but the magnitude is not great. In contrast, the auditory-visual scores show considerable growth, though not between the first and second groups. Note further that there is no significant effect of modality for the youngest group.

Once again, these data support the conclusion that the auditory-only score is primarily a measure of auditory capacity, unaffected by cognitive and linguistic status, while the auditory-visual score reflects steadily improving speech skills. The absence of a modality effect for the youngest group further

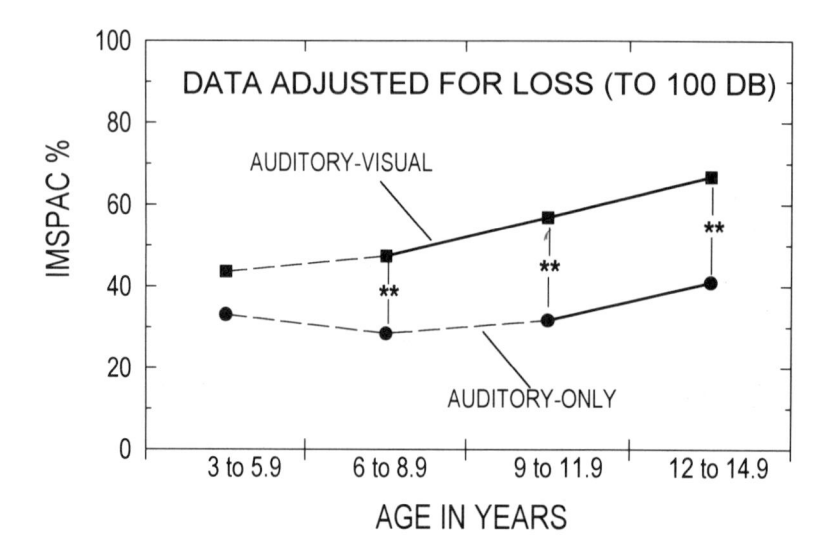

Figure 7. Auditory-visual and auditory-only IMSPAC scores of subjects grouped according to age in four-year intervals. The group means have been corrected for small differences of mean hearing loss using data from a linear regression analysis. Significant differences (p<0.05) between modalities are shown by asterisks, and significant differences between adjacent age groups by heavy lines. Note the much stronger age effect for the auditory-visual scores and the absence of a significant modality effect for the youngest age group. These are the only data that show a significant age effect for the auditory-only condition, but this appears only after age 10 years.

suggests that, at this age, auditory capacity is the primary determinant of speech production skills.

CONTRAST PROFILES

Figure 8 shows the group means for the ten contrasts under the two input conditions. The contrasts have been arranged in descending order of the mean auditory-only scores for the 90 to 99 dB group. These results are in keeping with those found in previous studies and summarized in the introduction. Note particularly that the suprasegmentals are among the most easily perceived via hearing and that the consonant place contrasts are the least easily perceived. The benefits of adding vision are greatest for the vowel and consonant place contrasts and least for the suprasegmentals. These data lend further support to the conclusion that performance on the IMSPAC test, under the auditory-only condition, provides a valid measure of auditory speech perception capacity at the level of the phonologically significant contrast. The fact that the subject must use speech skills to respond to the test does not appear to undermine its validity as a test of auditory speech perception capacity.

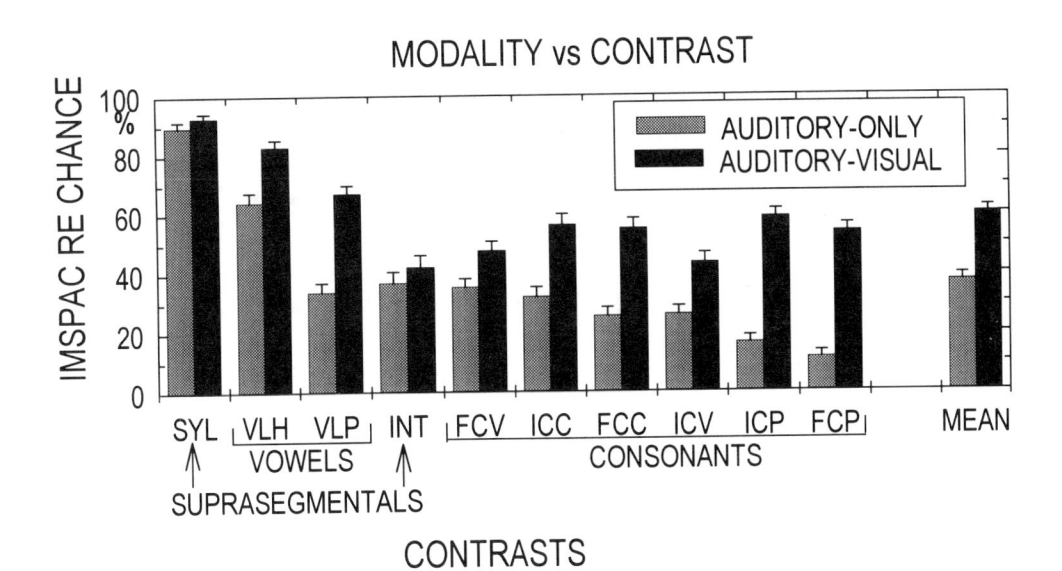

Figure 8. Group mean IMSPAC scores of 97 children who are severely and profoundly deaf as a function of contrast and input modality. The contrasts have been arranged in descending order of mean auditory-only score for the 90 to 99 dB group. Abbreviations are as follows: SYL = syllable number (1 vs. 2); VLH = vowel height; VLP = vowel place; INT = intonation (rise vs. fall); FCV = final consonant voicing; ICC = initial consonant continuance; FCC = final consonant continuance; ICV = initial consonant voicing; ICP = initial consonant place; FCP = final consonant place.

Figure 9 shows the auditory-only and auditory-visual contrast profiles for the five hearing loss groups. Because there were no significant effects of communication mode, and only minimal effects of age, the auditory-only data may be taken as a fair estimate of the probability of auditory perception of the various contrasts as a function of hearing loss. Note, however, that hearing loss accounted for only 50% of the variance in composite auditory-only IMSPAC scores. Hearing loss is not the only factor determining an individual's capacity for the auditory perception of speech pattern contrasts. The auditory-visual profiles show the benefit of adding visual to auditory input at all levels of hearing loss but especially for subjects who are more profoundly deaf. For each loss group, the special benefits of vision in providing information about vowel and consonant place of articulation are apparent. Note, however, that subjects who are more profoundly deaf also benefit considerably from visual information about vowel height and consonant continuance.

DISCUSSION

These data provide at least partial answers to some of the questions raised in the introduction. The sensation levels, for example, strongly suggest

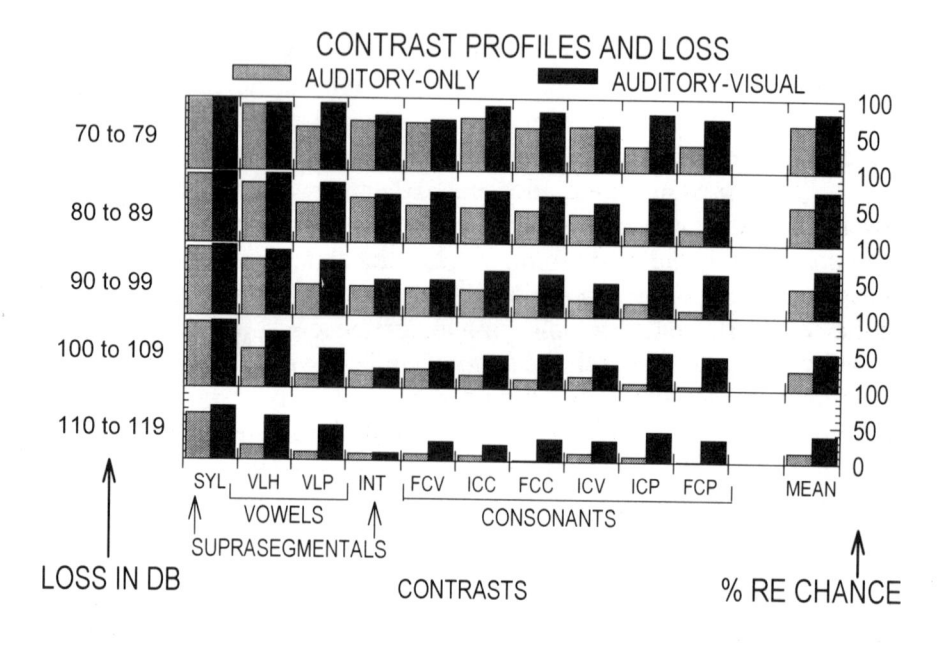

Figure 9. This figure shows the auditory-only and auditory-visual IMSPAC contrast profiles for five groups of subjects selected according to hearing loss in 10 dB steps. As in figure 8, the contrasts have been arranged in decreasing order of auditory-alone performance for the 90 to 99 dB group. (See figure 8 for key to contrast abbreviations.)

that empirical data on the auditory capacities of children who are profoundly deaf may, indeed, be influenced by electroacoustic properties of the amplification equipment. The present data suggest that a better match between the dynamic range of hearing and the intensity range of speech might produce better estimates of capacity. It is also possible, however, that attempts to improve the audibility of the speech signal by such things as amplitude compression, frequency transposition, and speech coding will generate compact acoustic patterns that overtax the limited resolving power of the damaged cochlea. There is still a need for research on this topic, preferably using multiple single subject designs.

These data suggest that the effects of age and maturation on measured auditory capacity are not serious, at least for a test of the type used here. As for the upper limit of hearing loss for which audition can remain useful, the present findings suggest something in the region of 120 dB. This observation could, however, be somewhat artificial. Subjects with losses in the region of 120 dB had sensation levels of only about 10 dB. This limit was set, in part, by the maximum undistorted output of the test equipment, which was 136 dB SPL for pure tones and 126 dB SPL for speech. In fact, subjects who were the most profoundly deaf were tested with their classroom amplification equipment, but that was unlikely to have added more than about 5 dB to the maximum available output. Thus, the 120 dB HL limit for usable hearing may, in part, reflect our inability to make sounds audible to subjects who are the most profoundly deaf. This should not, however, be interpreted as a plea for more powerful hearing aids. The extrapolation of results from subjects with lesser degrees of hearing loss also points to 120 dB HL as being an effective upper limit of usability.

The present data do not offer any information about the psychoacoustic correlates of auditory speech perception capacity in subjects who are severely and profoundly deaf (other than pure-tone threshold). It is reasonable to assume, however, that a portion of the 40% unexplained variance in the auditory-only data could be explained by psychoacoustic capacity. Previous research has generally failed to show such correlations, but the issue has usually been studied with speech perception tasks that are potentially confounded by lexical and other language factors. The present data do suggest that speech production ability was *not* a significant factor in determining perceptual performance—at least with these subjects and these tasks.

On the production side, the present data support Ling's assertion that measures of speech production in people who are profoundly deaf are likely to reveal as much about learning opportunity as about deafness (Ling 1976). The sensation level findings are also relevant to the question of amplification characteristics and their potential effects on the acquisition of speech production skills (Levitt 1982; Seewald, Hudson, Gagné, and Zelisko 1992).

The specific relationship between speech production and auditory speech perception was not examined here, but the fact that the two covary, and are correlated with degree of hearing loss, is self-evident. The profile data of figures 8 and 9 also testify to the fact that, for children who are profoundly deaf, audition alone cannot provide full access to the details of the speech signal and that speechreading can offer valuable supplementary information. On the strength of these data, it is difficult to justify instructional methods that require a child with profound deafness to acquire speech perception and production skills solely via the sense of hearing.

The use of the labels oral and TC to quantify learning opportunity is open to question. Both represent approaches or philosophies rather than specific instructional methods. Neither label offers information about the extent to which the philosophies are followed in practice or about the quality of instruction in general. Most of the oral subjects in the present study, however, attended traditional oral schools in which the development and everyday use of spoken language are given high priority. It seems reasonable to assume that this emphasis accounts for the higher scores under the auditory-visual condition. The possibility that self-selection might increase the chances of children with better auditory capacity entering oral programs is not supported by these data. Under the auditory-only conditions, the oral and TC groups did not perform differently.

The foregoing comments, and the data on which they are based, should not be taken as supportive of a specific educational philosophy. There is much more to the development of a competent, well-adjusted adult than the production of intelligible phonetic contrasts. These data do imply, however, that *if* the acquisition of speech production skills by children with profound deafness is a goal, then pursuit of that goal must be specifically addressed at an instructional level. They also show that efforts to teach children with profound deafness to produce intelligible speech can have measurable results.

The findings of this study argue for the validity of the IMSPAC test as a measure of auditory speech perception capacity that is unconfounded by current cognitive and linguistic status. This test is essentially a blending of the traditional clinical use of word repetition, as a measure of speech discrimination, with a forced-choice approach to assessing speech production. Previous research has shown that a forced-choice task can eliminate some of the effects of listener experience on measured speech intelligibility in children with deafness (Boothroyd 1985b). The use of syllables that are mostly nonwords removes potential effects of word familiarity. Moreover, the imitative task requires no reading ability, and it is both natural for young children and familiar to children with hearing impairment (Most 1985).

The IMSPAC procedure does have three drawbacks. One is that the contrast data do not address the issue of phoneme intelligibility. To develop intelligible speech, a child must not only contrast two targets but should also produce reasonable approximations of each one. We are currently exploring the relationship between contrast intelligibility and phoneme intelligibility in this population (Eran 1995). A second problem is that the test presupposes that the child has had the opportunity to develop speech production skills. The ideal candidate is the postlingually deafened child or the prelingually deafened child who has had experience with amplification and the opportunity to develop speech skills. The test is clearly not suitable for the prelingually deafened child who has not yet had these opportunities. To deal with this problem, we have been exploring the use of both video games (Boothroyd, Hanin, Yeung, and Chen 1992) and electrophysiological methods (Boothroyd 1991) in the assessment of auditory speech perception capacity. The third drawback is the expense and complexity of the editing and auditing procedure. The present data were collected under the auspices of a federal grant. It is difficult to imagine instructional or clinical programs being able to invest the time or money in setting up such an evaluation procedure. We have, however, developed an on-line version of this test in which a single auditor can respond to the child's imitations of recorded syllables (Boothroyd 1991). We plan to report on this system in the near future.

CONCLUSIONS

1. The ability of children with severe and profound deafness to produce intelligible phonetic contrasts by imitation of an auditory input is highly correlated with degree of hearing loss but not with age or communication mode.
2. The same ability, using an auditory-visual input, is *(a)* significantly better than with only an auditory input, *(b)* somewhat less dependent on degree of hearing loss, *(c)* improves with age, and *(d)* is greater in orally trained children.
3. The effects of communication mode on auditory-visual performance are present for children with profound deafness (losses >90 dB) but not for children with severe deafness.
4. The pattern of responses to various contrasts, found in the present study, is in agreement with previously published data and with the known acoustic and visual properties of speech.
5. The findings of this study support the use of an imitative procedure, with forced-choice evaluation of the responses, as a means of obtaining measures of auditory perception capacity that are unconfounded by cognitive and linguistic factors.

ACKNOWLEDGMENTS

The list of individuals who contributed to the work reported here is extensive. The hardware and software were designed and built by Eddy Yeung, Charlie Chen, and Gary Chant. Vardit Lichtenstein, Doron Milstein, Kim Meyer, Sarah Moore, and others edited the tapes and/or organized the auditing. We are especially grateful to the many professionals who collaborated in the administration of the IMSPAC test. These included Ann Geers, Jean Moog, and the staff of the Central Institute for the Deaf, Laura McKirdy and the staff of the Lakeshore program for the hearing impaired, Dennis Gjerdingen and the staff of the Clarke School for the Deaf, Joseph Fischgrund and the staff of the Pennsylvania School for the Deaf, Donald Nielsen, Lisa Tonakawa and the staff of the House Ear Institute, Jill Firszt and the staff of the Carle Clinic, Mary Rose McInerny and the staff of the Hackensack Medical Center, Diane Brackett and the staff of the New York League for the Hard of Hearing, and Susan Waltzman and the staff of the Bellevue Medical Center. This work was funded by grant number 17764 from NIDCD.

REFERENCES

Bilger, R.C., and Wang, M.D. 1976. Consonant confusions in patients with sensorineural hearing loss. *Journal of Speech and Hearing Research* 19:718-748.

Boothroyd, A. 1983. Evaluation of speech. In I. Hochberg, H. Levitt, and M.J. Osberger (eds.), *Speech of the hearing-impaired: Research, training, and personnel preparation.* Baltimore: University Park Press.

Boothroyd, A. 1984. Auditory perception of speech contrasts by subjects with sensorineural hearing loss. *Journal of Speech and Hearing Research* 27:134-144.

Boothroyd, A. 1985a. Auditory capacity and the generalization of speech skills. In J. Lauter (ed.), *Speech planning and production in normal and hearing-impaired children.* ASHA Reports 15:8-14.

Boothroyd, A. 1985b. Evaluation of speech production in the hearing-impaired: Some benefits of forced-choice testing. *Journal of Speech and Hearing Research* 28:185-196.

Boothroyd, A. 1986. Speech of deaf people. In *The Gallaudet encyclopedia of deafness and deaf people* (pp. 191-195). New York: McGraw Hill.

Boothroyd, A. 1991. Speech perception measures and their role in the evaluation of hearing aid performance in a pediatric population. In J.A. Feigin and P.G. Stelmachowicz (eds.), *Pediatric amplification* (pp. 77-91). Omaha: Boys Town National Research Hospital.

Boothroyd, A., Hanin, L., Yeung, E., and Chen, Q. 1992. Video-game for speech perception testing and training of young hearing-impaired children. Proceedings of the Johns Hopkins national search for computing applications to assist persons with disabilities. Baltimore: Johns Hopkins University.

Boothroyd, A., and Martin-Evans, B. 1990. Performance intensity functions for the perception of speech pattern contrasts. Paper presented at the annual conference of the American Speech-Language-Hearing Association.

Boothroyd, A., Springer, N., Smith, L., and Shulman, J. 1988. Amplitude compression and profound hearing loss. *Journal of Speech and Hearing Research* 31:362-376.

Braida, L.D., Durlach, N.I., DeGennaro, S.V., Peterson, P.M., and Bustamante, D.K. 1982. Review of recent research on multiband amplitude compression. In G.A. Studebaker and F.H. Bess (eds.), *The Vanderbilt hearing-aid report* (pp. 133-140). Upper Darby, Penn.: Contemporary Monographs in Audiology.

Braida, L.D., Durlach, N.I., Lippmann, R.P., Hicks, B.L., Rabinowitz, W.M., and Reed, C.M. 1980. Hearing aids: A review of past research on linear amplification, amplitude compression, and frequency lowering. *ASHA* Monographs, 19.

Eran, O. 1995. The effects of age and evaluation methods on measured speech perception and speech production capacities of profoundly hearing-impaired children. Paper presented at the 18th International Conference on Education of the Deaf, Tel Aviv, 1995.

Erber, N.P. 1969. Interaction of audition and vision in the recognition of oral speech stimuli. *Journal of Speech and Hearing Research* 12:423-425.

Erber, N.P. 1972. Auditory, visual, and auditory-visual recognition of consonants by children with normal and impaired hearing. *Journal of Speech and Hearing Research* 14:496-512.

Erber, N.P. 1974. Pure-tone threshold and word recognition abilities of hearing-impaired children. *Journal of Speech and Hearing Research* 17:194-202.

Erber, N.P. 1981. Speech perception by hearing impaired children. In F.H. Bess, B.A. Freeman, and J.S. Sinclair (eds.), *Amplification in education* (pp. 69-88). Washington, D.C.: Alexander Graham Bell Association for the Deaf.

Erber, N.P., and Alencewicz, C.M. 1976. Audiologic evaluation of deaf children. *Journal of Speech and Hearing Disorders* 41:256-267.

Hack, Z.C., and Erber, N.P. 1982. Auditory, visual, and auditory-visual perception of vowels by hearing-impaired children. *Journal of Speech and Hearing Research* 25:100-107.

Hudgins, C.V. 1949. A method of appraising the speech of the deaf. *Volta Review* 51:597-638.

Hudgins, C.V., and Numbers, F.C. 1942. An investigation of the intelligibility of the speech of the deaf. *Genetic Psychology Monographs* 25:289-392.

Levitt, H. 1982. Speech discrimination ability in the hearing impaired: Spectrum considerations. In G.A. Studebaker and F.H. Bess (eds.), *The Vanderbilt hearing-aid report* (pp. 32-43). Upper Darby, Penn.: Contemporary Monographs in Audiology.

Ling, D. 1976. *Speech and the hearing-impaired child: Theory and practice.* Washington, D.C.: Alexander Graham Bell Association for the Deaf.

McGarr, N.S. 1983. The intelligibility of deaf speech to experienced and inexperienced listeners. *Journal of Speech and Hearing Research* 26:451-458.

McGarr, N.S., and Harris, K.S. 1980. Articulatory control in a deaf speaker. *Haskins Laboratory Status Report* 63/64:45-66.

Monsen, R.B. 1978. Toward measuring how well hearing-impaired children speak. *Journal of Speech and Hearing Research* 21:197-219.

Most, T. 1985. Assessment of the perception of intonation by severely and profoundly hearing-impaired children. Ph.D. diss., City University of New York.

Nickerson, R.S. 1975. Characteristics of the speech of deaf persons. *Volta Review* 77:342-362.

Osberger, M.J., and McGarr, N.S. 1982. Speech production characteristics of the hearing impaired. *Speech and Language: Advances in Basic Research and Practice* 8:221-283.

Pickett, J.M., Martin, E.S., Johnson, D., Brandsmith, S., Daniel, Z., Willis, D., and Otis, W. 1972. On patterns of speech feature perception by deaf listeners. In G. Fant (ed.), *International symposium on speech communication ability and profound deafness* (pp. 119-134). Washington, D.C.: Alexander Graham Bell Association for the Deaf.

Risberg, A. 1976. Diagnostic rhyme test for speech audiometry with severely hard of hearing and profoundly deaf children. *Speech Transmission Laboratory Quarterly Progress and Status Report,* 2-3:40-55. Stockholm: Karolinska Technical Institute.

Ross, M., and Giolas, T.G. 1978. *Auditory management of hearing-impaired children.* Baltimore: University Park Press.

Rubin, J.A. 1984. *Static and dynamic information in vowels produced by the hearing impaired.* Ph.D. diss., City University of New York.

Seewald, R.C., Hudson, S.P., Gagné, J.P., and Zelisko, D.L. 1992. Comparison of two methods for estimating the sensation level of amplified speech. *Ear and Hearing* 13:142-148.

Smith, C.R. 1975. Residual hearing and speech production in deaf children. *Journal of Speech and Hearing Research* 18:795-811.

Stark, R.E., and Levitt, H. 1974. Prosodic feature reception and production in deaf children. *Journal of the Acoustical Society of America* 55:s63.

Subtelny, J.D. 1977. Assessment of speech with implications for training. In F.H. Bess (ed.), *Childhood deafness: Causation, assessment and management* (pp. 183-194). New York: Grune and Stratton.

Tyler, R.S. 1993. Speech perception by children. In R.S. Tyler (ed.), *Cochlear implants: Audiological foundations* (pp. 191-256). San Diego, Calif.: Singular Publishing Group.

Walden, B.E., and Montgomery, A.A. 1975. Dimensions of consonant perception in normal and hearing-impaired listeners. *Journal of Speech and Hearing Research* 18:444-455.

4

Binaural Auditory Processing and the Effects of Hearing Loss

Wayne O. Olsen

INTRODUCTION

"A listener's ability to perceive and organize his auditory environment depends strongly on the use of two ears and the neural interaction that occurs between the signals received at the two ears as they progress through the auditory pathway. . . . Such interaction contributes to the listener's ability to localize signal sources in space and to detect signals in backgrounds of interference" (Durlach, Thompson, and Colburn 1981, p. 181). In localizing sounds and ferreting out sounds of interest from other background noise, the auditory system takes advantage of subtle differences in the time of arrival of the stimuli at the two ears and differences in the acoustic spectra of the sounds at the two ears. "The importance of binaural interaction for these functions is indicated both by objective laboratory studies and by subjective reports from listeners who have lost their hearing in one ear" (Durlach et al. 1981, p. 181). Although the above quotation mentions hearing loss in one ear, these comments obviously also apply to persons who have bilateral hearing losses.

In considering the effects of hearing loss on binaural auditory processing, I have chosen to review a binaural phenomenon that is intriguing, is relatively robust, and has received a great deal of study since the work of Hirsh (1948) and Licklider (1948), the masking level difference (MLD). According to Pillsbury, Grose, and Hall (1991), "The MLD is a psychoacoustic measure of the sensitivity of the auditory system to subtle difference cues of time and amplitude and relates to the ability of the listener to detect and recognize signals in noisy backgrounds" (p. 718). Stubblefield and Goldstein state,

> The MLD resulting from binaural analysis requires a peripheral mechanism to preserve and transmit the temporal information in the stimulus received at each ear and also a central location mechanism where the two stimuli interact and are compared. . . . It is this processing of binaural temporal information which allows localization and permits the exceedingly important process of selective listening in noisy environments. (Stubblefield and Goldstein 1977, p. 420)

Hall and Grose further state,

> Whereas the anatomic stage of processing most critical for the MLD may have its locus at the level of the superior olivary complex (the most peripheral site of human binaural interaction), the MLD also hinges on more peripheral auditory processing and has been found to be reduced in cases where the site of lesion was conductive . . . , cochlear . . . , or neural/brainstem. . . . The MLD may therefore have importance as a gauge of peripheral/brainstem auditory development. (Hall and Grose 1990, p. 81)

Given the above quotations citing our use of binaural hearing to localize sounds and to detect stimuli in the presence of noise, and the necessity of intact peripheral and brainstem auditory systems, let us review conditions for measurement of masking level differences. Figure 1 shows six caricatures of unhappy and relatively happy listeners.

In figure 1A, the signal and noise are presented monaurally to the left ear. The SmNm designation on the forehead simply indicates signal monaural (Sm) and noise monaural (Nm). If the signal is maintained at just audible levels in the SmNm condition, but an identical noise is added to the opposite ear as in figure 1B, the signal suddenly becomes clearly audible, resulting in a somewhat happier listener. The No designation on this caricature indicates identical noise at both ears. Incongruously, the addition of more noise (i.e., noise at the second ear) yields better audibility of the signal barely heard when the noise and signal were in only one ear. However, if an identical signal is now added to the second ear as in figure 1C, the signal is barely heard again. Even though more signal is available to the listener in that the

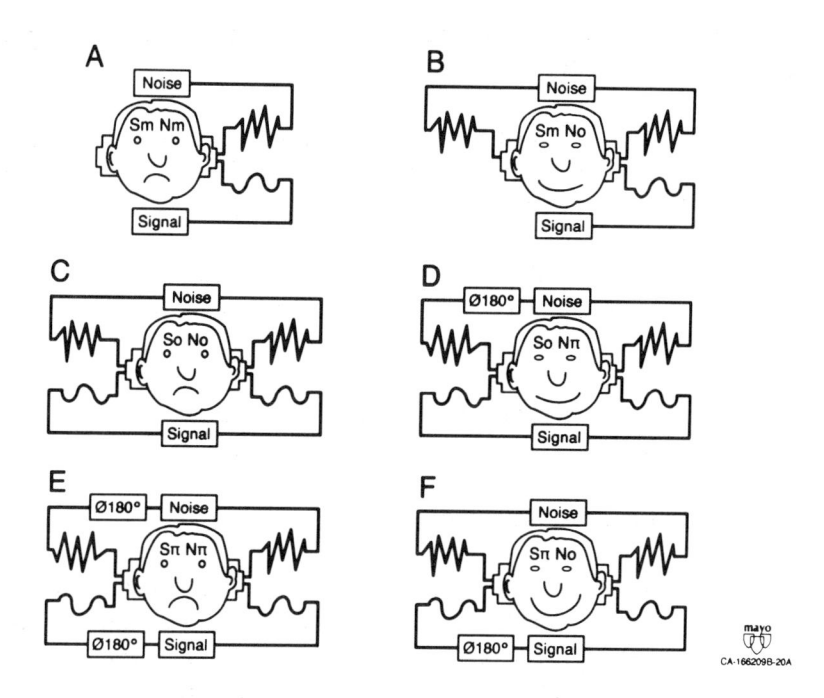

Figure 1. Stimulus conditions for MLD tests. S=signal, N=noise, m=monaural, o=in phase at two ears, π=180° out of phase at two ears. From Olsen and Noffsinger 1976. Reprinted by permission of *Annals of Otology, Rhinology and Laryngology*.

signal, along with the noise, is present at both ears, the signal is heard no better than when the signal and noise were presented to one ear. The SoNo label here indicates that the signal and noise each are identical at the two ears. But if the noise is altered so that it is 180° out of phase at the two ears (indicated by the π in figure 1D) while the signal remains identical (in phase, So) at both ears, the signal is easily heard again. On the other hand, if the phase of the signal is now also reversed at the ears (designated as Sπ in figure 1E) and the noise is also 180° out of phase bilaterally (Nπ), the signal reverts to near inaudibility again. The signal is most clearly audible when the signal is 180° out of phase (Sπ) with itself at the two ears, but the noise is in phase with itself (No) at the two ears.

Listening to these signal and noise combinations under earphones creates some unusual perceptual illusions. Obviously in the SmNm condition, signal and noise are lateralized to one ear. For SmNo, the noise image seems to be centered in the head rather than at the ears, and the signal is heard at the ear. Signal in phase, noise in phase (SoNo) results in both the noise and the signal being centered in the head. Reversing the phase of the noise at the ears while maintaining the signal in phase (SoNπ) produces a signal seemingly in the center of the head and a diffuse image of noise in the head or at the ears. When both the signal and the noise are out of phase with themselves bilaterally, both are heard diffusely throughout the head. The SπNo condition centers the noise in the head with signal being diffuse or at the ears.

Other like binaural listening conditions can be created under earphones; for example, the signal could be monaural and the noise could be out of phase with itself bilaterally, SmNπ; separate noise generators could be used for each ear to develop uncorrelated (u) noise stimuli at the two ears; the signal or the noise could be delayed in time slightly at one ear; the signal and the noise could be at different levels at one ear relative to the other ear; and so on. Regardless of the noise and signal conditions, those that create a binaural interaction within the auditory system that somehow separates, or localizes differently, the image of the signal and the noise allow easier detection of the signal. The conditions most commonly tested are those shown in figure 1, and of these, SoNo and SπNo are used most frequently because the largest MLD is observed for this comparison.

Masking level differences are determined by measuring thresholds for a signal in a constant level noise for two or more conditions and comparing the thresholds obtained. Thresholds for SmNm, SoNo, and SπNπ usually are very similar to one another, on average within 1 dB or so. SoNo usually serves as a single reference condition from which thresholds obtained in one or more of the less difficult conditions, for example, SπNo or SoNπ, are subtracted. The outcome of such comparisons is the MLD. In that the largest MLD is observed for SπNo, that condition is used more frequently than SoNπ.

Masking level differences are largest for low frequencies between 400 and 800 Hz, and very small for frequencies above 1000 Hz (Carhart, Tillman, and Dallos 1968). For this reason 500 Hz pure-tone stimuli, or very narrow band noise in this frequency region, presented against narrow band or wide band noise often serve as the stimuli. Spondees are the more commonly used stimuli for measurements of MLDs for speech. Recognition of spondees is more dependent on low-frequency information than is recognition of monosyllables (Carhart, Tillman, and Johnson 1966; Wilson, Civitello, and Margolis 1985). Most often the noise is maintained at levels in the neighborhood of 80 dB SPL. Smaller MLDs are observed for maskers below 80 dB SPL and sometimes for masking noise above 80 dB SPL (Carhart et al. 1968).

The following sections review some representative publications on masking level differences for low-frequency pure tones (or narrow band noise) and for speech (usually spondees) comparing results for subjects with normal hearing to those of subjects having hearing losses or other medical problems affecting the auditory system. MLDs for subjects with normal hearing are reviewed for each study since investigators routinely obtain normative MLD data specific to their stimuli and test conditions. This review is divided into a section on MLD results for adults followed by a section of MLDs for children, and finally a section on monaural and binaural hearing for speech in specific sound field conditions. To a large extent, the studies in each section are reviewed in chronological order.

MLD FOR ADULTS

Schoeny and Carhart (1971) provided early data on masking level differences for patients with a history and diagnosis of Ménière's disease. Patients having this diagnosis were selected because of the known low-frequency hearing loss associated with this disorder. Four signal monaural conditions (SmNm [right ear and left ear], SmNo, SmNπ) along with six binaural conditions (SoNo, SπNπ, SoNu, SπNu, SπNo, SoNπ) were tested, but in the interest of brevity only the SoNo versus SπNo comparison is considered here. The test stimulus was a 500 Hz pulsed pure tone presented in an 80 dB SPL narrow band noise 400 Hz in width. Twelve control subjects with normal hearing and 12 subjects with a diagnosis of unilateral Ménière's disease were tested.

Comparisons of mean thresholds and MLDs are shown in figure 2. Mean thresholds for the SoNo condition were 73.8 dB SPL for the control group, and 75.8 dB SPL for the sample with Ménière's disease, that is, 2 dB poorer for the latter group. Slightly elevated thresholds in noise are not uncommon for persons with sensorineural hearing losses. However, the SπNo thresholds for the two groups were quite different, 63.6 dB SPL for the group with normal hearing, yielding an MLD of 10.2 dB, and 72.2 dB SPL for the

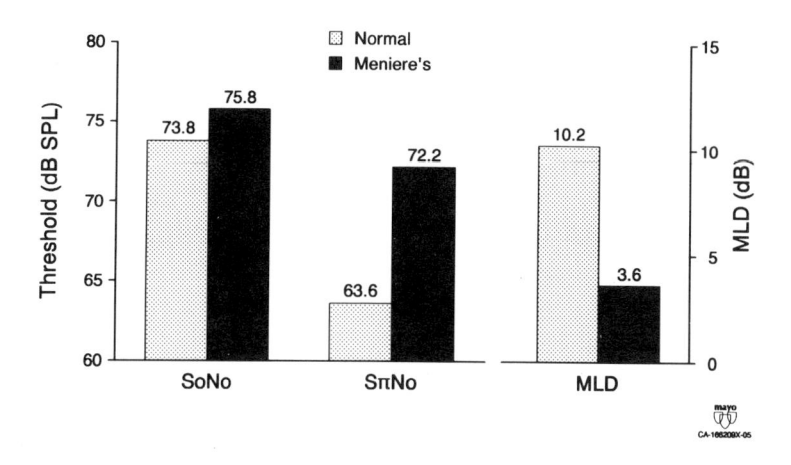

Figure 2. Mean 500 Hz masked thresholds and MLDs for people with normal hearing and for subjects with unilateral Ménière's disease. Adapted from Schoeny and Carhart (1971).

group with Ménière's disease, resulting in an MLD of only 3.6 dB. Three of the patients with Ménière's disease had normal hearing sensitivity ($\leq$ 15 dB Hearing Level [HL], see ANSI 1969) at 500 Hz at the time of the test, but they, too, had smaller MLDs ranging from 2.8 to 7.9 dB. Thus, even though hearing sensitivity had returned to normal for these three people, they were unable to take advantage of the SπNo condition as well as the group with normal hearing with no history of otologic pathology.

In a series of three publications from 1974 to 1978, Quaranta and colleagues (Quaranta and Cervellera 1974, 1977; Quaranta, Cassano, and Cervellera 1978) reported MLD data (SoNo versus SπNo) for a variety of patients having peripheral or central auditory disorders. The stimulus was a 500 Hz pure tone presented in broadband noise. The noise was presented at 60 dB sensation level (SL) to the poorer ear, and the level of the noise was adjusted at the opposite ear to achieve a median plane localization for the noise. Thus, the noise image was centered in the head for the SoNo and SπNo conditions despite hearing losses that were asymmetric for some of the patients.

Figure 3 shows the MLD results from the 1978 publication of Quaranta and colleagues that reported the larger sample sizes for the various groups. (Their two groups of patients with conductive hearing losses from different etiologies have been combined for this figure.) In descending order, the largest mean MLDs were observed for the group having normal hearing (N=20), followed by those with hearing losses due to conductive lesions

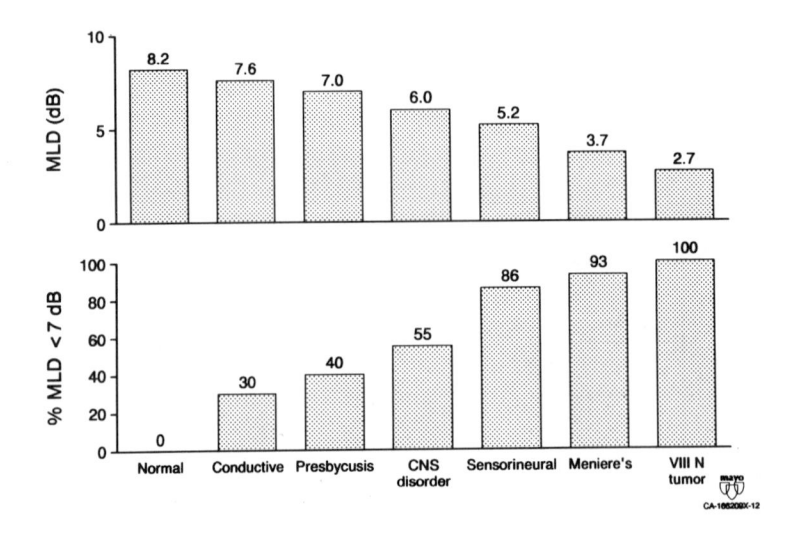

Figure 3. Mean 500 Hz MLDs for subjects with normal hearing and for patients with various medical diagnoses. Percentages with MLDs <7 dB also shown. Adapted from Quaranta, Cassano, and Cervellera (1978).

(N=27), presbycusis (N=20), normal hearing sensitivity but central nervous system (CNS) disorders due to vascular or neoplastic lesions (N=29), patients with sensorineural hearing losses of various etiologies (N=50), Ménière's disease (N=27), and VIIIth nerve tumors (N=5). Also shown in figure 3 are the percentages of MLDs smaller than 7 dB for these groups. Quaranta et al. (1978) considered MLDs of 6 dB or less as abnormal. On this basis, 30% of the patients with conductive hearing losses, 40% of those having hearing losses attributed to presbycusis, 55% of their sample of those with normal hearing sensitivity but CNS lesions, 86% of those with sensorineural hearing losses, 93% of their sample having Ménière's disorder, and all of the patients with VIIIth nerve tumors had abnormally small MLDs. These results demonstrate that masking level differences for 500 Hz tones are affected by a variety of hearing losses, particularly peripheral sensorineural hearing losses.

A publication by Tillman, Carhart, and Nicholls in 1973 described masking level differences for speech (spondees) obtained for a group of 10 young adult subjects (18 to 27 years of age) with normal hearing and for a group of 45 elderly subjects (63 to 88 years of age). For the latter group, the mean speech reception thresholds (SRT) in quiet were 8 dB and 10 dB HL (ANSI 1969) for the better and poorer ears, respectively, and no SRT was poorer than 30 dB HL. Although not reported, it seems safe to suspect that at least some of these elderly subjects had high-frequency sensorineural hearing losses.

The spondees were in phase bilaterally for all conditions, but numerous conditions were developed for a variety of masking stimuli. One of the maskers was white noise (N) modulated in level by 10 dB four times per second (50% duty cycle). Competing speech from two individual talkers presented singly (C) or together (CC) was used as a masker also, as were various combinations of modulated white noise and competing speech from one or both talkers. The maskers were in phase at the two ears, 180° out of phase, or the masker could be delayed to one ear by 0.8 ms. "The delay time of 0.8 msec was chosen since it corresponds roughly to the time required for an acoustic signal to travel over the head from one ear to the other" (Tillman et al. 1973, p. 154). With the masker delayed to one ear, the listener's perception was one of spondaic test items localized in the middle of the head and masker at the ear where the masker was leading in time. With combinations of maskers it was also possible to delay the maskers independently at the two ears. Tillman et al. labeled this condition as "opposed" time delay. In this listening condition the listeners perceived the spondees as being localized in the center of the head with different maskers at each ear. The individual maskers were maintained at 80 dB SPL for the competing speech, and the modulated white noise alone was at 78 dB SPL. For review purposes here, only the modulated white noise condition, single

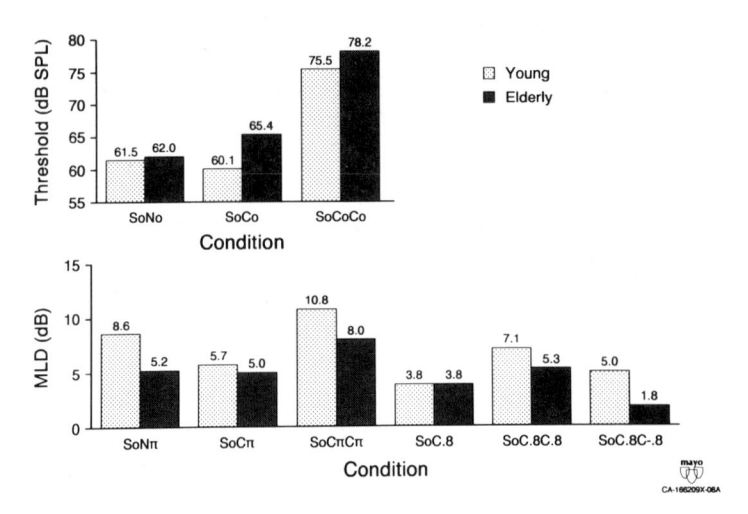

Figure 4. Mean masked spondee thresholds and MLDs for young subjects with normal hearing and for a group of elderly subjects. C=competing speech — single talker, CC=competing speech — two talkers, .8=0.8 ms time delay at one ear, .8 -.8 =opposed time delay at two ears. Adapted from Tillman, Carhart, and Nicholls (1973).

talker competing speech conditions (averaged across the two talkers), and two-talker competing speech conditions are considered.

Thresholds for the reference conditions SoNo, SoCo, SoCoCo and the masking level differences for SoNπ, SoCπ, SoCπCπ, SoC.8, SoC.8C.8, SoC.8C-.8 for the two groups are shown in figure 4. C.8C.8 indicates that the competition of both talkers was delayed to the same ear, and C.8C-.8 labels the "opposed" time delay in which the competing speech of one talker was delayed to one ear while the speech of the second talker was delayed to the opposite ear. Note that masked thresholds are similar for the two groups for the reference condition for modulated white noise (SoNo). However, masked thresholds for the elderly group are more than 5 dB poorer than for the younger subjects for the SoCo condition. When the competition of both talkers was combined, thresholds were elevated for both groups, more so for the elderly group of subjects, again demonstrating that speech masking was more detrimental to the older group of subjects than to the younger control subjects.

Masking level differences were largest for both groups for the SoCπCπ condition, but the MLD was 2.8 dB smaller for the elderly subjects; their MLDs also were 3.4 dB smaller when modulated white noise was the masker, and 3.2 dB smaller for competing speech in the opposed time delay condition. Based on these observations, the authors stated,

To the degree that this trend is representative, it may be taken as revealing one of the ways in which age reduces hearing efficiency. In this regard, it is particularly important to remember that this kind of deficit is not apparent through ordinary hearing tests, and that it represents a disadvantage in the most exacting type of every day listening task: namely, abstracting a desired message from among several competing sounds which are on the verge of masking the message. (Tillman et al. 1973, p. 159)[1]

Bocca and Antonelli (1976) also reported MLDs for speech (five-word sentences) in filtered noise presented to a group of persons with normal hearing and to persons with hearing losses due to symmetric or asymmetric conductive lesions, presbycusis, Ménière's disease, or unilateral cerebrovascular lesions. The noise was always in phase at the two ears, and the speech was either in phase bilaterally or delayed 0.8 ms at one ear. The latter condition resulted in a 7 dB improvement for people with normal hearing, and almost as large for those with conductive hearing losses and for the group of elderly persons. The latter group had normal hearing sensitivity through 2000 Hz, but 35 to 70 dB hearing losses at 4000 and 8000 Hz, respectively. MLDs were smaller for people having asymmetric hearing losses and led the authors to conclude, "Hearing asymmetry—of any type—seems to produce unfavorable conditions for binaural cooperation" (Bocca and Antonelli 1976, p. 486).

Also in 1976, Olsen, Noffsinger, and Carhart published data on MLDs for 500 Hz and for spondees for a control group of 50 subjects with normal hearing and for patients having unilateral conductive hearing losses (N=10), sensorineural hearing losses due to noise trauma (N=50), Ménière's disease (N=20), VIIIth nerve tumors (N=20), presbycusis (N=20), normal hearing sensitivity but central nervous system disorders attributed to multiple sclerosis (N=100), or to temporal lobe lesions (N=20). The age range for the sample with hearing loss due to presbycusis was 60 to 80 years; for the other groups the age range was 17 to 59 years.

A 600 Hz narrow band noise served as the masker for the 500 Hz pure-tone signal, and white noise masked the spondees for SoNo, SπNo, and SoNπ conditions. Both noises were maintained at 80 dB SPL bilaterally. Only SπNo MLDs are considered here.

---

[1] In 1994, Grose, Poth, and Peters reported MLD for 500 Hz and for spondees for a group of young subjects with normal hearing and for an elderly group of subjects. They, too, found MLDs to be about 3 dB smaller for the older subjects and suggested that the elderly subjects seemed to have a reduced ability to process subtle interaural difference cues.

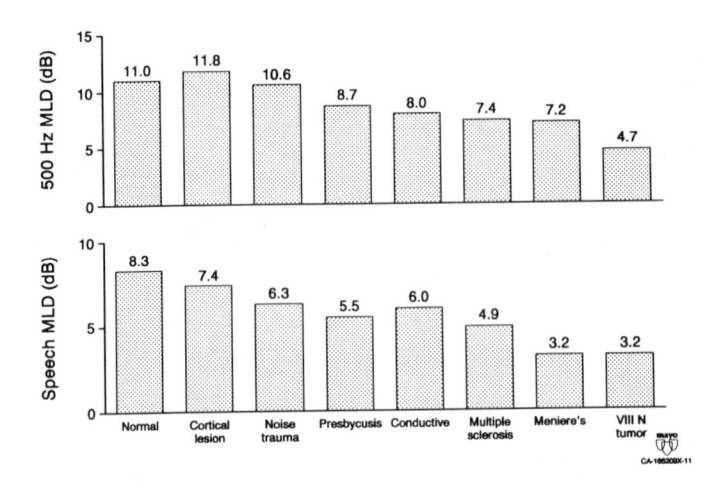

Figure 5. Mean 500 Hz and speech MLDs for subjects with normal hearing and for patients with various medical diagnoses. Adapted from Olsen, Noffsinger, and Carhart (1976).

The mean MLDs for these groups are reported in figure 5. MLDs for 500 Hz are on the order of 11 dB for the control group, for those with temporal lobe lesions, and for those with hearing loss due to noise trauma. In all likelihood subjects in the latter group had normal hearing sensitivity for 500 Hz as did the control group and those with temporal lobe lesions. The smallest MLDs for 500 Hz occurred for the patients with VIIIth nerve tumors, 4.7 dB; for the other groups the average MLDs were on the order of 7 to 8 dB. Mean MLDs for spondees were smaller for all groups but followed trends similar to the 500 Hz MLDs for these groups.

In reviewing their results, Olsen et al. (1976) noted that only 2 (4%) of their subjects with normal hearing yielded MLDs smaller than 8 dB for 500 Hz and only 3 (6%) had MLDs smaller than 6 dB for spondees. On this basis they considered MLDs 7 dB or smaller for 500 Hz and 5 dB or smaller for spondees as abnormal.[2]

Figure 6 shows the percentages of abnormal SπNo MLDs for the various groups. None of the patients with temporal lobe lesions, 6% of those with hearing loss due to noise trauma, and 20% of those with hearing loss

---

[2] In 1992, Harris, Brey, Miller, and Channell reported 500 Hz MLD data for 100 young adults with normal hearing sensitivity using conditions virtually identical to those used here. Their mean SπNo MLD was 11.3 dB, and their statistical analyses also established 8 dB as their lower limit of normal. In like manner, Wilson, Zizz, and Sperry (1994) reported MLDs for 120 subjects with normal hearing for ten selected spondees in 65 and 85 dB SPL noise. Their mean MLDs were 7.8 and 8.8 dB for the 65 and 85 dB SPL noise levels, respectively. Based on their data, they suggested that MLDs smaller than 5.5 dB be considered abnormal.

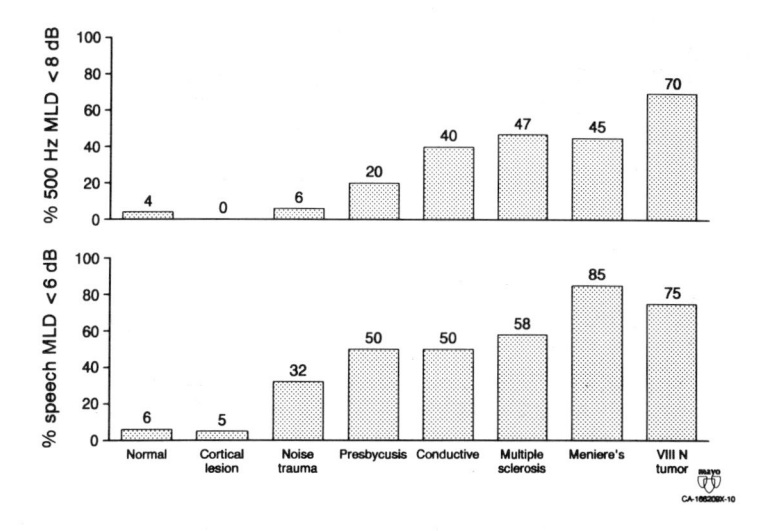

Figure 6. Percentages of abnormal MLDs for subjects with normal hearing and for patients with various medical diagnoses. Adapted from Olsen, Noffsinger, and Carhart (1976).

attributed to presbycusis had MLDs for 500 Hz smaller than 8 dB. Forty percent or more of the patients in the other groups had abnormally small MLDs. Particularly noteworthy is that 47 of the 100 patients with multiple sclerosis had abnormal MLDs despite the fact that hearing sensitivity was within normal limits (≤ 25 dB HL), and 500 Hz thresholds were within 10 dB at the two ears for all but three of them. Only one patient had 500 Hz thresholds differing by more than 15 dB interaurally. Obviously, the high incidence of abnormal MLDs for this group cannot be ascribed to peripheral hearing losses.

The incidence of abnormally small MLDs for spondees was higher for all groups. Note that only 5% (one patient) with a temporal lobe lesion attained an abnormal MLD for speech, but 32% of those with high-frequency hearing losses due to noise trauma did so. At least 50% of the patients in the other groups having medical problems had MLDs smaller than 6 dB for speech.

In the discussion of their results the authors pointed out that patients with conductive hearing losses who obtained small MLDs for 500 Hz had 50 dB HL thresholds at that frequency in one ear and normal hearing sensitivity in the other, that is, a large interaural disparity. Similarly, patients in this group who achieved less than normal-sized MLDs for speech had speech reception thresholds (SRTs) exceeding 25 dB HL and between ear differences in SRTs exceeding 15 dB. All the patients with high-frequency hearing losses due to noise exposure had SRTs of 25 dB HL or better, and none of them had interaural differences in SRTs exceeding 13 dB. Nevertheless, 32% of this sample failed to obtain normal MLDs for speech.

Larger mean 500 Hz MLDs were observed for the ten patients with Ménière's disease who had unmasked 500 Hz thresholds within 15 dB bilaterally on the day of the test than for those who did not, 10.2 dB and 4.3 dB, respectively. Speech MLDs for this group when differentiated on the basis of whether or not there was an interaural disparity of 15 dB for unmasked SRTs were on the order of 4 dB and 1 dB, respectively. In other words, differences in hearing sensitivity could not explain the reduced speech MLDs for these people. The authors agreed "with the view of Schoeny and Carhart (1971) that the reduction is an outcome of the distortion in signal transduction occurring at the cochlea on the affected side" (Olsen et al. 1976, p. 297).

Dividing the patients with VIIIth nerve tumors into subsamples according to hearing sensitivity or hearing symmetry versus asymmetry did not reveal any differences in MLD size. Their MLDs were uniformly small, on the order of 4 to 5 dB for 500 Hz, 3 dB for speech. Therefore, even though the VIIIth nerve tumor often did not cause loss of hearing sensitivity, it apparently did affect the transmission of the information to the central auditory nervous system such that subtle differences in the stimulus at the two ears for the SπNo condition could not be used to normal advantage.

As mentioned earlier, there was a high incidence of reduced MLDs for patients with multiple sclerosis (47% for 500 Hz, 58% for spondees) despite their almost uniform normal hearing sensitivity, even for high frequencies. The authors concluded that these patients had normal peripheral auditory function, but had lesions in the central nervous system that interfered with binaural processing necessary for attaining normal-sized MLDs. Lesions associated with multiple sclerosis have a known predilection for the paraventricular areas of the central nervous system, including those at the level of the brain stem and midbrain. Findings of normal masking level differences for patients having temporal lobe lesions also were of interest. In the words of the authors,

> These findings strongly suggest that unmodified participation of both cortical hemispheres is unnecessary for normal release from masking and, therefore, that MLDs are mediated at levels below the auditory cortex . . . . Hence, these results are evidence that reduced MLDs in tandem with normal hearing sensitivity are indicative of damage at lower levels of the central auditory nervous system and support the hypothesis . . . that small MLDs in

multiple sclerosis patients implicate lesions in the brainstem or midbrain, or both. (Olsen et al. 1976, p. 299)[3]

Further study of the effect of peripheral hearing losses on 500 Hz MLDs was reported by Jerger, Brown, and Smith in 1984. They presented 500 Hz tones in 80 dB SPL broadband noise in SoNo and SπNo conditions to 572 patients with cochlear hearing losses, 79 patients with conductive hearing losses, and 270 subjects with normal hearing sensitivity (thresholds no poorer than 20 dB HL from 250 through 8000 Hz). A portion of their data is summarized in figures 7 and 8.

Data from their normal hearing group revealed a mean MLD of 10.6 dB and 7 dB as the lower limit of normal. Jerger et al. also compared MLDs for a subset of subjects 10 to 19 years old and a subsample of subjects 61 to 69 years old in this group. The mean MLD was 1.1 dB smaller for the older subjects.

Data for the patients with hearing losses were analyzed as a function of hearing loss by frequency, and by asymmetry at 500 Hz. Mean MLDs decreased slightly and the lower limit of normal diminished to 6 dB when hearing sensitivity at 4000 Hz exceeded 20 dB HL, and remained relatively constant through hearing losses extending down to 2000 Hz. When hearing

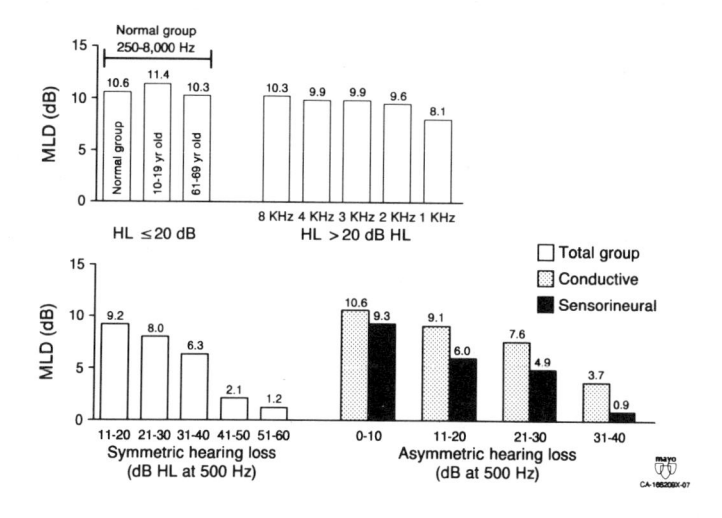

Figure 7. Mean 500 Hz MLDs for subjects with normal hearing and for patients with various degrees and configurations of hearing losses. Adapted from Jerger, Brown, and Smith (1984).

---

[3] Data for 12 subjects with normal hearing and for groups of 12 patients each with Ménière's disease, noise-induced hearing loss, or brain stem lesions seen at another institution were reported later in 1976 by Olsen and Noffsinger. Results corroborated findings summarized here.

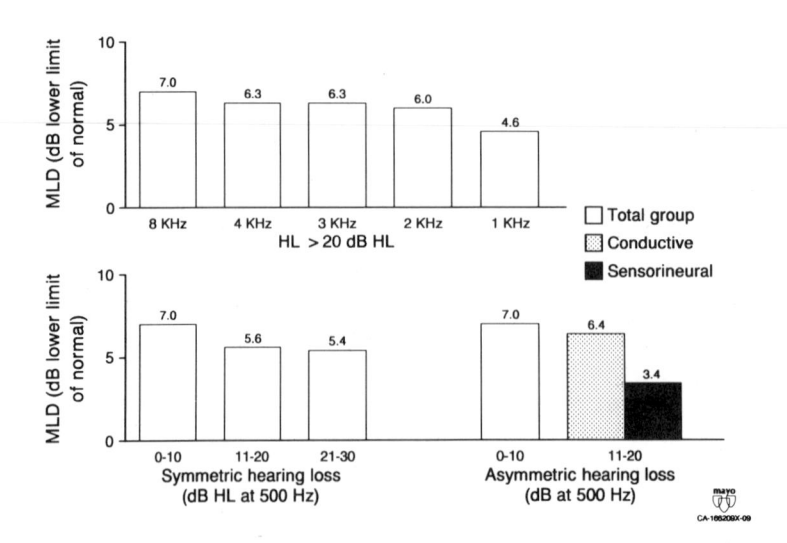

Figure 8. Lower limit of normal for 500 Hz MLDs for various degrees and configurations of hearing losses. Adapted from Jerger, Brown, and Smith (1984).

sensitivity at 1000 Hz was poorer than 20 dB HL, the mean MLD and lower limit of normal decreased by about 2 dB. Symmetric hearing losses through 30 dB at 500 Hz (differences between ears less than 10 dB) resulted in an average reduction in MLD size and lower limit of normal by about 2 dB, but a sharp drop occurred when hearing sensitivity at 500 Hz exceeded 30 dB HL bilaterally. The effect of asymmetric hearing losses was more dramatic. Threshold asymmetries of 11 to 20 dB at 500 Hz reduced the MLD by 1.5 dB for patients with conductive hearing losses, 3 dB for those with cochlear hearing losses; the lower limit of normal decreased to 6 dB for the former group, 3 dB for the latter group. They suggested that MLD testing is not appropriate when hearing asymmetry at 500 Hz exceeded 20 dB.[4]

These authors also noted that the masked thresholds across all subgroups remained relatively constant for the SoNo condition. However, SπNo thresholds increased rather systematically as a function of hearing loss, resulting in smaller MLDs.

Also in 1984, Hall, Tyler, and Fernandes reported results for a number of tests administered to six subjects with normal hearing and ten subjects with symmetrical cochlear hearing losses. Two of the tasks involved binaural stimulation, masking level differences, and an interaural time discrimination task. The signal was a 500 Hz tone in a noise band either 960

---

[4] In their evaluation of the influence of interaural level differences on MLDs for speech, Wilson, Civitello, and Margolis (1985) observed that interaural level differences exceeding 12 dB reduced the size of the MLD for spondees.

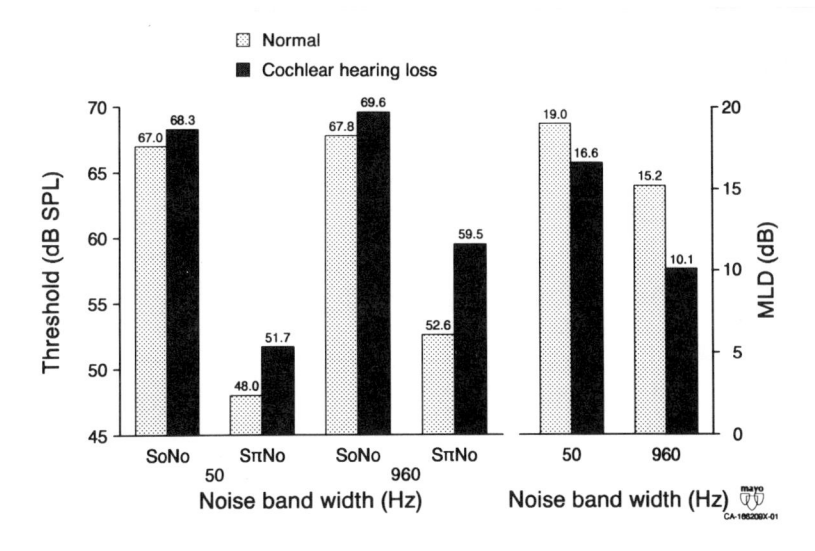

Figure 9. Mean 500 Hz masked thresholds and MLDs for subjects with normal hearing and for subjects with cochlear hearing losses. Adapted from Hall, Tyler, and Fernandes (1984).

Hz in width or 50 Hz in width. The other binaural task was detection of an interaural time delay (interaural Δt) (actually phase difference) for a 500 Hz tone at both ears.

Figure 9 shows the SoNo and SπNo thresholds and the MLDs for the two groups for both masker bandwidths. SoNo thresholds are similar for both groups and both maskers, but the SπNo thresholds and MLDs differ for the two maskers and two samples of subjects. The MLDs are larger for the 50 Hz noise masker than for the 960 Hz masking noise for both groups. Once again MLDs are smaller for the subjects with sensorineural hearing losses. The difference in MLD size between the two groups was larger for the 960 Hz masker than for the 50 Hz masking noise. The authors stated,

> One explanation of this is that, in wide band noise, the binaural analysis of the hearing impaired listeners was impaired by the relatively great amount of noise passed by abnormally wide auditory filters; in narrow band noise, . . . frequency resolution would be less important, because the masker is restricted to the center of the auditory filter. (Hall et al. 1984, p. 152)

Interaural time discrimination Δt also was larger, almost three times larger, for the people with cochlear hearing losses, averaging 64.6 μsec for those with normal hearing, 176.4 μsec for those with hearing losses. These observations led the investigators to conclude,

> The relatively poor performance of the hearing-impaired subjects on the MLD and interaural Δt both may result from poor temporal coding of the stimulus fine structure. This deficit in temporal coding could underlie disability in localization, and detection and discrimination in noise. (Hall et al. 1984, p. 153)

Hall and colleagues (Hall and Derlacki 1986, 1988; Hall and Grose 1993, 1994) have conducted a series of studies on MLDs for patients with conductive hearing losses. Only the 1993 Hall and Grose study is summarized here.

Hall and Grose (1993) investigated MLDs on three occasions for a control group of eight subjects with normal hearing and eight patients with otosclerosis. The patients with otosclerosis were tested shortly prior to middle ear surgery, one month after surgery, and again 11 months after the second test. The middle ear surgery decreased the interaural asymmetry at 500 Hz from about 50 dB prior to surgery to less than 5 dB after surgery. The test signal was a 500 Hz pure tone presented against an 80 dB SPL 100 Hz band of noise centered at 500 Hz.

Figure 10 shows the mean MLDs observed for the three test sessions. As expected, the average MLD remained quite constant for the subjects with

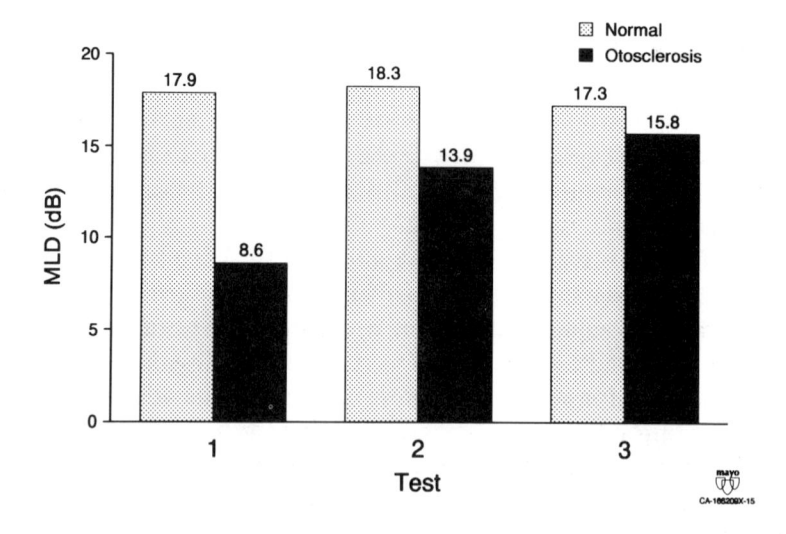

Figure 10. Mean 500 Hz MLDs for subjects with normal hearing and for patients with otosclerosis. Test 1=prior to surgery, Test 2=1 month after surgery, Test 3=11 months after Test 2. Adapted from Hall and Grose (1993).

normal hearing. However, the MLD improved considerably, 5.3 dB, after surgery for the patients with otosclerosis. Eleven months later, almost 2 dB of further improvement was observed. Thus, the decrease in interaural asymmetry resulted in a substantial increase in the size of the MLD, but not quite equal to the MLD for the control group.

Using two standard deviations of the MLD size for the control group as the lower limit of normal, Hall and Grose noted that the MLDs for all eight patients were abnormal prior to surgery, and although improved, seven of eight remained abnormal one month later. Eleven months later, however, MLDs were within normal limits for six of them. The authors suggested that a mechanical difference in the operated ear on the part of the surgical prosthesis could introduce a phase difference at the two ears, thereby producing slightly smaller MLDs one year postsurgery for the patients with otosclerosis. They also suggested that although it was possible that such mechanical anomalies could have changed between Tests 2 and 3, a more likely explanation for the further improvement in MLD size over a period of 11 months was that the central auditory nervous system was able to adapt favorably over time to the new set of peripheral cues.

From the above review it is clear that hearing losses, whether symmetric or asymmetric, sensorineural or conductive, and even when surgically corrected, disrupt binaural hearing function demonstrated by the masking level difference phenomenon for adults. In that the MLD task involves listening in noise, it would seem that the abnormally small MLDs achieved by persons with various types and degrees of hearing loss corroborate their complaints of hearing difficulty in noise.

MLD IN CHILDREN

Children with hearing losses encounter problems in noise, just as adults do. However, two other points of interest to be addressed here are: How early in life can the MLD phenomenon be observed? What is the influence of otitis media on MLD size?

MLDs for 7- to 8-month-old infants, 3.5- to 4.5-year-old preschool children, and adults were compared by Nozza, Wagner, and Crandell (1988). The stimulus was a synthetic /ba/ presented against a 300 to 3000 Hz noise band at 69 dB SPL. The adults were also tested with a 49 dB SPL masker. (The rationale for the second masking level for the adults is explained later.) Visual reinforcement audiometry, play audiometry, and conventional audiometric techniques were used for the infants, preschool children, and adults, respectively. Twelve subjects in each group completed the test protocol.

Figure 11 shows the mean SoNo and SπNo thresholds and MLDs for each group. Thresholds in noise and MLD size improved as a function of age.

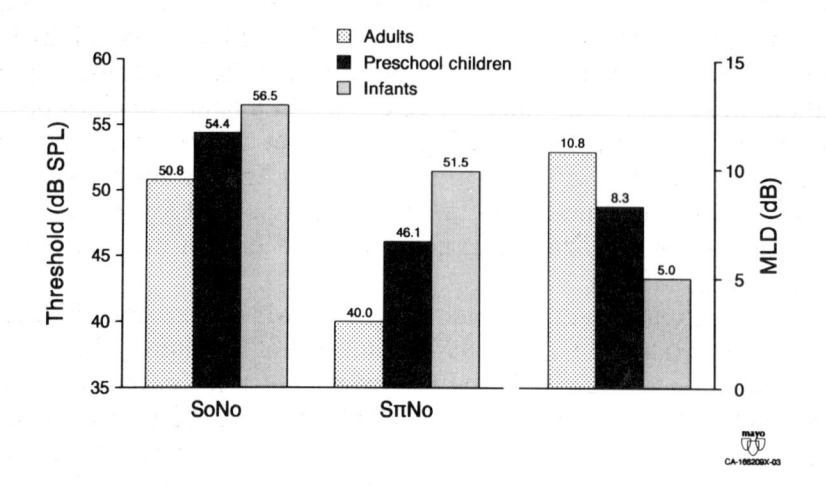

Figure 11. Mean masked speech thresholds and MLDs for adults, preschool children, and infants. Adapted from Nozza, Wagner, and Crandell (1988).

The difference in masked thresholds between the infants and the adults was almost 6 dB for the SoNo condition and more than 11 dB for the SπNo condition, yielding a difference in MLD size of almost 6 dB. The masked thresholds and MLDs for the preschool youngsters were intermediate.

As mentioned earlier, the adult group was also tested using a 49 dB SPL masker. The basis for the lower level was that the unmasked thresholds for the speech stimulus differed across groups. The mean unmasked threshold was 29.7 dB SPL for the infants, 20.7 dB SPL for the preschool children, and 13.0 dB SPL for the adults. Thus, the 69 dB SPL masking noise was at about 40 dB SL for the infants, 49 dB SL for the preschool youngsters, and 56 dB SL for the adults. The 49 dB SPL masker, on the other hand, was at about 36 dB SL for the adults. At this lower masking level, the mean MLD was 7.9 dB, slightly smaller than the MLD for the preschool children, but still almost 3 dB larger than the MLD for the infants.

To match more closely the sensation level of the noise experienced by the preschool children, another group of 12 adults was tested using 59 dB SPL noise. This group was also tested with 69 dB SPL noise for comparison purposes with the first group. The mean masked thresholds and MLDs for the two groups were within 0.5 dB of each other for the 69 dB SPL masker. For the 59 dB SPL masker, the MLD for the adults was 8.6 dB, very similar to the 8.3 dB obtained by the preschool youngsters. These results suggested that the difference in MLD size for the adults and preschool children in the 69 dB noise condition probably could be attributed to the difference in the hearing sensitivity of the two groups, that is, the lower sensation level of the noise and stimulus for the preschool children. These observations, in conjunction with their finding that the MLD was larger for adults than for infants even when adjusting for the difference in hearing sensitivity, led the authors to suggest "a developmental change in binaural analysis postnatally but probably not after 4 years of age" (Nozza et al. 1988, p. 216). They also stated that the small MLD for "infants below 12 months of age suggests that the analysis of interaural phase differences, important for selective listening in noise and for localization, is not developed fully in the first year of life" (Nozza et al. 1988, p. 212).

Additional data on the growth of MLD size for children were provided by Hall and Grose (1990). They tested 10 adults (19 to 35 years of age) and 26 children (3.9 to 9.5 years of age). In one part of their investigation the test stimulus was a 500 Hz tone in 300 Hz bandwidth noise centered at 500 Hz for SoNo and SπNo conditions. They also used 40 Hz bandwidth noise centered at 500 Hz as both signal and masker. For the latter stimulus arrangement, the noise band was added to itself, in phase, during the signal interval for the reference SoNo condition. For the SπNo condition, the signal was presented in phase with the masker in one ear and 180° out of phase with the masker at the other ear. This stimulus condition provided interaural amplitude difference cues. For the ear receiving the signal in phase with the masker, the effect of the signal was to add itself to the masker and thereby an increase in the overall amplitude of the combined signal and noise. For the ear receiving the signal out of phase, the effect of the signal was to decrease the amplitude of the masker. The net result was an interaural amplitude difference cue. They labeled the MLD derived from this SoNo-S$\pi\Delta$aNo comparison as MLDΔa.

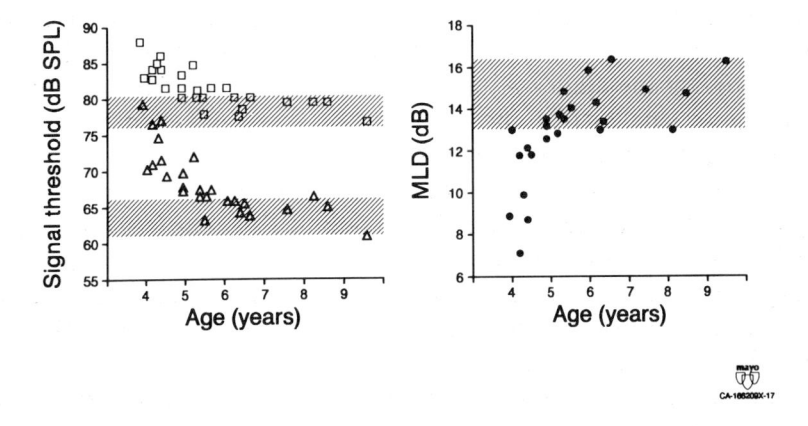

Figure 12. Masked 500 Hz thresholds and MLDs for children as a function of age. Shaded area encompasses 95% confidence interval for adults. □=SoNo, △=SπNo (Hall and Grose 1990).

In further manipulation of this stimulus paradigm the investigators delayed the Sπ signal by 500 μsec (90° at 500 Hz) with respect to the masker. According to the authors, this adjustment resulted in the same amount of amplitude increase at the two ears during the signal interval, but an interaural time difference was introduced, yielding an MLD labeled MLDΔt. The 10 adults and 16 of the children were tested with these 40 Hz stimuli. Figure 12 is taken from the publication of Hall and Grose (1990). It shows the children's thresholds for the 500 Hz tone in the SoNo and SπNo conditions and their MLDs as a function of age. The shaded area encompasses the 95% confidence interval derived from the data of the adult subjects. Note that the thresholds are elevated for children less than 6 years old, more so for the SπNo condition. Thresholds and MLDs are within the adult 95% confidence interval for children 6 years of age and older.

The results for the 40 Hz bandwidth signal and masker are shown in figure 13. The detection task for these conditions obviously was more difficult as reflected in the greater spread in the data points for the children and the wider 95% confidence interval for the adults, especially for the SπΔtNo condition.

Figures 14A and 14B show the mean thresholds and MLDs obtained by these groups of subjects. Mean thresholds were consistently higher and the

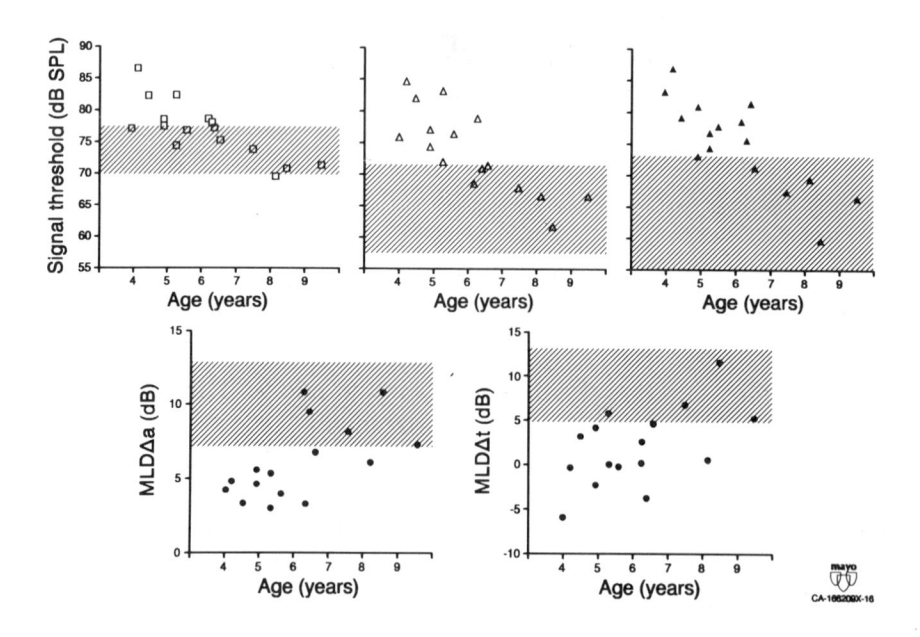

Figure 13. Masked thresholds and MLDs for 40 Hz bandwidth noise as a function of age. Shaded area encompasses 95% confidence interval for adults. □=SoNo, ▵=SπΔaNo, ▲=SπΔtNo (Hall and Grose 1990).

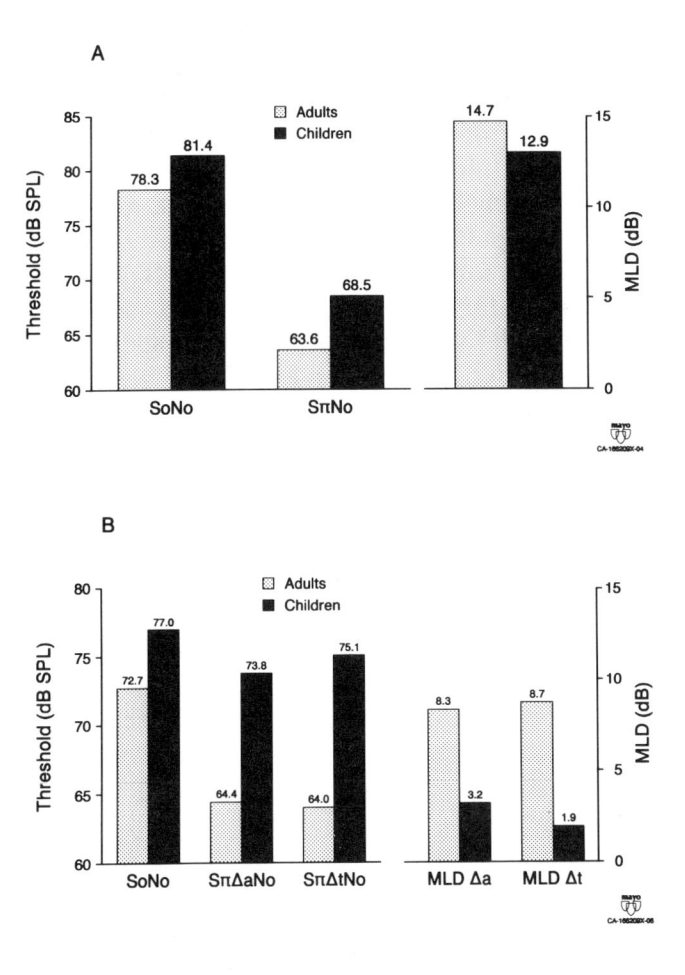

Figure 14A. Mean masked 500 Hz thresholds and MLDs for adults and children. **14B.** Mean masked 40 Hz bandwidth thresholds and MLDs for adults and children. Adapted from Hall and Grose (1990).

MLDs smaller for the children than for the adults. The differences were larger for the more complex stimulus paradigm.

In their discussion of the improvement in MLD size over the 4- to 6-year age range, the authors suggested, "Perhaps the most straightforward explanation is that the peripheral/brainstem auditory processes assumed to account for the MLD are not developmentally mature until an age of 5 or 6 years" (Hall and Grose 1990, p. 86). Later they went on to state,

> It is likely that the cues for detection are quite different in the NoSo and NoSπ conditions. In the NoSo case, as in monaural detection, the cue for

> signal detection is probably based largely on the energy increase due to the signal. However in the NoSπ case, detection is probably concerned primarily with the coding of binaural difference cues, although energy increase may also be an important factor.... Although there is no a priori reason why processing efficiency for both types of signal cues (NoSo and NoSπ) would not reach developmental maturity at about the same time, it would not be unreasonable to assume that the processing of binaural difference cues is more complex and could mature somewhat later in the developmental process. The present results would be consistent with an interpretation that processing efficiency for both NoSo and NoSπ detection improves over the ages 4 to 6 years, but that the processes accounting for NoSπ detection mature slightly later. (Hall and Grose 1990, p. 86)

The authors also noted, however, that MLDs for the narrow band signal and masker conditions seemed to improve over a wider age range. In explanation of these observations, the authors indicated,

> The MLD for a pure-tone signal presented in noise presumably depends on sensitivity to either interaural time differences, interaural amplitude differences, or to both kinds of interaural differences. Thus, if by age 5 or 6 the MLD for a pure tone presented in noise is comparable to that for adults, then it would follow that the MLD for the Δt cue or the Δa cue (or to both types of cue) would also be comparable to adult values; however, this is apparently not the case. One possible explanation for these results is that children, more than adults, require the simultaneous presence of both interaural amplitude and time cues for good binaural performance. (Hall and Grose 1990, p. 87)

Another possibility they suggested,

> In detecting an Sπ pure tone in a 300-Hz-wide No noise background, the tone is heard as being off midline and stands out as being different from the background noise both in terms of its pitch and its timbre. When the signal and masker are identical

narrow bands of noise, the Sπ signal again results in binaural difference cues that are associated with off-midline perception; however, neither a pitch nor timbre cue is available (since the signal has the same pitch and timbre as the masker), and the signal may not be heard out as readily from the masking noise. Under this circumstance, the binaural difference cue alone (without concomitant pitch and timbre cues) may be too subtle to allow good performance for the young listener. Both of the above hypotheses assume that cues for detection are available in the peripheral auditory system of the young children, but that detection is limited by the performance of a relatively central auditory process. (Hall and Grose 1990, p. 87)

Whatever the explanation, it would appear that MLD performance continues to improve during the first six years of life for relatively uncomplicated stimuli and probably over a longer period of time for more complex signal and noise conditions.

Whereas the investigations just reviewed tested children with normal hearing, Pillsbury, Grose, and Hall (1991) compared MLDs for a control group of 25 children 5.1 to 10.1 years of age with normal hearing and free of otitis media and a group of 30 children 5.1 to 13 years of age having otitis media with effusion (OME). The latter group was tested prior to placement of pressure equalization (PE) tubes, one month after surgery, and 22 of them were tested again three months after PE tube placement. The mean 500 Hz threshold for the poorer ear of the children in the otitis media group was 37.8 dB HL prior to surgery; for the children with normal hearing the 500 Hz threshold was 7.9 dB HL. The average asymmetry in hearing sensitivity at 500 Hz was 2.6 dB for the control group, 14.2 dB prior to surgery, and 2.6 dB and 2.7 dB at one month and three months, respectively, following surgery for the children in the otitis media group. The stimulus for the MLD testing was a 500 Hz tone in a 300 Hz bandwidth noise for SoNo and SπNo conditions.

SoNo thresholds were very similar for both groups with virtually all the pre- and postsurgery thresholds for the children with otitis media falling within the 95% confidence interval established with data from the control group. However, many of the SπNo thresholds for the children with otitis media fell outside the 95% confidence interval; 90% of their MLDs were abnormal prior to surgery, 70% remained abnormal one month later, and 64% were still abnormally small three months after placement of PE tubes.

Figure 15 shows the mean thresholds and MLDs for the two groups of subjects. All mean SoNo thresholds are within 1 dB of one another, but

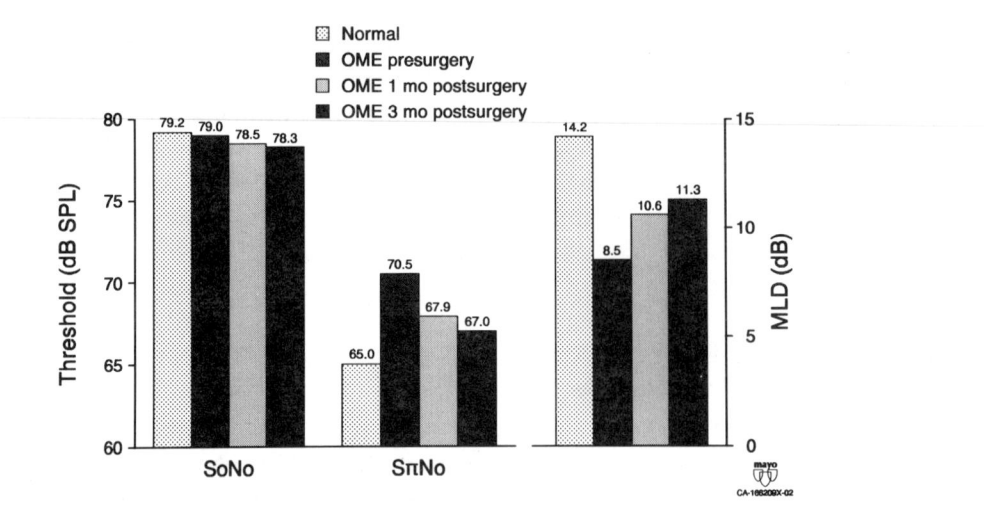

Figure 15. Mean masked 500 Hz thresholds and MLDs for children with normal hearing and for children with OME prior to surgery, 1 month and 3 months following PE tube placement. Adapted from Pillsbury, Grose, and Hall (1991).

SπNo thresholds are 5 dB to 2 dB higher presurgery to three months after surgery, respectively. Mean MLDs were about 5 dB to 3 dB smaller for the otitis media group over this time frame. These findings led the authors to comment,

> In some children the MLD continues to remain abnormally small after placement of PE tubes, even though the pure tone thresholds are within normal limits at the time of testing. Thus, both during and some time after the OME experience, these children can suffer loss in their ability to extract signals from noise on the basis of binaural difference cues. It is possible that this impairment, revealed by a psychoacoustical test, is associated with some degree of hearing disability in "real life" noisy environments. It is therefore possible to underestimate the hearing disability associated with OME from a consideration of only audiologic threshold data. (Pillsbury et al. 1991, p. 722)

These comments once again remind us that threshold tests in quiet do not and cannot reveal difficulties encountered by persons with hearing losses in noisy environments. One also wonders if the MLDs for children experiencing episodes of OME will continue to improve over time while free of OME in a manner similar to that observed by Hall and Grose (1993) following middle ear surgery for people with otosclerosis. Very likely such data will be forthcoming.

From the above review it is apparent that MLDs can be measured for 7- to 8-month old infants, that MLDs continue to grow at least through 6 years of age, and that hearing losses associated with otitis media with effusion can affect MLD size.

BINAURAL AND MONAURAL SOUND FIELD LISTENING

Obviously, the signal and noise conditions created for MLD testing under earphones cannot be duplicated in sound field conditions. Even though signal and noise directly in front of the listener might approach SoNo conditions at the two ears, slight displacements in the location of the signal or noise sources, or slight head movements will alter the time of arrival and the spectrum of the signal and noise at the two ears. Nevertheless, sound field conditions can be arranged such that differences in binaural listening can be measured.

If the signal and noise originate from a single loudspeaker directly in front of the listener (0° azimuth) and the listener's head movement is restricted as much as possible, the stimuli arriving at the two ears should be nearly identical. Then if a loudspeaker is moved to one side of the listener while another loudspeaker is maintained in front of the listener, differences will occur at the two ears for the signals or noise from the loudspeaker located to one side, but should remain relatively similar at the two ears from the loudspeaker directly in front of the listener. For example, if noise were delivered from a loudspeaker directly in front of the listener (0° azimuth) while speech is reproduced by a loudspeaker opposite the right ear of the listener (90° azimuth), the noise will be very similar at the two ears; but the speech will arrive about 0.8 ms later at the left ear than at the right ear, and the spectrum of the speech will be different at the two ears.

Figure 16A shows an estimate of the difference in spectra at the right and left ears for a stimulus generated at a 90° azimuth to the right of the listener relative to a stimulus originating directly in front at a 0° azimuth. This graph is adapted from a publication of Dirks and Moncur (1967) for one-third octave noise measurements on a dummy head with microphones located in its ear canals at a normal eardrum position. Care was taken in the fabrication of the head and ear canals to mimic the resonance characteristics of human ear canals. There is a slight increase in sound pressure level across the frequency range at the right ear (near ear) and a decrease in level at the left ear (far ear), greater for the midfrequencies and high frequencies. Figure

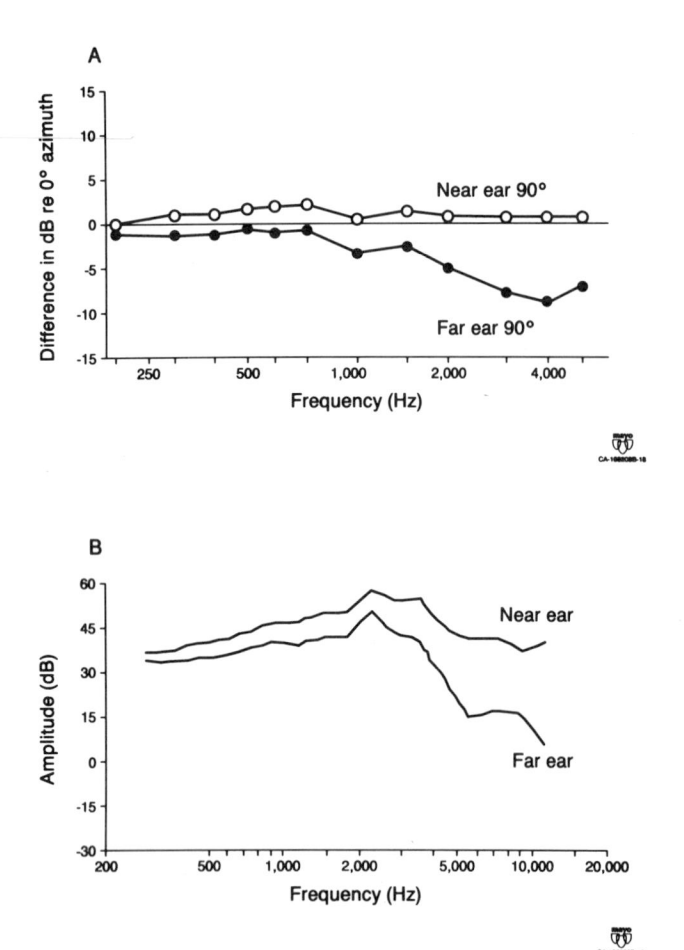

Figure 16A. Difference in spectra at near ear (90° azimuth) and far ear relative to spectra at 0° azimuth (adapted from Dirks and Moncur 1967). **16B.** Spectra at near ear (90° azimuth) and far ear measured near tympanic membrane. Adapted from Yost (1994).

16B is another representation of the differences in near and far ear spectra measured near the tympanic membranes of a human listener. Again, note the modest difference at the two ears for the low and midfrequencies, more pronounced at the high frequencies.

Dirks and Wilson (1969) used sound field conditions along these lines for presentation of spondees in noise to three young subjects (18 to 21 years of age) with normal hearing and to three subjects with sensorineural hearing losses (60, 67, and 70 years of age). Speech spectrum noise was maintained at 70 dB SPL while the level of the spondees was varied. The speech and noise originated from a single loudspeaker in front of the subject (0° azimuth)

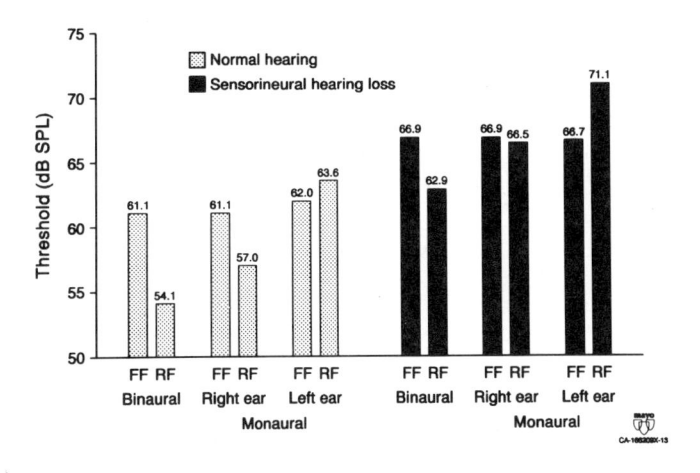

Figure 17. Mean masked spondee thresholds for young subjects with normal hearing and for elderly subjects with sensorineural hearing loss in monaural and binaural listening conditions. FF=speech and noise from single loudspeaker 0° azimuth; RF=speech from loudspeaker 90° azimuth, noise from loudspeaker 0° azimuth. Adapted from Dirks and Wilson (1969).

in a condition labeled "front front" (FF). With a second loudspeaker 90° to the right of the listener to reproduce the speech signal and the same loudspeaker still in front at 0° azimuth for the noise, the condition was called "right front" (RF). Head movement was restricted by a head rest and a strap assembly. The people responded to the spondees in binaural and monaural listening conditions. Either the right ear or the left ear was occluded for the monaural listening situations.

The results for the two groups are shown in figure 17. At first glance it is apparent that the subjects having sensorineural hearing losses needed 5 to 9 dB higher signal levels to attain 50% correct responses in the 70 dB SPL speech spectrum noise. The levels at which 50% of the spondees were heard correctly were quite consistent within each group when the speech and noise originated from a single loudspeaker in front of the people regardless of whether both ears were open for binaural listening or one ear was occluded for monaural listening. No binaural advantage was observed for either group in the FF condition.

Lower thresholds were obtained when the speech source was moved 90° to the right of the listeners. Subjects with normal hearing attained binaural thresholds that were 7 dB better for the RF condition than for the FF condition. With the right ear open and the left ear occluded the 50% response level was 4.1 dB lower in the RF condition than in its FF counterpart, but 1.6 dB higher when the left ear was open and the right ear occluded. The difference between monaural right ear and monaural left ear thresholds in the RF condition was 6.6 dB, attributable to the head shadow effect. Note that the monaural left ear threshold was 9.5 dB poorer than the binaural threshold in this listening situation. The RF versus FF advantage was less for the subjects with sensorineural hearing losses, but they, too, obtained binaural thresholds that were 4 dB better when binaural difference cues were available to them. The difference between right ear and left ear thresholds in the RF condition was 4.6 dB, and the monaural left ear threshold was 8.2 dB higher than the binaural threshold in this situation.

Thus, when the speech arrived at the left ear about 0.8 ms later, somewhat lower in level and altered in spectra, sufficient information from binaural difference cues was available to improve the binaural RF threshold by 7 dB for the young subjects with normal hearing and by 4 dB for elderly subjects with sensorineural hearing loss relative to their binaural FF thresholds. Moreover, their binaural thresholds were about 3 dB better than the best monaural threshold in the RF condition for both groups.

SUMMARY

The ability of the auditory system to take advantage of subtle differences in acoustic stimuli at the two ears is remarkable. Peripheral coding of the incoming stimuli is sufficiently precise and independent at the two ears that sound sources are localized rapidly. Further, differences in neural impulses from the two ears allow interactions within the central auditory nervous system that provide several dB of improvement in signal-to-noise ratio with binaural hearing. Ability to use binaural difference cues associated with binaural hearing can be demonstrated behaviorally within the first 7 to 8 months of life, and continues to improve during the first 6 years of life or longer. Clearly, there is an extremely delicate balance in the binaural interactions within the auditory system such that slight disturbances in the peripheral system seriously disrupt binaural hearing performance. Whether the hearing loss is unilateral or bilateral, conductive or sensorineural, in the frequency region of the stimulus or seemingly somewhat distant from it, evidence from studies on masking level differences demonstrate that binaural hearing often is impaired.

REFERENCES

American National Standards Institute. 1969. Specifications for audiometers. ANSI S3.6-1969. New York: American National Standards Institute.

Bocca, E., and Antonelli, A. 1976. Masking level differences: Another tool for the evaluation of peripheral and cortical defects. *Audiology* 15:480-487.

Carhart, R., Tillman, T., and Dallos, P. 1968. Unmasking for pure tones and spondees: Interaural phase and time disparities. *Journal of Speech and Hearing Research* 11:722-734.

Carhart, R., Tillman, T., and Johnson, K. 1966. Binaural masking by periodically modulated noise. *Journal of the Acoustical Society of America* 39:1037-1050.

Dirks, D.D., and Moncur, J.P. 1967. Interaural intensity and time differences in anechoic and reverberant rooms. *Journal of Speech and Hearing Research* 10:177-185.

Dirks, D.D., and Wilson, R.H. 1969. Binaural hearing of speech for aided and unaided conditions. *Journal of Speech and Hearing Research* 12:650-664.

Durlach, N.I., Thompson, C.L., and Colburn, H.S. 1981. Binaural interaction in impaired listeners. *Audiology* 20:181-211.

Grose, J.H., Poth, E.A., and Peters, R.W. 1994. Masking level differences for tones and speech in elderly listeners with relatively normal audiograms. *Journal of Speech and Hearing Research* 37:422-428.

Hall, J.W., and Derlacki, E.L. 1986. Effect of conductive hearing loss and middle ear surgery on binaural hearing. *Annals of Otology, Rhinology and Laryngology* 95:525-530.

Hall, J.W., and Derlacki, E.L. 1988. Binaural hearing after middle ear surgery. *Audiology* 27:89-98.

Hall, J.W., and Grose, J.H. 1990. The masking level difference in children. *Journal of the American Academy of Audiology* 1:81-88.

Hall, J.W., and Grose, J.H. 1993. Short-term and long-term effects on the masking level difference following middle ear surgery. *Journal of the American Academy of Audiology* 4:307-312.

Hall, J.W., and Grose, J.H. 1994. The effect of conductive hearing loss on the masking level difference: Insert versus standard earphones. *Journal of the Acoustical Society of America* 95:2652-2657.

Hall, J.W., Tyler, R.S., and Fernandes, M.A. 1984. Factors influencing the masking level difference in cochlear hearing-impaired and normal-hearing listeners. *Journal of Speech and Hearing Research* 27:145-154.

Harris, R.W., Brey, R.H., Miller, R.W., and Channell, R.W. 1992. Influence of masker bandwidth on binaural masking level differences. *Audiology* 31:196-204.

Hirsh, I.J. 1948. The influence of interaural phase on interaural summation and inhibition. *Journal of the Acoustical Society of America* 20:536-544.

Jerger, J., Brown, D., and Smith, S. 1984. Effect of peripheral hearing loss on the masking level difference. *Archives of Otolaryngology* 110:290-296.

Licklider, J.C.R. 1948. The influence of interaural phase relation upon the masking of speech by white noise. *Journal of the Acoustical Society of America* 20:150-159.

Nozza, R.J., Wagner, E.F., and Crandell, M.A. 1988. Binaural release from masking for a speech sound in infants, preschoolers and adults. *Journal of Speech and Hearing Research* 31:212-218.

Olsen, W.O., and Noffsinger, D. 1976. Masking level differences for cochlear and brain stem lesions. *Annals of Otology, Rhinology and Laryngology* 85:820-825.

Olsen, W.O., Noffsinger, D., and Carhart, R. 1976. Masking level differences encountered in clinical populations. *Audiology* 15:287-301.

Pillsbury, H.C., Grose, J.H., and Hall, J.W. 1991. Otitis media with effusion in children: Binaural hearing before and after corrective surgery. *Archives of Otolaryngology — Head and Neck Surgery* 117:719-723.

Quaranta, A., Cassano, P., and Cervellera, G. 1978. Clinical value of the tonal masking level difference. *Audiology* 17:232-238.

Quaranta, A., and Cervellera, G. 1974. Masking level differences in normal and pathological ears. *Audiology* 13:428-431.

Quaranta, A., and Cervellera, G. 1977. Masking level differences in central nervous system disease. *Archives of Otolaryngology* 103:482-484.

Schoeny, Z., and Carhart, R. 1971. Comparison of MLDs for normal hearing subjects and subjects with unilateral Ménière's disease. *Journal of the Acoustical Society of America* 50:1143-1150.

Stubblefield, J., and Goldstein, D. 1977. A test-retest reliability study on clinical measurement of masking level differences. *Audiology* 16:419-431.

Tillman, T., Carhart, R., and Nicholls, S. 1973. Release from masking in elderly persons. *Journal of Speech and Hearing Research* 16:152-160.

Wilson, R.H., Civitello, B.A., and Margolis, R.H. 1985. Influence of interaural level differences on the speech recognition masking level difference. *Audiology* 24:15-24.

Wilson, R.H., Zizz, C.A., and Sperry, J.L. 1994. Masking-level difference for spondaic words in 2000 msec bursts of broadband noise. *Journal of the American Academy of Audiology* 5:236-242.

Yost, W.A. 1994. New developments in the study of binaural and spatial hearing. *Audiology Today* 6(4):9-12.

PART II.

Issues in Pediatric Amplification

5

Fitting Hearing Aids in the Pediatric Population: A Survey of Practice Procedures

Andrea Hedley-Williams, Anne Marie Tharpe, and Fred H. Bess

INTRODUCTION

There are limited data available on current practice patterns of audiologists serving the pediatric population—especially with regard to the techniques employed in the selection, fitting, and verification of amplification. Ross (see chapter 1) has implied that the practice procedures of pediatric audiologists lag behind the available resources, both in terms of equipment and in clinical techniques employed. Indeed, the provision of quality hearing health care to children will be compromised if audiologists practice clinical procedures that are not supported by valid published data (Wiley, Stoppenbach, Feldhake, Moss, and Thordardottir 1995). In a time of health care reform, when emphasis is placed on cost containment, outcome, and efficacy, the need for evidence-based clinical procedures becomes increasingly important.

In this chapter, we report the findings from a nationwide survey designed to identify current hearing aid fitting practices employed by pediatric audiologists. The survey explored the selection, fitting, and verification practices commonly utilized and types of amplification devices recommended by audiologists serving infants and young children. In addition, it is relevant to review briefly throughout this chapter whether such practices are supported in the research literature.

DESCRIPTION OF THE PEDIATRIC AMPLIFICATION SURVEY

The survey instrument was a simple 57 item questionnaire that queried demographic information on the respondents and their hearing aid fitting practices by age group: birth to 6 months; 7 months to 4 years, 11

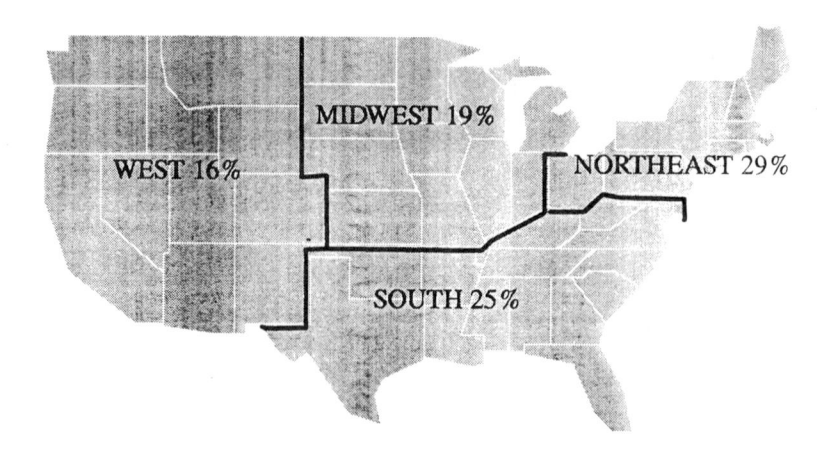

Figure 1. Distribution of response to the pediatric amplification survey by region across the United States.

months; 5 years to 11 years, 11 months; and 12 to 17 years. A random sampling of 1414 pediatric audiologists certified by the American Speech-Language-Hearing Association (ASHA) was selected and mailed the survey. Approximately four weeks later, the surveys were mailed again to the selected audiologists requesting that the surveys be returned in the provided envelopes (if not completed previously). This second mailing was designed to increase the response rate. As shown in figure 1, a wide distribution of response from across the United States was obtained. The final response rate was 38% (N=536).

In order to enhance response accuracy, respondents completed the questionnaire anonymously. To ensure that respondents routinely served a pediatric population, only audiologists performing a minimum of three new pediatric hearing aid fittings in a six-month period were requested to complete the fitting practices portion of the survey. Of the 536 surveys returned, 44% (N=237) met this criterion. As such, the findings are believed to reflect the clinical procedures of audiologists routinely serving the pediatric population.

PRACTICE PATTERNS OF PEDIATRIC AUDIOLOGISTS FITTING HEARING AIDS

For purposes of brevity, we report here only those findings believed to be of most interest. The data are categorized into five sections: fitting strategies, use of FM systems, use of new technology, recommendations in the 12- to 17-year-old population, and additional findings. The data are summarized in the accompanying figures (figures 2-8).

FITTING STRATEGIES

The following sections describe the hearing aid selection and verification strategies employed by the respondents. In addition, verification strategies used in the fitting of frequency modulated (FM) systems are discussed. Results are provided for different age groups including birth to 6 months; 7 months to 4 years, 11 months; and 5 years to 11 years, 11 months.

Selection Strategy

Prescriptive formulas are designed to specify the target frequency/gain and frequency/output values of hearing aids. Many of these formulas have been designed for use with an adult population but some may be adapted for use with children (Hawkins 1992). At least one prescriptive approach has been designed specifically for use with the pediatric population (Seewald 1992).

Respondents were asked the following question, "For what percent of your pediatric cases do you use the following methods to select hearing aid specifications?" Their options included "Your personal fitting strategy," "NAL-R," "POGO-II," "DSL," and "Berger" (Berger, Hagberg, and Rane 1988; Byrne and Dillon 1986; Schwartz, Lyregaard, and Lundh 1988; Seewald 1992). As depicted in figures 2A, B, and C it is evident that despite the availability of evidence-based fitting strategies, almost half of the respondents report always or frequently (75-100% of the time) using a personal fitting strategy when selecting amplification for children regardless of the child's age. Respondents reported that they rarely use prescriptive approaches to select amplification for children. In fact, greater than 90% of the responding audiologists indicated that they seldom (0-24% of the time) use the DSL (Seewald 1992) approach to assist in the selection of amplification, the one prescriptive approach specifically designed for use with young children!

Verification Strategy

It is well known that ear canal characteristics between children and adults vary greatly. The typical ear canal resonant peak response of an adult is considerably lower in frequency than that of an infant (Kruger 1987; Kruger and Ruben 1987). Additionally, smaller ear canal volumes as well as potential middle ear impedance differences in children can result in larger sound pressure levels in infants' and young children's ears than in adults (Bratt 1980; Feigin, Kopun, Stelmachowicz, and Gorga 1989). The use of probe-microphone measurements with children affords a reliable method for identifying these differences and verifying hearing aid fit.

**Selection Strategies
(Birth - 6 mos.)**

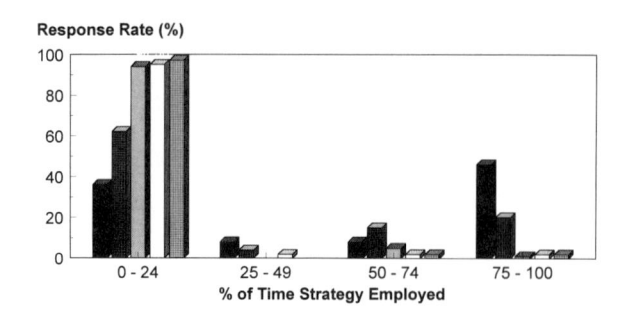

A

(7 mos. to 4 yrs., 11 mos.)

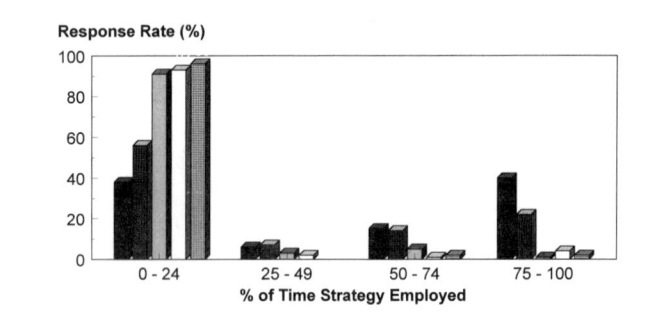

B

(5 yrs. - 11 yrs., 11 mos.)

C

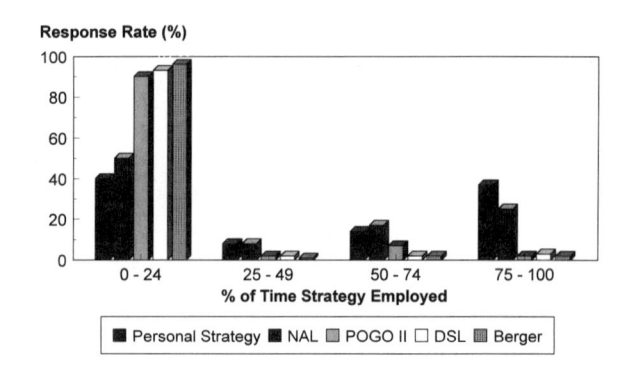

■ Personal Strategy ■ NAL ▨ POGO II ☐ DSL ▩ Berger

Figures 2A, B, C. Percentage of use of selection strategies across three age groups.

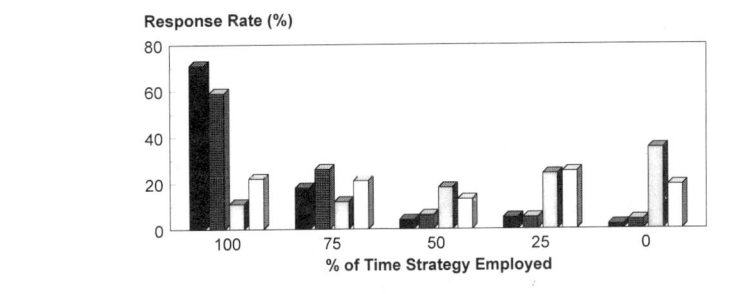

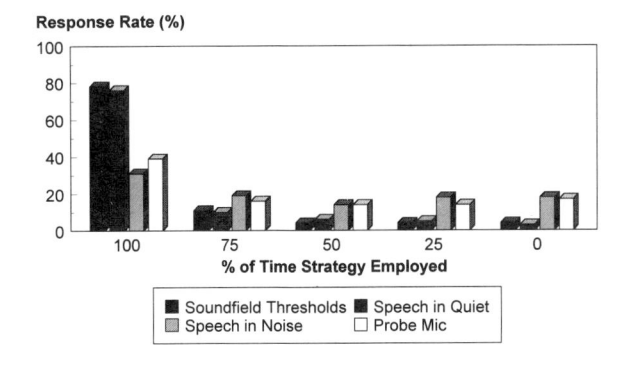

Figures 3A, B, C. Percentage of use of hearing aid fitting verification strategies across three age groups.

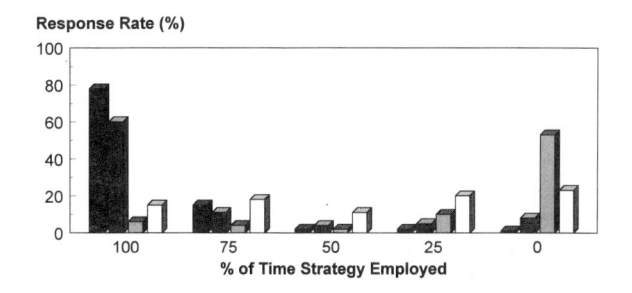

Survey respondents were asked, "How often do you use the following methods to verify your pediatric hearing aid fittings?" Their options included "aided sound field thresholds," "speech measures in quiet," "speech measures in noise," and "probe microphone measures." As demonstrated in figures 3A, B, and C between 15% and 39% of the audiologists surveyed *always* utilize probe-microphone assessment to verify pediatric hearing aid fittings. It is interesting to note that the older the child is, the more likely the respondents were to utilize probe microphone measures. Approximately 20% of the respondents reported that they *never* use probe-microphone measurements to verify the hearing aid fitting. Aided sound field threshold assessment clearly emerged as the verification method of choice with approximately 75% of the respondents reporting that they *always* use this procedure despite current research indicating that there are limitations to functional gain measures and that they are less reliable than real-ear gain measurement (Hawkins, Montgomery, Prosek, and Walden 1987; Humes and Kirn 1990; Macrae 1982).

Aided sound field speech testing in quiet and noise is a useful counseling tool to demonstrate to teachers or parents the benefits and limitations of amplification, particularly for a given environment. It is important to realize, however, that aided speech testing has long been discarded as a means of reliably detecting differences between hearing aids (Mueller and Grimes 1983; Shore, Bilger, and Hirsh 1960; Walden, Schwartz, Williams, Holum-Hardegen, and Crowley 1983). Nonetheless, as observed in figures 3A, B, and C, between approximately 60% and 80% of the audiologists surveyed report *always* using speech in quiet as a method of verifying hearing aid fit.

FM Verification Strategy

Several published guidelines and procedures for assessment of FM systems have appeared in recent years (ASHA 1994; Hawkins 1987; Lewis, Feigin, Karasek, and Stelmachowicz 1991). These publications have consistently advocated the use of systematic procedures preferably utilizing probe-microphone technology and have discouraged sound field behavioral measures. As seen in figure 4, however, some type of sound field assessment is the test of choice among our respondents for verifying the fit of FM systems with approximately 50% of responding audiologists *always* utilizing sound field thresholds, speech in quiet measures, or both. These audiologists are less likely to use probe microphone measures to verify FM fittings than they are to verify hearing aid fittings. Approximately half of these audiologists *never* utilize probe microphone measures in verifying the fitting of FM systems on children.

FM Verification Strategies

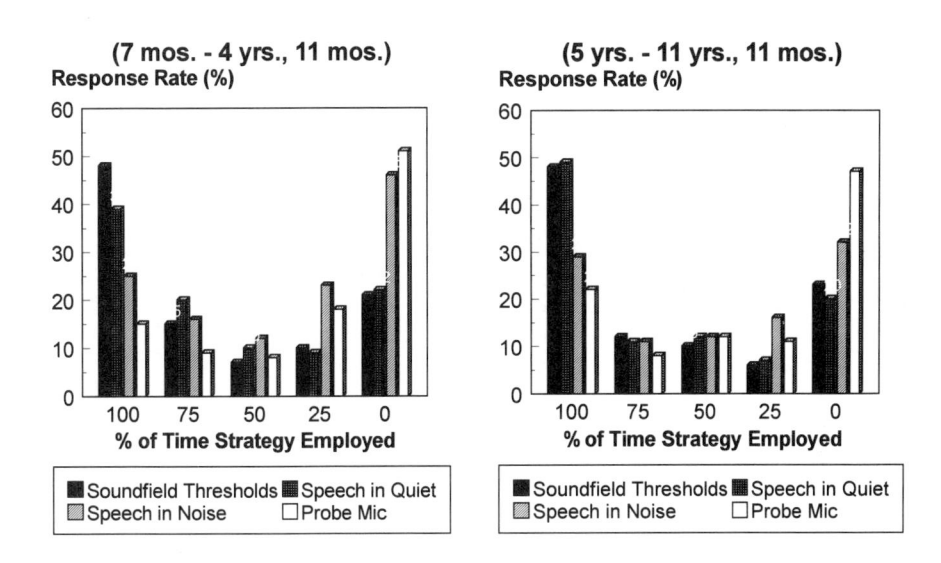

Figure 4. Percentage of use of FM fitting verification strategies for two age groups.

USE OF FM SYSTEMS

It is well recognized that individuals with hearing loss do not perform well in noisy and reverberant environments (Finitzo-Hieber and Tillman 1978; Nabelek and Pickett 1974; Olsen 1988). FM systems have been advocated for educational and noneducational settings (Benoit 1989; Ross 1992; Vaughn, Lightfoot, and Teter 1988). Survey respondents were asked, "How often do you recommend an individual FM system, sound field FM system, or BTE FM combination for children in classroom or therapy settings?" They were also asked the same question for FM use *outside* the classroom or clinical setting. These questions were repeated for minimal-to-mild, moderate, and severe-to-profound hearing losses. Responses are summarized in figures 5A, B, and C as a function of varying degrees of hearing loss and two age groups (7 months–4 years, 11 months; 5 years–11 years, 11 months). The respondents more often recommend an FM system for a severe-to-profound hearing loss than for a mild hearing loss. Further, little difference was seen between the FM recommendation practices for the younger preschool population and the older school-age population.

114 • ISSUES IN PEDIATRIC AMPLIFICATION

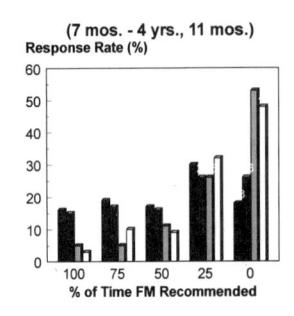

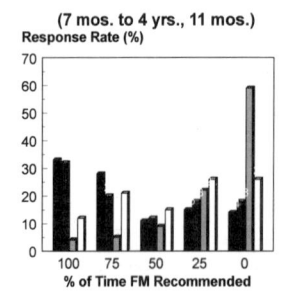

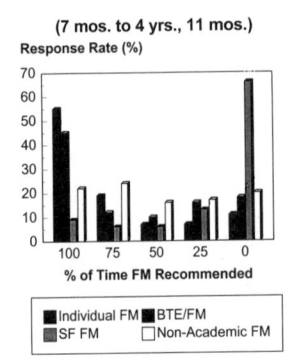

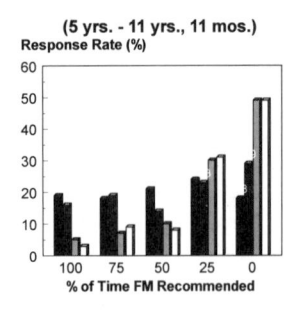

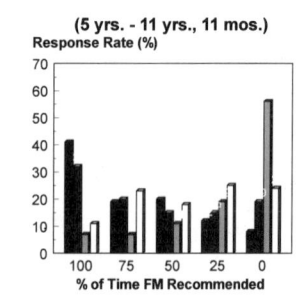

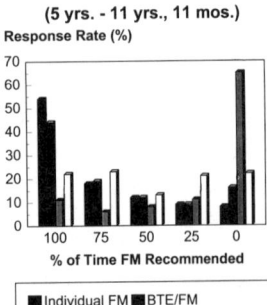

Figures 5A, B, C. Percentage of different FM recommendations for two age groups and varying degrees of hearing loss.

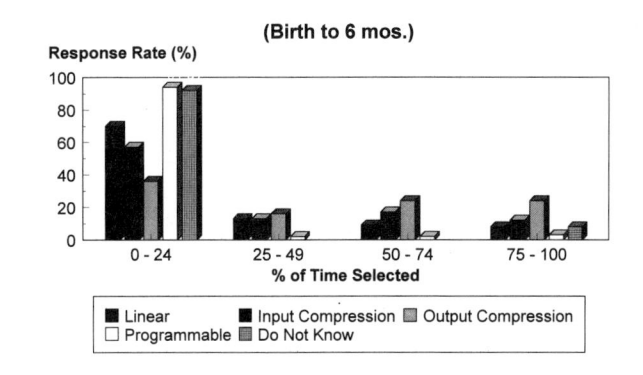

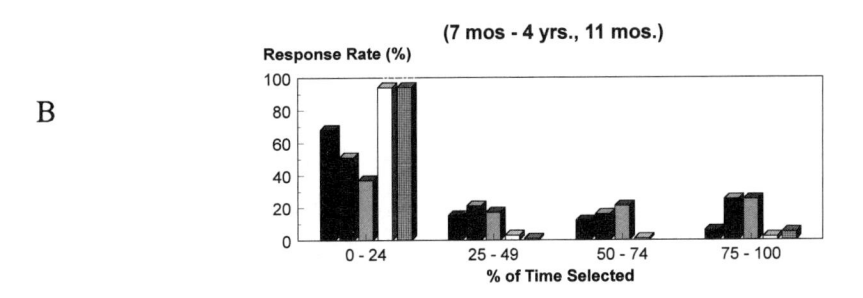

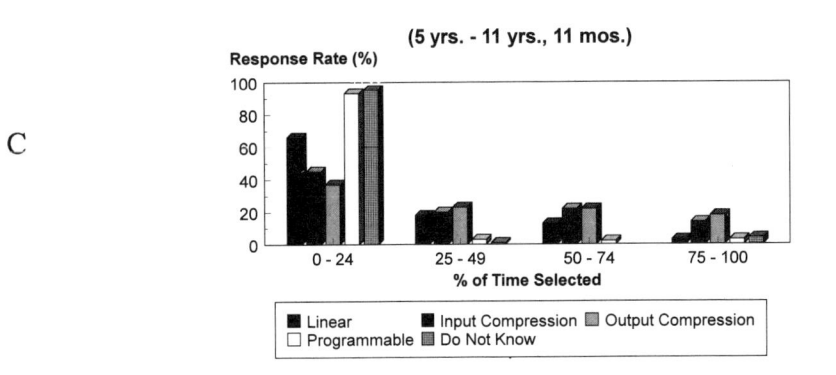

Figures 6A, B, C. Percentage of hearing aid circuitry recommendations across three age groups.

The recommendation of an FM system for listening environments outside the classroom/therapy setting was not routinely made by our respondents. As was seen with the other FM recommendations, the more severe the hearing loss, the more likely an FM recommendation for non-academic settings was made.

The sound field FM system represents a relatively new development in the amplification marketplace. This unit increases the signal-to-noise ratio for the entire classroom, benefiting those with and those without hearing impairment (see chapter 11). As depicted in figure 5A, 5% of responding audiologists *always* recommend a sound field system for children with mild-to-moderate hearing impairment (the population for which this system was primarily designed) and approximately 50% *never* recommend this system for use with this population.

USE OF NEW TECHNOLOGY

Recent advances in hearing aid circuitry have made compression circuits readily available. Designed to improve sound fidelity while minimizing tolerance problems, compression circuits offer some advantages over traditional linear circuits (Mueller and Hawkins 1992). A summary of the type of circuitry recommended by the respondents as a function of age can be seen in figures 6A, B, and C. Little difference between recommendations of input versus output compression was evident.

Many programmable aids allow the audiologist to adjust the frequency response with more flexibility than nonprogrammable aids. This increased flexibility could appear to be an ideal option for fitting pediatric patients. As more information about the hearing loss is obtained or a change in hearing sensitivity is measured, an adjustment to the gain and frequency response of the hearing aid can be easily made. Very little published information, however, is available on the use of programmable hearing aids with children. As is evident in figures 6A, B, and C, programmable hearing aids are seldom recommended by the survey respondents. More than 90% of the respondents reported that they rarely or never (0-24% of the time) recommend programmable hearing aids.

RECOMMENDATIONS IN THE 12- to 17-YEAR-OLD POPULATION

In the 12- to 17-year-old age group, the survey focused on whether hearing aid and FM recommendations were influenced by social or cosmetic concerns. That is, were audiologists willing to sacrifice optimum amplification because of personal concerns expressed by their teenage clients? For example, the flexibility of a behind-the-ear (BTE) hearing aid may be

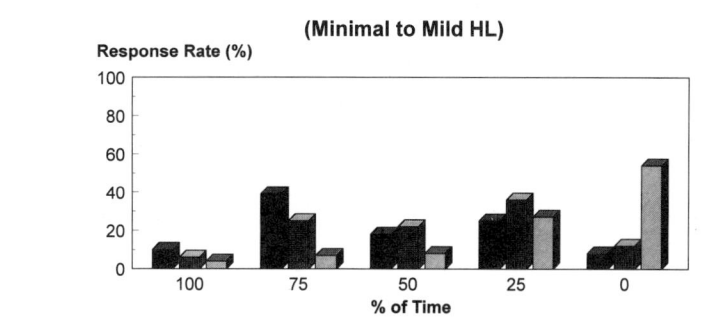

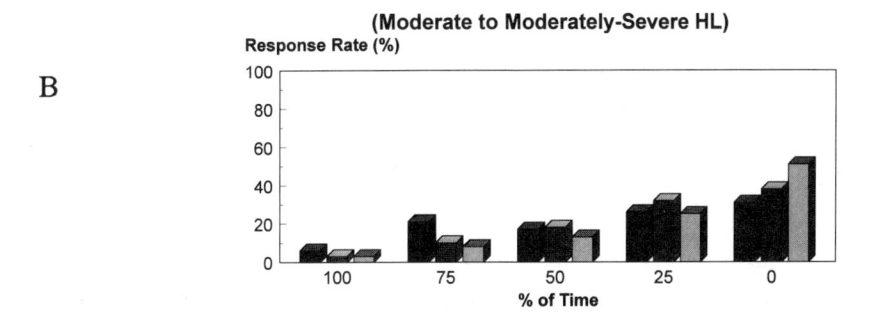

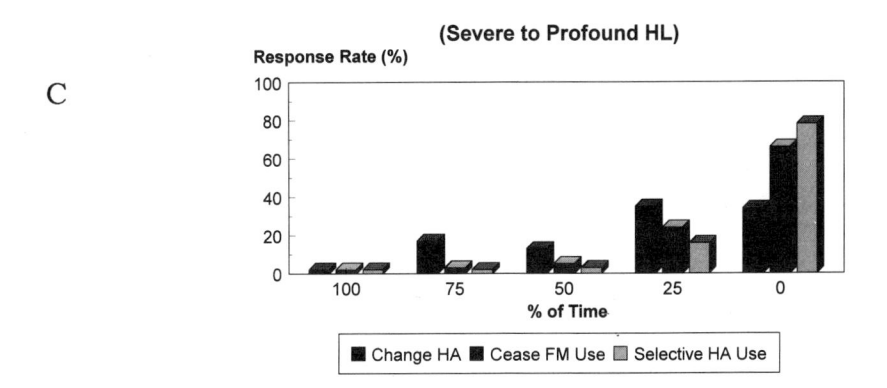

Figures 7A, B, C. Percentage of changes in amplification recommendations due to social/cosmetic concerns of teenage clients as a function of degree of hearing loss.

118 • ISSUES IN PEDIATRIC AMPLIFICATION

Fitting Considerations
(Birth to 6 mos.)

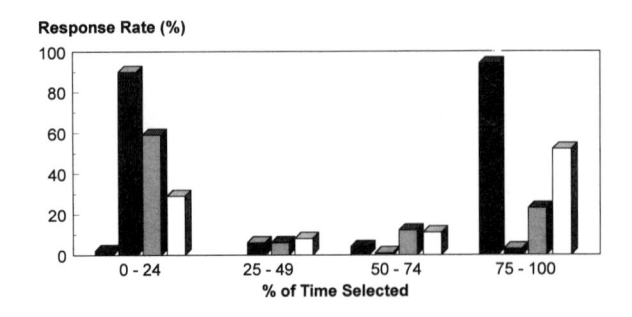

A

(7 mos. - 4 yrs., 11 mos.)

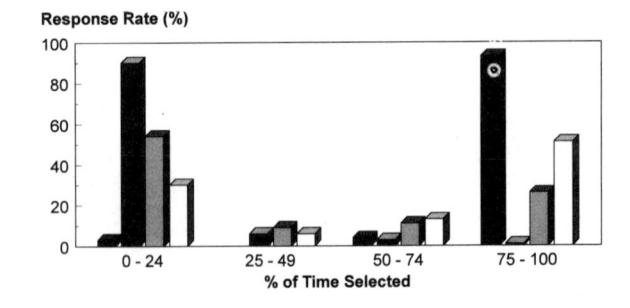

B

(5 yrs. - 11 yrs., 11 mos.)

C

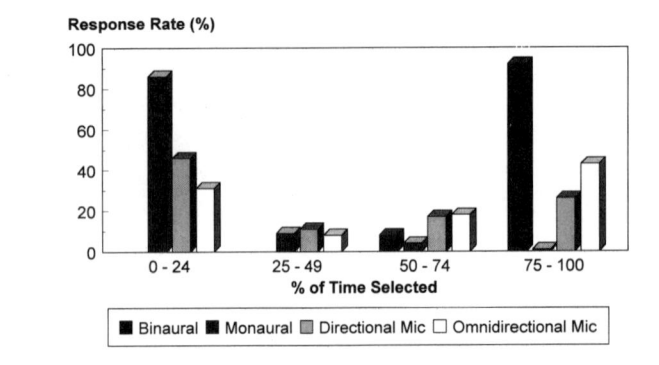

■ Binaural ■ Monaural ■ Directional Mic □ Omnidirectional Mic

Figures 8A, B, C. Percentage of various fitting considerations across three age groups.

sacrificed for a more cosmetically appealing canal hearing aid. The respondents were asked, "How often do you change your hearing aid recommendation based on cosmetic/social concerns of children 12 to 17 years of age?" This question was asked for each hearing loss category of minimal-to-mild, moderate-to-moderately-severe, and severe-to-profound. Figures 7A, B and C summarize these findings. Approximately 40% of the respondents frequently (75% of the time) change hearing aid recommendations for cosmetic/social concerns of teenagers with minimal or mild losses. In contrast, less than 20% frequently change hearing aid recommendations for those with severe-to-profound losses.

Similarly, approximately 25% of the respondents indicated that they are frequently willing to cease FM use for cosmetic/social reasons for children with minimal-to-mild losses. Less than 5% of the respondents were frequently willing to cease FM use for children with severe-to-profound hearing losses. Of the audiologists surveyed, 54% *never* recommend selective use of amplification for children with minimal-to-mild hearing losses compared to 78% who *never* recommend selective use of amplification for those with severe-to-profound losses.

ADDITIONAL FINDINGS

In 1981, Smaldino and Hoene reported the results of a survey of audiologists who fit children and adults with amplification. They found that none of their respondents always fit binaurally and only 27% fit binaurally 50-75% of the time. Approximately 15 years later, things have changed. Figures 8A, B, and C reveal that most respondents routinely recommend binaural over monaural hearing aid fittings. Of the audiologists surveyed, greater than 90% *always* recommend binaural amplification across all age groups. This finding is consistent with standard accepted practice of binaural amplification unless a clear contraindication is present (Bess, Chase, Gravel, Hedley-Williams, Seewald, Stelmachowicz, and Tharpe 1996).

Although the desirability of directional microphones on hearing aids for children with mild-to-moderate hearing loss has been demonstrated (Hawkins 1984), little additional evidence has appeared in the literature, particularly for varying degrees of loss. As seen in figures 8A, B, and C, omnidirectional microphones were selected more frequently than directional microphones across all age ranges by our respondents.

SUMMARY AND CONCLUSIONS

The purpose of this chapter was to review the findings of a survey that queried pediatric audiologists about their hearing aid selection, fitting, and verification procedures for use with infants and children. The results of the survey suggest that no systematic procedures are being consistently used with the pediatric population. There may be several reasons for this finding. First, reports of research findings in support of systematic hearing aid procedures for children may not be reaching the clinical professionals. Second, clinicians may be aware of the research findings but may not have access to the equipment needed to conduct these procedures. Third, clinicians may find that these procedures are not as easy or efficient as they appear in the literature and subsequently reject them. It is most likely that all of these reasons contribute to the lack of consistent usage of evidence-based, systematic hearing aid fitting procedures for children. Effective communication between clinical practitioners and researchers is essential in solving these problems.

As audiologists, we must be accountable to our patients. As noted by Wilson and Margolis (1983): "If patients are expected to spend their time and money in the audiology clinic, then they deserve the benefit of an ongoing critical evaluation of clinical procedures." To this end, a position statement was developed by a pediatric working group to offer audiologists a guideline for providing quality, systematic hearing health care to the pediatric population (Bess et al. 1996). There is a need to combine our current knowledge of equipment and effective assessment techniques with our standard practice procedures "to read and to learn, and to practice what we have learned" (Wiley et al. 1995). Incorporating this knowledge into our clinical practice will help us to provide consistent quality services in the fitting and evaluation of amplification to the pediatric population.

REFERENCES

American Speech-Language-Hearing Association. 1994. Guidelines for fitting and monitoring FM systems. *Asha* 36(Suppl. 12):1-9.

Benoit, R. 1989. Home use of FM amplification systems during the early childhood years. *Hearing Instruments* 40:8-12.

Berger, K.W., Hagberg, E.N., and Rane, R. 1988. *Prescription of hearing aids: Rationale, procedures, and results*. Kent, Ohio: Herald Publishing.

Bess, F.H., Chase, P.A., Gravel, J.S., Hedley-Williams, A., Seewald, R.C., Stelmachowicz, P.G., and Tharpe, A.M. 1996. Amplification for infants and children with hearing loss. *American Journal of Audiology*. 5(1):53-68.

Bratt, G. 1980. *Hearing aid receiver output in occluded ear canals of children*. Ph.D. diss., Nashville, Tenn.: Vanderbilt University.

Byrne, D., and Dillon, H. 1986. The National Acoustics Laboratories' (NAL) new procedure for selecting the gain and frequency response of a hearing aid. *Ear and Hearing* 7:257-265.

Feigin, J.A., Kopun, J.G., Stelmachowicz, P.G., and Gorga, M.P. 1989. Probe-tube microphone measures of ear-canal sound pressure levels in infants and children. *Ear and Hearing* 10:254-258.

Finitzo-Hieber, T., and Tillman, T. 1978. Room acoustics effects on monosyllabic word discrimination ability for normal and hearing-impaired children. *Journal of Speech and Hearing Research* 21:440-458.

Hawkins, D.B. 1984. Comparisons of speech recognition in noise by mild-to-moderately hearing-impaired children using hearing aids and FM systems. *Journal of Speech and Hearing Disorders* 49:409-418.

Hawkins, D.B. 1987. Assessment of FM systems with probe tube microphone system. *Ear and Hearing* 8(5):301-303.

Hawkins, D.B. 1992. Prescriptive approaches to selection of gain and frequency response. In H.G. Mueller, D.B. Hawkins, and J.L. Northern (eds.), *Probe microphone measurements* (pp. 91-112). San Diego: Singular Publishing Group.

Hawkins, D.B., Montgomery, A.A., Prosek, R.A., and Walden, B.E. 1987. Examination of two issues concerning function gain measurements. *Journal of Speech and Hearing Disorders* 52:56-63.

Humes, L. and Kirn, E. 1990. The reliability of functional gain. *Journal of Speech and Hearing Disorders* 55:193-197.

Kruger, B. 1987. An update on the external ear resonance in infants and young children. *Ear and Hearing* 8:333-336.

Kruger, B., and Ruben, R.J. 1987. The acoustic properties of the infant ear: A preliminary report. *Acta Otolaryngologica* 103:578-585.

Lewis, D., Feigin, J.A., Karasek, A., and Stelmachowicz, P.G. 1991. Evaluation and assessment of FM systems. *Ear and Hearing* 12(4):268-280.

Macrae, J. 1982. Invalid aided thresholds. *Hearing Instruments* 33(9):20-22.

Mueller, H.G., and Hawkins, D.B. 1992. Assessment of fitting arrangements, special circuitry, and features. In H.G. Mueller, D.B Hawkins, and J.L. Northern (eds.), *Probe microphone measurements* (pp. 201-226). San Diego: Singular Publishing Group.

Mueller, H.G., and Grimes, A. 1983. Speech audiometry for hearing aid selection. *Seminars in Hearing* 4(3):255-272.

Nabelek, A., and Pickett, J. 1974. Monaural and binaural speech perception through hearing aids under noise and reverberation with normal and hearing-impaired listeners. *Journal of Speech and Hearing Research* 17:724-739.

Olsen, W.O. 1988. Classroom acoustics for hearing-impaired children. In F.H. Bess (ed.), *Hearing impairment in childhood.* (pp. 266-277). Parkton, Md.: York Press.

Ross, M. 1992. Room acoustics and speech perception. In M. Ross (ed.), *FM auditory training systems: Characteristics, selection and use.* Timonium, Md.: York Press.

Schwartz, D.M., Lyregaard, P.E., and Lundh, P. 1988. Hearing aid selection for severe-to-profound hearing loss. *Hearing Journal* 41(2):13-17.

Seewald, R.C. 1991. Hearing aid output limiting considerations for children. In J.A. Feigin and P.G. Stelmachowicz (eds.), *Pediatric amplification: Proceedings of the 1991 national conference.* Omaha: Boys Town National Research Hospital.

Seewald, R.C. 1992. The desired sensation level method for fitting children: Version 3.0. *The Hearing Journal* 45(4):36-41.

Shore, I., Bilger, R.C., and Hirsh, I.J. 1960. Hearing aid evaluation: Reliability of repeated measurements. *Journal of Speech and Hearing Disorders* 25(2):152-170.

Smaldino, J., and Hoene, J. 1981. Part 1: A view of the state of hearing aid fitting practices. *Hearing Instruments* 32(1):14, 15, 38.

Vaughn, G., Lightfoot, R., and Teter, D. 1988. Assistive listening devices and systems (ALDs) enhance the lifestyles of hearing-impaired persons. *American Journal of Otology* (Suppl.) 9:101-106.

Walden, B.E., Schwartz, D.M., Williams, D.L., Holum-Hardegen, L.L., and Crowley, J.M. 1983. Test of the assumptions underlying comparative hearing aid evaluations. *Journal of Speech and Hearing Disorders* 48:264-273.

Wiley, T.L., Stoppenbach, D.T., Feldhake, L.J., Moss, K.A., and Thordardottir, E.T. 1995. Audiologic practices: What is popular versus what is supported by evidence. *American Journal of Audiology* 4(1):26-34.

Wilson, R.H., and Margolis, R.H. 1983. Measurements of auditory thresholds for speech stimuli. In D.F. Konkle and W.F. Rintelmann (eds.), *Principles of speech audiometry* (pp. 79-126). Baltimore: University Park Press.

6

Initiating Early Amplification: *TIPS* for Success

Allan O. Diefendorf, Patricia S. Reitz, Michelle W. Escobar, and Michael K. Wynne

INTRODUCTION

Moving from making a diagnosis of hearing loss to fitting appropriate amplification in infants and young children depends on the audiologist's implementation of a parallel process model of service delivery (see figure 1). In this model, the audiologist should concurrently and successfully integrate

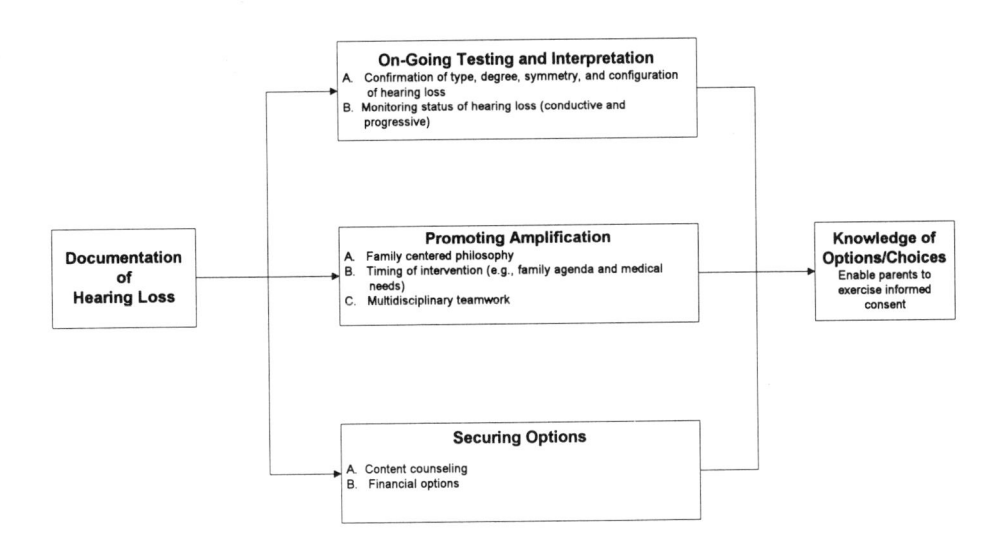

Figure 1. Parallel process of service delivery delineating components that must be considered ongoing.

three elements into the service delivery program: (1) ongoing *Testing* and *Interpretation* of auditory function, (2) *Promoting* amplification within the framework of a family-centered philosophy, and (3) *Securing* options that lead to desired outcomes. By developing intervention goals and strategies using this parallel process model for service delivery, the audiologist can establish positive, proactive attitudes toward intervention programs, improve the family's satisfaction with the delivery of hearing health services, and facilitate team building in the habilitation process.

Winton and Bailey (1990) describe several central themes underlying approaches to successful intervention with families of children with disabilities. One of these themes is family empowerment and equal partnerships with professionals. They stress that the intervention program should incorporate and capitalize on family strengths and resources. Families must be involved from the initiation of any decision process, that is, when intervention programming is planned rather than when it is implemented. No persons are more influential than the parent(s) in the habilitative process of a child with hearing loss.

The successful application of this model is paramount when one considers the factors that influence the family's behaviors after a hearing loss has been first documented. The audiologist is often trying to initiate amplification intervention during a time when the family is reacting emotionally to the diagnosis. In many instances, these emotions will be intense and may not be equally shared by different members within the family. Therefore, the development of an intervention plan that supports, rather than supplants, the caregiving role of family is critical to the success of the habilitation process. Furthermore, the audiologist's relationship with the family has changed. The audiologist now plays a central role in family dynamics. This role requires the audiologist to achieve a delicate balance between acquiring information from the family and providing information to the family related to the habilitation process.

The purpose of this chapter is to recognize factors that influence and impact identification of and intervention for congenital and early onset hearing loss. Subsequent to the confirmation of hearing loss, the provision of information (sometimes referred to as content counseling) is intended to enable and empower families as they invite early intervention programs into their lives. Content counseling provides information that promotes and secures strategies that facilitate amplification intervention for families inclined to pursue amplification options. This chapter promotes a parallel approach to service delivery with families guiding the process. This approach is consistent with the Joint Committee on Infant Hearing (1994), which emphasizes "habilitation of the child with hearing loss may (and should) begin while the audiologic portion of the diagnostic evaluation is in process." The use of the word *TIPS* (*T*esting-*I*nterpretation-*P*romoting-*S*ecuring) in this chapter's title is intended to provide the framework that leads to the successful use of amplification by children with hearing loss and their families.

TESTING AND INTERPRETATION

Accurate testing of hearing status and/or auditory function and appropriate interpretation of test results are essential before a diagnosis of hearing loss can be conferred. When achieved, audiologic findings allow intervention services to be initiated, be they communicative, medical, prosthetic, or educational. Both electrophysiologic and behavioral test approaches are viewed as appropriate and complementary, yet test selection must be based on the child's developmental level and physical capabilities.

AUDITORY BRAINSTEM RESPONSE (ABR) AUDIOMETRY

The auditory brainstem response (ABR) is an effective means of assessing auditory function in newborns and infants with developmental delays. The ABR assumes two important roles in the management of infants and children who might sustain hearing loss. First, the ABR identifies and quantifies hearing loss when behavioral techniques cannot be used because of a person's age or developmental level. Second, ABR results can be used to select hearing aid characteristics.

Traditionally, supra-aural earphones (TDH-49 or TDH-50) have been used for air-conducted stimuli in both ABR and behavioral audiometric assessments. Standardized calibration procedures are available, and supra-aural earphones provide a broad frequency response and wide dynamic range. Insert receivers coupled to an appropriately sized ear tip can also be used (Galambos and Wilson 1994). Insert earphones have a frequency response similar to that of supra-aural earphones. Several advantages of insert earphones include increased comfort, decreased likelihood of ear canal collapse, increased interaural attenuation, and reduced stimulus artifact. After a correction for tubing length is applied to specific waveform latency, results obtained with insert earphones are essentially equivalent to those obtained with a supra-aural transducer.

Clicks are commonly used stimuli in ABR assessments. Useful information can be extracted from click-evoked responses (e.g., ABR thresholds, absolute latencies, and interpeak latency differences), which have predictive value for degree, type, and configuration of hearing loss. Click-evoked ABR thresholds agree with behavioral audiometric thresholds in the 2000 to 4000 Hz range, and the shape of the wave V latency-intensity function may have some relation to configuration of hearing loss.

Table 1

Three examples demonstrating how the 500 Hz tone-burst ABR and a click-evoked ABR response provide information about degree, symmetry, and configuration of hearing loss.

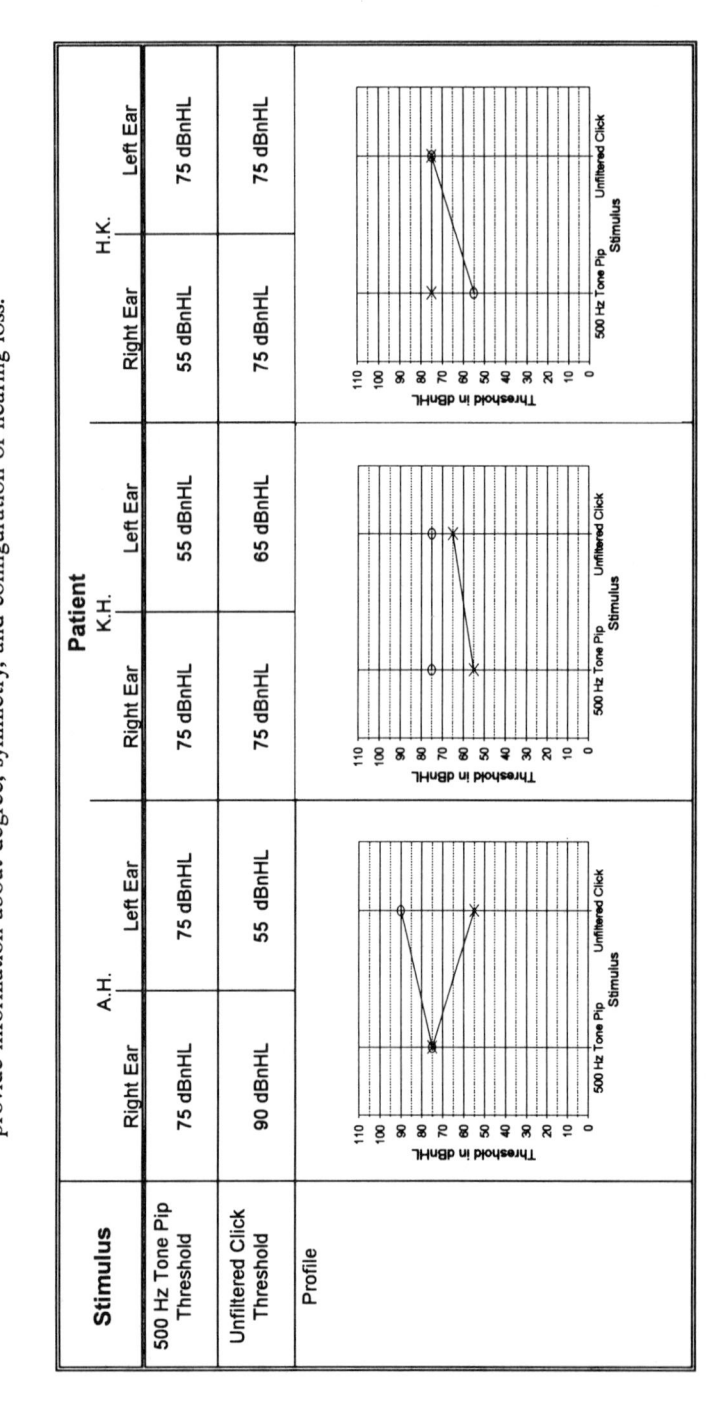

Stimulus	Patient A.H. Right Ear	A.H. Left Ear	K.H. Right Ear	K.H. Left Ear	H.K. Right Ear	H.K. Left Ear
500 Hz Tone Pip Threshold	75 dBnHL	75 dBnHL	75 dBnHL	55 dBnHL	55 dBnHL	75 dBnHL
Unfiltered Click Threshold	90 dBnHL	55 dBnHL	75 dBnHL	65 dBnHL	75 dBnHL	75 dBnHL
Profile						

Although clicks can provide accurate information about hearing loss, at least for high-frequency hearing, these results should be supplemented with as many frequency-specific thresholds as are practical. In general, responses to tone bursts provide relatively accurate predictions of the pure-tone audiogram, depending somewhat on the test parameters (Werner, Folsom, and Mancl 1994). Normal thresholds and wave V latencies for a wide range of frequencies (250 to 8000 Hz) are described elsewhere (Gorga, Kaminski, Beauchaine, and Jesteadt 1988; Stapells, Picton, Perez-Abalo, Read, and Smith 1985).

The limiting factors for achieving a tone-burst ABR audiogram usually are time and the child's sleep state. Minimally, a low-frequency threshold (500 Hz) should supplement the click threshold (ASHA 1991; Gravel 1994). As demonstrated in table 1, the use of a 500 Hz tone burst provides audiologists with information about degree of hearing loss, ear symmetry, and configuration that otherwise would not be available on the basis of a click-evoked ABR only. These ABR thresholds, in conjunction with clinical observations and parental reports of the infant's auditory behaviors, provide a baseline from which to make recommendations for amplification.

BEHAVIORAL AUDIOMETRY

Once an infant has achieved a developmental age of 5 to 6 months, audiometric information can be obtained efficiently using a behavioral technique based on the principles of operant conditioning. Visual reinforcement audiometry (VRA) is a behavioral test method that capitalizes on the natural interests and developmental abilities of children.

Normally developing infants make head turns toward a sound source in the first few months of life. The localization response represents a behavioral window through which many aspects of auditory behavior can be studied. Although there is an obvious tendency for infants to turn initially toward interesting or novel auditory stimuli, there is a limit to the number of times a child will respond (Moore, Thompson, and Thompson 1975; Moore, Wilson, and Thompson 1977). However, it is possible to increase the rate of response if a positive reinforcer is used. Since typical test stimuli (i.e., pure tones, warbled tones, filtered noise) are known to have little reinforcing value in children, it is best to use a test procedure in which the signal and reinforcer are separate and the signal only cues the youngster that a correct response will result in reinforcement. The success of VRA is certainly related to the fact that the response (head turn) and reinforcer (animated toy) are well suited to the developmental level of children between 6 and 24 months of age.

Accurate VRA assessment depends in large part on the ability of an examiner to keep an infant appropriately attentive during the stages of

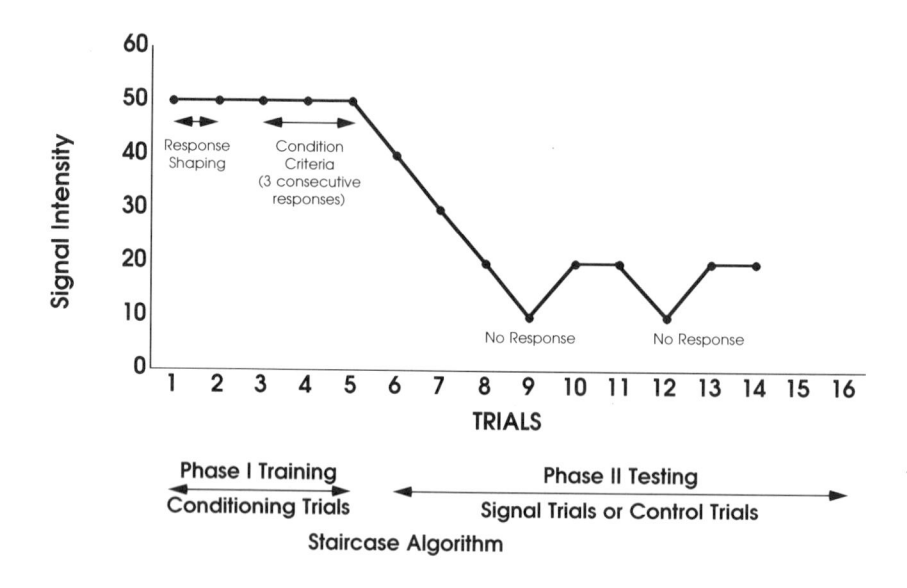

Figure 2. Adaptive test procedure with 10 dB step size; threshold (minimum response level) is based on the mean of the four reversals. In this child, the MRL was 20 dB HL.

operant conditioning and response acquisition. Whether one examiner or two are used to shape response behavior, the child's behavior is enhanced by the examiner's ability to maintain the child's head in a midline position.

The first phase of VRA is the conditioning process. Response shaping is critical to the success of the operant procedure. This phase of testing is completely under the examiner's control. Thus, the examiner must be skilled in response training and sensitive to the various stages of response acquisition. Two approaches that can be attempted in the first phase of VRA are (1) pairing the stimulus with the reinforcer and (2) observing a spontaneous response from the infant followed by reinforcement. Following several training trials, a criterion of several consecutive head turn responses must be met prior to moving to the second phase of actual test trials (figure 2). Successful completion of training occurs when the infant is making contingent responses and random head turning is at a minimum. If criterion is not reached, phase one retraining must occur until criterion is met. The number of training trials needed before phase two trials begin differs among infants. However, the training phase is usually brief.

Following training, the test phase of VRA begins. Depending on response outcome during the test phase, signal intensity is either attenuated after every "yes" response or increased after every "no" response. An adaptive threshold search is initiated until a stopping criterion (four reversals) is met.

Threshold (minimum response level) is then defined as the mean of the reversal points (figure 2).

A critical feature of the VRA procedure is that the reward (reinforcement) for correct responding be highly appealing. Maintaining response behavior over repeated trials depends on the child's continued interest in viewing the reinforcement. Visual stimuli containing movement, color, and contour (animated toys) are more effective reinforcers than less-dimensional visual stimuli.

In general, a 100% reinforcement schedule results in more rapid conditioning, yet more rapid habituation. Conversely, an intermittent reinforcement schedule produces slower conditioning but also a slower rate of habituation. Consequently, most clinicians recommend a protocol that begins with a 100% reinforcement schedule and then gradually shifts to an intermittent reinforcement schedule.

The use of novelty in a reinforcement protocol is an effective technique for improving responses. The availability of multiple visual reinforcers (stacked and housed in separate compartments) in VRA enhances novelty and, therefore, the impact of reinforcement. The primary benefits of novel reinforcement in VRA are an increased amount of information gathered about hearing in a single test session and an extended age range for success with VRA. Children 2 years of age and slightly older can be successfully tested.

Reinforcement duration is also a factor influencing response outcome from children in the 2-year age range (Culpepper and Thompson 1994).

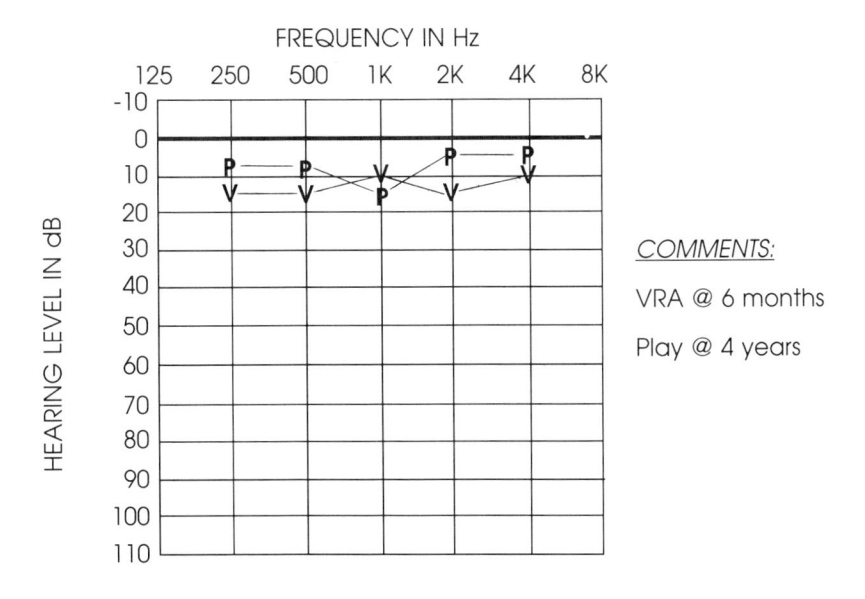

Figure 3. Longitudinal comparison between VRA and play audiometry.

Decreasing the duration of a child's exposure to the visual reinforcer (e.g., 4 seconds to .5 second) results in an increase in response behavior and a decrease in habituation. Clinicians may increase the amount of audiometric information obtained from older children by decreasing their exposure to the visual reinforcer.

Clinical reports shared among clinicians as well as reports in the literature reveal highly consistent findings from different settings. That is, for infants with normal hearing, thresholds are consistently obtained within a conservative definition of normal hearing (<15 dB HL), and reliability over time (figure 3) is impressive. These reports support the accuracy of the VRA procedure in correctly identifying normal hearing, thereby resulting in an excellent test operating characteristic for specificity. Figures 4 and 5 present audiograms representative of those that may be obtained from infants on one test day using the visually reinforced head turn procedure. They provide audiometric information that is specific to frequency, ear, degree of hearing loss, symmetry, and configuration of hearing loss. Figure 4 illustrates two points: (1) sound field responses (V) reflect the hearing in the better ear and demonstrate that ear symmetry cannot be assumed until an earphone or insert phone assessment has been completed; and (2) aided thresholds (A) can be successfully determined at different audiometric frequencies. Figure 5 illustrates the success of VRA testing during a single test session. Initially, the insert earphone tubing is coupled to the child's own earmolds and

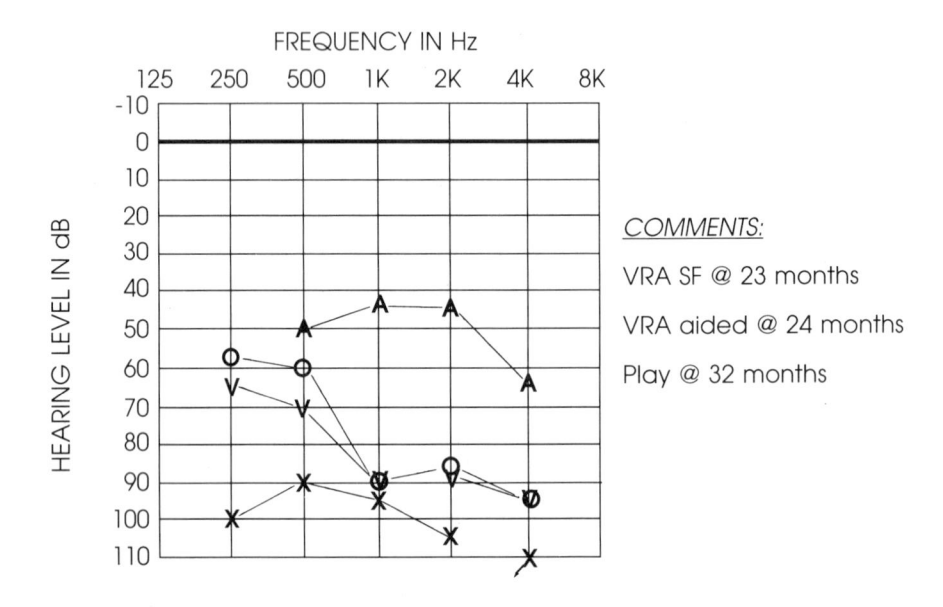

Figure 4. Sample audiogram from VRA assessment. V = sound field responses; A = aided responses; X = left ear; O = right ear.

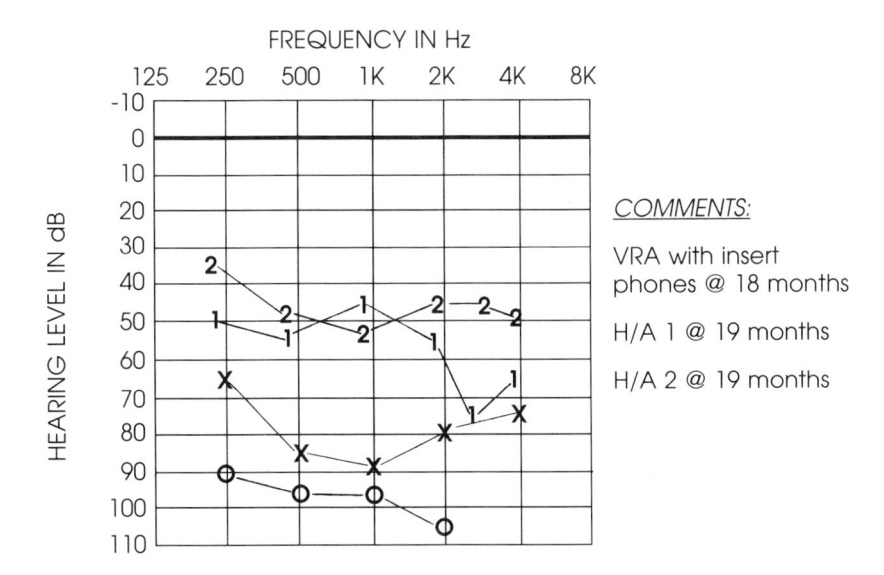

Figure 5. Sample audiogram from VRA assessment; unaided and aided results. X = left ear; O = right ear.

unaided thresholds are obtained. Subsequently, hearing aids are coupled to the earmolds and aided thresholds are obtained.

PROMOTING AMPLIFICATION

The *P* of the *TIPS* acronym represents *Promoting* amplification within the framework of a family-centered philosophy. When a hearing loss is initially identified, the habilitation process may begin. If the hearing loss is sensorineural, one goal of the habilitation process is the selection and fitting of appropriate personal amplification. Even by providing the best possible hearing aid, the audiologist cannot provide a successful hearing aid fitting if the child does not wear the hearing aid consistently. The provision of amplification must therefore coincide with the family's readiness to pursue this option.

Adults with hearing aids, while influenced by their peers and families, are ultimately responsible for using their personal hearing aids. Infants and young children, however, depend upon the involvement of others for the proper use of hearing aids on a regular basis. The practical problems associated with daily hearing aid use for children are detailed in chapter 10. Audiologists working with families of children with newly identified hearing loss must recognize the range of difficulties that will be encountered on a daily basis. A personal and individualized family focus is essential for the successful use of amplification by their children.

Pediatric audiology has historically held a *child-centered* focus, where the perceived needs of the child were addressed. Early intervention services focused on recommendations and treatments specific to those needs. In recent years, a *family-centered* philosophy has steadily gained acceptance in early intervention. As Trivette, Dunst, Deal, Hamer, and Propst (1990) point out, the goal of intervention should be viewed not so much as the professional providing needed services as much as strengthening the functioning of families so that they will ultimately be less dependent on the professional for help. With respect to hearing aids, families can be much more effective in the vigilance required for ensuring the consistent use and monitoring of personal amplification devices. Moreover, clinicians currently involved in providing early intervention services recognize that by educating and empowering the families of these children, compliance with recommendations for communicative, medical, prosthetic, and educational services will be enhanced (Matkin 1988; Schuyler and Rushmer 1987; Thompson 1992).

The following discussion on promoting amplification and intervention services is divided into three sections of equal importance: family-centered services, timing of intervention, and multidisciplinary teamwork.

FAMILY-CENTERED SERVICES

Services that are family-centered involve a philosophy that families have the right to retain as much control as they desire over the intervention process for their children. The child's needs will best be served by meeting the family's needs first. Bernheimer, Gallimore, and Weisner (1990) stress the importance of embracing what they refer to as an ecocultural theory as a framework for designing intervention for children with disabilities. Ecocultural theory refers to consideration of the sociocultural environment of the child and family. Professionals working with children in the first three years of life must be sensitive to whoever makes up the child's family social support network. The definition of family should go beyond the traditional family and should include primary caregivers and others who assume important roles in the child's daily life such as grandparents, cousins who live in the same house, trusted neighbors, or longtime caregivers. By accepting each family's diversity, the strengths and competencies within that family will be drawn upon, and a support network between the family and audiologist (or other professional) will be established. This support network will enable progress at home and in the clinical setting.

What affects one family member affects all family members (Rushmer 1994). The introduction of a hearing aid on a child within a family will affect all people close to that child, from correctly inserting an earmold to recognizing and dealing with feedback problems to budgeting the family finances for hearing aid and battery purchases. Issues related to communication with the child will also affect the whole family. Thus, the family must guide the process toward amplification and communication options that, in turn, allows the child to function successfully within the family.

Parents should be empowered to make decisions that they believe are right for their child and their family. Empowerment is both a process and an outcome that takes different forms in different families. Empowering families for early intervention does not mean giving or bestowing power to families—the power is theirs by right. Rather, it means interacting with families in such a way that they maintain or acquire a sense of control over their daily family life and attribute positive changes that result from early intervention to their own strengths, abilities, and actions (Dunst, Trivette, and Deal 1988).

Family goals should drive the habilitation program. Parents need to know that the professionals working with them will support them in their decisions, even if the professionals do not agree with the decisions. This acceptance leaves a door open if families decide later to reconsider their original plan.

The family-centered service model has its foundation in a federally mandated plan, first defined in 1986 by Public Law 99-457. This law guarantees early intervention services to children and their families. It is one of several legislative mandates influential in directing services provided to children with special needs. The laws and regulations implemented at both the state and the federal levels provide guidelines regarding the access and implementation of services for children with hearing loss. Individuals who encounter institutional barriers can refer to these laws, regulations, and policies to gain an understanding of how they can acquire and promote intervention services for these children.

In 1975, the Education of All Handicapped Children Act (P.L. 94-142) was passed. This law guaranteed free and appropriate education to all school-age children and stated that education should be provided in the least restrictive environment. The child's educational plan was to be outlined in the Individualized Education Plan (IEP). The evolution of public laws since that time has taken clinicians and educators from a child-centered plan with considerable emphasis placed on the written document (the IEP) to a family-centered plan, now required through the Individualized Family Service Plan (IFSP).

The IFSP is a written plan developed by a multidisciplinary team, including the parent(s) or guardian(s) of the child. In addition to the child-centered components required in the IEP, the IFSP must include documentation of family strengths and needs, specification of expected family outcomes, a description of services to be provided for the family, and the name of the family service coordinator who will assist the family in implementing the plan and coordinate services with other agencies and persons. With the introduction of the IFSP, families became essential members of the multidisciplinary team.

P.L. 99-457 amended P.L. 94-142 to include *mandatory* special education services for children ages 3 through 5 years. Additionally, Part H of P.L. 99-457 provided funding to states to develop a system of services for infants and toddlers (ages birth through 2 years) with developmental delays, physical disabilities, or at-risk conditions. States are not required to participate in Part H, but those electing to must develop and implement this system as a statewide plan. As of October 1, 1994, all states and territories had fully phased-in early intervention services. Federal regulations do not require screening of every child determined to be at risk. Part H of P.L. 99-457 mandates that states are required only to provide early intervention services for children who have already been determined to be eligible.

In 1990, P.L. 101-476 was introduced. This law reauthorized P.L. 94-142 and changed its name to Individuals with Disabilities Education Act (IDEA). Terminology used to refer to eligible recipients of services was changed. In 1991, P.L. 102-119 reauthorized Part H of 99-457 and included specific requirements for every aspect of the IFSP. This reauthorization of Part H added a new IFSP requirement; all IFSPs must now address the provision of services to children in their natural environments including the home and community settings in which children without disabilities also participate. The IFSP embodies a promise to children and families, a "promise that their strengths will be recognized and built on, that their beliefs and values will be respected, that their choices will be honored, and their hopes and aspirations will be encouraged and enabled" (McGonigel and Johnson 1991).

TIMING OF INTERVENTION

The diagnostic process is often a period of extreme anxiety for most family members, and confirmation that an infant or toddler has a permanent hearing loss can elicit a wide range of emotions (Matkin 1988). Once a hearing loss is confirmed, family members must deal with their own emotional responses. For some families or family members, the identification of a permanent hearing loss confirms a set of beliefs and allows them the opportunity to deal directly with the child's challenges. For others, the identification of a hearing loss may trigger anger and denial responses, similar to the same stages of grieving when a family has lost a loved one in death. In all cases, the audiologist must be prepared to provide extensive counseling to help family members address their own emotional needs. Team planning regarding communication options and the introduction of amplification options should be presented only at a time when the family is ready to consider these options. The *timing of intervention* for each child and family must be considered according to their own state of readiness and in relation to their set of agendas. Listening, understanding the family's perspectives, establishing mutually agreed upon goals and strategies, and coming to agreement are essential components to the successful promotion of amplification.

Throughout this process, the audiologist must consider the priority of amplification in relation to the global needs of the child and family. Some infants and children with multiple disabilities as well as some medically at-risk children have so many problems, some of which may be life threatening, that a hearing aid is not the top priority for the family at the time the hearing loss is identified. The successful promotion of amplification depends on the audiologist's ability to accommodate the needs and priorities of the family and child.

Communication with the child's primary care physician, nurses, and social workers is also paramount if the audiologist is working with a child who is an in-patient within a hospital setting. The introduction of amplification should occur at a time when the amplification fits in relative to the overall needs of the child or a time that is not incompatible with the needs of health care professionals trying to stabilize medically compromised conditions. In addition, the audiologist does not want to provide any sense of false hope regarding the ultimate prognosis of a severely involved child or inadvertently negate the work of a pediatrician who may be working with a family to help members accept realistic outcomes.

MULTIDISCIPLINARY TEAMWORK

The third component essential to promoting amplification and intervention for the young child with hearing loss is *multidisciplinary teamwork*. No one agency or discipline can meet the diverse and complex needs of infants and toddlers with special needs and their families. Therefore, a team approach to planning and implementing the IFSP is necessary. Furthermore, effective teamwork can assist the audiologist in keeping the big picture in focus.

From an educational viewpoint, the enactment of P.L. 99-457 brings new opportunities for the audiologist as a multidisciplinary team player in the early intervention process. Audiology is one of the ten disciplines specifically identified in this legislation that can contribute to the successful integration of special education services. By participating as a member of a team, the audiologist can provide input regarding ongoing family education and the development of an audiologic management plan. In addition, the audiologist can contribute to the team by providing access to resources regarding hearing loss and management, by facilitating open and frequent communication, and by encouraging flexibility and innovation. After the initiation of an action plan, the child's progress should be monitored and documented on an ongoing basis. Documentation must include the following: unaided and aided audiometric information; family's satisfaction with and understanding of amplification systems; communication milestones, including objective test scores; and documentation about ongoing management of amplification for the child. The audiologic management plan should be evaluated in terms of the processes used to develop and provide services, and the extent to which outcomes are achieved or needs are met. Any system of accountability must provide multiple opportunities and methods for families and other team members to evaluate the plan.

SECURING OPTIONS FOR COUNSELING AND AMPLIFICATION

The *S* of the *TIPS* acronym represents *Securing* strategies for counseling and amplification planning for children and their families. While public laws provide the mandate entitling services for children and families, securing strategies for initiating counseling and pursuing amplification is required if services are to be effectively implemented. As part of a family-centered philosophy to service provision, professionals must be willing to go beyond the narrow boundaries of their disciplines or agencies and reach out to others who are also planning or providing services to these children and their families. Within the framework of securing services, families will need guidance in the following areas: content counseling intended to facilitate amplification intervention, and financial options for implementing intervention recommendations.

PARENT COUNSELING

For a child with hearing loss, chances for successful communication, academic achievement, and personal satisfaction are greatly enhanced when the child's parents can emotionally accept the child and are dedicated to maximizing the child's potential. From the initial diagnosis of hearing loss through the school-age years, parent counseling is a powerful habilitative tool that should receive priority consideration from professionals who work with children and their families.

Given the mandate by P.L. 99-457 for dramatically increased family involvement in intervention services for infants and toddlers with disabilities, as well as the increasing awareness of the importance of the family to the overall development of the child with a hearing loss, it is incumbent on professionals to approach counseling with parents' input. This approach supports the concept of family empowerment, with intervention goals as well as strategies guided by parental input.

Williams and Darbyshire (1982) stated that effective management during and after the time of diagnosis is critical to the acceptance of a permanent hearing loss and subsequent involvement in rehabilitation. Thus, the important role of counseling during this time cannot be underestimated. Parents' acceptance, attitudes, beliefs, and motivation regarding amplification will be impacted by their knowledge of hearing loss, hearing aids, and the range of intervention alternatives available. Our team at the medical center approaches content counseling by making use of a family interview scheduled early in the intervention process. The family is asked to complete a Family Needs Questionnaire (table 2) prior to the family interview. Parents are asked to rate a variety of topics on a scale of 1 to 4. Content areas include hearing loss, hearing aids, listening skills, communication skills, general development, behavior management, educational resources, and financial assistance and funding. During the family interview, each area is discussed, and the family's choices and specific needs are addressed. This questionnaire is used frequently in the course of the child's program as family needs and concerns change.

Schuyler and Rushmer (1987) have identified six needs that parents of infants or toddlers with hearing loss have expressed or demonstrated as they learn about their child's hearing loss and as they begin to deal with their emotions that were elicited from the confirmation of the hearing loss. First, parents need to be able to express their feelings in an environment in which these feelings are acknowledged and accepted. A subsequent study by Bernstein and Barta (1988) indicated that parents want to have more opportunities to inform professionals of their own needs as parents of children with hearing loss. Second, therefore, parents need to be able to talk to individuals with whom they have established mutual trust so that it is safe to express their feelings. Third, parents need empathic and objective feedback about their fears and expectations related to their child's hearing loss. Fourth, parents need a sense of community, a sense that others really understand their problems because of shared experiences or feelings. Fifth, parents require information regarding their child's communication needs and assistance in finding an interaction style with their child to promote the development of communication skills. Finally, parents need assistance in identifying, defining, and sorting out all of the options related to their child's needs. A repeated theme from interviews with parents of children with special needs is the parental desire to become more knowledgeable about their children's needs and the services available to address these needs (Able-Boone, Sandall, and Frederick 1990).

Table 2
Family Needs Questionnaire

INDIANA UNIVERSITY MEDICAL CENTER
JAMES WHITCOMB RILEY HOSPITAL FOR CHILDREN

Name of Child: _____
Name of Person Completing Form: _____   Date: _____

FAMILY NEEDS QUESTIONNAIRE

Please rate each question on a 1-4 scale of your need or desire to know:
    1 — Information you would like to know now.
    2 — Information you would like to know sometime.
    3 — Don't know or undecided.
    4 — Don't need to know or already know.

Hearing Loss

__ 1. What is my child's hearing loss?
__ 2. Will my child's hearing change?
__ 3. What caused my child's hearing loss?

Hearing Aids

__ 1. How do I get my child to wear the hearing aids?
__ 2. How does a hearing aid work?
__ 3. Can a hearing aid be too loud?
__ 4. How do I know if the hearing aids are not working?
__ 5. What do I do if the hearing aids should not be worn?
__ 6. Are there times when the hearing aids should not be worn?
__ 7. Are there devices other than hearing aids that may help my child to hear?
__ 8. How often does my child have to wear the hearing aids?
__ 9. To what degree do the hearing aids improve my child's ability to hear speech?

Learning How to Listen

__ 1. What sounds should my child be able to hear without hearing aids? With hearing aids?
__ 2. How can I encourage my child to listen for sounds/speech?
__ 3. What do I do if my child isn't responding to sound?
__ 4. How can I help my child alert to warning sounds in the environment?
__ 5. What devices are available to help my child alert to sounds in the environment?

Communication

__ 1. How will the hearing loss affect my child's ability to learn to talk?
__ 2. How will it affect my child's ability to learn language?
__ 3. How can I communicate with my child?
__ 4. How will my child be able to communicate with others?
__ 5. What are the different methods of communication for the hearing impaired?

Table 2 (continued)

General Development

   __ 1.   Is my child's motor development (coordination) appropriate for his age?
   __ 2.   Is my child's social development (interaction with others) appropriate for his age?
   __ 3.   How can I help my child learn daily routines?

Behavior Management

   __ 1.   What can I do when my child misbehaves?
   __ 2.   What do I do when my child runs from me and can't hear me when I call?
   __ 3.   How do I set limits and rules for my child?

Educational Resources

   __ 1.   Does my child need a special program or special services?
   __ 2.   What kind of daycare/developmental center would be appropriate for my child?
   __ 3.   What kind of preschool/school would be appropriate for my child?
   __ 4.   How can I help my child be ready for school?

Financial Assistance/Funding

   __ 1.   What state and federal funding is available to help pay for therapy and hearing aids?

I have concerns regarding my child's . . . .
| __ vision | __ weight gain | __ ear infections |
| __ coordination | __ eating | __ behavior |

Please describe other concerns:

What do you see are the most important issues or needs that you have right now? Try to think of 2 or 3.

There may be times when the expertise of other professionals will be necessary to address specific concerns. Referral to these professionals will be discussed with you.

Securing amplification figuratively means getting the family to accept amplification; getting the family to accept amplification means meeting the family's needs by providing timely, comprehensive, and effective parent counseling.

FINANCIAL OPTIONS

Securing services for children with hearing loss and their families may often be difficult due to the financial commitment involved. Not all families are able to absorb the financial burden of transportation, child care, hearing aids, earmolds, batteries, and other expenses related to the total habilitative effort. Resources may be available to these families. The family service coordinator or social worker may guide families through the myriad of options. The role the audiologist takes in this challenge will enhance the family's ability to follow through with recommendations and will demonstrate the audiologist's commitment to team building with the family.

Insurance coverage for hearing services will vary with specific policies and providers. It should not always be assumed that a private insurance carrier *will not* pay for services, especially when dealing with the pediatric population. For example, individuals who receive benefits from Champus may be eligible for Champus's Program for the Handicapped. Those who qualify will receive reimbursement for services such as hearing aids, hearing aid repairs, earmolds, and audiologic evaluations.

Traditional financial options for families with limited financial resources may include state or federal assistance programs such as Medicaid or Services for Children with Special Health Care Needs (formerly Crippled Children's Services). Additional federally funded programs include the Medicaid Disability Program for children deemed eligible by Medicaid. Supplemental monthly income from the Social Security Administration (SSI) may also be an option.

Providers who receive funds from organizations such as Easter Seals and the United Way offer financial assistance to families of children with disabilities. Benefits for eligible recipients will be determined on an individual basis and may include sliding fee scales or generous payment plans. Selected hearing aid manufacturers may also be consulted regarding hearing aid donations for young children.

Local philanthropic organizations such as Sertoma and Psi Iota Xi may be contacted with specific requests for families with children residing in local communities. In 1971, Lions International adopted Hearing and Speech Action and Work with the Deaf as a major Lions activity. For example, the Indiana Lions Speech and Hearing, Inc. Trustees and the Indiana University Medical Center have developed a loaner hearing aid bank that can be accessed by audiologists throughout the state. The loaner hearing aid bank can be used for a short term during initial fitting stages or over a longer term while other financial alternatives are being explored. Moreover, the Lions provide funding for the purchase of new hearing aids when needed, for repair services, for hearing aid batteries, and for other support services.

In addition, there are charitable organizations that are dedicated to providing funding assistance exclusively to children with hearing loss. *HEAR NOW* is a national nonprofit organization based in Denver, Colorado. *HEAR NOW* raises funds to provide hearing aids, cochlear implants, and related services to children and adults with hearing loss who are without the financial resources to purchase devices. Eligibility is based on financial need and a bilateral hearing loss with the pure-tone average no better than 55 dB HL in the better ear. This organization may conduct individualized fund-raising campaigns on behalf of applicants in their own communities. Additionally, *HEAR NOW* loans hearing aids nationally through its recently established National Hearing Aid Bank.

The Hearing Impaired Kids Endowment fund (HIKE) is a charitable project supported by the International Order of Job's Daughters. Its purpose is to assist children with hearing loss, from birth through 20 years, to achieve improved communication skills. Grants from the HIKE fund are considered on an individual basis for hearing aids and other assistive devices. Applications must be completed by the families and the audiologist prior to being presented to the HIKE fund board of directors for consideration.

According to a recent interpretation of the Individuals with Disabilities Education Act (IDEA) by the U.S. Office of Special Education Programs (OSEP), a hearing aid is considered a covered device under the definition of *assistive technology device*. Therefore, some school districts may provide hearing aids under IDEA (Peters-Johnson 1994). Specifically, where a district has determined that a child with a disability requires amplification in order to receive a fair and appropriate public education, and the need for amplification is specified in the child's IEP, the district is responsible for providing the hearing aid at no cost to the child or the child's family. Although this interpretation can help families gain access to amplification for their children while their children attend school, the actual implementation of this policy must be made cautiously. Many school districts do not have access to comprehensive audiology services, and appropriate personnel must be identified to provide these services. Accordingly, school personnel must be better educated regarding the acquisition, dispensing, use, care, and repair of hearing aids.

Identifying and securing financial options for the families of children with hearing loss are not easy. Indeed, many audiologists have some discomfort even discussing the financial needs and options with families. However, the risks inherent in failing to address these issues are too great to ignore. The best diagnostic services in the world become meaningless if benign neglect is the course of treatment. It is paramount that the audiologist is informed about the financial options that are available and is committed to tapping into those resources to secure amplification.

CONCLUSION

The *TIPS* acronym used in the title of this chapter is intended to underscore a dynamic parallel process and transition that moves from diagnosis of hearing loss to amplification intervention. The process includes age-appropriate test selection, commitment to follow-up, intervention in accordance with P.L. 102-119, immediate access to resources (including amplification), and an IFSP consistent with family needs and input. Professionals must have specialized information and skills regarding assessment and amplification to meet the specific needs of infants and toddlers with hearing loss. However, the success of an early intervention program is directly related to the effectiveness of the partnership between parents and skilled professionals.

REFERENCES

Able-Boone, H., Sandall, S.R., and Frederick, L.L. 1990. An informed, family-centered approach to Public Law 99-457: Parental views. *Topics in Early Childhood Special Education* 10(1):100-111.
American Speech-Language-Hearing Association. 1991. Guidelines for the audiologic assessment of children from birth through 36 months of age. *Asha* 33:37-43.
Bernheimer, L.P., Gallimore, R., and Weisner, T.S. 1990. Ecocultural theory as a context for the Individual Family Service Plan. *Journal of Early Intervention* 14:219-233.
Bernstein, M.E., and Barta, L. 1988. What do parents want in parent education? *American Annals of the Deaf* 133:235-246.
Culpepper, B., and Thompson, G. 1994. Effects of reinforcer duration on the response behavior of preterm 2-year-olds in visual reinforcement audiometry. *Ear and Hearing* 15:161-167.
Dunst, C.J., Trivette, C.M., and Deal, A.G. 1988. *Enabling and empowering families: Principles and guidelines for practice.* Cambridge, Mass.: Brookline Books.
Galambos, R., and Wilson, M. 1994. Newborn hearing thresholds measured by both insert and earphone methods. *Journal of the American Academy of Audiology* 5:141-145.
Gorga, M.P., Kaminski, J.R., Beauchaine, K.A., and Jesteadt, W. 1988. Auditory brainstem responses to tone bursts in normally hearing subjects. *Journal of Speech and Hearing Research* 31:87-97.
Gravel, J.S. 1994. Auditory assessment of infants. *Seminars in Hearing* 15:100-113.
Joint Committee on Infant Hearing. 1994. 1994 position statement. *Asha* 36:38-41.
Matkin, N.D. 1988. Key considerations in counseling parents of hearing-impaired children. *Seminars in Speech and Language* 9:209-221.
McGonigel, M.J., and Johnson, B.H. 1991. An overview. In M.J. McGonigel, R.K. Kaufmann, and B.H. Johnson (eds.), *Guidelines and recommended practices for the*

individualized family service plan, 2d ed. (pp. 1-5). Bethesda, Md.: Association for the Care of Children's Health.

Moore, J.M., Thompson, G., and Thompson, M. 1975. Auditory localization of infants as a function of reinforcement conditions. *Journal of Speech and Hearing Disorders* 40:29-34.

Moore, J.M., Wilson, W.R., and Thompson, G. 1977. Visual reinforcement of head-turn responses in infants under 12 months of age. *Journal of Speech and Hearing Disorders* 42:328-334.

Peters-Johnson, C. 1994. Action: School services. *Language, Speech, and Hearing Services in Schools* 25:273-280.

Rushmer, N. 1994. Supporting families of hearing-impaired infants and toddlers. *Seminars in Hearing* 15:160-171.

Schuyler, V., and Rushmer, N. 1987. *Parent-infant habilitation: A comprehensive approach to working with hearing-impaired infants and toddlers and their families.* Portland, Oreg.: IHR Publications.

Stapells, D.R., Picton, T.W., Perez-Abalo, M., Read, D., and Smith, A. 1985. Frequency specificity in evoked potential audiometry. In J.T. Jacobson (ed.), *The auditory brainstem response* (pp. 147-177). San Diego: College-Hill Press.

Thompson, M. 1992. Birth to five: The important early years. In F.H. Bess and J.W. Hall III (eds.), *Screening children for auditory function* (pp. 399-434). Nashville, Tenn.: Bill Wilkerson Center Press.

Trivette, C.M., Dunst, C.J., Deal, A.G., Hamer, A.W., and Propst, S. 1990. Assessing family strengths and family functioning style. *Topics in Early Childhood Special Education* 10(1):16-35.

Werner, L.A., Folsom, R.C., and Mancl, L.R. 1994. The relationship between auditory brainstem response and behavioral thresholds in normal hearing infants and adults. *Hearing Research* 68:131-141.

Williams, D.M., and Darbyshire, J.O. 1982. Diagnosis of deafness: A study of family responses and needs. *Volta Review* 84:24-30.

Winton, P.J., and Bailey, D.B., Jr. 1990. Early intervention training related to family interviewing. *Topics in Early Childhood Special Education* 10(1):50-62.

7

Amplification Selection Considerations in the Pediatric Population

Kathryn Laudin Beauchaine and Kris Frisbie Donaghy

INTRODUCTION

The objective of fitting any amplification device is to maximally enhance communication in the majority of listening situations that the young child with hearing loss encounters. Although similar decisions about amplification characteristics must be made for the young child as for the adult, the information on which these decisions are based and the needs of these two groups are quite different. At the simplest level, infants' and children's ears are smaller than those of adults: a difference that significantly impacts amplification-fitting decisions. Moreover, audiometric information (behavioral and electrophysiologic) that is available to the audiologist from a 4-month-old infant differs greatly from that of a 14- or 40-year-old listener. The communication needs of an infant who has congenital hearing loss also are distinct from those of an adult who has gradually progressive, late-onset hearing loss. These topics will be explored below in the context of amplification selection considerations, in particular practical aspects. Case studies will be used to highlight the discussion topics.

PRESELECTION CONSIDERATIONS

STYLE CHOICES

The first consideration in choosing amplification is the style of the hearing aid. The options are behind-the-ear (BTE), in-the-ear (ITE), in-the-canal (ITC) devices, and body-worn style. In addition to the decision about style, decisions must be made about which options to request: off-on switches, telecoil option, potentiometers, and direct-audio input capabilities. The choices depend on the child's anticipated educational placement and communication needs.

BTE hearing aids accounted for approximately 20% of hearing aid sales between 1987 and 1993 (Kirkwood 1993). For young children, BTEs are the most common style of hearing aids. These devices are relatively small in size, have electroacoustic flexibility, have options for telecoils and direct-audio input, are available as programmable and frequency-modulated (FM) listening systems, and are relatively sturdy compared to ITE/C devices.

ITE/C styles, however, are not generally recommended for infants or very young children for several reasons. Housing the needed components in an infant ITE/C casing would be challenging if there were more than minimal power requirements. The need for frequent recasing is another reason not to use ITE/C hearing aids in young children. Although several manufacturers offer extended warranties that include recasing, the child would be left without amplification for many days each time a new casing is fabricated (unless a BTE loaner is available). Additionally, these devices tend to be more fragile than BTE devices, and may require even more frequent repair when used by active children. Safety is also an issue. There is danger of the casing breaking in the ear canal. We follow a young patient who has been fitted with an ITE. One day at school, another child hit her on the side of the head, fracturing the ITE case in her ear canal. Pieces of the device had to be removed from her eardrum. The parents did have the ITE remade after healing. If ITE/C is recommended, a choke-precaution label would be in order for infant and toddler fittings.

In adults, the ITE and ITC microphone location provides a boost in the high frequencies of at least 5 dB, between approximately 2 to 5 kHz (Fikret-Pasa and Revit 1992; Skinner 1988). This potential high-frequency boost provided by the ITE/C microphone locations is attributed to pinna effects and might serve the acoustic needs of some children. The amount of high-frequency boost, which would presumably vary with pinna size, has not been reported in the young ear.

An option for children with severe-to-profound hearing loss is a body-style hearing aid (Ross and Madell 1988). A body-worn device provides the potential benefit of a low-frequency boost from the body-baffle effect, estimated to be 3 dB from 250 to 750 Hz. However, a high-frequency decrease of approximately 4 dB from 1000 to 2500 Hz also is present (Skinner 1988). Thus, the trade-offs for this style unit are size, bulk of the device, and the chest microphone location rather than an ear-level microphone location. With these devices, acoustic feedback is reduced because of the separation between the body-worn microphone and the external receiver. Body-style devices account for only a small portion of total hearing aid sales. Although sales of body-style devices increased 6.6% during the first three quarters of 1993 compared to the same time frame of the previous year, they accounted for less than 0.5% of the overall market (Kirkwood 1993).

The gain requirements for some children who have little or no residual hearing may not be adequately met with conventional body aids. These children may be candidates for low-frequency emphasis, frequency transposer hearing aids, vibrotactile units, or cochlear implants. The specific candidacy requirements and fitting protocols for these devices will not be covered in this chapter.

ACOUSTIC FEEDBACK MANAGEMENT

Although BTEs have less likelihood of acoustic feedback compared to ITEs, for children who have severe-to-profound hearing loss, BTE devices may provide acoustic feedback challenges. There are several ways to reduce or eliminate acoustic feedback when a well-fitting earmold with superthick tubing is not sufficient. One option is to use a microphone that is distanced from the receiver. BTEs with hardwired remote microphones, wireless power-CROS aids, body-style hearing aids, and FM systems meet this criterion. Of course, the option that involves removing the microphone from the child reduces the extent to which the child can monitor his or her own voice.

Other options include BTEs with some sort of feedback suppression circuitry (Engebretson, French-St. George, and O'Connell 1993; Henningsen, Dyrlund, Bisgaard, and Brink 1993). The purpose of these circuits is to decrease acoustic feedback without decreasing high-frequency gain. Using a digital feedback suppression circuit (DFS), Henningsen et al. (1993) reported an additional 5 to 10 dB of usable gain across frequencies without acoustic feedback in a group of ten children.

An antifeedback microphone (Dyrlund and Lundh 1990) is another option. Some of these options sacrifice high-frequency gain. Some tone hooks can eliminate feedback problems by altering the shape of the hearing aid's frequency response. For children with corner audiograms, where there is no possibility of adequately amplifying frequencies above 1 kHz, a low-pass tone hook is an option. On a practical level, however, these tone hooks are fragile and may require frequent replacement.

It has been shown that bulkier earmold styles do not increase the amount of usable insertion gain (Kuk 1994). Even a pressure relief vent, often ordered for children who have pressure equalization tubes, can reduce usable insertion gain because of acoustic feedback (Kuk 1994).

BINAURAL VERSUS MONAURAL FITTING

There are obvious exceptions to binaural fittings, including atresia, chronic ear drainage, extreme threshold asymmetry, unilateral losses, and demonstrated cases of binaural interference. Still, our clinical protocol is to provide binaural amplification on children until it is shown that this is detrimental or of limited benefit.

The binaural advantage in challenging listening conditions has been established (Hawkins and Yacullo 1984). In addition to the reported improvements in signal-to-noise ratios when binaural amplification is used, improved sound localization has been reported (Punch, Jenison, Allan, and Durrant 1991). These studies lend empirical support to the fitting of binaural amplification over monaural amplification.

There have been some reports suggesting that monaural amplification on children may lead to detrimental effects on the word recognition abilities in the unaided ear. These effects have been attributed to auditory deprivation. For example, Hattori (1993) reported findings for a group of children with bilateral, symmetrical moderate-to-profound hearing loss. Those who were fitted monaurally had poorer nonsense syllable test scores in the unaided ear as compared to the aided ear than those who were fitted binaurally or who wore a monaural aid, alternated weekly between ears. In another retrospective study, Gelfand and Silman (1993) noted that children who had been fitted monaurally, with amplification to the better-hearing ear, showed significant differences between the aided and unaided ears using open-set monosyllabic words (unaided ear poorer). This was attributed to auditory deprivation effects in the unaided ear. Recovery from such auditory deprivation has been demonstrated in adults (Burkey and Arkis 1993; Silverman and Emmer 1993) but has not been reported in children.

Binaural interference refers to the phenomenon of the poorer ear interfering with speech recognition when the signal is delivered to both ears. Although it was initially discussed in relation to adults (e.g., Jerger, Silman, Lew, and Chmiel 1993), we have observed the phenomenon in children as well. A case is presented below of a child who demonstrated fluctuating and progressive hearing loss and fluctuating word recognition scores.

Figure 1 displays the initial audiogram (obtained at 3 years, 10 months of age), an audiogram at 9½ years, and the most current audiogram (at 13 years of age) from a boy who has a diagnosis of perilymph fistula and ossicular deformity bilaterally. The hearing loss is mixed below 750 Hz, but primarily sensorineural at higher frequencies. Fistula repairs were done for the right ear at 6 years of age and for the left ear at 7 years of age. The child had used binaural amplification successfully until, at 9 years, 6 months, he reported that one ear sounded "junky." At that visit, speech recognition was tested, and the right ear had significantly poorer (Thornton and Raffin 1978)

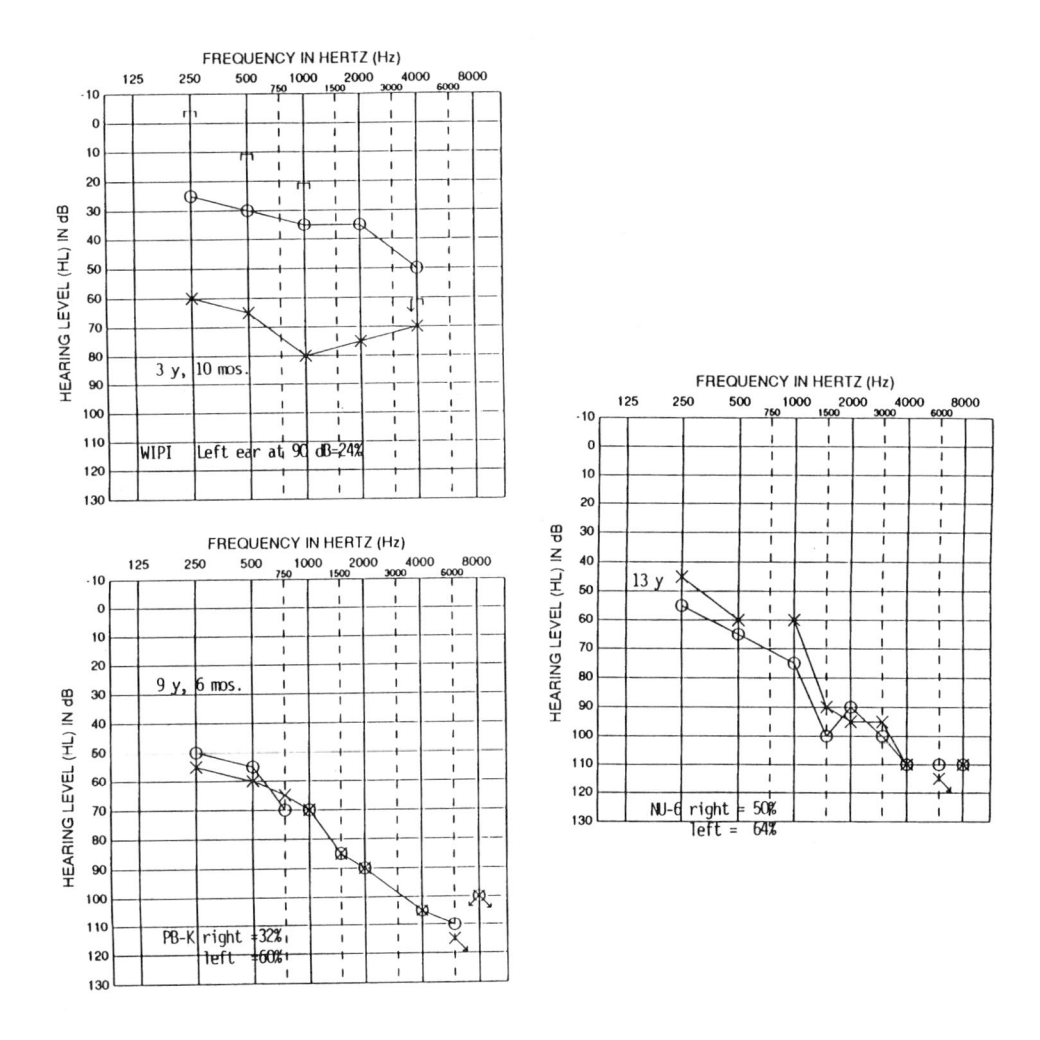

Figure 1. Right ear (o) and left ear (x) air conduction and unmasked bone conduction (⊓) thresholds are noted for three different test dates. Down-pointing arrows attached to these symbols indicate no response at that level, which is at the equipment limits. Word recognition scores are reported within each audiogram for the test given: the Phonetically Balanced-Kindergarten (PB-K), the Word Intelligibility by Picture Identification (WIPI), and the Northwestern University-6 (NU-6).

aided (36% right, 64% left) and unaided (32% right, 60% left) speech recognition scores, using taped presentations of Phonetically Balanced-Kindergarten (PB-K) word lists. His binaural aided speech recognition score was poorer at 48% than his monaural, better-ear aided score of 64%; this difference was not significant. Amplification was, however, discontinued in the ear with the poorer speech recognition score because of the child's complaints. Eventually, the score improved, and the child returned to binaural hearing aid use. Though this case is not typical because of the fluctuating and progressive hearing loss, it does address the issue that two hearing aids are not always better than one, and that what appears to be an unaidable ear at one session may be aidable at a later date. This may occur whether or not hearing thresholds for pure tones are symmetrical.

DIRECTIONAL MICROPHONE VERSUS OMNIDIRECTIONAL MICROPHONE

Hawkins and Yacullo (1984) showed that a 3 to 4 dB S/N (signal-to-noise) advantage is provided by a directional microphone. Certainly, many manufacturers offer the option to include a directional microphone, but it is not a standard feature on the majority of hearing aids. The use of directional microphones may depend on each child's unique listening environment. As a child matures from infancy to toddlerhood to school age, listening needs and typical listening positions change. Communication with an infant is often completed at a close range as food, clothing, and care are provided. An infant is often transported in the arms of a parent/caregiver, held close, and spoken to at close range. In most of these situations communication is face-to-face and at a 0° azimuth, suggesting that directional microphones would be well suited to these situations. As the child starts to crawl, the floor is often close to the baby's face, and a directional microphone may not serve the child's communication needs when primary care adults are offering encouragement or advice from behind. An active toddler moving around a house, playroom, lobby, or mall might be better served with an omnidirectional or even a remote microphone. Preschoolers and school-agers, who assert increasing independence, are often not face-to-face at critical times. A switchable omni-unidirectional microphone might be a good option under these circumstances. This option is available on a few conventional BTEs, and it now is available on at least one programmable hearing aid. Other proximity issues are discussed in the following section.

AGE-RELATED FITTING CONSIDERATIONS

EAR CANAL RESPONSE

Developmental changes in ear canal resonance suggest that the newborn external ear has a high resonant frequency (approximately 6000 Hz) that decreases with age and reaches adult values (approximately 2700 Hz) by the second year of life (Kruger 1987; Kruger and Ruben 1987). Bentler (1989) investigated external ear characteristics in children 3 to 13 years of age and made comparisons with published adult data. She found that the average resonance curve obtained by Shaw (1974) was similar but not identical to that obtained in her group of children; however, peak resonance in the children varied widely. Additionally, Dempster and Mackenzie (1990) investigated ear canal resonance in children who were 3 to 12 years of age. In contrast to Bentler (1989), these authors found further maturation of the ear canal resonance; adult values were reached at 7 years of age. The apparent discrepancy between the two latter studies may be attributable to the small differences shown by Dempster and Mackenzie, with considerable overlap between age groups. Regardless, there are differences in ear canal resonance that change with age, and large variations exist even among subjects of the same age.

The practical application of these ear canal resonance data suggests that the audiologist must take into account the real-ear unaided response (REUR) changes at least during the first two years of life and perhaps for a longer period. As the peak of the REUR moves downward in frequency, the insertion loss will change. In some cases of severe hearing loss, this loss may make the difference in the audibility of some speech components. Consequently, individual real-ear measurements provide the most valid estimates of REUR because of the aforementioned large intersubject differences.

REAL-EAR-TO-COUPLER DIFFERENCE (RECD)

When traditional probe microphone measurements cannot be obtained because of lack of cooperation from a child, real-ear-to-coupler differences (RECD) can be used to obtain accurate predictions of real-ear sound pressure level (SPL). After an RECD is obtained from a child, all further hearing aid manipulations can be completed in a test box without the need for further cooperation from the child. These RECD values can be applied to 2-cm^3 coupler values to assure that targets for gain and output are obtained and to estimate the audibility of the speech spectrum (Moodie, Seewald, and Sinclair 1994).

Clinical use of average RECD values for adults has been found to be inadequate because of large individual differences (Fikret-Pasa and Revit 1992). The same is true for average children's RECD values (Feigin, Kopun, Stelmachowicz, and Gorga 1989). Indeed, larger RECD values are obtained from children as compared to adults (except at 250 Hz). These real-ear-to-coupler differences are not predictable from equivalent ear canal volume (Feigin et al. 1989; Nelson Barlow, Auslander, Rines, and Stelmachowicz 1988). Feigin et al. (1989) found that in early life mean RECD values for children differed from the mean adult RECD values. Children's RECD values, however, approach the adult mean (within 1 standard deviation) by 7.7 years of age.

Given that RECD values show large individual variability and can exceed 20 dB (Feigin et al. 1989), it is critical to consider them when choosing amplification characteristics based on 2-cm^3 coupler measures. The RECD values are reliable in infants and young children with the possible exception of the 13- to 18-month age group (Sinclair, Beauchaine, Moodie, Feigin, Seewald, and Stelmachowicz 1994). For probe-tube microphone measurements, including RECD or other real-ear measures, Stelmachowicz and Seewald (1991) recommend an insertion depth 10 mm past the ear canal entrance for children under 5 years of age and 15 mm past the entrance for those over 5 years of age. These insertion depths should minimize measurement errors at and above 4000 Hz where the risk of errors related to the probe's proximity to the tympanic membrane is greatest.

LEVEL AND PROXIMITY ISSUES

Prescriptive targets for the amplified speech spectrum might differ for infants and young children as compared to adults because of the differing communication experiences and needs of the developing child. The work of Nozza, Rossman, and Bond (1991) suggested that infants 7 to 11 months of age required greater stimulus intensity levels than adult listeners in order to reach criterion performance on a speech discrimination task. Indeed, as much as 25 to 28 dB greater levels were necessary. Nozza et al. (1991) speculated that was evidence that an infant's phonologic development is more susceptible to minimal hearing loss than would be predicted from adult normative performance. Allen and Wightman (1994) investigated detection thresholds for tones in noise in 3- to 5-year-olds and in adults, and they showed that there was greater variability in the performance of children. However, the children showed poorer thresholds in noise compared to adults, some as much as 20 dB. They suggested that there may be several reasons for this difference, such as wider auditory filters or attention factors. Regardless of the reason, the implication is that children require a greater signal level or a more advantageous signal-to-noise ratio for detection compared to adults.

Stelmachowicz, Mace, Kopun, and Carney (1993) investigated the effects of speaker-listener distance on the long-term and short-term characteristics of speech, and they showed that some of the typical close listening positions of infants and young children could result in a 20 dB increase in the input signal compared to adult listening situations. Therefore, the level of speech delivered to a hearing aid microphone at close proximity might place the hearing aid in saturation (assuming a linear circuit) more frequently than expected. This listening condition might have impact on how gain and output are set.

The extent to which the wearer's own voice is amplified by the hearing aid is also of concern. The assumption that the signal of interest (amplified speech) is originating in front of the person wearing the hearing aid is inaccurate when one considers how the hearing aid user receives his or her own voice. The user's own voice contains more low-frequency (below 1 kHz) energy and less high-frequency (above 2.5 kHz) energy than if the source were directly in front of him or her (Cornelisse, Gagné, and Seewald 1991). The implication for children is that high-frequency components of their own voices will be less audible than otherwise might be presumed. The deleterious effect of this circumstance on self-monitor and self-correction will increase with greater hearing loss. The use of a remote microphone held at a 0° azimuth during speech training might enhance the audibility of high-frequency components.

PRACTICAL DETAILS

EARMOLDS

The earmold style that is used will depend on the degree and configuration of hearing loss. Typically, the goal is to provide adequate amplification without acoustic feedback. Size constraints in the pediatric population limit acoustic earmold modifications, such as bore size and venting. Thus, the hearing aid's electroacoustic parameters may play a larger role in frequency shaping than would be true for adults.

Earmold materials have evolved so that there are numerous choices in soft materials and brilliant colors. Still, for the infant ear, venting options and bore size are limited. A diagonal vent, which is often the only venting option when working with infant-sized earmolds, may cause a decrease in the low and high frequencies. See Skinner (1988) for a summary of earmold effects.

Temporary options, such as foam earmolds (e.g., Comply™) and preshaped stock earmolds (e.g., Doc's™ earmolds), should be considered during periods when the child is waiting for new or replacement earmolds. Because the ear canal portion of these earmolds may vary from the child's custom earmold, matching the temporary mold to the child's more typical earmold should be accomplished electroacoustically if possible. RECD measures could be used to identify any needed changes.

Wire retention attachments to earmolds can help maintain the earmold in the ear. This is useful in cases such as a ten-pound girl who was recently seen at our clinic. Her petite concha was misshapen and almost absent. Use of the wire retention attachment and some tape helped to keep an earmold coupled to a BTE hearing aid in her case.

Insertion loss is a consideration when fitting patients who have regions of normal hearing in the high frequencies. Kopun, Stelmachowicz, Carney, and Schulte (1992) obtained estimates of the attenuation characteristics of

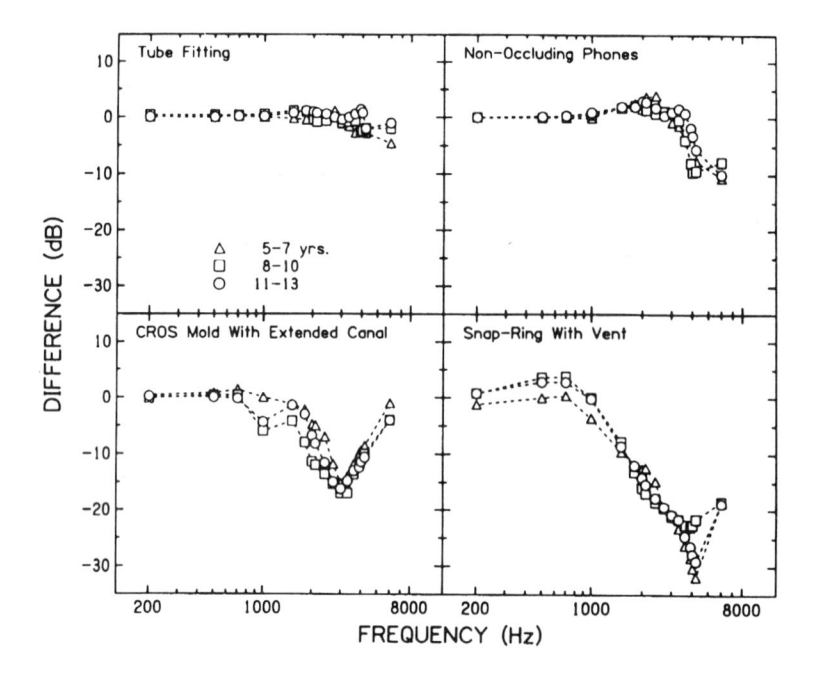

Figure 2. Difference (in dB) between open-ear response and response with four different sound delivery options as a function of frequency for 15 children in three age groups (open triangles represent 5 children 5-7 years, open squares for 5 children 8-10 years, and open circles for 5 children 11-13 years of age). From Kopun et al. (1992). Used with permission of author.

different types of coupling options for a group of children and adults. They found that the least occluding option for children who had regions of normal hearing or minimal hearing loss was a tube fitting, followed by a lightweight headphone (for use with FM systems) (figure 2).

RETENTION OF THE HEARING AID

Babies and young children tend to put things in their mouths: fingers, thumbs, Cheerios, hearing aids, batteries, and so on. Perhaps the biggest practical challenge in fitting amplification on babies and young children is keeping the devices on their ears and out of their mouths and their siblings' mouths. This section will be devoted to such details and cover other considerations that may enhance use, safety, and longevity of hearing aids.

Tamper-resistant battery compartments are available on hearing aids. This feature and information regarding actions to take if there is an accidental ingestion of batteries should be standard offerings to parents during hearing aid orientations.

Retention of hearing aids has been approached from many angles. Even the best-fitting earmolds do not stay in place if tugged by a persistent small hand. Wire retention features, built into the earmold and mentioned above, may help in some cases. A device called a Huggie-Aid™ may help an active toddler keep a hearing aid in place behind the ear. Toupee tape between the mastoid area and hearing aid has been successful for some children. If the hearing aid is removed, however, some fishing line or dental floss tied to the tone hook on one end and to a safety pin on the other (pinned to the back of the child's shirt) can help to prevent loss of the hearing aid.

Adults typically can adjust their volume-control wheels, but for most children, we recommend a specific volume-control setting. Tape, a version of plastic wrap (e.g., Moisture Guard™), or volume-control covers can be used to fix volume controls in place. Any of these are feasible options for children. To offer protection from moisture and to cover all of the controls, there is a hearing aid cover called Super Seals™. These come in a variety of colors and shapes and fit snugly to enclose the hearing aid.

After the hearing aids are in place on the child's ears, they are subject to loss and damage. Manufacturer warranties vary, and some offer extended warranties. After warranties expire, hearing aid insurance is advisable.

SPECIAL CIRCUITS

THE FM OPTION

The young child who is in a day care, preschool, or regular classroom has distinct amplification needs because of time spent in noisy listening conditions, which can interfere with the reception of speech. In classrooms, FM listening devices (auditory trainers) are used to provide a more optimal S/N ratio. An FM system, with use of the remote microphone, can improve the S/N ratio by as much as 10 dB (Fabry 1994). These FM devices also may be considered as an alternative or adjunct to conventional hearing aids outside the classroom (Benoit 1989; Frisbie, Beauchaine, Carney, Lewis, Moeller, and Stelmachowicz 1991).

Audiologists recommending FMs as an option need to provide extensive parent training regarding the complexity of the device, including the modes of operation (FM only, environmental microphone [EM] + FM, or EM only). Several factors need to be considered when selecting the mode of operation. The FM only mode will preserve the optimal S/N ratio; however, this mode will allow the child to hear only the speech of the primary speaker. For a child to monitor his or her own voice or hear the speech of others, the FM + EM mode would need to be selected. This mode, however, may reduce the S/N by 3 to 7 dB. The advent of voice-activated microphones may alleviate this drawback associated with combined FM + EM use (Fabry 1994). The availability of BTE FM systems may make more acceptable the use of FM systems outside academic environments. Minimally, parents should be made aware of the pros and cons of FM use outside the classroom.

PROGRAMMABLE DEVICES

With some constraints, programmable hearing aids currently provide the greatest fitting flexibility. Before deciding on a programmable device for a young child, however, it is important to remember that there are extremely flexible electroacoustic characteristics in many analog BTE devices. A programmable, multiband, multimemory device might be chosen for a young child who has fluctuating hearing loss, a hearing loss with a unique configuration, and/or extreme differences in daily listening environments.

One issue that has not been well addressed when using multimemory devices with children is the issue of accommodation time. Adults may require 8 to 16 weeks to accustom themselves to a new hearing aid response (Gatehouse 1993). The implications of such acclimatization periods when changing hearing aid memories for young children who are just learning to listen and understand are unknown. Moreover, questions such as how parents decide which memory best serves a given situation when the child is unable (because of age or language limitations) to communicate or how many program options should be available remain unanswered.

The cost-benefit issues also must be considered when recommending programmable hearing aids for very young children. The development of a programmable, multimemory, BTE FM unit with a voice-activated microphone and a switchable omni/unidirectional microphone might cover all possible permutations (at least for the moment), but not without significant cost. Finally, affordability of this most ideal solution would be an issue for many families purchasing such a device for their child.

A SERIES OF CHOICES

Parenting a child with a hearing loss increases the number of choices that must be made: choices related to hearing aids, communication mode, and educational programming. The following is a case study of triplets who were born prematurely at a local hospital. They were screened for hearing loss early in life using auditory brainstem response (ABR) techniques and were referred for further testing. A follow-up ABR assessment did not show any recordable response to the limits of the equipment (90 dB nHL). The parents had noted that one of the triplets seemed unresponsive to sound, but they felt that the other infants were responsive. The triplets were referred to our facility at 5 months of age (each weighing 10 to 12 pounds), where our test findings confirmed the suspicion of significant hearing loss in all three infants. There were no observable ABRs at 90 dB nHL and no observable response to stimuli presented in the sound field at the limits of the equipment. All three infants were progressing well, but were still on apnea monitors as a precaution.

The following options for amplification were presented to the parents as possibilities: ear-level hearing aids, body-style hearing aids, or FM units. Body-style hearing aids were not chosen because they had all of the drawbacks (cords, bulk) of the FM unit with none of its advantages. The family initially chose FM systems because of the availability of the remote microphone. The family was loaned three FM receivers with two transmitters/microphones. This afforded the parents the flexibility of using all receivers on the same channel or having two separate channels for more individualized use. Button receivers were used, and each child's earmolds were color coded. The local education agency soon purchased FM units for the children's use. Although the FM system had the most logical appeal, the family did not keep the system for long because all three babies typically were awake at the same time, and they all enjoyed yanking each other's cords. The next option was ear-level hearing aids. Adjustment to ear-level hearing aids has been somewhat poor. Only one of the children wears amplification consistently; the other two children frequently remove theirs. Purchase of any single device has been deferred until more definite behavioral audiologic information can be obtained. Current estimates of hearing loss are in the profound hearing loss range, and these responses may be vibrotactile.

Typically, we pursue purchase of amplification soon after confirmation of hearing loss; however, because any of our decisions will be multiplied by six for this family, we are keeping these children in loaner hearing aids and vibrotactile units until additional aided and unaided information can be obtained. The family is pursuing a total communication program at this time and receives support services from the local educational area.

SUMMARY

There are numerous considerations when fitting amplification on infants and young children. Information gathered from adults with hearing loss is useful but not always applicable with children. Advances in technology and prescriptive fitting procedures in the past five years have provided options and methods that greatly enhance our ability to make amplification decisions for this population. However, many unanswered questions remain.

"It's a very humbling situation to be in . . . because the more you find out, the more complex it gets. But what's that old saying—we're confused on a much higher level" (Zwingle 1993, p. 109). Although this quote is from a geologist as he describes the challenge of managing the High Plains aquifer, it could have easily come from an audiologist who is fitting amplification on children. Indeed, we have come a long way from hardwired FM systems and from peak clipping body-style hearing aids fitted with Y cords as the only option for children with hearing loss. However, we have a long way to go to adequately address all of the issues pertinent to the selection of hearing aids for infants and young children. New options will undoubtedly continue to be introduced into the marketplace. We must continue to examine these advances and their suitability for infants and young children with hearing loss.

ACKNOWLEDGMENTS

The authors gratefully acknowledge the editorial contributions of Michael Gorga and Judy Kopun, and also Skip Kennedy and LaVon Bowman for preparation of the figures. This work was supported in part by NIH.

REFERENCES

Allen, P., and Wightman, F. 1994. Psychometric functions for children's detection of tones in noise. *Journal of Speech and Hearing Research* 37:205-215.

Benoit, R. 1989. Home use of FM amplification systems during the early childhood years. *Hearing Instruments* 40:8-12.

Bentler, R. 1989. External ear resonance characteristics in children. *Journal of Speech and Hearing Disorders* 54:265-268.

Burkey, J.M., and Arkis, P.N. 1993. Word recognition changes after monaural, binaural amplification. *Hearing Instruments* 44:8, 10.

Cornelisse, L.E., Gagné, J.P., and Seewald, R.C. 1991. Ear level recordings of the long-term average spectrum of speech. *Ear and Hearing* 12:47-54.

Dempster, J.H., and Mackenzie, K. 1990. The resonance frequency of the external auditory canal in children. *Ear and Hearing* 11:296-298.

Dyrlund, O., and Lundh, P. 1990. Gain and feedback problems when fitting behind-the-ear hearing aids to profoundly hearing-impaired children. *Scandinavian Audiology* 19:89-95.

Engebretson, A.M., French-St. George, M., and O'Connell, M.P. 1993. Adaptive feedback stabilization of hearing aids. *Scandinavian Audiology* Suppl. 38:56-64.

Fabry, D. 1994. Noise reduction with FM systems in FM/EM mode. *Ear and Hearing* 15:82-86.

Feigin, J.A., Kopun, J.G., Stelmachowicz, P.G., and Gorga, M.P. 1989. Probe-microphone measures of ear-canal sound pressure levels in infants and children. *Ear and Hearing* 10:254-258.

Fikret-Pasa, S., and Revit, L.J. 1992. Individualized correction factors in the preselection of hearing aids. *Journal of Speech and Hearing Research* 35:384-400.

Frisbie, K.A., Beauchaine, K.L., Carney, A.E., Lewis, D., Moeller, M.P., and Stelmachowicz, P.G. 1991. Longitudinal study of FM use in non-academic settings. In J.A. Feigin and P.G. Stelmachowicz (eds.), *Pediatric amplification: Proceedings of the 1991 national conference.* Omaha: Boys Town National Research Hospital.

Gatehouse, S. 1993. Role of perceptual acclimatization in the selection of frequency responses for hearing aids. *Journal of American Academy of Audiology* 4:296-306.

Gelfand, S.A., and Silman, S. 1993. Apparent auditory deprivation in children: Implications of monaural versus binaural amplification. *Journal of American Academy of Audiology* 4:313-318.

Hattori, H. 1993. Ear dominance for nonsense-syllable recognition ability in sensorineural hearing-impaired children: Monaural versus binaural amplification. *Journal of American Academy of Audiology* 4:319-330.

Hawkins, D.B., and Yacullo, W.S. 1984. Signal-to-noise advantage of binaural hearing aids and directional microphones under different levels of reverberation. *Journal of Speech and Hearing Disorders* 49:278-286.

Henningsen, L.B., Dyrlund, O., Bisgaard, N., and Brink, B. 1993. Digital feedback suppression (DFS): Clinical experiences when fitting a DFS hearing instrument on children. *Scandinavian Audiology* 23:118-122.

Jerger, J., Silman, S., Lew, H.L., and Chmiel, R. 1993. Case studies in binaural interference: Converging evidence from behavioral and electrophysiologic measures. *Journal of American Academy of Audiology* 4:122-131.

Kirkwood, D.H. 1993. The economy + FDA + the media add up to an off year for hearing aid sales. *Hearing Journal* 46:7-14.

Kopun, J.G., Stelmachowicz, P.G., Carney, E., and Schulte, L. 1992. Coupling of FM systems to individuals with unilateral hearing loss. *Journal of Speech and Hearing Research* 35:201-207.

Kruger, B. 1987. An update on the external ear resonance in infants and young children. *Ear and Hearing* 8:333-336.

Kruger, B., and Ruben, R.J. 1987. The acoustic properties of the infant ear: A preliminary report. *Acta Otolaryngologica* 103:578-585.

Kuk, F.K. 1994. Maximum usable real-ear insertion gain with ten earmold designs. *Journal of American Academy of Audiology* 5:44-51.

Moodie, K.S., Seewald, R.C., and Sinclair, S.T. 1994. Procedure for predicting real-ear hearing aid performance in young children. *American Journal of Audiology* 3:23-31.

Nelson Barlow, N.L., Auslander, M.C., Rines, D., and Stelmachowicz, P.G. 1988. Probe tube microphone measures in hearing-impaired children and adults. *Ear and Hearing* 9:243-247.

Nozza, R.J., Rossman, R.N., and Bond, L.C. 1991. Infant-adult differences in unmasked thresholds for the discrimination of consonant-vowel syllable pairs. *Audiology* 30:102-112.

Punch, J.L., Jension, R.L., Allan, J., and Durrant, J.D. 1991. Evaluation of three strategies for fitting hearing aids binaurally. *Ear and Hearing* 12:205-215.

Ross, M., and Madell, J.R. 1988. Premature demise of body worn hearing aids. *Asha* 30:29-30.

Shaw, E.A.G. 1974. Transformation of sound pressure level from the free field to the eardrum in the horizontal plane. *Journal of Acoustical Society of America* 56:1848-1861.

Silverman, C.A., and Emmer, M.B. 1993. Auditory deprivation and recovery in adults with asymmetric sensorineural hearing impairment. *Journal of American Academy of Audiology* 4:338-346.

Sinclair, S.T., Beauchaine, K.L., Moodie, J.A., Feigin, J.A., Seewald, R.C., and Stelmachowicz, P.G. 1994. Repeatability of a real-ear to coupler difference measurement as a function of age. Poster presented at American Academy Audiology Sixth Annual Convention, April, Richmond.

Skinner, M.W. 1988. *Hearing aid evaluation.* New Jersey: Prentice-Hall.

Stelmachowicz, P.G., Mace, A.L., Kopun, J.G., and Carney, E. 1993. Long-term and short-term characteristics of speech: Implications for hearing aid selection for young children. *Journal of Speech and Hearing Research* 36:609-620.

Stelmachowicz, P.G., and Seewald, R.C. 1991. Probe-tube microphone measurements in children. *Seminars in Hearing* 12:62-72.

Thornton, A.R., and Raffin, M.J.M. 1978. Speech-discrimination scores modeled as a binomial variable. *Journal of Speech and Hearing Research* 21:507-518.

Zwingle, E. 1993. Ogallala aquifer: Wellspring of the high plains. *National Geographic* 183:80-109.

8

Traditional and Theoretical Approaches to Selecting Amplification for Infants and Young Children

Richard C. Seewald, K. Shane Moodie, Sheila T. Sinclair, and Leonard E. Cornelisse

INTRODUCTION

Regardless of the specific approach taken in selecting amplification for infants and young children, pediatric audiologists would likely agree that there should be some relationship between a child's unique auditory characteristics and the amplification characteristics that are subsequently recommended. Beyond this, however, there is presently no consensus among professionals regarding most aspects of this clinical process. For example, pediatric audiologists have yet to agree on (1) which type of audiometric data are considered to be both valid and sufficient for the purposes of electroacoustic selection and fitting with this population; (2) what constitute appropriate amplification characteristics for a given audiometric profile; (3) which of the available electroacoustic and audiometric measurement options are best suited to verifying and evaluating hearing aid performance; and (4) how the hearing aid selection process for infants and young children is both conceptualized and implemented within the general context of the habilitative program.

Support for these observations can be derived from survey data on current clinical practices in the United States (e.g., Martin and Gravel 1989; Martin and Morris 1989; see chapter 5). For example, Martin and Morris (1989) reported that of 417 pediatric audiologists surveyed, only one-third rated auditory brainstem response (ABR) testing as highly reliable for threshold estimation in infants and young children. Furthermore, the majority

Table 1

Saturation sound pressure level (SSPL90) recommended by responding audiologists (n=172) for children with profound hearing impairment, with whom complete audiometric results are unobtainable. From Martin and Gravel (1989).

SSPL90 Setting	Audiologists Responding	%
115 dB SPL	22	12.8
120 dB SPL	63	36.6
125 dB SPL	51	29.7
130 dB SPL	35	20.3
135 dB SPL	6	3.5
Other	13	7.6

(68.5%) of these clinicians reported that they would not fit hearing aids to infants and young children on the basis of ABR test results. Clinician attitudes such as these are noteworthy in light of recent statements concerning infant hearing screening such as the Joint Committee on Infant Hearing 1994 Position Statement in which it is recommended that "all infants with hearing loss should be identified before three months of age, and receive intervention by six months of age" (p. 6). Either clinician attitudes changed dramatically between 1989 and 1994 or, from our perspective, something is both confusing and troubling about this situation.

In a survey conducted by Martin and Gravel (1989), a sample of pediatric audiologists were asked to state the maximum hearing aid output they would recommend for a young child with profound hearing impairment with whom complete unaided results could not be obtained. The findings obtained from 172 clinicians are presented in table 1. From these results it can be seen that, depending on which of the 172 pediatric audiologists had been consulted, the maximum hearing aid output that would be recommended for the same child could range from anywhere between 115 and 135 dB sound pressure level (SPL). Because this theoretical fitting was for a young child or infant, it is of particular importance to note that the maximum hearing aid output levels that the clinicians were asked to consider were measured/defined in a conventional 2cc coupler. It is known that the SPLs delivered by a hearing aid into the ear canal of an infant or young child can be 15 to 20 dB higher at some frequencies relative to the SPLs measured in a 2cc coupler (Feigin, Kopun, Stelmachowicz, and Gorga 1989).

Consequently, in terms of *real-ear hearing aid performance*, the maximum hearing aid output levels recommended by this sample of clinicians potentially range between 130 and 155 dB SPL!

Practice variations such as those illustrated in table 1 are relatively unimportant unless they are known to lead to true differences in treatment effectiveness or outcome. To our knowledge, no data unequivocally prove that a 20 dB range in the recommended output limiting levels will subsequently lead to a difference in outcome. However, based on available knowledge concerning this electroacoustic variable and its relationship to audibility, comfort, and safety, it is likely that a 20 dB range in output limiting exceeds the limits for what could be considered an appropriate and/or scientifically defensible fitting for the same child (Seewald 1991). If data such as those shown in table 1 provide a true reflection of current fitting practices with infants and young children, there is a clear need to develop and agree upon more informed and uniform approaches to this clinical problem.

A substantial body of knowledge related to hearing aid selection for infants and young children has accumulated over the past 25 years that can be (but is not) uniformly applied in routine clinical practice. Therefore, the purpose of this chapter is to provide a review of approaches to hearing aid electroacoustic selection that have been applied to and/or proposed for application with infants and young children and where possible to discuss the relative strengths and limitations that are known to be associated with each.

Historically, two approaches to selecting amplification characteristics for young children emerge from the literature, each with its own theme and numerous variations. Throughout this chapter, these two approaches will be referred to as (1) the traditional approach and (2) the theoretical approach. These differ in several ways. First, the selection process itself is conceptualized differently depending on which approach is taken. Second, the audiometric and electroacoustic measurement options that are presently available to clinicians are applied and interpreted differently. Finally, the two approaches differ with respect to how willing one is to explicitly state the desired relationship between the auditory characteristics of children and the amplification characteristics of hearing aids.

THE TRADITIONAL APPROACH

Our conceptualization of the traditional hearing aid selection process for infants and young children is illustrated in figure 1. The selection process is initiated with an assessment stage. This is the one aspect of the selection process that is common to both traditional and theoretical approaches. At this initial stage the clinician collects as much information as possible about the child and the family constellation before attempting to construct and

```
    ASSESSMENT
         ↓      ←——  CLINICAL EXPERIENCE
    PRESELECTION
         ↓
    EVALUATION
         ↓
    SELECTION
```

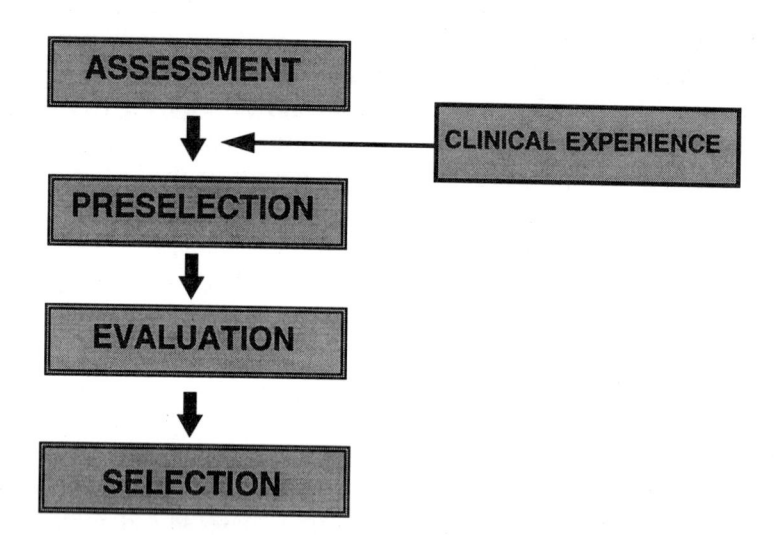

Figure 1. Conceptualization of the traditional approach to hearing aid selection.

implement a relevant habilitation program. For most children with sensorineural hearing impairment, the habilitation program will include a recommendation for use of a conventional hearing aid or FM system.

When a clinician is working with infants in particular, it is unlikely that a complete audiometric profile will be available at the conclusion of a single assessment session. Nonetheless, once sufficient information has been collected to confirm the presence of a hearing impairment and to provide some estimate of the degree of hearing loss, the process continues into the next stage.

With the assessment data in hand, the clinician applies her or his clinical experience to preselect several instruments and earmold couplings that are judged to be appropriate for the child under consideration. In most situations time is provided for fabrication of custom earmolds, and the child subsequently returns to the hearing clinic for what can be considered the centerpiece of the traditional approach—the comparative hearing aid evaluation.

At the evaluation stage, audiometric measurements are performed with the hearing aids that have been preselected for the child. For infants and young children, this most likely includes the measurement of sound field aided thresholds with each preselected option. For older children, repeated measures of speech reception with the preselected instruments are also commonly applied. In view of the relative importance of the evaluation component in the traditional approach, an in-depth discussion of the procedures that are applied at this stage will be provided within the following section of this chapter.

As illustrated in figure 1, the traditional approach concludes with the selection stage at which point a hearing aid is selected from among the preselected instruments on the basis of the hearing aid evaluation test findings. In other words, the option that results in the "best" performance (either in terms of the sound field aided thresholds or word recognition performance scores) is the one selected for use.

Any reader who is knowledgeable about the historical evolution of hearing aid selection methods should see the relationship between this conceptualization of the traditional approach to selection for infants and young children and the comparative hearing aid evaluation process that was applied for so many years with adults (Carhart 1946). In fact, the only major difference between the two relates to the measurement procedures that are performed within the evaluation stage. For adults, the comparison between preselected hearing aids was performed on the basis of repeated measures of word recognition primarily, whereas for infants and young children, sound field aided thresholds provide the basis upon which the selection-related decisions are made. In view of the key role the evaluation component plays in the traditional approach to hearing aid selection, we will now consider the specific procedures applied at this stage. This includes a description of how they have been used and interpreted for the purposes of clinical decision making and, where possible, a discussion related to what is known about these procedures in terms of their relative strengths and limitations.

TRADITIONAL HEARING AID EVALUATION PROCEDURES FOR INFANTS AND YOUNG CHILDREN

Historically, two types of hearing aid evaluation procedures have been applied with infants and young children: (1) the measurement of sound field aided thresholds and (2) either formal or informal measures of speech reception. As we consider each, we need to keep in mind the purpose for which these measurements are performed. Specifically, the results obtained from these audiometric test procedures are used subsequently to decide which of several alternative amplification options will be selected for the child under consideration. The present discussion has been developed with this specific purpose in mind.

Sound Field Aided Threshold Measures

For many years, sound field aided threshold measures have been the primary means for evaluating hearing aid performance with infants and young children. Over time, clinicians have used the results of sound field aided threshold testing in a variety of ways. For example, sound field aided thresholds have been used to (1) directly measure some quantity of interest (e.g., detection level by frequency); (2) compare aided performance under different amplification conditions (e.g., hearing aid A versus hearing aid B); and (3) predict the levels at which amplified speech will be received within the aided condition. In reality, the evaluation of aided performance with infants and young children is often approached with some unique combination of all of the above purposes simultaneously.

Assuming that a valid measurement of aided thresholds can be obtained, the results of these measurements provide clinicians with an estimate of the level of sound that can be detected within the audiometric test environment and offer at least two advantages relative to alternative measurement options (e.g., probe microphone measures). First, the results of this testing provide information about the child's auditory performance in terms of the ability to detect the presence of sound within the aided condition. Second, the findings of sound field aided threshold testing are presented on a conventional audiogram, a context that is familiar to relevant professionals and parents.

Direct Measures of Aided Performance

As we consider using sound field aided threshold measures for the purpose of selecting an amplification device for an infant or young child, we need to acknowledge several limitations that are known to be associated with these measures as well as any potential threats to the validity of the test results we obtain. The first and perhaps most obvious limitation of these measures for the purposes of selection-related decision making is that a reliable behavioral response is required. As pediatric audiologists know, this is not a trivial requirement. Second, even when reliable aided thresholds can be measured, we need to acknowledge that the real-ear frequency response of the hearing aid under evaluation is being sampled at a very limited number of test frequencies. Third, when sound field aided thresholds are used exclusively in choosing among the preselected instruments, several important electroacoustic characteristics of the options under consideration are virtually ignored, including, for example, the input/output (i/o) characteristics and the output limiting characteristics of the hearing aid across frequencies. This is rapidly becoming a more serious limitation of sound field aided threshold testing as we begin to work with a new generation of hearing instruments that embody more sophisticated automatic signal processing capabilities (e.g., Killion 1988).

Macrae (1982) and Haskell (1987) have described a potential threat to the validity of sound field aided threshold measures that is particularly relevant in the testing of young children who have mild hearing loss.

Specifically, on the basis of his study, Macrae (1982) concluded that one potential cause of invalid aided thresholds is the masking produced either by the internal noise output of the hearing aid or by ambient noise that is present within the test environment and subsequently amplified by the hearing aid or by some combination of both factors. The potential for this "noise floor" problem to influence the validity of sound field aided test findings is greatest for children with mild hearing loss and particularly for those who have regions of normal or near-normal hearing sensitivity at some frequencies.

We have attempted to illustrate this problem in figures 2A and 2B. In figure 2A we have plotted both the unaided and the sound field aided test results for the right ear of this theoretical child. On the basis of the sound field aided test results shown, it might be concluded that the hearing aid under evaluation provides essentially no gain at 250 to 1000 Hz and approximately 25 dB of real-ear gain at 2000 and 4000 Hz. However, by examining figure 2B, in which the noise floor for this hearing aid/test environment combination is shown, it can be seen that it is not possible to know if the aided thresholds at 250 to 2000 Hz provide valid estimates of the real-ear gain provided by this hearing aid. That is because test signals presented at lower HLs would be masked by the noise that is present under these specific measurement conditions. To avoid this potential problem, Macrae (1982) has recommended that clinicians not attempt aided threshold testing at frequencies where the *unaided threshold is better than 30 dB HL*.

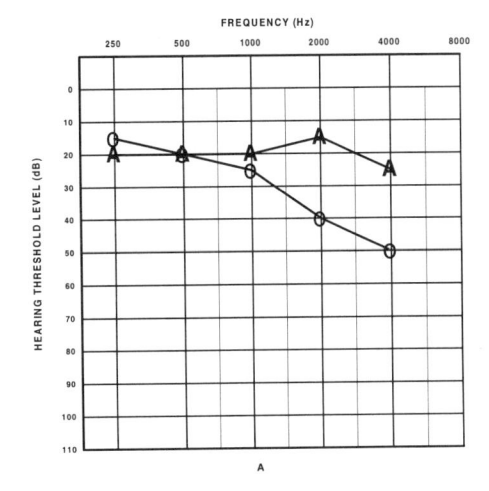

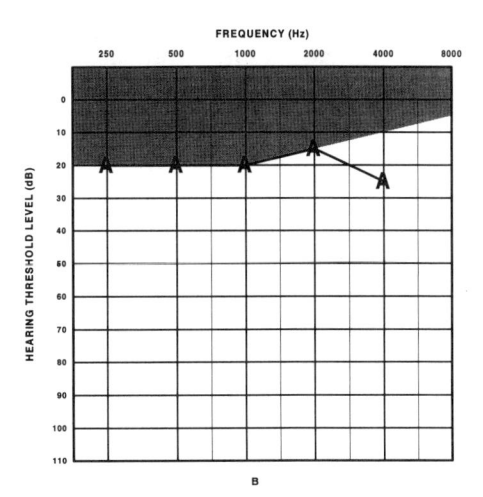

Figure 2. Illustration of the noise floor problem, which can influence the validity of sound field aided thresholds. A child's unaided (O) and sound field aided (A) thresholds are shown in **2A**. In figure **2B** the same aided thresholds are shown in relation to the noise floor that was present for these measures.

Comparing Amplification Conditions

As noted previously, one common use of sound field aided threshold measures in a traditional approach to hearing aid selection is to compare the test results obtained under two or more different amplification conditions. For example, a clinician might preselect two different instruments and obtain sound field aided thresholds with each. The instrument that yields the "best" aided thresholds consequently would be selected as the instrument of choice. Similarly, comparisons between different earmold coupling systems, different tone control settings, or different types of amplification devices (e.g., hearing aid versus FM system) are sometimes performed with children using the results of sound field aided threshold testing.

Whenever such comparisons are made, it is necessary to know something about the variability associated with the measurement procedure used. We want to know that a difference observed in the test findings is a true reflection of the variable under consideration (e.g., earmold type) and not simply a result of the test-retest variability associated with the measurement procedure itself. Studies have been performed with both adults and school-age children to derive estimates of the test-retest variability associated with sound field aided threshold testing (Hawkins, Montgomery, Prosek, and Walden 1987; Humes and Kirn 1990; Stuart, Durieux-Smith, and Stenstrom 1990). Despite some procedural differences among these studies, the findings support the following conclusions. First, test-retest variability is somewhat greater for aided than for unaided sound field threshold measures. For example, Humes and Kirn (1990) found that the simple removal and reinsertion of a hearing aid introduced variability into the sound field aided threshold measurement process. Second, the test-retest variability associated with sound field threshold-based estimates of real-ear gain (i.e., functional gain) is greater than it is for the alternative real-ear gain measurement procedure (i.e., insertion gain), which is performed with a computerized probe-tube microphone system. Specifically, Humes and Kirn (1990) estimated that the test-retest variability associated with functional gain measures is roughly 150% of the test-retest variability that has been reported for insertion gain measures. Finally, at present, we do not have solid estimates of the test-retest variability associated with aided sound field measures with preschool children. It is reasonable to assume, however, that the variability will not be less than and will, in all likelihood, be greater than the values reported for adults and school-age children. This will most certainly be the case in situations where the step size applied in sound field aided threshold testing with infants and young children is increased beyond the conventional 5 dB.

On the basis of their findings, Hawkins and colleagues (Hawkins et al. 1987) calculated critical difference values, in dB, for repeated sound field

Table 2
Critical differences in dB for sound field aided thresholds at a probability level of .05.
From Hawkins et al. (1987).

	Frequency (kHz)					
p	.25	.5	1	2	3	4
.05	12	16	15	15	16	17

threshold measures. The critical difference values shown in table 2 were calculated for a probability level of .05 and can be used to determine when the dB difference between two aided thresholds, obtained at the same frequency, can be interpreted as significantly different from each other. For the purposes of routine clinical decision making, it can be generally concluded from the findings reported by Hawkins et al. (1987) that *two sound field aided thresholds obtained at the same frequency must differ by more than 15 dB to be considered significantly different from each other.* Again, in repeated measures testing with infants and young children, the critical difference values shown in table 2 may, at least in some cases, underestimate the test-retest variability associated with sound field aided threshold measures (Hawkins 1991).

Predicting Amplified Speech Reception

One additional way in which sound field aided threshold measures have been used to evaluate the relative performance among hearing aids in infants and young children is illustrated in figure 3. Note that a graphic representation of the levels associated with average conversational speech is shown on this audiogram along with a set of aided thresholds. Typically, on the basis of this type of visual comparison, a prediction is made regarding how much of the speech spectrum will be audible to the child or at what levels above threshold speech will be received by the child within the aided condition. For example, on the basis of the aided threshold values plotted in figure 3, it would be concluded that most of the speech spectrum will be audible to this child within the aided condition. The sound field aided test results obtained with alternative amplification options would be subsequently evaluated in the same manner, and the option that provides the child with the greatest proportion of the amplified speech spectrum would be selected for use.

It has been known for many years that this approach to evaluating aided performance in children will be invalid in some cases (Schwartz and

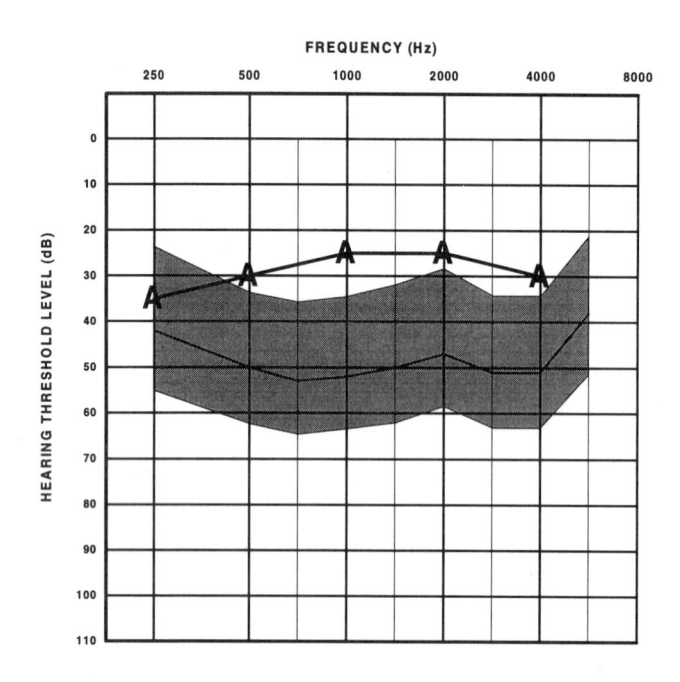

Figure 3. Sound field aided thresholds (A), in dB HL, shown in relation to an idealized graphic representation of the acoustic characteristics associated with conversational speech.

Larson 1977). The primary problem relates to the fact that aided thresholds are measured in response to audiometric test signals that are low in level relative to the SPLs associated with average conversational speech. Consequently, the sound field aided thresholds do not provide a valid indication of how a given hearing aid will operate in response to speech under everyday listening conditions. Thus, in many cases, the sound field aided thresholds will tend to overestimate the available gain and, consequently, the levels at which amplified speech will be received by the child within the aided condition (Hawkins 1991; Schwartz and Larson 1977; Seewald, Hudson, Gagné, and Zelisko 1992; Seewald, Ross, and Stelmachowicz 1987; Stelmachowicz and Lewis 1988).

Two studies have been reported in which the sound field aided threshold-based approach to predicting amplified speech sensation levels (SLs) has been compared with alternative electroacoustically based procedures (Schwartz and Larson 1977; Seewald et al. 1992). The results of both studies confirm that under certain electroacoustic conditions, sound field aided thresholds provide unrealistically high estimates of the SLs at which amplified speech will be received. On the basis of their findings, Schwartz and Larson concluded (nearly 20 years ago!) that "the traditional sound-field audiogram is inappropriate for determining usable amplification for severe and profoundly hearing impaired children" (p. 406). Furthermore, Schwartz and Larson strongly advised pediatric audiologists to consider alternative electroacoustic-based procedures (e.g., Erber 1973) to the traditional sound field audiogram when evaluating the performance of hearing aids in children.

Measures of Speech Reception

Repeated speech reception measures have been and continue to be applied in some clinical settings to evaluate the relative performance of hearing aids with older children. With this comparative approach to hearing aid evaluation, word recognition scores are obtained with each of the preselected options, and the hearing aid that results in the highest performance score is selected for the child. To use conventional monosyllabic word recognition measures in this way, it is again necessary to account for the variability associated with these measures so that a valid interpretation of the findings can be made.

We have known for more than ten years that conventional monosyllabic word recognition measures are not sufficiently reliable to detect true differences among electroacoustically similar hearing aids (Walden, Schwartz, Williams, Holum-Hardegen, and Crowley 1983). Nonetheless, evidence suggests that this approach to hearing aid evaluation is still applied in some settings with children. For example, in a clinical report we received recently it was stated that "the child's speech discrimination score improved from 60% correct with her own hearing aid to 72% correct with a new (brand X) instrument." Unfortunately, this is not a valid interpretation of these findings. In this particular case, 25-item word lists were applied in the testing. With a score of 60% correct for the child's current hearing aid, the performance score obtained with the new instrument would have to be less than 36% correct or greater than 84% correct to be interpreted as a significant difference (Thornton and Raffin 1978). Thus, the score of 72% correct obtained with the new hearing aid cannot be considered to be significantly different from the score this child obtained with her own hearing aid. Skinner (1988) has provided a "user friendly" table in which the lower and upper limits of the 95% critical differences for percentage scores are shown. Those who wish to continue to take this comparative approach to hearing aid evaluation are strongly encouraged to consult this table before drawing conclusions about the relative performance of hearing aids on the basis of repeated measures word recognition testing.

Some recent findings reported by Gatehouse (1992, 1993) raise additional questions regarding the routine clinical application of repeated speech perception measures in evaluating a child's relative performance with different hearing aids or different amplification strategies. In one experiment,

Gatehouse (1992) studied both the time course and the magnitude of improvements in aided speech perception that followed the fitting of amplification in four adult listeners. He found that a period of "perceptual acclimatization" was required before the benefits of amplification for speech perception were fully realized.

In a second study, Gatehouse (1993) measured the speech perception performance of 36 full-time hearing aid users on three occasions after refitting them with instruments that provided more high-frequency gain. Specifically, speech perception measures were performed at the time of the refitting (week 0) and at 8 and 16 weeks following the introduction of more high-frequency gain. No significant difference was observed in performance on the Four Alternative Auditory Feature (FAAF) Test between the old and the new fitting at the time of the refit. However, significant improvements in speech perception were evident at postfitting weeks 8 and 16 for the instruments that provided greater high-frequency gain. On the basis of his findings, Gatehouse (1992) has concluded that "any evaluation concerning the overall effectiveness of a hearing aid prescription should only be made after the process of acclimatization is substantially complete" (p. 1267).

In light of the findings reported by Gatehouse (1992, 1993), we may need to question the validity of some of our conventional applications of speech perception testing with children. How reasonable is it to assume that the potential benefits of a particular electroacoustic manipulation will be revealed instantaneously through conventional measures of speech perception? Furthermore, what period of time is required before we can expect to measure the true benefits of one signal processing strategy (e.g., wide dynamic range compression amplification) in comparison to some alternative (e.g., linear gain)? Unfortunately, these questions can be answered only through future systematic investigation. In the meantime, it would be advisable for clinicians who use speech perception measures for the purpose of comparing one amplification condition to another without providing for some learning or "perceptual acclimatization" to occur to interpret their findings with caution.

SUMMARY OF THE TRADITIONAL APPROACH TO SELECTION

For many years the traditional approach has been the most popular method for hearing aid selection in children. When this approach is taken, it is assumed that the test findings obtained during the evaluation stage are both valid and sufficient for the purposes of informed clinical decision making. However, issues presented within this section suggest that this assumption can be questioned for several reasons. First, it is known that repeated sound field aided threshold and conventional word recognition measures are too variable to allow clinicians to detect meaningful differences among amplification options that would be reasonable for the same child.

Second, aided sound field thresholds provide a simplistic, limited and, under some electroacoustic conditions, invalid characterization of how a hearing aid or FM system will perform within everyday listening conditions. This is not to suggest that the measurement of sound field aided thresholds with children should be discontinued completely. The measurement made with a child should be determined by the specific clinical question that is being asked. Thus, if the purpose in performing the measurement is to quantify the lowest level of sound a child can detect within the aided condition, the measurement of sound field aided thresholds would be the procedure of choice. However, for most of the other clinical applications for which aided sound field threshold measurements have been used in the past, there are now more reliable and valid options available to the pediatric audiologist.

Finally, as we have noted earlier, with this general approach to hearing aid selection, the assumption is that it will always be possible to obtain valid behavioral test results with the target population. Unfortunately, when this requirement cannot be met, the usefulness of this general approach to hearing aid selection is severely compromised.

THEORETICAL APPROACH

As noted earlier, one of the major differences between traditional and theoretical approaches to this clinical problem relates to how the selection process itself is conceptualized. Our present conceptualization of the theoretical approach is presented in figure 4 and is modified only slightly from one proposed by Denis Byrne at the 1979 Vanderbilt Conference on Amplification in Education (Byrne 1981). As illustrated in this figure, the selection process is initiated with the audiologic assessment. This is the one characteristic shared by both traditional and theoretical approaches (figure 1). It can be seen in figure 4, however, that once the relevant assessment data have been collected, a theoretical rationale or prescriptive strategy is applied to the data to select appropriate amplification characteristics. In other words, on the basis of the theoretical rationale applied at this stage, a "best fit" prescription is derived for the relationship between the known auditory characteristics of a given child and the electroacoustic characteristics of a theoretically appropriate hearing aid (Byrne 1981, 1982). As Byrne (1982) has observed, a major advantage of theoretical selection procedures, relative to the more traditional (empirically based) approach, is that the theoretical basis on which the selection is made has been explicitly stated and is therefore accessible to critical examination.

ASSESSMENT → SELECTION → VERIFICATION → EVALUATION
(with THEORETICAL RATIONALE feeding into SELECTION)

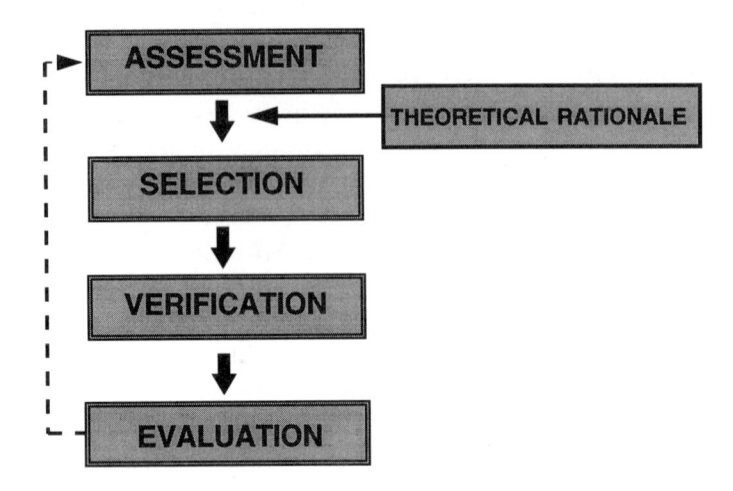

Figure 4. Conceptualization of the theoretical approach to hearing aid selection. Adapted from Byrne (1981).

The end result of the selection stage of the process is a set of electroacoustic performance criteria that are, at least in theory, considered to be appropriate for the child under consideration. The manner in which these criteria are stated will depend on the specific theoretical approach that is applied. For example, the desired hearing aid performance may be expressed in terms of target sound field aided thresholds (e.g., Matkin 1987), target insertion gain values (e.g., Byrne and Dillon 1986), or target real-ear aided response and real-ear saturation response values (e.g., Seewald, Ramji, Sinclair, Moodie, and Jamieson 1993). However, regardless of the manner in which the electroacoustic performance criteria are stated, the fact that a set of explicitly stated criteria are developed for the individual child is one of the major factors differentiating the theoretical from the more traditional approach to this clinical process.

Skinner (1988) has commented on this key difference between the two alternative approaches to hearing aid selection. Specifically, she has observed that with a traditional approach

> the criteria for preselecting and adjusting the aids are not specified but are rather based on the experience and judgement of the clinician. When criteria are not specified, it is difficult to develop the needed experience and impossible to verify whether a hearing aid has met criteria. With prescriptive approaches,

there are specified criteria for preselecting and adjusting aids that can be followed by any clinician. For these reasons, a prescriptive approach is recommended. (p. 150)

As shown in figure 4, once a hearing aid with appropriate earmold coupling has been identified for the child, which should provide a reasonable approximation to the performance criteria, the process continues to the verification stage. The fundamental question to be addressed at the verification stage of the process is: To what extent does the measured performance of a specific instrument meet the theoretical set of criteria that were developed for a given child? To answer this question, two requirements must be met. First, a set of electroacoustic performance criteria must exist for the child under consideration. Otherwise, there is no basis upon which to assess the adequacy of the fitting. Second, the type of measurement employed within the verification stage must provide the clinician with a valid answer to the question being asked. Naturally, the type of measurement procedure that is applied at this stage will depend on the manner in which the selection criteria have been stated (e.g., target sound field aided thresholds, target insertion gain values). Thus, a clear and logical relationship exists between the selection and verification stages of the process (Seewald 1994).

Regardless of the specific approach to verification, once the clinician has determined that the hearing aid fitting provides the child with both physical comfort and appropriate amplification characteristics, the final stage of the process is initiated wherein the child's auditory performance with amplification is evaluated. Relative to the other stages of the hearing aid selection process, the evaluation of aided auditory performance is viewed as long term in nature rather than a single event in time and should include both clinic-based and reality-based indexes of the child's performance with amplification.

Finally, we have attempted to illustrate the recursive nature of the theoretical selection process in figure 4. Specifically, if the child's auditory performance with amplification is unimpressive relative to the expected performance, there is then a need to recycle through all stages of the process to identify any sources of error that could potentially affect the all-important outcome with amplification.

During the 15-year period from approximately 1970 to 1985, a number of theoretical selection procedures were developed specifically for application with infants and young children (Byrne 1978; Erber 1973; Gengel, Pascoe, and Shore 1971; Ross 1975; Schwartz and Larson 1977; Seewald, Ross, and Spiro 1985). For the most part, these procedures were greeted by the audiologic community with what might be described as something less than wild enthusiasm and, to our knowledge, are not currently applied with any measurable frequency in routine clinical practice. There are several possible reasons for this.

First, for each of the theoretical methods identified above, it was recommended that the conventional audiogram be replaced with a dB SPL graphic presentation of results. For both conceptual and practical reasons, this recommendation has been generally unpopular. Second, clinical implementation of these methods requires that some modification be made to conventional audiometric and/or electroacoustic instrumentation systems. Finally, it our hypothesis that developments related to hearing aid selection and fitting with adults, which took place during the late 1970s, have had a significant impact on the natural evolution of selection methods for young children. Specifically, around this time customized in-the-ear (ITE) instruments became generally available. With these instruments, manufacturers began to accept the predominant role in selecting amplification characteristics on the basis of the submitted audiometric data. Consequently, clinicians had to think less about how they wanted hearing instruments to perform for their clients electroacoustically. In many hearing centers children comprise a relatively small proportion of hearing aid candidates. Perhaps it has been easier to continue to apply the more traditional approaches to hearing aid selection with this population than to consider a substantial conceptual and procedural overhaul for this relatively small segment of the routine audiologic caseload.

It was noted earlier that one difference among theoretical selection procedures relates to the form in which the electroacoustic performance criteria are specified. Theoretical selection procedures developed for application with children can be classified either as *audiometric-based*, where the performance criteria are specified in terms of an audiometric variable (i.e., target sound field aided thresholds), or as *electroacoustic-based*, where the performance criteria are specified in terms of how a hearing aid should perform in a child's ear or a 2cc coupler.

AUDIOMETRIC-BASED METHODS

The specification of desired hearing aid performance characteristics in terms of target sound field aided thresholds is not unique to procedures developed specifically for young children with hearing impairment. In fact, many of the theoretical procedures developed in the 1970s (e.g., Byrne and Tonisson 1976) recommended the use of sound field aided threshold testing as the primary means for verifying the adequacy of real-ear hearing aid performance. For the most part, this approach to verification has been subsequently replaced by real-ear insertion response measures using computerized probe microphone systems.

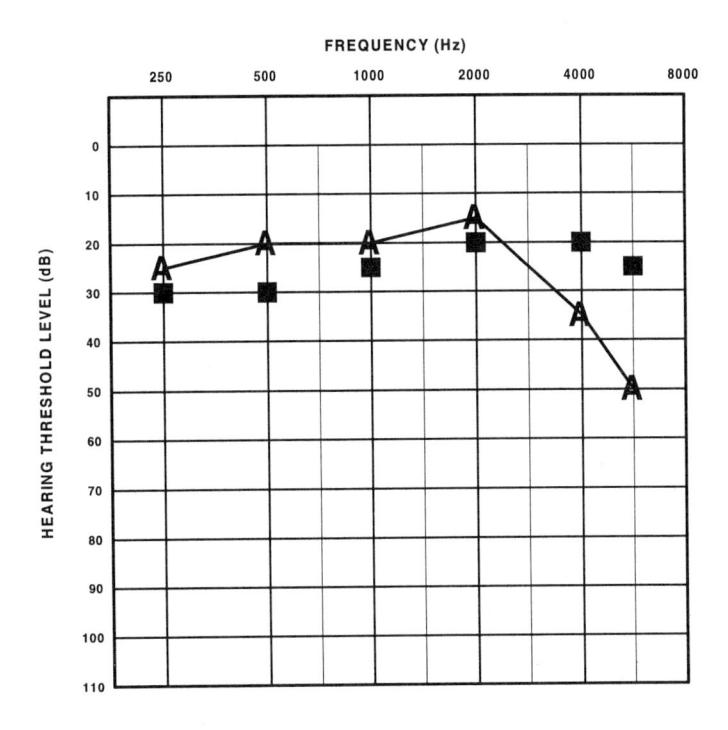

Figure 5. Sound field aided thresholds (A), in dB HL, plotted relative to the "optimal aided thresholds" (■) for children with sensorineural hearing loss proposed by Matkin (1987).

An audiometric-based theoretical procedure developed specifically for application with young children was described by Matkin in 1987. This approach to hearing aid selection is graphically illustrated in figure 5. Specifically, Matkin developed a set of real-ear hearing aid performance criteria for young children that were expressed in terms of target sound field aided thresholds. These "optimal aided thresholds," for children with sensorineural hearing loss, are shown in figure 5 along with a set of measured sound field aided thresholds. Note that because hearing aid performance criteria have been stated, it is possible to objectively assess the adequacy of a given electroacoustic fitting. Thus, in a relatively simple form and familiar audiometric context, the information presented in figure 5 illustrates the essence of the theoretical approach to selecting amplification characteristics for children. The previous observations concerning the interpretation of statistically significant differences between sound field aided thresholds obtained with different devices are equally applicable in this context.

ELECTROACOUSTIC-BASED METHODS

Over the years, it has been acknowledged that several limitations are associated with theoretical audiometric-based approaches to selecting amplification characteristics for infants and young children. One potentially serious limitation with this type of approach that can be particularly troublesome with the pediatric population is related to the form in which the performance criteria are specified (i.e., target aided thresholds). Unfortunately, when a purely audiometric-based approach is taken to the selection problem, it is not possible to verify that the desired electroacoustic characteristics have been provided to the child without valid/reliable behavioral test results. Consequently, for many infants and for some young children, this approach will be of limited use when important selection-related decisions need to be made.

Second, a review of the information presented in figure 5 indicates that the frequency/gain characteristic is the only amplification-related variable for which performance criteria are stated. There are, of course, additional electroacoustic characteristics of hearing aids that should be considered within the selection process. At an absolute minimum, consideration should be given also to output limiting in any selection approach developed for this particular population. In addition, the new generation of hearing instruments requires that we consider a host of additional variables such as compression thresholds, compression ratios, crossover frequencies between multiple bands, and so forth. When electroacoustic performance criteria have been specified in terms of sound field aided thresholds only, it is as if these additional electroacoustic variables are nonexistent.

Finally, a problem that we confront routinely in clinical hearing aid selection is related to how the variables we are working with are measured and defined. Unfortunately, the manner in which audiometric and electroacoustic variables are defined has often led to confusion, misinterpretations and, perhaps in some cases, inappropriate fittings.

In amplification-related work with infants and young children, we are often dealing with what can be described as a quintessential "apples and oranges" problem. In fact, in some situations we find ourselves working with several varieties of apples (i.e., HLs) and several varieties of oranges (i.e., SPLs) simultaneously. For example, audiometric data may be collected in dB HL using a conventional audiometric earphone, insert earphone, or sound field loudspeaker. Each of these transducers is calibrated using different instrumentation and a different set of sound pressure level reference values. By some means, the audiometric findings collected in dB HL need to be interfaced with the electroacoustic variables associated with hearing aids that are quantified in dB SPL in a 2cc coupler (of which there are several varieties) or as measured in the real ear. The simultaneous manipulation of these variables is not trivial and, unfortunately, can all too easily result in fitting error. In response to the limitations and/or problems associated with conventional audiometric-based approaches to hearing aid selection, several alternative electroacoustic-based methods have been developed over the years for application with children (Byrne 1978; Erber 1973; Gengel et al. 1971; Ross 1975; Schwartz and Larson 1977; Seewald 1992; Seewald et al. 1985).

In an attempt to circumvent the variable definition/measurement problem described above, Erber (1973) developed a hearing aid selection procedure for school-age children in which all variables were measured/defined using a common reference (i.e., the SPL developed in a 2cc coupler). Specifically, Erber measured the child's thresholds with narrow bands of noise transduced by a button-type hearing aid receiver attached to the child's custom earmold. The receiver was calibrated such that the threshold levels could be expressed in terms of the equivalent SPL in a 2cc coupler. Subsequently, narrow bands of noise were presented in the sound field at one-third octave band levels corresponding to the long-term average spectrum of speech. The hearing aid output was measured by connecting the hearing aid button receiver to the 2cc coupler. The level of the resulting hearing aid output was then compared with the 2cc coupler-defined threshold levels to develop frequency-specific estimates of the sensation levels at which average conversational speech would be received by the child.

Erber (1973) also advocated that the maximum linear output of each child's hearing aid be measured, as a function of frequency, by using the same procedures employed to define thresholds and the aided speech levels. Therefore, the procedure described by Erber provided the means to make direct comparisons among the frequency specific levels associated with thresholds, amplified speech, and the output limiting characteristics of the hearing aid using a common (i.e., 2cc coupler) reference. The stated goal of Erber's hearing aid selection procedure was to deliver amplified speech to levels between approximately 10 and 25 dB SL (depending on the degree of hearing loss) and yet maintain the amplified speech output to levels that were at least 5 dB below the maximum linear output of the hearing aid.

The results Erber (1973) obtained with one child using this electroacoustic-based approach to hearing aid selection are shown in figure 6. With the exception of the average speech levels that were measured/defined in the undisturbed field, all other relevant variables are defined in dB SPL as measured in a 2cc coupler including (1) the child's detection thresholds, (2) the aided speech levels, (3) the maximum hearing aid output, and (4) the child's discomfort thresholds.

There appear to be at least two advantages to the hearing aid selection procedure described by Erber (1973) relative to a more conventional audiometric-based approach. First, by virtue of the fact that the output limiting characteristic is measured and plotted (figure 6), this variable is

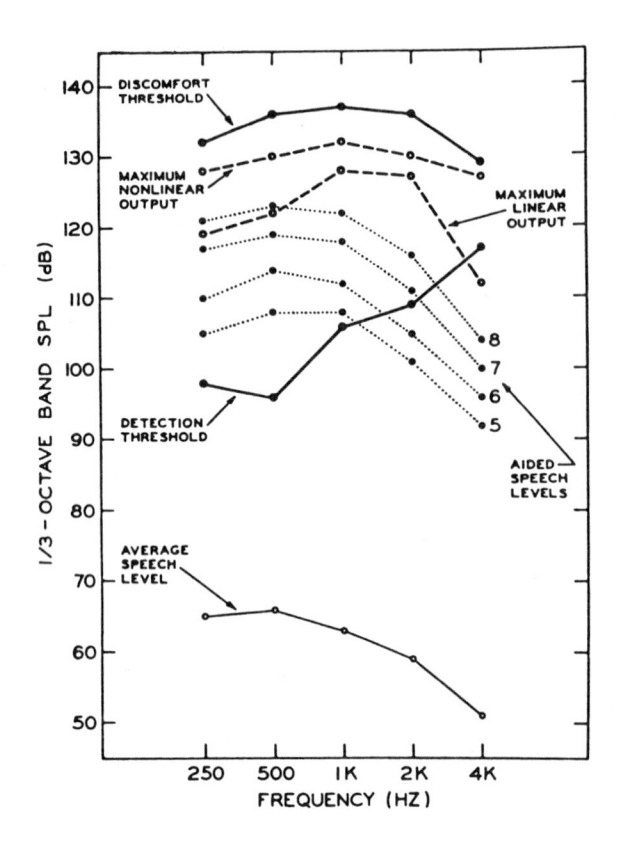

Figure 6. Results of a hearing aid evaluation plotted in dB SPL. The average speech levels were measured in the undisturbed field. The one-third octave band levels of all audiometric and electroacoustic variables were measured using a common point of reference (i.e., 2cc coupler). The aided speech levels were obtained at four different volume control wheel settings (#5-8) with the tone control position held constant. Reproduced from Erber 1973, with permission.

considered to be important in the selection and fitting process. This is in marked contrast to the more conventional sound field aided audiogram approach used with infants and young children in which the upper end of the selection/fitting problem (i.e., loudness discomfort and output limiting) is notably absent. Second, Erber's method allows for a direct comparison among all auditory and electroacoustic variables of interest and thereby eliminates several potential sources of error that are commonly associated with more conventional clinical procedures. Finally, as early as 1973, Erber proposed that "a more meaningful clinical procedure would be to define both thresholds and hearing aid output in terms of sound pressures generated in each patient's own ear canal" (p. 229). With the general availability of computerized probe microphone systems, it is now possible to implement a real-ear version of Erber's electroacoustic-based approach to hearing aid selection with infants and young children. Several such procedures have been described in the literature for application with children (Hawkins, Morrison, Halligan, and Cooper 1989; Seewald et al. 1987; Seewald et al. 1993; Stelmachowicz and Seewald 1991).

Two theoretical selection procedures that are currently applied with children (see chapter 5) include the National Acoustic Laboratories' (NAL) revised procedure (Byrne and Dillon 1986) and the Prescription of Gain and Output (POGO) procedure (McCandless and Lyregaard 1983). It is important for those who currently use these procedures with children, and particularly important for clinicians who apply these procedures with children with severe and profound hearing impairment, to know that both procedures have been modified for individuals with severe and profound hearing impairment (Byrne, Parkinson, and Newall 1991; Schwartz, Lyregaard, and Lundh 1988). Unfortunately, these modifications are not yet incorporated into software implementations of these procedures on some clinical real-ear measurement systems. We hope this situation will be remedied within the near future. In the meantime, clinicians who wish to apply either the NAL or the POGO procedure with children with severe and profound hearing impairment should determine in advance that the appropriate real-ear gain equations will be applied in the electroacoustic selection process. The interested reader may find it helpful to know that the appropriate modifications in the NAL procedure for severe and profound hearing loss are fully implemented in an excellent electroacoustic selection software system that is available through the National Acoustic Laboratories in Chatswood, Australia (Battaglia, Dillon, and Byrne 1991).

The most recent of these electroacoustic-based selection procedures for children is version 3.1 of the desired sensation level (DSL) method (Seewald 1992; Seewald et al. 1993). The general goal of this method is to provide children with amplified speech that is audible, comfortable, and undistorted across the broadest relevant frequency range possible (Seewald et al. 1987). Version 3.1 of this method is fully implemented in a PC-based software system and uses the following sequential steps in electroacoustic selection with children:

1. Both audiometric and relevant acoustic data are collected for the individual child. The assessment measures applied in the DSL method include detection thresholds; loudness discomfort levels (when possible); and real-ear-to-coupler difference (RECD) values across frequencies (see Moodie, Seewald, and Sinclair [1994] concerning the measurement of the RECD with infants and young children).
2. All audiometric variables are transformed from dB HL to dB SPL (ear canal level) regardless of which signal transducer was

used in the audiometric testing (e.g., sound field loudspeaker, Telephonics TDH series earphones). The preferred procedure for audiometric assessment in the DSL method is to attach the child's custom earmold to an insert earphone. With this approach, the measured coupler to real-ear transfer function can be used to derive an accurate prediction of the ear canal SPLs associated with audiometric variables (Zelisko, Seewald, and Whiteside 1992). Alternatively, the ear canal levels at threshold can be measured directly using a probe microphone (Gagné, Seewald, Zelisko, and Hudson 1991; Zelisko, Seewald, and Gagné 1992).

3. On the basis of the measured/predicted ear canal levels at threshold, real-ear electroacoustic performance criteria are derived for the individual child including target real-ear aided response (REAR) and real-ear saturation response (RESR) values across frequencies.

4. The RECD values measured for the individual child are applied to the target REAR and RESR values to derive a set of target 2cc coupler-based values for both gain and output limiting across frequencies. When RECD values have not been measured, age-appropriate default values are automatically applied by the software system in deriving the 2cc coupler target values.

5. The hearing aid response characteristics are shaped in a 2cc coupler until a best fit to the coupler-based performance criteria has been achieved.

6. Electroacoustic performance of the hearing aid is verified in the 2cc coupler and subsequently in the real ear using a probe microphone (when possible).

The following case example is presented to illustrate how in general the DSL strategy for selection and fitting is applied with an individual child. The air conduction thresholds for the right ear of this 26-month-old child with a bilateral sensorineural hearing impairment are plotted on a conventional audiogram in figure 7. In addition, the RECD values that were measured for this child are shown in figure 8. All positive values shown in figure 8 indicate the amount by which the SPL measured within the child's ear canal exceeded the SPL measured in an HA-2 coupler. These RECD values were measured using the child's own custom earmold in accordance with the RECD measurement procedure described recently by Moodie et al. (1994).

The next step in the process is to transform all audiometric variables to dB SPL (ear canal level) and to derive a set of real-ear electroacoustic performance criteria on the basis of the predicted ear canal level at threshold

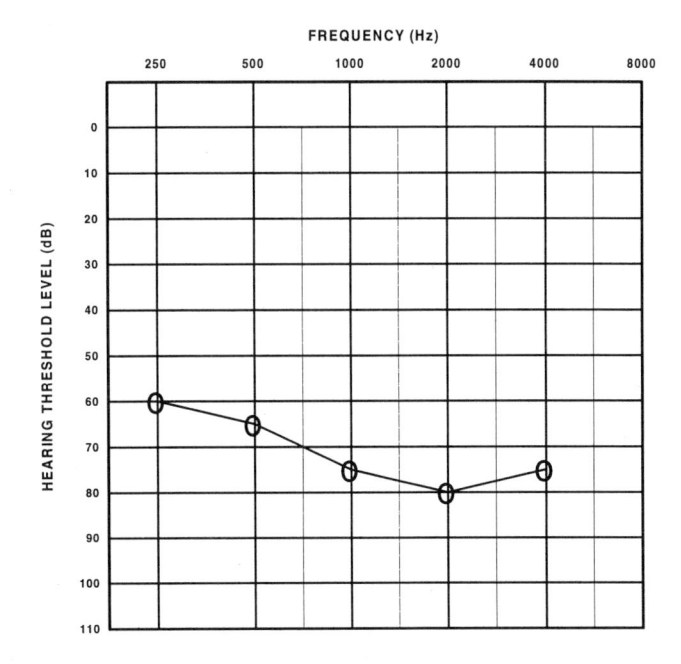

Figure 7. Air conduction thresholds plotted in dB HL for the right ear of a 26-month-old child with bilateral sensorineural hearing impairment.

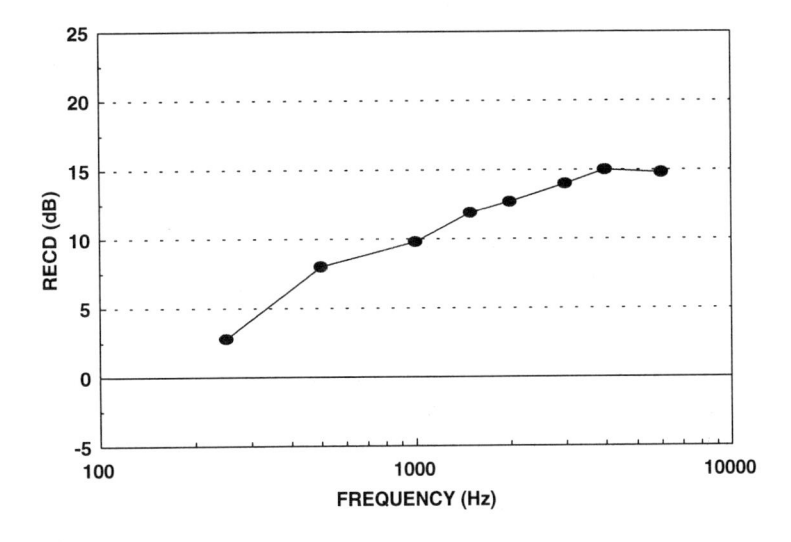

Figure 8. The real-ear-to-coupler difference (RECD) values measured for a 26-month-old child using the procedure described by Moodie et al. (1994). All positive values indicate the extent to which the SPLs measured in the child's ear canal exceeded those that were measured in an HA-2 coupler.

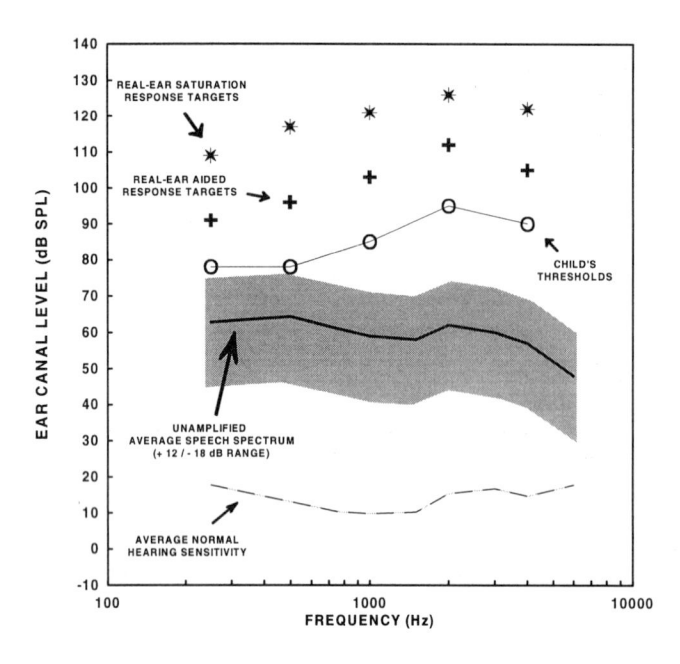

Figure 9. The unaided SPL-O-GRAM for the case example. All variables including average normal hearing sensitivity, the long-term average speech spectrum, the child's air conduction thresholds, the real-ear aided response, and the real-ear saturation response target values are plotted in dB SPL (ear canal level).

across frequencies. The transformed threshold values in dB SPL (ear canal level) for this child are shown in figure 9 along with several other relevant variables. All of the variables shown in figure 9 are plotted in an SPL-O-GRAM format (i.e., dB SPL in the ear canal as a function of frequency). These variables include (1) average normal hearing sensitivity; (2) the unamplified long-term average spectrum of speech (including the 30 dB intensity range associated with conversational speech) that is applied in the current version of DSL method; (3) the child's air conduction thresholds; (4) the target REAR values; and (5) the target RESR values for this child across frequencies.

Once real-ear hearing aid performance criteria have been developed, the appropriate transfer functions and correction factors are applied to these values to derive a corresponding set of performance criteria for 2cc coupler-based measures. The target 2cc coupler gain and SSPL values developed for a behind-the-ear (BTE) hearing aid fitting are shown in figures 10A and 10B, respectively. These figures also illustrate the match that was achieved between the set of desired amplification characteristics and the measured performance of the instrument that was subsequently fitted.

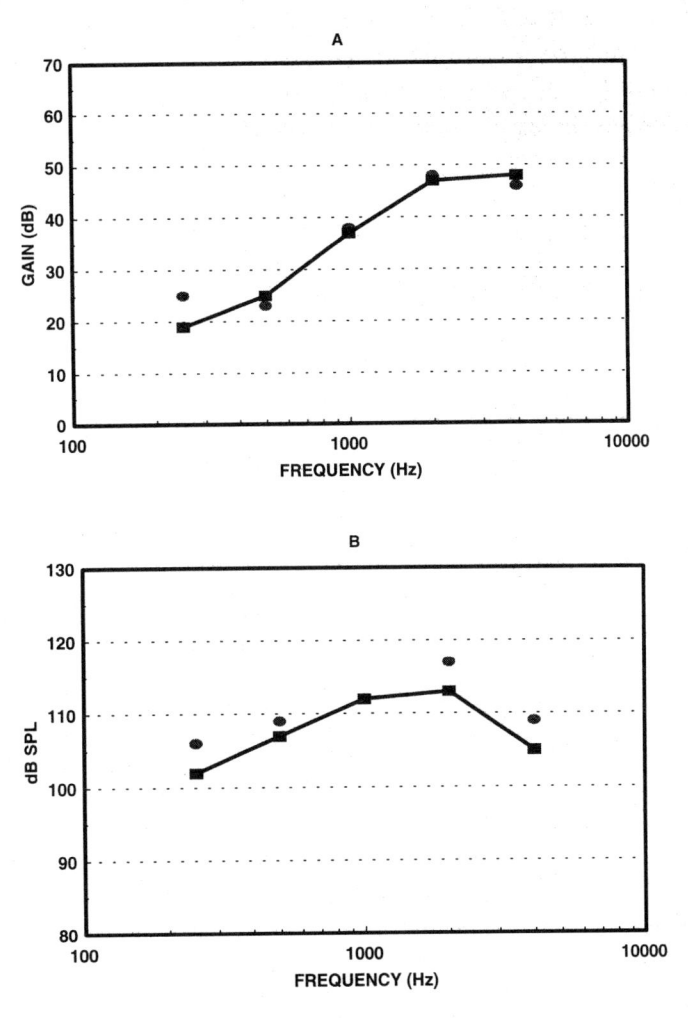

Figure 10. Target (●) and measured (■) 2cc coupler gain (**10A**) and saturation response (**10B**) values for the case example.

In this particular case, probe microphone measurements of real-ear hearing aid performance were not obtained. However, because the RECD values had been measured, it was possible to accurately predict real-ear performance on the basis of the 2cc coupler-based measures shown in figure 10 (Seewald, Sinclair, and Moodie 1994). The results of this prediction, performed by the current version of the DSL software system, are presented in figure 11. Specifically, this figure shows the predicted amplified speech spectrum and the predicted real-ear saturation response of this hearing aid based on the results of the 2cc coupler verification measures plus the coupler to real-ear transfer function measured for this child. A reasonable

186 • ISSUES IN PEDIATRIC AMPLIFICATION

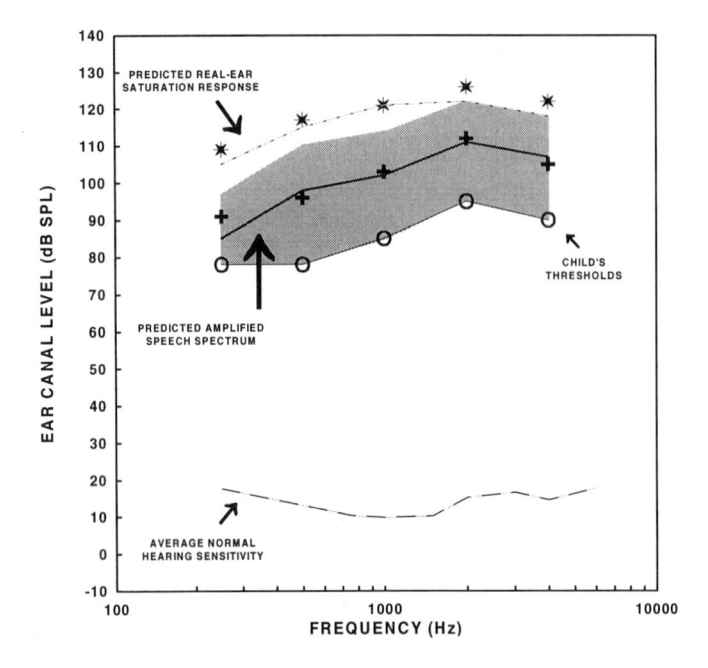

Figure 11. The aided SPL-O-GRAM for the case example. All variables including average normal hearing sensitivity, the child's air conduction thresholds, the predicted amplified spectrum of speech, and the predicted real-ear saturation response are plotted in dB SPL (ear canal level).

approximation to the theoretical performance criteria has been accomplished with this instrument. In line with the conceptualization of the theoretical approach to selection shown in figure 4, it is at this point that evaluation of the child's performance with amplification is initiated.

SUMMARY OF THE THEORETICAL APPROACH TO SELECTION

From our perspective, the theoretical electroacoustic-based selection procedures described in this section offer the following advantages relative to the traditional audiometric-based approach:

1. Electroacoustic performance criteria are formally stated for both gain and output limiting across frequencies.
2. A common reference is used that facilitates direct comparison among audiometric and electroacoustic variables that are relevant in the hearing aid selection process.
3. Electroacoustic performance of hearing aids is characterized under the highly controlled conditions of the hearing aid test

chamber at levels that are more representative of everyday speech across the entire frequency spectrum.
4. Active cooperation, in terms of a behavioral response, is not required from the child to proceed through electroacoustic selection and verification stages of the process. For practical reasons, this may be the most important advantage of theoretical electroacoustic-based procedures, particularly in selecting hearing aids for infants.

In their current form, theoretical selection approaches are not without limitations. First, to implement the electroacoustic-based procedures in routine clinical practice, some procedural modifications are required. Second, the current versions of theoretical approaches that have been developed for application with children (e.g., DSL version 3.1) are of only limited assistance in the fitting of the new generation of automatic signal processing hearing aids. For this reason, the development of a device-independent enhancement of the DSL method for fitting wide dynamic range compression instruments is in process (Cornelisse, Seewald, and Jamieson 1994, 1995).

Finally, we are unaware of any theoretical hearing aid selection method for which validation evidence has been collected on all aspects with infants and young children. Consequently, it is not yet possible to state unequivocally that one procedure (e.g., POGO) is better than another (e.g., NAL-R) for application with this population. With regard to the issue of validating hearing aid selection methods in general, Denis Byrne (with tongue in cheek) observed in 1984, "One reason for the comparative dearth of validation studies may be that it is more fun to dream up a plausible procedure than it is to find out that it doesn't work! However, another reason is that it is very difficult to obtain useful validation evidence."

Byrne's acknowledgment of the difficulties associated with obtaining validation evidence is particularly relevant for methods specifically developed for application with infants and young children. At the present time our own approach to this problem has been to work systematically and sequentially through the procedures applied at each stage of the selection and fitting process (figure 4). Our working assumption in taking this approach to validation has been this: If you don't get it right from the beginning, the error will haunt you through the rest of the process. Our first series of studies have focused on collecting validation data for procedures we have developed for the assessment stage of the process (Moodie et al. 1994; Seewald et al. 1994; Sinclair, Beauchaine, Moodie, Feigin, Seewald, and Stelmachowicz 1994; Zelisko, Seewald, and Gagné 1992; Zelisko, Seewald, and Whiteside 1992). With this work on assessment procedures now largely completed, we have begun to shift the focus of our studies to the second (i.e., electroacoustic selection) stage of the process. Unfortunately, validation work of this nature is both slow and resource intensive. Nonetheless, whatever can be done in this regard should be given high priority in the future.

CONCLUSIONS

In this chapter, we have focused attention on alternative processes and procedures that can be applied in selecting hearing aids for infants and young children. Recent evidence suggests that, despite the availability of new and potentially useful technologies as well as some alternative electroacoustic selection strategies, the majority of pediatric audiologists in the United States take essentially the same approach to hearing aid selection as they did more than 25 years ago (see chapter 5). For several reasons, it is both important and timely to reevaluate how we have been approaching this clinical problem.

First, we now have a new generation of hearing aids that, at least in theory, bring with them performance capabilities particularly attractive for application with infants and young children. If we are to ensure that these instruments are applied in valid ways, we will need to employ electroacoustic selection strategies that account for the relative complexity these new technologies incorporate.

Second, the conventional hearing aid is no longer the only amplification option available to young children. To a certain extent, candidacy for alternative devices (e.g., cochlear implants) is determined by the degree of success a child demonstrates with a conventional hearing aid. Unfortunately, a hearing aid is not a hearing aid is not a hearing aid . . . That is, the degree of success a child achieves with a hearing aid will result from several interacting factors that include, for example, (1) the child's residual auditory capacity; (2) the quality and quantity of therapy the child receives; (3) the level of support from the parents and other managing adults for the habilitation program; and (4) the quality of the hearing aid fitting. Before serious consideration is given to more elaborate alternatives for any child, we need to ensure that the child's experiences with a conventional hearing aid have been of the highest quality possible.

Finally, a renewed interest in the early identification of hearing impairment has particular relevance to the topic of this chapter. We began the chapter by observing that we have yet to reach consensus regarding most aspects of the hearing aid selection process for infants and young children. Simultaneously, our profession is recommending that universal hearing screening be implemented so that appropriate and comprehensive habilitation programming can be initiated by 6 months of age. It is, of course, one thing to identify a problem and yet another to know what to do about it in an informed and scientifically defensible way. Clearly, as we work collectively toward implementing universal hearing screening programs, there is an equally pressing need to devote attention toward ensuring access to effective habilitation that naturally includes the selection of appropriate amplification for these children.

REFERENCES

Battaglia, D., Dillon, H., and Byrne, D. 1991. *HASP: Version 2 user's manual*. Chatswood, Australia: National Acoustic Laboratories.

Byrne, D. 1978. Selection of hearing aids for children with severe deafness. *British Journal of Audiology* 12:9-22.

Byrne, D. 1981. Selective amplification: Some psychoacoustic considerations. In F.H. Bess, B.A. Freeman, and J.S. Sinclair (eds.), *Amplification in education*. Washington, D.C.: Alexander Graham Bell Association for the Deaf.

Byrne, D. 1982. Theoretical approaches for hearing aid selection. In G.A. Studebaker and F.H. Bess (eds.), *The Vanderbilt hearing-aid report*. Upper Darby, Penn.: Monographs in Contemporary Audiology.

Byrne, D. 1984. Validation of the National Acoustic Laboratories' hearing aid selection procedure. Paper read at the Sixth National Conference of the Audiological Society of Australia, May, Coolangatta.

Byrne, D., and Dillon, H. 1986. The National Acoustic Laboratories' (NAL) research for hearing aid gain and frequency response selection strategies. In G.A. Studebaker and I. Hochberg (eds.), *Acoustical factors affecting hearing aid performance*. 2d ed. Boston: Allyn and Bacon.

Byrne, D., Parkinson, A., and Newall, P. 1991. Modified hearing aid selection procedure for severe-profound hearing losses. In G.A. Studebaker, F.H. Bess, and L.B. Beck (eds.), *The Vanderbilt hearing-aid report II*. Parkton, Md.: York Press.

Byrne, D., and Tonisson, W. 1976. Selecting the gain of hearing aid for persons with sensorineural hearing impairments. *Scandinavian Audiology* 5:51-59.

Carhart, R. 1946. A practical approach to the selection of hearing aids. *Transactions of the American Academy of Ophthalmology and Otolaryngology* Jan.-Feb.:123-131.

Cornelisse, L.E., Seewald, R.C., and Jamieson, D.G. 1994. Wide-dynamic-range compression hearing aids: The DSL[i/o] approach. *Hearing Journal* 47(10):23-29.

Cornelisse, L.E., Seewald, R.C., and Jamieson, D.G. 1995. The input/output formula: A theoretical approach to the fitting of personal amplification devices. *Journal of the Acoustical Society of America* 97(3):1854-1864.

Erber, N.P. 1973. Body-baffle and real-ear effects in the selection of hearing aids for children with deafness. *Journal of Speech and Hearing Disorders* 38:224-231.

Feigin, J.A., Kopun, J.G., Stelmachowicz, P.G., and Gorga, M.P. 1989. Probe-tube microphone measures of ear-canal sound pressure levels in infants and children. *Ear and Hearing* 10:254-258.

Gagné, J.P., Seewald, R.C., Zelisko, D.L., and Hudson, S.P. 1991. Procedure for defining the auditory area of adolescents with hearing impairment with a severe/profound hearing loss: I — Detection thresholds. *Journal of Speech-Language Pathology and Audiology* 12(3):13-20.

Gatehouse, S. 1992. The time course and magnitude of perceptual acclimatization to frequency responses: Evidence from monaural fitting of hearing aids. *Journal of the Acoustical Society of America* 92:1258-1268.

Gatehouse, S. 1993. Role of perceptual acclimatization in the selection of frequency responses for hearing aids. *Journal of the American Academy of Audiology* 4:296-306.

Gengel, R., Pascoe, D.P., and Shore, I. 1971. A frequency-response procedure for evaluating and selecting hearing aids for children with severe hearing impairment. *Journal of Speech and Hearing Disorders* 36:341-353.

Haskell, G.B. 1987. Functional gain. *Ear and Hearing* 8(Suppl. 5):95S-99S.

Hawkins, D.B. 1991. Acoustic measures of hearing aid performance. In G.A. Studebaker, F.H. Bess, and L.B. Beck (eds.), *The Vanderbilt hearing-aid report II*. Parkton, Md.: York Press.

Hawkins, D.B., Montgomery, A.A., Prosek, R.A., and Walden, B.E. 1987. Examination of two issues concerning functional gain measurements. *Journal of Speech and Hearing Disorders* 52:56-63.

Hawkins, D.B., Morrison, T.M., Halligan, P., and Cooper, W.A. 1989. Use of probe tube measurements in hearing aid selection for children: Some initial clinical experiences. *Ear and Hearing* 10:281-287.

Humes, L.E., and Kirn, E.U. 1990. The reliability of functional gain. *Journal of Speech and Hearing Disorders* 55:193-197.

Joint Committee on Infant Hearing. 1994. Position statement. *Audiology Today* 6(6):6-9.

Killion, M.C. 1988. An "acoustically invisible" hearing aid. *Hearing Instruments* 39(10):40-44.

Macrae, J. 1982. Invalid aided thresholds. *Hearing Instruments* 33(9):20, 22.

Martin, F.N., and Gravel, K.L. 1989. Pediatric audiology practices in the United States. *Hearing Journal* 42(8):33-48.

Martin, F.N., and Morris, L.J. 1989. Current audiologic practices in the United States. *Hearing Journal* 42(4):25-44.

Matkin, N.D. 1987. Hearing instruments for children: Premises for selecting and fitting. *Hearing Instruments* 38(9):14-16.

McCandless, G.A., and Lyregaard, P.E. 1983. Prescription of gain and output (POGO) for hearing aids. *Hearing Instruments* 34:16-17, 19-21.

Moodie, K.S., Seewald, R.C., and Sinclair, S.T. 1994. Procedure for predicting real-ear hearing aid performance in young children. *American Journal of Audiology* 3(1):23-31.

Ross, M. 1975. Hearing aid selection for preverbal hearing-impaired children. In M.C. Pollack (ed.), *Amplification for the hearing-impaired*. Orlando, Fla.: Grune and Stratton.

Schwartz, D.M., and Larson, V.D. 1977. A comparison of three hearing aid evaluation procedures for young children. *Archives of Otolaryngology* 103:401-406.

Schwartz, D.M., Lyregaard, P.E., and Lundh, P. 1988. Hearing aid selection for severe-to-profound hearing loss. *Hearing Journal* 41(2):13-17.

Seewald, R.C. 1991. Hearing aid output limiting considerations for children. In J.A. Feigin and P.G. Stelmachowicz (eds.), *Pediatric amplification: Proceedings of the 1991 national conference*. Omaha: Boys Town National Research Hospital.

Seewald, R.C. 1992. The desired sensation level method for fitting children: Version 3.0. *Hearing Journal* 45(4):36-41.

Seewald, R.C. 1994. Current issues in hearing aid fitting. In J.P. Gagné and N. Tye-Murray (eds.), Research in audiological rehabilitation: Current trends and future directions. *Journal of the Academy of Rehabilitative Audiology Monograph* 27 (suppl.):93-112.

Seewald, R.C., Hudson, S.P., Gagné, J.P., and Zelisko, D.L. 1992. Comparison of two procedures for estimating the sensation level of amplified speech. *Ear and Hearing* 13(3):142-149.

Seewald, R.C., Ramji, K.V., Sinclair, S.T., Moodie, K.S., and Jamieson, D.G. 1993. *Computer-assisted implementation of the desired sensation level method for electroacoustic selection and fitting in children: User's manual.* London, Ontario: University of Western Ontario.

Seewald, R.C., Ross, M., and Spiro, M.K. 1985. Selecting amplification characteristics for young children with hearing impairment. *Ear and Hearing* 6(1):48-53.

Seewald, R.C., Ross, M., and Stelmachowicz, P.G. 1987. Selecting and verifying hearing aid performance characteristics for young children. *Journal of the Academy of Rehabilitative Audiology* 20:25-38.

Seewald, R.C., Sinclair, S.T., and Moodie, K.S. 1994. Predictive accuracy of a procedure for electroacoustic fitting in young children. Presented at the Twenty-second International Congress of Audiology, July, Halifax.

Sinclair, S.T., Beauchaine, K.L., Moodie, K.S., Feigin, J.A., Seewald, R.C. and Stelmachowicz, P.G. 1994. Repeatability of a real-ear to coupler difference measurement as a function of age. Presented at the American Academy of Audiology sixth annual convention, April, Richmond.

Skinner, M.W. 1988. *Hearing aid evaluation.* Englewood Cliffs, N.J.: Prentice Hall.

Stelmachowicz, P.G., and Lewis, D. 1988. Some theoretical considerations concerning the relation between functional gain and insertion gain. *Journal of Speech and Hearing Research* 31:491-496.

Stelmachowicz, P.G., and Seewald, R.C. 1991. Probe-tube microphone measures in children. *Seminars in Hearing* 12(1):62-72.

Stuart, A., Durieux-Smith, A., and Stenstrom, R. 1990. Critical differences in aided sound field thresholds in children. *Journal of Speech and Hearing Research* 33:612-615.

Thornton, A.R., and Raffin, M.J.M. 1978. Speech-discrimination scores modeled as a binomial variable. *Journal of Speech and Hearing Research* 21:507-518.

Walden, B.E., Schwartz, D.M., Williams, D.L., Holum-Hardegen, L.L., and Crowley, J.M. 1983. Test of assumptions underlying comparative hearing aid evaluations. *Journal of Speech and Hearing Disorders* 48:264-273.

Zelisko, D.L., Seewald, R.C., and Gagné, J.P. 1992. Signal delivery/real ear measurement system for hearing aid selection and fitting. *Ear and Hearing* 13(6):460-463.

Zelisko, D.L., Seewald, R.C., and Whiteside, S. 1992. Comparing three procedures for predicting the ear canal SPL at LDL. Presented at the annual convention of the American Speech-Language-Hearing Association, November, San Antonio.

9

Situational Hearing Aid Response Profile (SHARP)

Patricia G. Stelmachowicz, Ann Kalberer, and Dawna E. Lewis

INTRODUCTION

Technological advances have provided the means for identifying hearing loss in children at very young ages. As a result, amplification and habilitation can begin early in an attempt to maximize a given child's potential for speech, language, and psychosocial development. Recent advances in hearing aid technology have the potential to improve the amplification these young children receive. However, the application of new hearing aid technology to the pediatric population has been limited.

In the selection and fitting of hearing aids, a relatively large number of decisions must be made to optimize parameters. One approach to the decision-making process is to use one of the numerous prescriptive procedures designed to provide target values for gain and/or maximum output based on auditory threshold, most comfortable listening levels (MCL), upper limit of comfortable loudness (ULCL), uncomfortable loudness levels (UCL), or some combination of these measures (Berger, Hagberg, and Rane 1984; Byrne and Dillon 1986; Cox 1988; McCandless and Lyregaard 1983; Seewald and Ross 1988; Skinner, Pascoe, Miller, and Popelka 1982).

A prescriptive approach may appear ideal for use with young children, but there are limitations. First, the majority of these approaches assume an idealized speech spectrum at a single input level so only one gain value and one maximum output value are specified at each frequency. In reality, speech is not static. Factors such as distance, vocal effort, and direction of the signal relative to the hearing aid microphone will affect the level and frequency composition of the speech signal. In addition, to adequately specify the electroacoustic characteristics of a nonlinear hearing aid, gain must be determined over a wide range of input levels. Recently, two approaches have been described for use with nonlinear systems (Cornelisse, Seewald, and Jamieson 1994; Killion 1995). However, these fitting strategies have not yet been validated on either adults or children.

A second limitation to many of the prescriptive procedures is that they are based on preferred gain and frequency response characteristics of adult hearing aid users. For young children with hearing loss, linguistic cues and world knowledge are not likely to facilitate the perception of speech in the same way as for adults (Nittrouer and Boothroyd 1990). Other studies also suggest that children may differ from adults in their ability to use various kinds of acoustic information. It appears that young children tend to use slowly changing dynamic or temporal cues whereas adults rely more on static spectral cues (Morrongiello, Robson, and Best 1984; Nittrouer 1992; Nittrouer and Studdert-Kennedy 1987). A less than optimal hearing aid fitting for an adult may not affect the perception of speech as much as it would a child who is attempting to learn speech and language through audition. For highly contextual materials, such as continuous discourse, low frequencies contribute more to intelligibility than do high frequencies (Studebaker, Pavlovic, and Sherbecoe 1987). Conversely, for low-context materials, such as nonsense syllables, the contribution of the high-frequency region to intelligibility is much greater (ANSI S3.5-1969). If young children are limited in their ability to use contextual cues, the optimal frequency/gain characteristics of a hearing aid may differ from the preferred values for adults.

An alternative approach to hearing aid selection and fitting is to require subjective judgments on the part of the listener. Measures such as loudness scaling and paired comparison judgments of quality, comfort, pleasantness, or perceived intelligibility have been used to modify a variety of hearing aid characteristics on an individual basis. For adults, these subjective judgments have been shown to correlate reasonably well with objective measures of speech perception as long as the hearing aids being compared differ substantially in frequency/gain characteristics (Levitt, Sullivan, Neuman, and Rubin-Spitz 1987; Sullivan, Levitt, Hwang, and Hennessey 1988). However, the subjective measures that have been described in the literature require a certain degree of cognitive skill and often a relatively high language level. It is unlikely that young children would be able to provide extensive and reliable subjective input into the hearing aid fitting process. Because the subjective measures have no obvious objective correlates, this approach does not seem feasible with young children.

The purpose of this chapter is to describe a new approach to viewing the audibility of the amplified long-term average speech spectrum (LTASS) that will allow a comparison across different amplification systems and different listening conditions. The Situational Hearing Aid Response Profile

(SHARP) is a PC-based computer program designed to assist clinicians with the process of selecting and fitting hearing aids to children and to provide information to parents, educators, and therapists on signal audibility under typical listening conditions. In the following sections, theoretical issues involved in the development of SHARP will be described along with cases illustrating its practical application.

OVERVIEW OF SHARP

SHARP provides a graphic display of the audibility of the amplified LTASS in a variety of listening situations. Figure 1 illustrates a typical display from SHARP for a child with a severe-to-profound hearing loss. In this figure, the circles represent auditory thresholds, the solid line depicts the amplified LTASS, the dotted lines illustrate the 30 dB range of speech, and the asterisks represent the real-ear saturation response (RESR). The crosshatched region shows the portion of the signal that is audible to the child. In this case, raised voice (figure 1A) is audible over a wide range of frequencies, but average conversation at 4 meters (figure 1B) is almost completely inaudible. To display aided results in this manner, the following information is needed: auditory thresholds; hearing aid input/output characteristics; frequency/gain responses as a function of intensity; saturation sound pressure level (SSPL90) as a function of frequency; and the overall level and spectral characteristics of the speech input. The following sections describe the various components of SHARP.

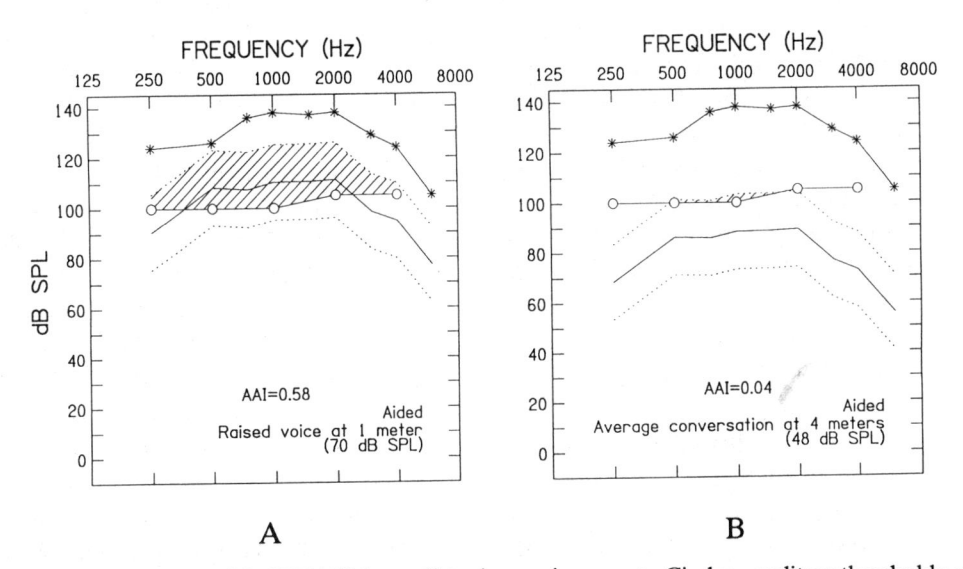

Figures 1A and 1B. Amplified LTASS in two listening environments. Circles=auditory thresholds; solid line=amplified LTASS; dotted lines= +15/-15 dB range of speech; crosshatched region=audible portion of signal; asterisks=RESR.

AUDITORY THRESHOLDS

To provide maximum flexibility, SHARP is designed to accept audiometric data obtained with the range of transducers typically used with a pediatric population (TDH-49/50 earphones, ER-3A insert phones, sound field loudspeakers). Age-related transforms are applied to these values to provide an estimate of the sound pressure level (SPL) at the tympanic membrane at auditory threshold (Stelmachowicz, Lewis, Karasek, and Creutz 1994). Alternatively, the SPL in the ear canal at auditory threshold can be measured directly using a clinical probe-tube microphone system. Hawkins, Morrison, Halligan, and Cooper (1989) and Gagné, Seewald, Zelisko, and Hudson (1991) provide a complete description of this method. Theoretically, any type of transducer can be used and should produce equivalent results when values are transformed to the SPL at the tympanic membrane. In practice, the sound field option is least desirable because head movement can affect test-retest reliability, particularly in the high frequencies (Hawkins, Montgomery, Prosek, and Walden 1987).

HEARING AID PARAMETERS

Because the overall level of the speech spectra available in SHARP varies over a range of intensities, it is necessary to consider the nonlinear characteristics of the hearing aid being evaluated. Each hearing aid must be classified into one of three types based on its input/output (i/o) characteristics. For SHARP, a linear peak-clipping hearing aid is characterized by an equal increase in output for a given change in input below saturation.

Instruments using "soft-peak clipping" or "diode clipping" also are classified as linear. A full dynamic range compression (FDRC) hearing aid is characterized by a low-compression threshold (usually < 65 dB SPL at 500 or 2000 Hz). Typically, compression ratio is low (< 5:1) and the release time is < 200 ms (Dillon 1988; Fabry 1991; Walker and Dillon 1983). Finally, compression limiting is defined as a circuit with a high-compression threshold (> 65 dB SPL) and a high compression ratio (> 5:1). Usually, the release time for compression limiting hearing aids is < 200 ms (Dillon 1988; Fabry 1991; Walker and Dillon 1983). Figure 2 shows examples of input-output curves for each of the three types of circuits described.

In addition to this classification, two additional hearing aid characteristics must be determined by the user. The first, the point of nonlinearity, is defined as the input level at which gain has decreased by 2 dB relative to the gain measured with a 50 dB input signal at either 500 or 2000 Hz. Because even linear instruments can become nonlinear below 90 dB SPL, the point of nonlinearity will determine how many gain curves (from 1 to 4)

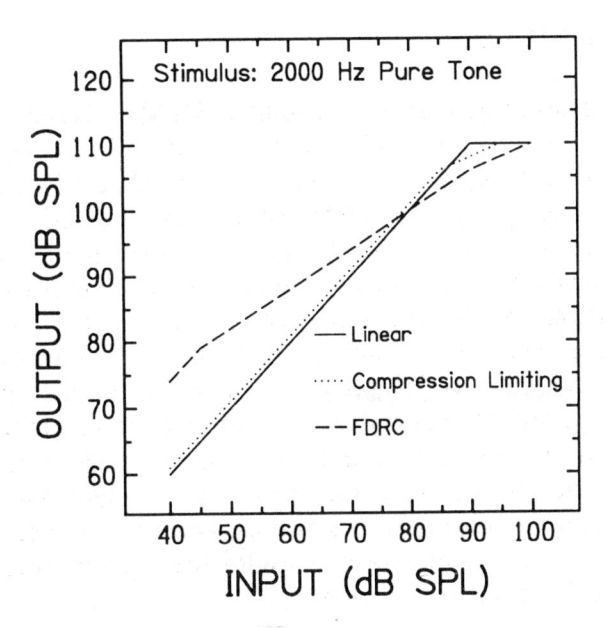

Figure 2. Output as a function of input at 2000 Hz for a linear hearing aid (solid line), a compression limiting hearing aid (dotted line), and an FDRC hearing aid (dashed line).

must be obtained to characterize the processing of the hearing aid. Thus, for a linear peak-clipping hearing aid that does not saturate until 90 dB SPL, only a single gain curve is necessary because the gain will be similar at all input levels below saturation. When the point of nonlinearity is lower, however, additional curves must be obtained. For full dynamic range compression hearing aids, it is also necessary to determine the compression ratio (CR) of the system at 2000 Hz (ANSI S3.22-1987). Numerous investigators have shown, however, that the CR computed from steady-state signals will overestimate the effective CR for speech (Bustamante and Braida 1987; DeGennaro, Braida, and Durlach 1986; Stone and Moore 1992). Therefore, an additional modification is applied to the CR to account for this discrepancy (Stelmachowicz et al. 1994), and the modified CR is used to rescale the normal 30 dB range of speech to a narrower range.

HEARING AID GAIN AND SSPL90

Hearing aid gain and maximum output may be entered either as 2-cm^3 coupler values or as real-ear values, using in situ gain as a metric (real-ear aided response minus input). Gain may be measured with swept pure tones or a complex stimulus, but the SSPL90 curve is obtained with swept pure tones. Depending on the hearing aid input/output characteristics, gain curves may be needed over a range of intensities (50 to 80 dB SPL). If 2-cm^3

coupler measures are entered, values are transformed to estimated real-ear values by age-related average values (Feigin, Kopun, Stelmachowicz, and Gorga 1989) or by the real-ear-to-coupler difference (RECD) as a function of frequency measured for each individual.

The RECD method, as described by Seewald (1991) and Moodie, Seewald, and Sinclair (1994), is an innovative method for obtaining real-ear measures in the difficult-to-test population. The method is based on the assumption that the real-ear aided response = 2-cm^3 coupler response + RECD. The RECD can be obtained easily using a clinical probe-tube microphone system (see Moodie et al. [1994] for a detailed review of the procedure). Briefly, the signal from the real-ear measurement system is directed to an insert earphone (Etymotic, ER-3A), which is attached to a 2-cm^3 coupler as shown in figure 3. A complex stimulus is presented and the response is stored. The probe tube is placed in the child's ear canal, and the earphone then is attached to the tubing of the child's earmold, which is coupled to the ear. The complex stimulus is presented again and a second response is stored; the difference between these two responses is the RECD. Test time for both ears with the child present is usually less than ten minutes. All subsequent hearing aid measures can be made in a 2-cm^3 coupler. The RECD then can be added to the appropriate 2-cm^3 coupler measures to estimate both the real-ear gain and the real-ear saturation response. In some real-ear systems, multiple memories allow these computations to be made automatically. This procedure has been found to provide a valid estimate of real-ear hearing aid performance across frequency for both children and adults with moderate-to-severe hearing losses (Seewald, Sinclair, and Moodie

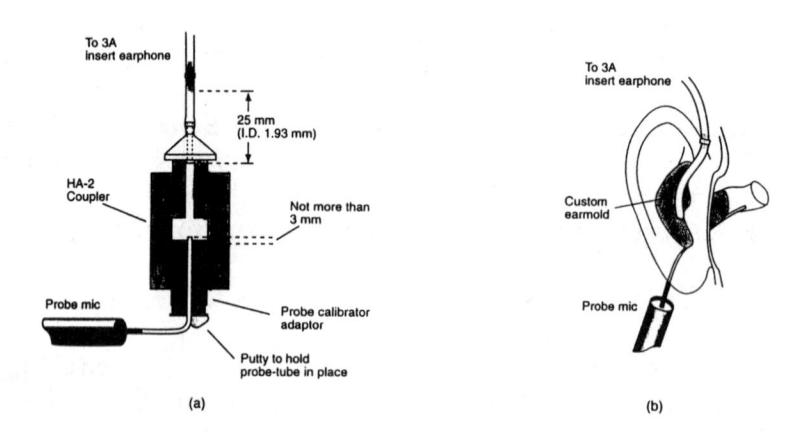

Figure 3. Apparatus for determining the real-ear-to-coupler difference (RECD). **3A:** insert earphone (Etymotic, ER-3A) in an A-2, 2-cm^3 coupler. **3B:** insert earphone in the ear of a child. From Moodie et al. 1994, reproduced with permission.

1994). Sinclair, Beauchaine, Moodie, Feigin, Seewald, and Stelmachowicz (1994) have shown good test-retest reliability for this procedure for children in the 1 month to 7 year age range. In their study, the highest intrasubject variability was seen for children in the 13 to 18 months age range, who were often very active and difficult to test.

Although the RECD originally was intended to extend the feasibility of real-ear measures to younger children and infants, the procedure also can be useful with active older children and other individuals who demonstrate a limited attention span.

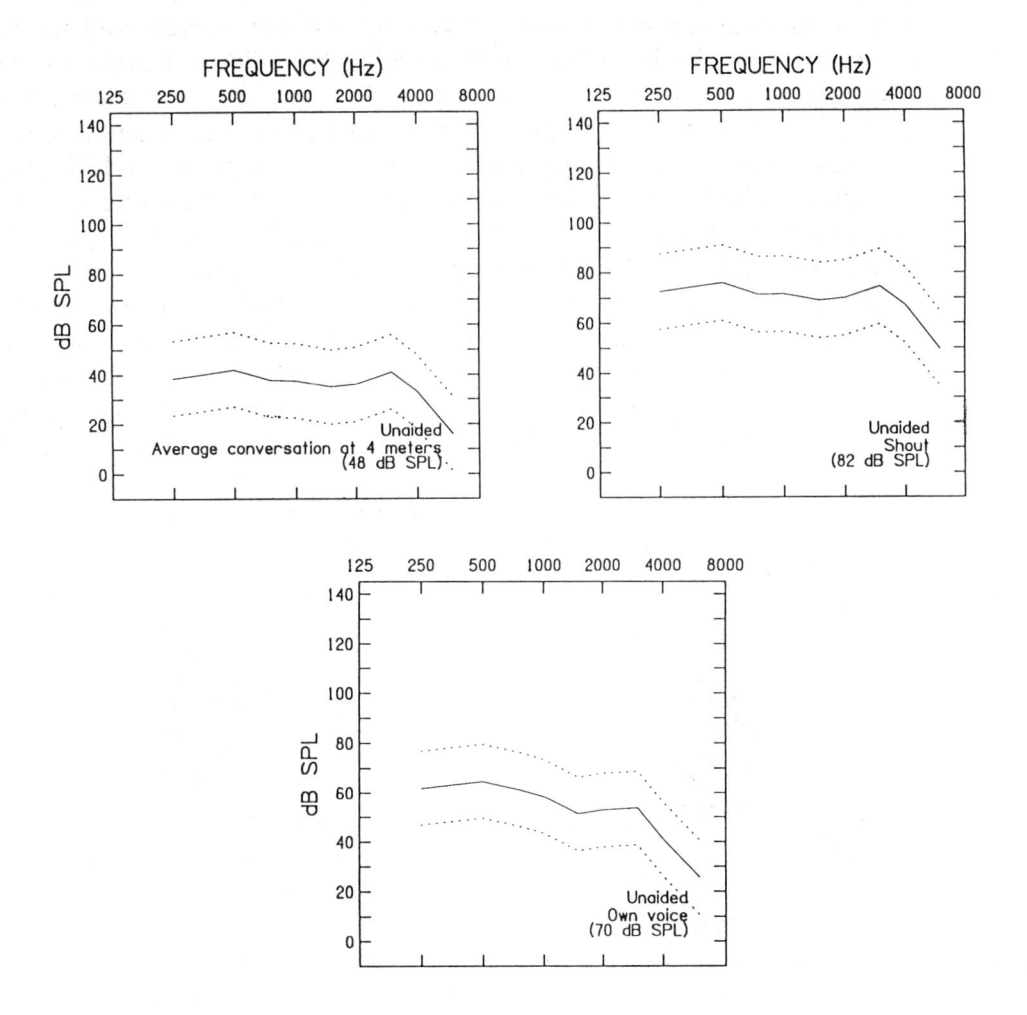

Figure 4. One-third octave band levels for three different speech spectra. The solid line represents the LTASS and the dotted lines represent the +15/-15 dB range of speech.

SPEECH SPECTRA

Currently, 13 speech spectra are available in SHARP. The rms levels of these spectra range from a low of 48 dB SPL to a high of 82 dB SPL. Figure 4 shows examples of three spectra chosen to represent differences related to distance, vocal effort, and speaker-listener azimuth. The upper left panel displays the spectrum for average conversation at 4 meters. To obtain this spectrum, 12 dB was subtracted from the Cox and Moore (1988) spectrum for average conversation at 1 meter, representing a change from 1 meter to 4 meters based on the inverse square law. This assumes conversation in a nonreverberant field such as outdoors or in a large indoor area (gymnasium). The upper right panel displays the spectrum of a shout with an overall level of 82 dB SPL (Pearsons, Bennett, and Fidell 1977). The bottom panel displays the spectrum for one's own voice, with an overall level of 70

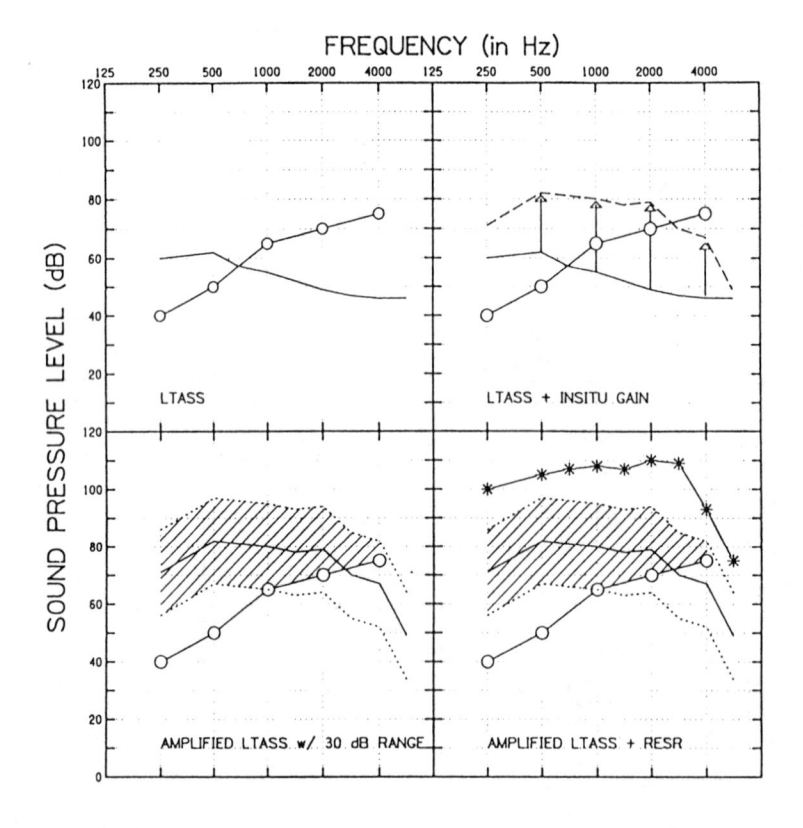

Figure 5. Top left: Circles indicate auditory thresholds and solid line shows Cox and Moore (1988) LTASS; Top right: arrows denote that in situ gain of hearing aid is added to the LTASS; Lower left: +15/-15 dB range of speech is added to the amplified LTASS and the audible portion of the spectrum is crosshatched; Lower right: asterisks denote the RESR. From Stelmachowicz et al. 1994, reproduced with permission.

dB SPL (Cornelisse, Gagné, and Seewald 1991). For each spectrum selected, the overall level is used to select the appropriate gain curve for subsequent computations.

COMPUTATION OF THE AMPLIFIED SPEECH SPECTRUM

For each speech spectrum, the amplified LTASS is computed by adding the appropriate hearing aid gain curve to the presumed input spectrum. Figure 5 illustrates the steps involved in this process. The top left panel shows auditory thresholds plotted in relation to the LTASS (Cox and Moore 1988), which is depicted by the solid line. In the top right panel, the arrows denote that the in situ gain of the hearing aid has been added to the LTASS. Corrections for hearing aid microphone location effects also are applied (Bentler and Pavlovic 1989). In the lower left panel, the ±15 dB

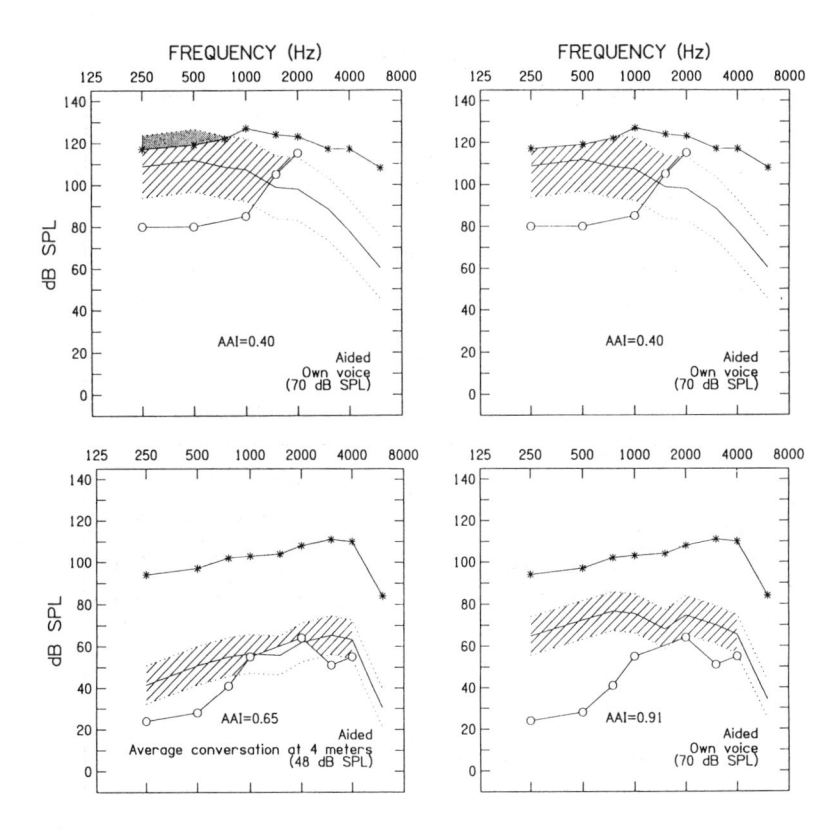

Figure 6. Effect of type of signal processing on the amplified LTASS in different listening environments following the convention used in figure 1. Top two panels show a comparison of a linear peak-clipping hearing aid (left) and a compression limiting hearing aid (right). The shaded region (left) represents the portion of the signal that has been peak clipped. Lower two panels show amplified spectra in two listening conditions for an FDRC hearing aid.

range of speech (ANSI S3.79 in revision) is added to the amplified LTASS, and the audible portion of the spectrum is crosshatched. In the lower right panel, asterisks denote the real-ear saturation response (RESR). Although not shown in figure 5, peak clipping is denoted as a shaded area above the RESR curve. Because both compression limiting and FDRC are assumed to reduce distortion, shading is omitted when this type of output limitation is used.

SHARP allows the user to assess the effects of different types of signal processing on the amplified LTASS and the calculated Aided Audibility Index (AAI). The top two panels in figure 6 show a comparison of a linear peak-clipping hearing aid (top left) and a compression limiting hearing aid (top right). These hearing aids were matched to provide approximately the same gain and maximum output. For the linear peak-clipping hearing aid, the low-frequency components of the speech signal are in saturation for this stimulus (one's own voice at 70 dB SPL). In addition, audibility of a portion of the spectrum is limited by peak clipping (e.g., the 30 dB range is reduced in the low frequencies). For the compression limiting hearing aid, the audibility of the low-frequency components of speech also is reduced by the maximum output of the hearing aid. However, no shading is present for the compression limiting circuit because it is assumed that this type of processing will not produce distortion in the same way as a peak-clipping hearing aid. In this example, the AAI (discussed in the next section) for the two spectra is the same. Peak clipping can degrade signal quality resulting in a lower AAI, but in this example, the amount of peak clipping produced was not sufficiently high to reduce the AAI.

The lower two panels of figure 6 depict two listening conditions with an FDRC hearing aid. The left panel illustrates the audibility of speech at 4 meters, and the right panel shows the audibility of one's own voice. The configuration of the amplified LTASS differs across these two panels because the overall level of speech determines the operating point of the instrument. Thus, in the left panel, the 50 dB gain curve is added to the speech spectrum to derive the amplified LTASS, while in the right panel, the 70 dB gain curve is used. Note also that the 30 dB range of speech has been rescaled to approximately 20 dB based on the input/output characteristics of the instrument.

COMPUTATION OF THE AIDED AUDIBILITY INDEX (AAI)

The Articulation Index (AI) (French and Steinberg 1947) is a model that originally was developed to predict the speech recognition of listeners with normal hearing based on the portion of the average speech spectrum that is audible under less than optimal listening conditions. For listeners with normal hearing, performance is well predicted by knowledge of auditory thresholds, level and spectrum of both speech and interfering noise, and the speech materials. Results have been more variable, however, when the AI is applied to listeners with sensorineural hearing loss (Dirks, Bell, Rossman, and Kincaid 1986; Humes, Dirks, Bell, Ahlstrom, and Kincaid 1986; Kamm, Dirks, and Bell 1985; Pavlovic 1984). Factors such as widened critical bands, level-dependent upward spread of masking, intraspeech masking, abnormally rapid response growth as a function of stimulus level, and changes in temporal resolution have been suggested as possible causes for the poorer correlations (Pavlovic, Studebaker, and Sherbecoe 1986).

A number of investigators have modified the AI to apply the model to performance under aided conditions (Engebretson, Popelka, Morley, Niemoeller, and Heidbreder 1986; Hou and Thornton 1994; Humes 1991; Mueller and Killion 1990; Pavlovic 1988, 1989, 1991; Pavlovic and Studebaker 1984; Rankovic 1991; Studebaker and Marincovich 1989). Some of these modifications were designed to provide easy computation of the AI under clinical conditions, whereas others have attempted to account for factors such as cochlear distortions, upward spread of masking, and masking by speech across bands. With one exception (Hou and Thornton 1994), these approaches have focused on measures of audibility in relation to the LTASS at a single input level, and none have included provisions for nonlinear processing.

Numerous permutations of the mathematical formula for computing the AI have been reported in the literature. The basic formula (Pavlovic 1989) describes the AI as an algebraic sum:

$$AI = (\sum_{i=1}^{n} I_i W_i)/30$$

In this formula, i (varying from 1 to n) refers to each of the frequency bands chosen for use in the formula. Historically, octave or one-third octave bands have been used. Pavlovic (1988) has described an approach in which the audiometric frequencies can be used. The term I_i represents the band importance function for the ith band and denotes the contribution of a particular frequency region to overall intelligibility. The band importance weights were derived from extensive speech intelligibility measures completed under varying conditions of high- and low-pass filtering. The importance of a particular band will vary, depending on the type of speech materials used for testing (Studebaker et al. 1987). Thus, different importance functions are used for different speech materials (e.g., monosyllables, continuous discourse). W_i, the band-weighting function, represents the audibility of speech within each band, taking into account the presumed 30 dB range over which the short-term components of speech vary.

The computations used in SHARP to provide an AAI are based on a composite of information gathered from many sources. The mathematical model for AI has been modified to account for the effects of different types of hearing aid signal processing on the audibility of speech. For linear peak-clipping hearing aids, the clipping is assumed to cause a reduction in the sensation level (SL) of speech as well as the introduction of distortion. It is assumed that the SL of speech may be reduced by compression limiting, but corrections for distortion will not be necessary, as is the case for linear peak-clipping hearing aids. An additional modification is needed for FDRC circuits. Presumably, the 30 dB range of speech will be reduced depending on the CR of the hearing aid. As stated previously, the nominal CR of an FDRC hearing aid will overestimate the magnitude of compression for real speech. This occurs because the time constants of the system may not allow full recovery of gain between words or syllables. Thus, the nominal compression ratio is modified (Stelmachowicz et al. 1994) and the ±15 dB range of speech is rescaled accordingly. This modified range is substituted for the presumed 30 dB range of speech in the AAI computations.

PRACTICAL APPLICATIONS

In this section, three case examples illustrating the application of SHARP will be presented. Cases 1 and 2 demonstrate the use of SHARP to determine signal audibility in various listening environments. In Case 3, SHARP is used to compare the audibility of speech for two different hearing aid signal processing schemes.

Case 1 is an 11-month-old girl with a profound, bilateral hearing loss. Her hearing loss was identified at 6 months of age, and she was aided two months later with binaural high-gain, ear-level hearing aids (linear peak-clipping circuit). She was referred to our facility for evaluation at 11 months of age to determine the adequacy of her hearing aid fitting and to assist in decisions regarding mode of communication. At that time, her parents reported that although she was responding to sounds when wearing her hearing aids, she was not as responsive as they had hoped. Figure 7 shows the audibility of speech for this child (better ear only) under various listening conditions with her hearing aid as it was set originally. All data were obtained using traditional probe-tube microphone measures. For average conversation at 1 meter (upper left), only the peak energy of the low-frequency components of speech is audible. For the remaining three panels, the overall level of speech is higher and better audibility is achieved in the midfrequencies, but the low-frequency components of speech are in saturation. This is particularly apparent for the child's own voice (upper right) and for the common position in which the child is carried at the parent's hip (lower right).

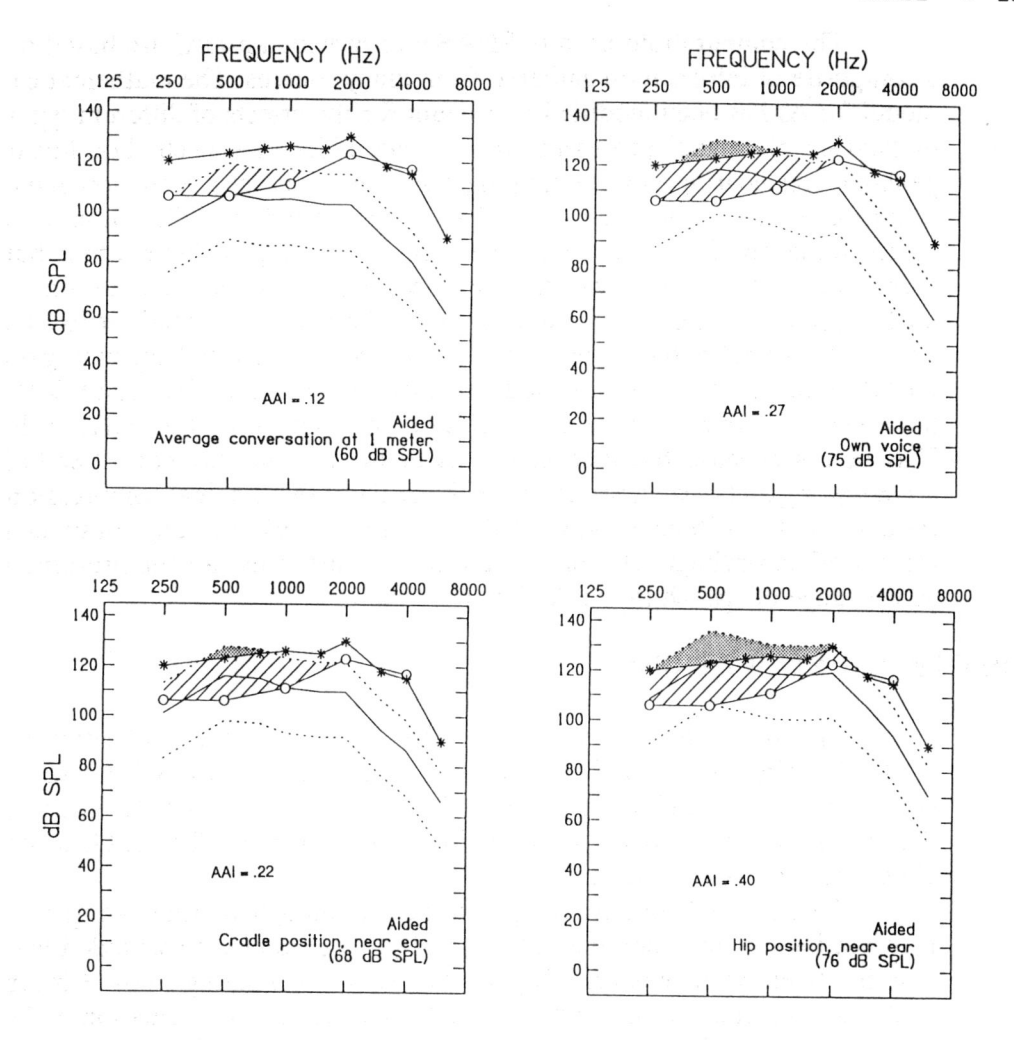

Figure 7. Following the convention used in figure 6, amplified LTASS in four listening environments for a listener with a profound hearing loss.

This information raises questions regarding the type of output limitation that should be used in this case. Given that high-level speech is likely to drive this hearing aid into saturation, a compression limiting circuit might be considered because distortion would be minimized. On the other hand, Boothroyd (1986, 1987) and Dawson, Dillon, and Battaglia (1991) have shown that speech perception for some listeners with profound hearing loss may be reduced due to the loss of envelope cues associated with high-compression ratios. Thus, the choice between peak clipping and compression limiting may not be straightforward. In this case, another alternative is possible. The RESR is 120 to 127 dB SPL in the low frequencies. Assuming an average RECD for a child of this age to be 10 to 13 dB from 500 to 1000 Hz (Feigin et al. 1989), the coupler output of this hearing aid would be no more than 114 dB SPL in the low frequencies. Because this child's unaided thresholds in the low to midfrequencies are in the 107 to 111 dB SPL range, the maximum output of this hearing aid appears to be set too low. Damping the peak at 1000 Hz and increasing the maximum output of the hearing aid improved the audibility of the low-frequency components of speech for this child.

Case 2 is a 2-year-old girl with a symmetrical, moderate-to-severe hearing loss. This child was aided initially with a monaural loaner hearing aid at 21 months of age and with binaural high-gain, ear-level hearing aids (linear

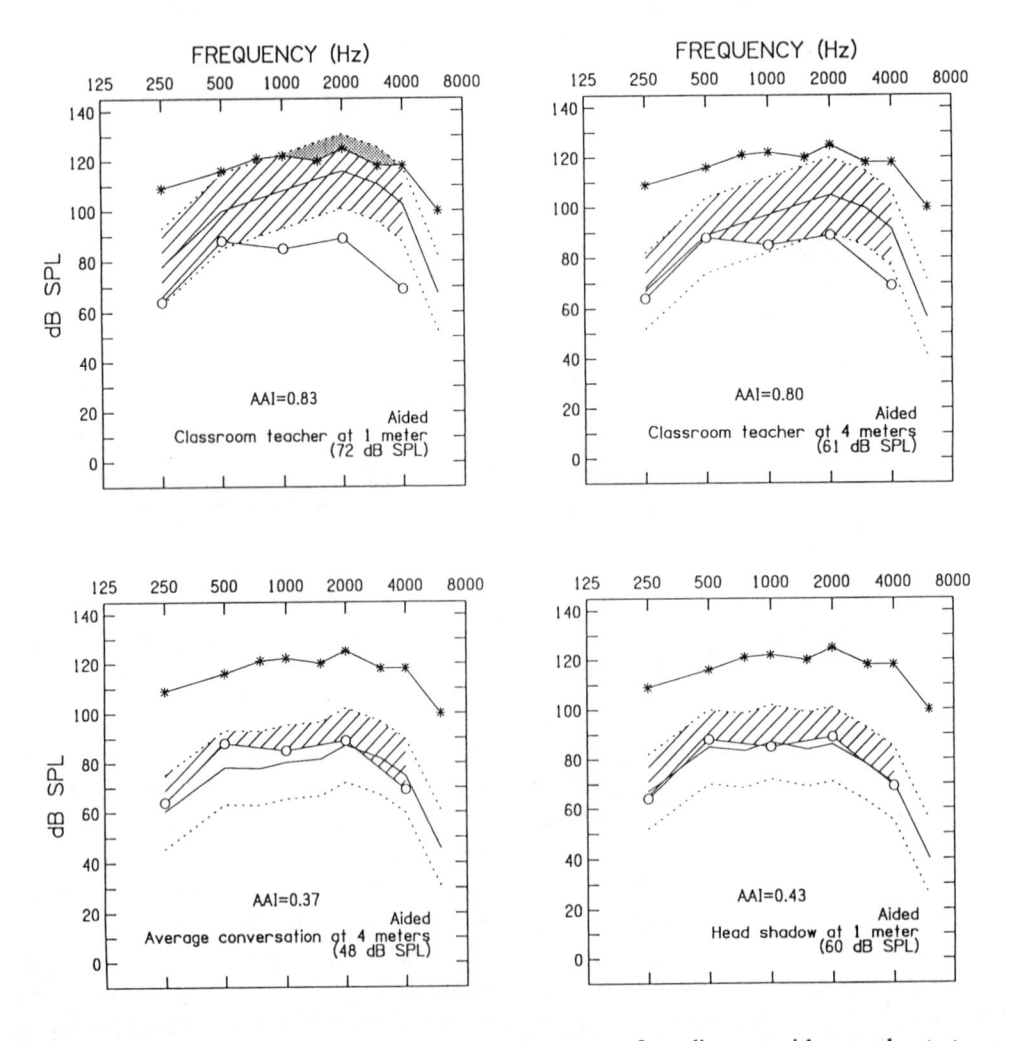

Figure 8. Amplified LTASS in four listening environments for a listener with a moderate-to-severe hearing loss.

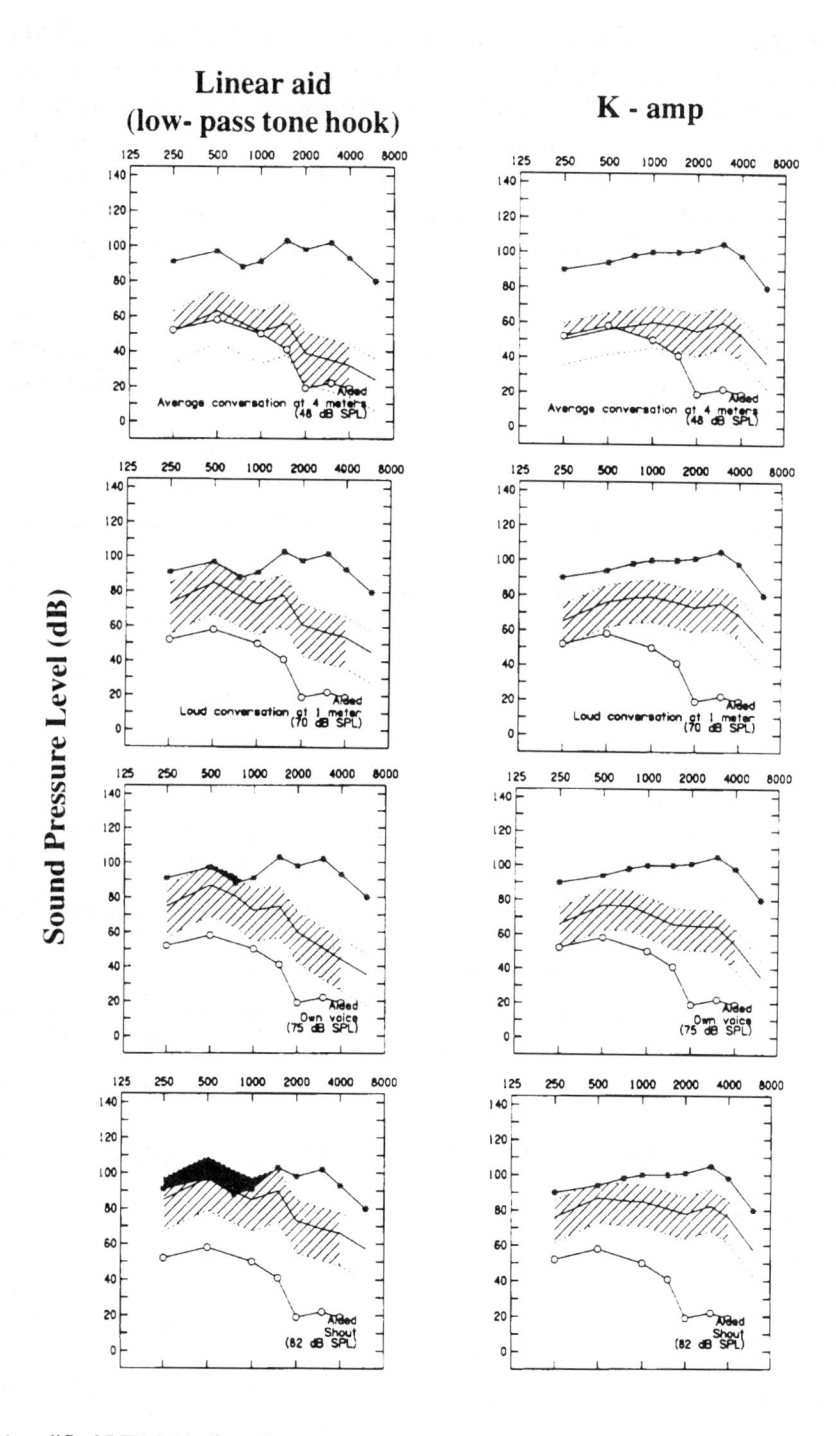

Figure 9. Amplified LTASS in four listening environments for a listener with a rising hearing loss. The left column represents the effects of a linear hearing aid, and the right column represents the effects of an FDRC hearing aid.

peak-clipping circuit) at 26 months. This child was enrolled in a total-communication toddler classroom two mornings a week. The parents questioned the benefit of binaural versus monaural amplification as well as the need for an FM system in the educational setting.

The information shown in figure 8 was used to illustrate to the parents how audibility might be affected by both distance and monaural versus binaural amplification. The top two panels suggest that in quiet, most of the speech spectrum will be audible in classroom conditions where the teacher's voice is assumed to be at a 0° azimuth. However, at higher input levels, the peaks of speech will be in saturation. The lower left panel suggests that at a distance of 4 meters (e.g., in a gymnasium or outdoors), only the loudest components of speech will be audible, even when aided binaurally. The lower right panel depicts the audibility of speech, at an azimuth of 180°, when aided monaurally (head shadow effect at 1 meter). In this instance, much of the speech spectrum will be inaudible even in quiet situations. In a typical classroom, this type of listening situation may occur frequently as the teacher moves around the room or as other students answer questions or interact with this child.

Obviously, even with an appropriate hearing aid fitting, this child can be expected to have difficulty hearing in many situations. Furthermore, the effects of noise and/or reverberation, which have not been considered here, would be expected to limit audibility further. Because there are no contraindications for binaural amplification, this child should be aided binaurally, and an FM system should be considered for use in educational settings.

Case 3 is a 10-year-old boy with an asymmetrical hearing loss. The audiometric configuration is unusual, showing a rising loss with regions of normal hearing from 2000 to 4000 Hz in the right ear and a severe loss in the left ear. Speech recognition ability in the left ear is extremely poor, so this child has been aided in the right ear only, with limited success. It is often difficult to achieve a successful hearing aid fitting for this type of low-frequency hearing loss. In quiet, the high-frequency components of speech will be audible even without a hearing aid. Listening in noise may not alter intelligibility markedly, since the low-frequency components of noise often may be below threshold. Furthermore, when regions of normal hearing exist in the high frequencies, as in this case, the amplification options are somewhat limited. In figure 9, two types of signal processing are compared to determine which might provide better signal audibility in a variety of listening conditions. The left column shows results for a linear hearing aid with a low-pass filtered tone hook, and the right column shows the results for an FDRC hearing aid under the same listening conditions. Each row represents a different listening condition, with overall levels ranging from 48 to 82 dB SPL.

For low-level inputs, greater audibility is achieved with the FDRC circuit. For the linear hearing aid, the shape of the amplified LTASS is somewhat irregular, and virtually no gain is provided in the high frequencies where hearing is normal. For the compression hearing aid, approximately 40 dB of gain is provided despite the normal thresholds. As the level of speech increases to 70 dB SPL, audibility becomes more similar for the two circuits as shown by the calculated AAI. At 75 dB SPL, the linear hearing aid has begun to operate in saturation in the low frequencies. At the highest level shown (82 dB SPL), the peaks of speech in the low frequencies are clipped with the linear circuit, and the AAI has decreased slightly compared to the FDRC hearing aid. Changes in the overall level of the amplified LTASS are less dramatic for the compression hearing aid compared to the linear circuit. Stated differently, although 40 dB of high-frequency gain exists for low-level inputs, the gain decreases as the input increases so that loudness discomfort and/or potential overamplification is not a concern. Thus, for this type of hearing loss, FDRC appears to be a reasonable option because amplified speech should fit within the child's dynamic range across a wide range of listening levels.

SUMMARY AND CONCLUSIONS

The hearing aid fitting approach described has the potential to improve the ability to apply advanced signal processing technology to the pediatric population. The RECD procedure can be implemented easily in most clinical settings and often can provide more reliable estimates of real-ear hearing aid gain and output than traditional probe-tube microphone measures in very young children. In addition, the procedure requires minimal cooperation from the child and can be accomplished in a fraction of the time required for traditional testing.

SHARP can provide a comparative evaluation of the audibility of speech across different hearing aids and/or different listening situations that may be relevant to a particular child. When target values cannot be met during the hearing aid fitting, this information can help the clinician weigh alternative strategies and make decisions about a sensible compromise of hearing aid parameters. A comparison of audibility and dynamic range across different hearing aids may influence decisions regarding methods of output limitation, and the AAI can provide a relative measure of audibility across different listening situations or different hearing aids. This information can be very useful for parents, educators, and therapists.

There are, however, a number of limitations inherent in the current version of SHARP. Pilot data in our laboratory suggest that, for some hearing aids, neither swept pure-tone stimuli nor speech-weighted noise provides a valid estimate of hearing aid gain for real speech. With advances in signal processing such as nonlinear multiband systems, combined input and output controlled circuits, adaptive release times, frequency-dependent compression thresholds and CRs, the ability to predict speech gain from simpler stimuli has become increasingly problematic. Additional studies are needed to determine whether alternative stimuli can provide a better estimate of how hearing aids process running speech. The issue of stimulus choice is a problem not only for the approach described here but also for any hearing aid fitting strategy that relies on target gain/output values.

A second limitation is related to the computation of the AAI. In the current algorithm, a number of assumptions were made regarding effective versus nominal CR, the negative consequences of peak clipping, and the effects of compression limiting. To date, this approach has not been validated on either adults or children, and many of the assumptions underlying the AAI are based on limited data or assumptions that have not been tested. Clearly, additional studies are needed to address these unresolved issues and to validate the efficacy of this approach.

Finally, in its current form the user must enter hearing aid gain/output curves into the program manually. In addition, the system does not categorize the specific type of hearing aid processing; rather, the user must define the type of processing (linear, FDRC, compression limiting), and the program assumes that the processing is similar across all frequencies. For many types of hearing aids, this will not be the case. Additional studies currently are under way to address this problem and to automate the approach.

ACKNOWLEDGMENTS

The authors wish to acknowledge Richard Seewald for many helpful discussions during the development of this program and Rene Brandemuehl, Joellen Henriksen, and Donna Neff for beneficial comments on an earlier draft of this paper. This work was supported by NIH-NIDCD Grant P-60 DC00982.

REFERENCES

American National Standards Institute. *Methods for the calculation of the speech intelligibility index.* Draft V3.0, 12/17/92. ANSI S3.79 in revision. New York: American National Standards Institute.

American National Standards Institute. *Methods for the calculation of the articulation index.* ANSI S3.5-1969. New York: American National Standards Institute.

American National Standards Institute. *Specification of hearing aid characteristics.* ANSI S3.22-1987. New York: American National Standards Institute.

Bentler, R., and Pavlovic, C.V. 1989. Transfer functions and correction factors used in hearing aid evaluation and research. *Ear and Hearing* 10:58-63.

Berger, K.W., Hagberg, E.N., and Rane, R. 1984. *Prescription hearing aids: Rationale, procedures, and results.* 4th ed. Kent, Ohio: Herald Press.

Boothroyd, A. 1986. Compression-limited amplification for the profoundly deaf. Paper read at the RESNA Rehabilitation Technology Ninth Annual Conference, June, San Jose, California.

Boothroyd, A. 1987. Experiments with a two-channel compression-limiting amplification system designed for profoundly deaf subjects. Paper read at the RESNA Rehabilitation Technology Tenth Annual Conference, June, San Jose, California.

Bustamante, D.K., and Braida, L.D. 1987. Principal-component amplitude compression for the hearing impaired. *Journal of the Acoustical Society of America* 82:1227-1242.

Byrne, D., and Dillon, H. 1986. The National Acoustic Laboratories' (NAL) new procedure for selecting the gain and frequency response of a hearing aid. *Ear and Hearing* 7:257-265.

Cornelisse, L.E., Gagné, J.P., and Seewald, R.C. 1991. Ear level recordings of the long-term average spectrum of speech. *Ear and Hearing* 12:47-54.

Cornelisse, L.E., Seewald, R.C., and Jamieson, D.G. 1994. Fitting wide dynamic range hearing aids: The DSL [i/o] approach. *Hearing Journal* 47:23-29.

Cox, R.M. 1988. Distribution of short-term RMS levels in conversational speech. *Journal of the Acoustical Society of America* 84:1100-1104.

Cox, R.M., and Moore, J.N. 1988. Composite speech spectrum for hearing aid gain prescriptions. *Journal of Speech and Hearing Research* 31:102-107.

Dawson, P., Dillon, H., and Battaglia, J. 1991. Output limiting compression for the severe-profoundly deaf. *Australian Journal of Audiology* 13:1-12.

DeGennaro, S., Braida, L.D., and Durlach, N.I. 1986. Multichannel syllabic compression for severely impaired listeners. *Journal of Rehabilitation Research and Development* 23:17-24.

Dillon, H. 1988. Compression in hearing aids. In R.E. Sandlin (ed.), *Handbook of hearing aid amplification,* vol. 1. San Diego: College Hill Press.

Dirks, D.D., Bell, T.S., Rossman, R.N., and Kincaid, G.E. 1986. Articulation index predictions of contextually dependent words. *Journal of the Acoustical Society of America* 80:82-92.

Engebretson, A.M., Popelka, G.R., Morley, R., Niemoeller, A., and Heidbreder, A. 1986. A digital hearing aid and computer-based fitting procedure. *Hearing Instruments* 37:8-12.

Fabry, D. 1991. Hearing aid compression. *American Journal of Audiology* 1:11-13.

Feigin, J.A., Kopun, J.G., Stelmachowicz, P.G., and Gorga, M.P. 1989. Probe-tube microphone measures of ear-canal sound pressure levels in infants and children. *Ear and Hearing* 10:254-258.

French, N.R., and Steinberg, J.C. 1947. Factors governing the intelligibility of speech sounds. *Journal of the Acoustical Society of America* 19:90-119.

Gagné, J.P., Seewald, R.C., Zelisko, D.L., and Hudson, S.P. 1991. Procedure for defining the auditory area of hearing-impaired adolescents with a severe/profound hearing loss: I—Detection thresholds. *Journal of Speech Language Pathology and Audiology* 15:13-20.

Hawkins, D.B., Montgomery, A.A., Prosek, R.A., and Walden, B.E. 1987. Examination of two issues concerning functional gain measurements. *Journal of Speech and Hearing Disorders* 52:56-63.

Hawkins, D.B., Morrison, T.M., Halligan, P.L., and Cooper, W.A. 1989. Use of probe tube microphone measurements in hearing aid selection for children: Some initial clinical experiences. *Ear and Hearing* 10:281-287.

Hou, Z., and Thornton, A.R. 1994. A model to evaluate and maximize hearing aid performance by integrating the articulation index across listening conditions. *Ear and Hearing* 15:105-112.

Humes, L.E. 1991. Understanding the speech-understanding problems of the hearing impaired. *Journal of the American Academy of Audiology* 2:59-69.

Humes, L.E., Dirks, D.D., Bell, T.S., Ahlstrom, J., and Kincaid, G.E. 1986. Application of the articulation index and the speech transmission index to the recognition of speech by normal-hearing and hearing-impaired listeners. *Journal of Speech and Hearing Research* 29:447-462.

Kamm, C.A., Dirks, D.D., and Bell, T.S. 1985. Speech recognition and the articulation index for normal and hearing-impaired listeners. *Journal of the Acoustical Society of America* 77:281-288.

Killion, M.C. 1995. Talking hair cells: What they have to say about hearing aids. In C.I. Berlin (ed.), *Hair cells and hearing aids.* San Diego: Singular Press.

Levitt, H., Sullivan, J.A., Neuman, A.C., and Rubin-Spitz, J.A. 1987. Experiments with a programmable master hearing aid. *Journal of Rehabilitative Research and Development* 24:29-54.

McCandless, G.A., and Lyregaard, P.E. 1983. Prescription of gain/output (POGO) for hearing aids. *Hearing Instruments* 34:16-21.

Moodie, K.S., Seewald, R.C., and Sinclair, S.T. 1994. Procedure for predicting real-ear hearing aid performance in young children. *American Journal of Audiology* 3:23-31.

Morrongiello, B.A., Robson, R.C., and Best, C.T. 1984. Trading relations in the perception of speech by 5-year-old children. *Journal of Experimental Clinical Psychology* 37:231-250.

Mueller, H.G., and Killion, M.C. 1990. An easy method for calculating the articulation index. *Hearing Journal* 43:14-17.

Nittrouer, S. 1992. Age-related differences in perceptual effects of formant transitions with syllables and across syllable boundaries. *Journal of Phonetics* 20:1-32.

Nittrouer, S., and Boothroyd, A. 1990. Context effects in phoneme and word recognition by young children and older adults. *Journal of the Acoustical Society of America* 87:2705-2715.

Nittrouer, S., and Studdert-Kennedy, M. 1987. The role of coarticulatory effects on the perception of fricatives by children and adults. *Journal of the Acoustical Society of America* 30:319-329.

Pavlovic, C.V. 1984. Use of the articulation index for assessing residual auditory function in listeners with sensorineural hearing impairment. *Journal of the Acoustical Society of America* 75:1253-1258.

Pavlovic, C.V. 1988. Articulation index predictions of speech intelligibility in hearing aid selection. *Asha* 30:63-65.

Pavlovic, C.V. 1989. Speech spectrum considerations and speech intelligibility predictions in hearing aid evaluations. *Journal of the Acoustical Society of America* 54:3-8.

Pavlovic, C.V. 1991. Speech recognition and five articulation indexes. *Hearing Instruments* 42:20-23.

Pavlovic, C.V., and Studebaker, G.A. 1984. Evaluation of some assumptions underlying the articulation index. *Journal of the Acoustical Society of America* 75:1606-1612.

Pavlovic, C.V., Studebaker, G.A., and Sherbecoe, R.L. 1986. An articulation index based procedure for predicting the speech recognition performance of hearing-impaired individuals. *Journal of the Acoustical Society of America* 80:50-57.

Pearsons, K., Bennett, R., and Fidell, S. 1977. Speech levels in various noise environments. Project report on contract 68 01-2466. Washington D.C.: U.S. Environmental Protection Agency.

Rankovic, C.M. 1991. An application of the articulation index to hearing aid fitting. *Journal of Speech and Hearing Research* 34:391-402.

Seewald, R.C. 1991. Hearing aid output limiting considerations for children. In J.A. Feigin and P.G. Stelmachowicz (eds.), *Pediatric amplification: Proceedings of the 1991 national conference*. Omaha: Boys Town National Research Hospital.

Seewald, R.C., and Ross, M. 1988. Amplification for young hearing-impaired children. In M.C. Pollack (ed.), *Amplification for the hearing-impaired*. Orlando: Grune and Stratton.

Seewald, R.C., Sinclair, S.T., and Moodie, K.S. 1994. Predictive accuracy of a procedure for electroacoustic fitting in young children. Paper read at the American Academy of Audiology convention, April, Richmond.

Sinclair, S.T., Beauchaine, K.L., Moodie, K.S., Feigin, J.A., Seewald, R.C., and Stelmachowicz, P.G. 1994. Repeatability of a real-ear to coupler difference measurement as a function of age. Poster presented at the American Academy of Audiology convention, April, Richmond.

Skinner, M.W., Pascoe, D.P., Miller, J.D., and Popelka, G.R. 1982. Measurements to determine the optimal placement of speech energy within the listener's auditory area: A basis for selecting amplification characteristics. In G.A. Studebaker and F.H. Bess (eds.), *The Vanderbilt hearing-aid report*. Upper Darby, Penn.: Monographs in Contemporary Audiology.

Stelmachowicz, P.G., Lewis, D., Karasek, A., and Creutz, T. 1994. *Situational Hearing Aid Response Profile (SHARP, version 2.0) user's manual*. Omaha: Boys Town National Research Hospital.

Stone, M.A., and Moore, B.C. 1992. Syllabic compression: Effective compression ratios for signals modulated at different rates. *British Journal of Audiology* 26:351-361.

Studebaker, G.A., and Marincovich, P.J. 1989. Importance weighted audibility and the recognition of hearing aid-processed speech. *Ear and Hearing* 10:101-108.

Studebaker, G.A., Pavlovic, C.V., and Sherbecoe, R.L. 1987. A frequency importance function for continuous discourse. *Journal of the Acoustical Society of America* 81:1130-1138.

Sullivan, J.A., Levitt, H., Hwang, J.Y., and Hennessey, A. 1988. An experimental comparison of four hearing aid prescription methods. *Ear and Hearing* 9:22-32.

Walker, G., and Dillon, H. 1983. Compression in hearing aids: An analysis, a review and some recommendations. Report no. 90. Sydney, Australia: National Acoustic Laboratories.

10

Monitoring and Management of Amplification Systems for Children

Jackson Roush

INTRODUCTION

The past quarter century has witnessed remarkable advances in the design and manufacture of hearing aids and other sensory devices. Improvements in hearing instruments have been accompanied by the development of innovative software and instrumentation to assist in the selection and fitting process. Hearing aids offering electroacoustic flexibility combined with probe-tube microphone measurements and selection strategies appropriate for children allow unprecedented accuracy and control in the pediatric amplification fitting process. But how long do our carefully selected and verified electroacoustic characteristics exist in the child's day-to-day listening environment? When this question has been asked empirically, the answer has not been encouraging. In fact, the results of several studies have been uniformly disappointing with regard to the functional condition of children's hearing aids. The following discussion will review past and present monitoring and management practices as well as recommended strategies for improving the functional status of amplification in children.

HISTORICAL PERSPECTIVE

Gaeth and Lounsbury, in a classic study published in 1966, evaluated the hearing aids worn by 134 school-age children. Based on a combination of parent survey, comparison of aided and unaided evaluations, and electroacoustic analysis, they found a hearing aid failure rate ranging from 55% to 69%, depending on the severity of the problem. Only 16% of the hearing aids evaluated met all the requirements for adequate hearing aid use. Even by the most lenient standards, only 50% of the children were judged to be getting any benefit at all from their hearing aids. They also found that parents seemed to know little about the care and use of their children's hearing aids.

Fourteen years later, Robinson and Sterling (1980) studied the same metropolitan population and found only moderate improvement. Specifically, 38% of a total of 102 hearing aids did not meet electroacoustic performance specifications and 4% were missing completely. Thus, 42% of the instruments worn by children in this study were malfunctioning or missing. As shown in table 1, numerous investigators have reported similar findings over a period spanning a quarter century.

Elfenbein, Bentler, Davis, and Niebuhr, in a more recent study, examined several issues relevant to the ongoing monitoring and management of amplification systems (1988). Data were gathered for three groups of children with hearing impairment: 248 children in public schools receiving services from itinerant specialists, 43 children who were seen at a university clinic for day-long, comprehensive evaluations, and 10 who attended a six-week residential treatment program where hearing aids were checked twice each day. The first group (public schools) was studied to determine (1) the frequency of hearing aid checks, (2) the person responsible for performing those checks, and (3) assumptions of school personnel regarding the functional status of children's hearing aids. At the elementary level, it was found that many hearing aids were rarely or never checked. Only 60% of the children had their instruments checked at least once each week, and 20% received no assistance. At the middle and high school levels, children were expected to assume significantly more independence in monitoring their hearing instruments. At those grade levels, fewer than one-third had their hearing aids monitored at least once each week, and 44% reported never having them checked. The person most frequently responsible for hearing aid monitoring was the itinerant specialist; however, the investigators found that classroom teachers and others in frequent contact with the child were unaware of the high incidence of hearing aid malfunction. For the second study group, which consisted of children seen for a comprehensive evaluation at the university clinic, Elfenbein and colleagues reported that 14 of 56 hearing aids (22%) had major malfunctions of which the parents were unaware. Over 60% of binaurally aided children had malfunctioning instruments while only 10% of children aided monaurally had hearing aids that were not working properly. The third group, children enrolled in a summer residential program, allowed the examiners to investigate the functional status of children's hearing aids twice each day over the course of the six-week program. Routine problems (low voltage or missing batteries, earmold and tubing problems, etc.) occurred during 85% of the therapy

Table 1
Data on malfunction of hearing aids worn by children (adapted from Elfenbein et al. 1988, with permission).

Investigators	No. of Hearing Aids	Evaluation Procedure[1]	% Malfunction
Gaeth & Lounsbury (1966)	134	V, L, E	55-69
Zink (1972)	195 (year 1)	E	59
	92 (year 2 follow-up)	E	45
	75 (new aids)	E	47
	35 (loaner aids)	E	92
Coleman (1972)	25	V, L, E	40-50
Northern et al. (1972)	138	V, L, E	69
Findlay & Winchester (1973)	109	V, L, E	60
Porter (1973)	82	V, L, E	51
Schell (1975)	120-150	V, L, E	57
Bess (1977)	121	V	27
	35	E[2]	38a, 80b, 25-30c
Kemker et al. (1979)	836 (year 1)	V, L	28
	589 (year 2)	V, L	29
	709 (year 3)	V, L	27
	980 (year 4)	V, L	12
	1473 (year 5)	V, L	14
Robinson & Sterling (1980)	102	E	38
Potts & Greenwood (1983)	66	V, L, E	25
Elfenbein et al. (1988)	43 (clinic evals.)	V, L, E	22
	10 (residential prog.)	V, L, E	67-85[3]

[1] V: visual inspection; L: listening check; E: electroacoustic evaluation.
[2] a, did not meet specification for gain; b, did not meet specification for frequency response; c, did not meet specification for SSPL90.
[3] 67% of the hearing aids worn by children during a six-week residential program required manufacturer's repair. On 84.6% of the treatment days, at least one hearing aid malfunctioned.

period. Of even greater concern was the finding that 67% of the hearing aids worn by these children had to be returned to the manufacturer for repair at least once during the study period.

The findings of Elfenbein and colleagues, although reported several years ago and confined to a single midwestern state, typify the problems that continue to exist nationwide. These investigators recommend that the children themselves be encouraged to assume a more active role in hearing aid management. Indeed, the user is in the best position to judge the functional status of the hearing aid. Given a well-organized hearing aid management program that permits correction of minor problems when they occur and loaner instruments when more serious problems arise, older children can assume primary responsibility for monitoring and management of their hearing instruments. For younger children, involvement of family members and others who come in frequent contact with the child is critical to successful hearing aid management.

FAMILY AND INTERDISCIPLINARY ISSUES

Family members and professionals who work closely with the family are generally in the most advantageous position to observe the effects of amplification in the child's day-to-day listening environment and to ensure that the devices are used and properly maintained (Roush and Gravel 1994). But as Elfenbein and colleagues have shown, these individuals may not be aware of how frequently hearing aid problems occur or even when an instrument is malfunctioning. The audiologist must be certain that family members and others in frequent contact with the child are thoroughly instructed in the operation and care of the hearing instruments. This process can be facilitated by expanding the traditional hearing aid orientation to include multiple family members and significant others. A family-centered approach to hearing aid management has the practical advantage of increasing the number of resident troubleshooters, and it reduces the pressures on one person, usually the mother, to assume the role of family expert on such matters.

Even with careful instruction on hearing aid care and use, conscientious monitoring is unlikely unless family members have come to accept the child's hearing loss and need for amplification. Based on more than 25 years of experience directing a family-centered preschool, Luterman (1979) has observed that the condition of the child's hearing aids may serve as an indicator of how far the family has progressed in this regard, noting that hearing aid use and maintenance often improve as the parents move toward greater acceptance of their child's hearing loss. Indeed, it would appear that parent groups and other support systems contribute not only to the family's emotional well-being but to the accomplishment of practical matters as well.

In addition to accepting the hearing loss and need for amplification, parents and professionals working with the family must recognize the *benefits* of amplification. This can be accomplished through sound field demonstration combined with an explanation of test data delivered at a level appropriate for the family. We have found the graphic displays generated by the DSL method (Seewald, Zelisko, Ramji, and Jamieson 1991) to be particularly effective in this regard (chapter 8). Using the DSL software and video displays, even the unsophisticated observer can gain a conceptual understanding of how acoustic amplification provides greater access to speech and other acoustic signals.

Once oriented, people responsible for hearing aid management must have the necessary equipment to provide ongoing monitoring. Although many audiologists provide the family with a battery tester, a stethoscope, a wax loop, and other accessories, a recent report by Elfenbein (1994) indicates that approximately one-third of the families in her sample did not own these basic items. Among those who did, major signs of hearing aid malfunction were still undetected. It is clear that in addition to providing the necessary equipment for monitoring, follow-up is needed on return visits to ensure regular and appropriate use of these devices.

The delivery of consistent, high-quality amplification requires daily inspection and listening checks. Careful observation of the child's progress with amplification is also needed. Since it is not feasible for the audiologist to be involved in day-to-day management, professionals from other disciplines who interact with the child must play a key role. School personnel and early intervention specialists are often able to accompany family members to audiology appointments. For infants and young children with newly identified hearing losses, follow-up visits should occur at intervals of at least every three months. During the early stages, parents and professionals, in addition to monitoring hearing aid function, can provide valuable input regarding the child's progress with amplification. As the child gets older and audiologic follow-up visits occur less frequently, it is equally important that family members and professionals be capable of judging the adequacy of the child's amplification system so that hearing aid malfunction or changes in aided performance can be noted and reported to the audiologist. In particular, appropriate hearing aid settings must be clearly communicated, preferably in writing, to parents and caretakers. The all-too-common practice of lowering the volume when feedback is a problem defeats whatever efforts may have gone into the selection of appropriate electroacoustic characteristics. Those in frequent contact with the child need clear guidelines for troubleshooting and systematic procedures for follow-up when routine efforts are unsuccessful.

FM units are particularly prone to misuse, especially when proper settings are not clearly indicated. Indeed, an FM unit used inappropriately will be less beneficial to the child than conventional amplification. Unfortunately, school-age children may have their personal amplification managed by a clinic-based audiologist while FM selection, fitting, and adjustment occur with minimal audiologic involvement. When school-based audiology services are not available, parents should be encouraged to bring the child's FM unit to the audiology clinic for electroacoustic analysis and fitting (see Ross 1992 for an excellent review of FM evaluation and fitting strategies).

Specific activities for early interventionists or school personnel can be written into the Individualized Education Plan (IEP) or Individualized Family Service Plan (IFSP). These can include monitoring and maintenance of the child's amplification system. As noted below, instrumentation needs can also be included in the written plan.

THE ACOUSTIC ENVIRONMENT

In addition to monitoring the functional status of hearing aids, it is equally important to monitor the auditory environment where the devices are used. It is well known that adverse acoustic conditions (the interaction of noise, distance, and room reverberation) are more detrimental to listeners with impaired hearing than to children with normal hearing (chapter 11). Even carefully fitted and maintained hearing instruments are of little benefit in a poor acoustic environment. Site visits by an audiologist are necessary to ensure that the acoustic environment has been optimized to the fullest extent possible (chapter 19). The audiologist needs to consult with family members and professionals involved with the child to evaluate the listening environment and make whatever acoustic modifications are feasible.

LEGISLATIVE ISSUES

Ideally, educational personnel and others involved with the family will be thoroughly familiar with the hearing instruments and conscientious about daily monitoring. Since this is not always the case, audiologists responsible for the management of children's amplification systems should be familiar with relevant federal and state laws and how these laws can be used to facilitate monitoring and maintenance of hearing instruments.

Individuals with Disabilities Education Act, 1990. Federal regulations, originally established under Public Law 94-142 and reauthorized in subsequent legislation, require states to demonstrate their compliance with federal regulations by establishing guidelines for implementation at the local level. States have tremendous latitude in determining how they will comply with federal regulations. Hearing aid monitoring is among the many requirements of these regulations that must be managed at the state and local levels. If comprehensive guidelines are developed at the state level, they can result in better monitoring and management of hearing aids in the educational setting. Conversely, a "token" policy may be sufficient to achieve compliance with federal regulations but will do little to improve the status of children's hearing.

Federal regulations currently existing under Part B of the Individuals with Disabilities Education Act (IDEA) and published in the *Federal Register* on September 29, 1992, *require* states to develop procedures for proper monitoring and maintenance of amplification systems at the local level. Section 300.303, entitled "Proper Functioning of Hearing Aids," reads as follows: "Each public agency shall ensure that hearing aids worn by children with hearing impairments including deafness in school are functioning properly" (*Federal Register*, vol. 57, no. 189, p. 44812).

Again, note that federal regulations do not set standards for how states should meet this requirement. Rather, state departments of education are charged with establishing policies and guidelines for use by school systems to ensure proper hearing aid function. As with many other federal regulations, there is enormous variability among states in how they choose to set policy and ensure compliance. For example, some states require only the annual performance of an electroacoustic evaluation. Others have taken a more comprehensive approach. The state of North Carolina has adopted a hearing aid policy that aims to ensure proper monitoring and maintenance of amplification systems, but within reasonable boundaries of time and cost-effectiveness. It is described here for the benefit of readers who wish to review and compare existing policies in their own states.

The North Carolina Hearing Aid Monitoring Policy, summarized in table 2, was developed by the North Carolina Department of Public Instruction in cooperation with audiologists from around the state (D. Mills, personal communication). Important features include daily battery checks, daily listening checks, filing of a monthly report documenting these activities, annual electroacoustic evaluation, and in-service training for teachers and staff. The North Carolina Department of Public Instruction, through its *Hearing Conservation Guide,* recommends that staff in-services, conducted by an audiologist, occur prior to the beginning of the school year or, if not, on the first teacher work day. An amplification checklist (see appendix) is provided for classroom monitoring. The North Carolina program has been successful, in part, because written documentation is required when local education agencies are audited by state compliance officers. The implications of noncompliance can be serious. Local education agencies lacking

Table 2
Example of how one state, North Carolina, has used the federal regulations for P.L. 102-119 (IDEA) to establish a cost-effective model for ongoing monitoring of children's amplification devices.

Federal Legislation

Federal Regulations for P.L. 102-119, Individuals with Disabilities Education Act (IDEA), Section 300.303: "Proper Functioning of Hearing Aids."

State Legislation

N.C. State Law: Amendments to Article 9 require the state to enact policies for compliance with federal regulations.

State Policy, North Carolina Department of Public Instruction

The N.C. Hearing Aid Monitoring Policy is set forth in the *Hearing Conservation Guide*, N.C. Department of Public Instruction.

Requirements at the Local Level

The following activities are required at the local level to satisfy state guidelines established to ensure compliance with federal regulations:

Activity	When	By Whom
Battery Check	Daily	Teacher/Designee
Listening Check	Daily	Teacher/Designee
Summary Report	Monthly	Teacher/Designee
Electroacoustic Check	Annually	Audiologist
Training and In-Service	Annually	Audiologist

compliance with federal regulations, including appropriate documentation of hearing aid monitoring, must complete a corrective action plan. Failure to complete a corrective plan and assure implementation can result in potential loss of funding for the local education agency. Since the state audit serves as a report card for the education agency, administrators are generally quite willing to cooperate with the educational audiologist to ensure that the necessary activities are carried out and properly documented. Comprehensive guidelines must exist at the *state* level, however, so that activities required for compliance result in better aided hearing for children. Although there are no statewide data allowing comparison of North Carolina to other states with less-comprehensive guidelines, audiologists report excellent follow-through with daily monitoring procedures as well as conscientious record keeping (J. Sexton, personal communication). Likewise, officials responsible for ensuring that federal regulations are implemented at the state level report nearly 100% compliance (M. Meany, personal communication).

Audiologists are encouraged to examine and evaluate the hearing aid monitoring policies in their states. If guidelines are insufficient or if they lack appropriate enforcement, it may be possible to form a task force of audiologists, parents, and officials from the state department of education to collaborate on revising or expanding policies for hearing aid management. Even with careful hearing aid monitoring, however, the delivery of consistent, high-quality amplification remains an enormous challenge. Comprehensive monitoring does not prevent hearing aid malfunctions from occurring. It can, however, ensure that problems are identified soon after they arise so that corrective steps can be taken in a timely manner.

REPAIRS AND FINANCIAL CONSIDERATIONS

Improved hearing aid monitoring inevitably results in a larger number of hearing aids needing repair. Although the financial implications can be substantial, it makes little sense to establish comprehensive monitoring practices unless there are efficient mechanisms for follow-up. Traditionally, school systems have absorbed the expense of purchasing and maintaining group amplification systems (e.g., FM transmitters/receivers) while families or applicable third parties have been responsible for purchase and maintenance of personal amplification. In November 1993, the Office of Special Education Programs of the U.S. Department of Education ruled that *for children over 3 years of age:*

> A hearing aid is considered a covered device under the definition of "assistive technology device." Thus, where a district has determined that a child with a disability requires a hearing aid in order to receive a free and appropriate public education and the child's I.E.P. specifies that the child needs a hearing aid, the district is responsible for providing the hearing aid at no cost to the child and his or her parents in accordance with 34 CFR 300.308. *(Individuals with Disabilities Education Law Report,* vol 20, pp. 1216-1217).

Although the issue of repairs was not specifically addressed in this ruling, it can be assumed that the local education agency would be responsible for maintenance of that instrument as well.

Schools are required by federal regulation to assure that each child with a hearing loss, beginning at age 3, has appropriate amplification. Schools are not required to assure such for children *under* the age of 3 unless the state education agency has a state law mandating services for children under 3 or has been given responsibility for the implementation of Part H (Infant and Toddler Program, birth to age 3) of P.L. 102-119 (an amendment to P.L. 99-457, the federal special education law that provides funding and requirements for early intervention services to children with disabilities from birth through age 5).

The advent of ear-level FM systems raises some interesting new questions. Although local education agencies are not required to purchase a particular *type* of hearing instrument, many are now choosing this option. Ear-level FM instruments incorporate features of both group and personal amplification. If the local education agency purchases an ear-level FM unit, should the child be permitted to use the instrument outside the school setting? And if so, who is responsible for the management and repair of this instrument if problems arise outside the school setting? Audiologists will be called upon to resolve these and other questions related to the provision and maintenance of hearing aids as state and federal regulations change or undergo further interpretation.

CONCLUSIONS

Nearly all children, regardless of age, degree of hearing loss, or educational setting, derive substantial benefit from hearing aids and other sensory devices. Regardless of how carefully and accurately these instruments are selected and fitted, however, their benefits will be minimal without rigorous monitoring and management. Parents, other professionals, and the youngsters themselves can and must play an active role in this process. The desired outcome is most likely to occur if systematic procedures are established at the state level and successfully implemented at the local level. This requires the audiologist to encourage family members and professionals from other disciplines to acquire the knowledge and skills needed to successfully operate and maintain the child's hearing instruments. It also requires the audiologist to assume an active role in the development of the child's educational or early intervention plan. For children under 3 years of age, the "multidisciplinary team evaluation" required in conjunction with the development of an IFSP under Part H of Public Law 102-119 (IDEA) is the appropriate mechanism for involvement. For children over the age of 3, these issues are addressed in the Individualized Education Plan (IEP) under Part B of this law.

The following general recommendations are made in an effort to improve the functional status of children's amplification systems:

1. Older children should be thoroughly familiar with their hearing instruments and encouraged to assume primary responsibility for their operation and maintenance. For younger children, family members and related professionals need a comprehensive orientation as well as the basic necessities for ongoing management (battery testers, listening devices, etc.). Verification of regular and appropriate use of these devices must occur at each follow-up appointment.

2. The traditional hearing aid orientation and subsequent follow-up visits will be more effective if they include as many family members and other relevant individuals as possible. If acceptable to the family, significant others can include early intervention personnel or itinerant specialists who work with the child. Specific roles for these professionals can be written into the IEP or IFSP. Family members and professionals should be encouraged to play an active role not only in hearing aid monitoring but also in providing input to the audiologist regarding the child's progress with amplification.

3. Hearing aids and related equipment (FM transmitters, etc.) must be checked at least once each day. This goal is most easily accomplished if daily monitoring is required by state guidelines for compliance with section 300.303 of the federal regulations. Audiologists are encouraged to review their state policies regarding hearing aid monitoring and to pursue revision or expansion of these guidelines where needed.

4. Specific procedures must be established to deal with hearing aid malfunctions when they occur. Mechanisms must exist for immediate correction of minor problems and timely follow-up for instruments needing outside repairs. Loaner instruments must be available during these periods.

Nearly three decades have passed since Gaeth and Lounsbury first reported on the functional status of children's hearing aids (1966). Although some improvements have occurred, progress has been minimal in comparison to technological advances in the design and fitting of hearing aids. Only through systematic monitoring and management procedures, combined with well-informed family members and professionals, will technological advances in the design and fitting of hearing instruments translate into better hearing for the children who use them.

ACKNOWLEDGMENTS

The author gratefully acknowledges the contributions of Mr. David Mills, Chief Consultant for the Areas of Exceptionality Section, Exceptional Children Support Team, North Carolina Department of Public Instruction, Raleigh, North Carolina.

REFERENCES

Bess, F.H. 1977. Condition of hearing aids worn by children in a public school setting. Publication no. OE 77-05002. Washington, D.C.: Department of Health, Education, and Welfare.

Coleman, R.F. 1972. Stability of children's hearing aids in an acoustic preschool. Final Report, Project 522466, Grant no. 6-4-71-00. Washington, D.C.: Department of Health, Education, and Welfare.

Elfenbein, J. 1994. Monitoring preschoolers' hearing aids: Issues in program design and implementation. *American Journal of Audiology*, July, 65-70.

Elfenbein, J., Bentler, R., Davis, J., and Niebuhr, D. 1988. Status of school children's hearing aids relative to monitoring practices. *Ear and Hearing* 9(4):212-217.

Findlay, R.C., and Winchester, R. 1973. Defects in hearing aids worn by preschool and school-age children. Paper presented at the convention of the American Speech and Hearing Association, Detroit, Michigan.

Gaeth, J.H., and Lounsbury, E. 1966. Hearing aids and children in elementary schools. *Journal of Speech and Hearing Disorders* 31:283-289.

Kemker, F.J., McConnell, F., Logan, S.A., and Green, B.W. 1979. A field study of children's hearing aids in a school environment. *Language, Speech and Hearing Services in the Schools* 10(1):47-53.

Luterman, D. 1979. *Counseling the parents of hearing impaired children*. Boston: Little, Brown.

Meany, M. April 1994. Personal communication.

Mills, D. January 1994. Personal communication.

Northern, J.L., McChord, W., Fischer, E., and Evans, P. 1972. Hearing services in residential schools for the deaf. *Maico Audiology Library* 11(4):16-18.

Porter, T.A. 1973. Hearing aids in a residential school. *American Annals of the Deaf* 118:31-33.

Potts, P.L., and Greenwood, J. 1983. Hearing aid monitoring: Are looking and listening enough? *Language, Speech and Hearing Services in Schools* 14:157-163.

Robinson, D.O., and Sterling, G.R. 1980. Hearing aids and children in school: A follow-up study. *Volta Review* 82:229-235.

Ross, M. 1992. Room acoustics and speech perception. In M. Ross (ed.), *FM auditory training systems: Characteristics, selection, and use*. Baltimore: York Press.

Roush, J., and Gravel, J.S. 1994. Acoustic amplification and sensory devices for infants and toddlers. In J. Roush and N.D. Matkin (eds.), *Infants and toddlers with hearing loss: Family-centered assessment and intervention.* Baltimore: York Press.

Schell, V. 1975. A program for the electroacoustic evaluation of hearing aids. Paper presented at the convention of the American Speech and Hearing Association, Washington, D.C.

Seewald, R.C., Zelisko, D.L., Ramji, K.V., and Jamieson, D.G. 1991. *DSL user's manual.* London, Ontario: University of Western Ontario.

Sexton, J. February 1994. Personal communication.

Zink, G.D. 1972. Hearing aids children wear: A longitudinal study of performance. *Volta Review* 74:41-52.

Appendix
Amplification Checklist Used in the North Carolina Public Schools

Amplification Checklist

School Year: _____
Date: _____

Student: _____ School: _____
Amplification: _____
_____

Hearing Aid Serial Numbers: Right: _____
Left: _____

Auditory Trainer Serial Number: _____

Date	Hearing Aid: Right	Hearing Aid: Left	Auditory Trainer: Right	Auditory Trainer: Left	5 Sound Test AH EE U SH S	Comments

Key:
- √ Aids are working
- H Student left aids at home
- NW Not working: **Notify Teacher of the Hearing Impaired or the Audiologist**
- A Student was absent
- R Sent for repair

11

Sound-Field Amplification in the Classroom: Applied and Theoretical Issues

Carl C. Crandell and Joseph J. Smaldino

INTRODUCTION

The acoustic conditions of a classroom are important factors in the psychoeducational and psychosocial achievement of children with normal hearing and children with hearing impairment. Inappropriate levels of classroom reverberation and/or noise can compromise not only speech perception but also behavior, concentration, attention, reading/spelling ability, and academic achievement (Bess and Tharpe 1986; Blair, Peterson, and Viehweg 1985; Crandell 1991, 1993a; Crandell and Bess 1986; Crandell and Smaldino 1992, 1995b; Crandell, Smaldino, and Flexer 1995; Davis, Elfenbein, Schum, and Bentler 1986; Finitzo-Hieber 1988; Finitzo-Hieber and Tillman 1978; Leavitt and Flexer 1991; Ross 1978; Ross and Giolas 1971). Reduced teacher performance, including increases in teacher stress and vocal fatigue, has also been shown to be related to classroom acoustics (Crandell, Smaldino, and Flexer 1995; Flexer 1989; Gilman and Danzer 1989). Research has demonstrated that acceptable speech communication is possible in a classroom if reverberation times (RTs) do not surpass 0.4 seconds, signal-to-noise (S/N) ratios are at least +15 dB, and ambient noise levels do not exceed 30 to 35 dBA (Bess and McConnell 1981; Crandell and Bess 1986, 1987; Crandell and Smaldino 1992, 1995a, 1995b; Crum and Matkin 1976: Finitzo-Hieber 1988; Finitzo-Hieber and Tillman 1978; Fourcin et al. 1980; Gengel 1971; McCroskey and Devens 1975; Niemoeller 1968; Olsen 1977, 1981, 1988). An examination of the literature, however, indicates that it is uncommon for these acceptable acoustic conditions to exist in typical educational settings. Specifically, the range of reverberation times for classrooms is typically reported to be from 0.4 to 1.2 seconds, while classroom S/N ratios range from +5 to -7 dB (Blair 1977; Crandell 1991; Crandell, Smaldino, and Flexer 1995; Finitzo-Hieber 1988; Finitzo-Hieber and Tillman 1978; Kodaras 1960; Markides 1986; McCroskey and Devens 1975; Paul 1967; Pearsons, Bennett, and Fidell 1977; Ross 1978; Sanders 1965). In a recent investigation, Crandell and Smaldino (1995a) reported that only 7 of 32 classrooms (22%) used for children with hearing impairment actually met recommended criteria for RTs. Even more discouraging, none of the classrooms achieved recommended criteria for ambient noise levels.

One strategy to decrease the deleterious influences of impoverished classroom acoustics is the utilization of a sound-field frequency modulation (FM) amplification system. With such a system, speech is picked up via a wireless microphone located near the teacher's mouth, amplified, and delivered to the students via a room loudspeaker system. It has been reported that the use of sound-field FM systems in the educational environment can significantly augment not only perceptual ability in pediatric listeners, but also psychoeducational/psychosocial achievement (Berg 1987, 1993; Crandell and Bess 1987; Crandell and Smaldino 1992, 1995a,b; Flexer, Millin, and Brown 1990; Jones, Berg, and Viehweg 1989; Ray 1987; Ray, Sarff, and Glassford 1984; Sarff 1981; Sarff, Ray, and Bagwell 1981). The present chapter will examine several applied and theoretical issues concerning the use of sound-field FM amplification in the classroom. The following areas will be addressed: (1) description and current availability of commercially available sound-field FM amplification systems; (2) pediatric populations considered appropriate for use of sound-field amplification; (3) effects of FM sound-field amplification on speech perception and psychoeducational/psychosocial development; (4) comparative analysis of commercially available sound-field FM amplification systems; (5) cost-effectiveness of sound-field FM amplification systems; and (6) comparison of sound-field amplification with other forms of classroom amplification. The reader is directed to additional sources (Beranek 1954; Bess and McConnell 1981; Crandell and Bess 1986, 1987; Crandell and Smaldino 1992, 1995a,b; Crandell, Smaldino, and Flexer 1995; Finitzo-Hieber 1988; Finitzo-Hieber and Tillman 1978; Knudsen and Harris 1978; Niemoeller 1968; Olsen 1977, 1981, 1988; Ross 1978) for discussions pertaining to other strategies, such as acoustic modifications, to enhance speech perception in the classroom.

DESCRIPTION/CURRENT AVAILABILITY OF SOUND-FIELD FM AMPLIFICATION SYSTEMS

The components of a sound-field FM system are presented in figure 1. A sound-field FM system is essentially a room public address system, in

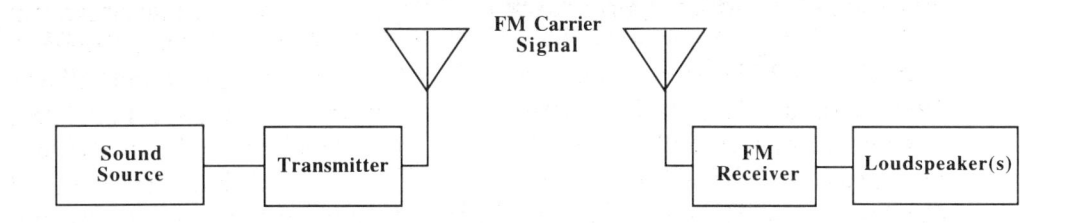

Figure 1. Block diagram of sound-field amplification system.

which speech is picked up via an FM wireless microphone located near the speaker's mouth (thus decreasing the speaker-listener distance), where the detrimental effects of reverberation and noise are minimal. The acoustic signal is then converted to an electrical waveform and transmitted via an FM signal to a receiver. The electrical signal is then amplified, converted back to an acoustic waveform, and conveyed to listeners in the room via one or more strategically placed loudspeakers. The objectives when placing a sound-field FM system in a classroom are twofold: (1) to amplify the speaker's voice by approximately 8 to 10 dB, thus improving the S/N ratio of the listening environment; and (2) to provide amplification uniformly throughout the classroom regardless of teacher or student position. Sound-field systems vary from compact, portable, battery-powered single-speaker units to more permanently placed, alternating current (AC)-powered speaker systems that use multiple (usually four) loudspeakers. Several companies manufacture sound-field FM amplification systems that range in price from approximately $600 to $1700. Information concerning companies that manufacture sound-field systems can be found at the end of this chapter.

APPROPRIATE POPULATIONS FOR UTILIZATION OF SOUND-FIELD AMPLIFICATION

For optimal learning to occur in the academic environment, the teacher's voice must be highly intelligible to all children. Consequently, sound-field FM amplification is appropriate for all children who experience perceptual difficulties under typical classroom listening conditions. While it is well known that listeners with sensorineural hearing loss (SNHL) experience greater perceptual deficits in noise and/or reverberation than children with normal hearing, a number of children with normal hearing sensitivity also experience significant difficulties understanding noisy or reverberated speech (Bess 1985; Boney and Bess 1984; Crandell 1991, 1992: Crandell and Smaldino 1992, 1995b; Crandell, Smaldino, and Flexer 1995;

Nabelek and Nabelek 1985). These listeners include children with fluctuating conductive hearing loss, learning disabilities, articulation disorders, central auditory processing deficits, language disorders, attention deficits, minimal degrees of SNHL (pure-tone sensitivity from 15 to 25 dB HL), unilateral hearing loss, and developmental delays. Crandell (1993a) examined the speech-recognition abilities of children with minimal degrees of sensorineural hearing loss at commonly reported classroom S/N ratios ranging from +6 to -6 dB. Then children with minimal hearing impairment exhibited pure-tone averages (.5 to 2 kHz) from 15 to 25 dB HL. Speech recognition was assessed with the Bamford-Koval-Bench (BKB) Standard Sentence Test (Bench, Koval, and Bamford 1979). The multitalker babble from the Speech Perception to Noise (SPIN) Test was utilized as the noise competition (Kalikow, Stevens, and Elliott 1977). Mean sentential recognition scores for children with minimal hearing impairment and a control group of children with normal hearing, as a function of varying S/N ratios, are presented in figure 2. Trends from these data are similar to those reported in children with more pronounced degrees of SNHL (Finitzo-Hieber and Tillman 1978). That

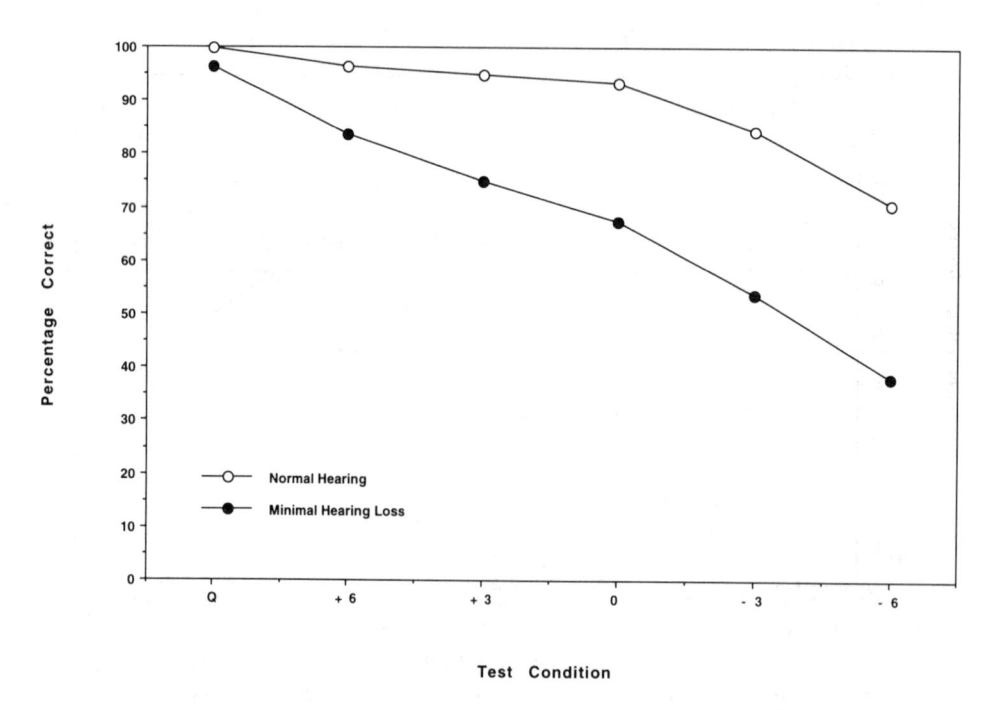

Figure 2. Mean sentential recognition scores, in percentage correct, as a function of signal-to-noise ratio for children with normal hearing sensitivity (indicated by the open circles) and children with minimal hearing impairment (indicated by the closed circles). Reprinted with permission from Crandell, C., Smaldino, J., and Flexer, C. 1995. *Sound field FM amplification: Theory and practical applications.* San Diego: Singular Press.

is, children with minimal degrees of SNHL performed poorer than children with normal hearing across most listening conditions. Moreover, the differences in recognition scores between the two groups increased as the listening environment became more unfavorable. For example, at an S/N ratio of +6 dB, both groups obtained recognition scores in excess of 80%. At an S/N ratio of -6 dB, however, the group with minimal hearing impairment obtained less than 50% correct recognition compared to approximately 75% recognition ability for the children with normal hearing.

In a similar investigation, Crandell (1994) examined the speech recognition of 20 native English-speaking children and 20 non-native English-speaking children under classroom SNRs of +6, +3, 0, -3, and -6 dB. Speech recognition was assessed by BKB sentences, while the SPIN multibabble was used as the noise competition. Results from this investigation are shown in figure 3. Note that the same trends in speech recognition as demonstrated for the children with minimal hearing impairment are shown for these populations. That is, although both groups obtained essentially equivalent speech-recognition scores in quiet, the non-native English-speaking group performed significantly poorer as the listening environment became less favorable.

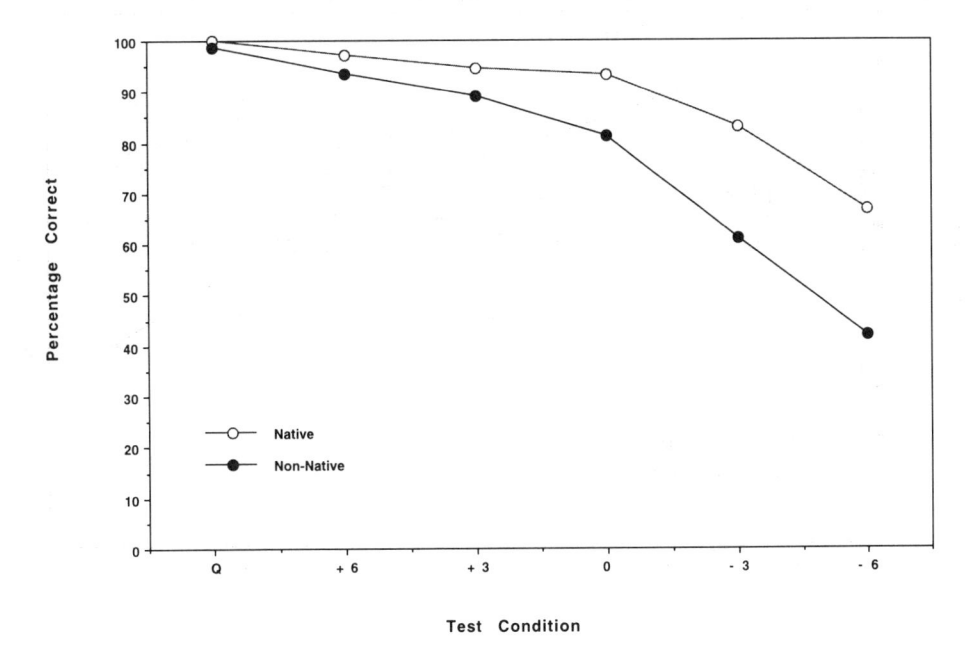

Figure 3. Mean sentential recognition scores, in percentage correct, as a function of signal-to-noise ratio for native English-speaking children (indicated by the open circles) and non-native English-speaking children (indicated by the closed circles). Reprinted with permission from Crandell, C., Smaldino, J., and Flexer, C. 1995. *Sound field FM application: Theory and practical applications*. San Diego: Singular Press.

Further, young listeners (<13 to 15 years old) require higher S/N ratios than adult listeners to achieve equivalent recognition scores (Crandell and Bess 1987; Elliott 1979, 1982; Elliott, Connors, Kille, Levin, Ball, and Katz 1979; Finitzo-Hieber and Tillman 1978; Nabelek and Robinson 1982). Elliott (1982) and Nabelek and Robinson (1982) reported that young listeners require an additional 10 dB of signal strength to produce equivalent recognition scores to those of adults. Presumably, the additional signal is necessary to provide adequate acoustic cues to the immature auditory and linguistic system. It is thus reasonable to assume that commonly reported levels of classroom reverberation and noise have the potential of adversely affecting speech recognition in many pediatric listeners. To support this assumption, let us examine speech-recognition data from the seminal article by Finitzo-Hieber and Tillman (1978). In this investigation, the authors evaluated monosyllabic word recognition at various S/N ratios (S/N ratios = +12 dB, +6 dB, 0 dB) and reverberation times (RTs = 0.0, 0.4, and 1.2 seconds). Subjects included 12 children with SNHL and 12 children with normal hearing, ages 8 to 12 years. Results for the children with normal hearing sensitivity and hearing impairment are presented in table 1. Note that at an S/N ratio of +6 dB and an RT of 0.4 seconds (acoustic conditions rarely found in a classroom), the children with normal hearing obtained mean

Table 1
Mean speech-recognition scores, in percentage correct, of children with normal hearing and hearing impairment for monosyllabic words across various signal-to-noise ratios and reverberation times (adapted from Finitzo-Hieber and Tillman 1978).

Test Condition	Normal Hearing	Hearing Impaired
RT = 0.0 Seconds		
Quiet	94.5	83.0
+12 dB	89.2	70.0
+ 6 dB	79.7	59.5
0 dB	60.2	39.0
RT = 0.4 Seconds		
Quiet	92.5	74.0
+12 dB	82.8	60.2
+ 6 dB	71.3	52.2
0 dB	47.7	27.8
RT = 1.2 Seconds		
Quiet	76.5	45.0
+12 dB	68.8	41.2
+ 6 dB	54.2	27.0
0 dB	29.7	11.2

[Figure: graph showing Percentage Correct vs Speaker-Listener Distance (Feet), with points approximately at 6 ft ≈ 89%, 12 ft ≈ 55%, 24 ft ≈ 36%]

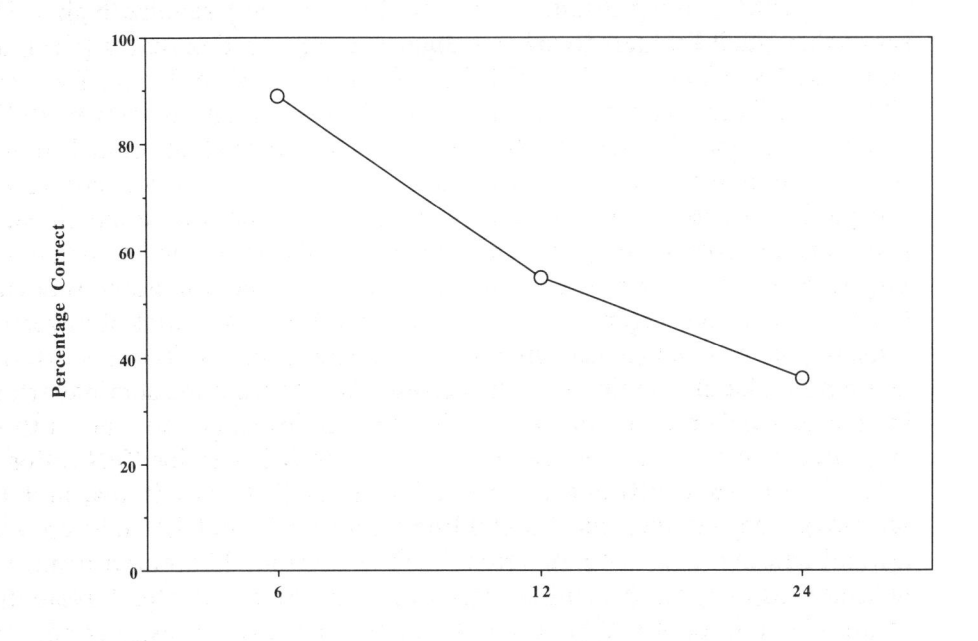

Figure 4. Mean sentential recognition scores, in percentage correct, as a function of speaker-listener distance for children with normal hearing in a typical classroom (signal-to-noise ratio = +6 dB; reverberation time = 0.45 seconds). Reprinted with permission from Crandell, C., Smaldino, J., and Flexer, C. 1995. *Sound field FM amplification: Theory and practical applications.* San Diego: Singular Press.

recognition scores of 71.3%. At more commonly reported classroom conditions, recognition scores were considerably poorer. For example, at an S/N ratio of 0 dB and an RT of 1.2 seconds, mean recognition scores decreased to 29.7%.

Crandell and Bess (1986) also examined the speech recognition of young children with normal hearing under difficult classroom listening conditions (S/N ratio = +6 dB; RT = 0.45 seconds). Sentential materials were recorded through the Knowles Electronics Mannequin for Acoustic Research (KEMAR) manikin at speaker-listener distances often encountered in the classroom (6, 12, and 24 feet). Subjects consisted of children 5 to 7 years of age. Results from this investigation are presented in figure 4. As can be noted, there was a systematic decrease in speech-recognition ability as a function of increased speaker-listener distance. Specifically, mean recognition scores of 89%, 55%, and 36% were obtained at 6, 12, and 24 feet, respectively. Overall, these results suggest that children with normal hearing seated in the middle to rear of a typical classroom setting have greater difficulty understanding speech than has traditionally been suspected.

Certainly, such decreased perceptual ability would not be appropriate for optimal learning in the classroom setting.

EFFECTS OF SOUND-FIELD AMPLIFICATION IN CHILDREN

Numerous investigations have shown that when sound-field amplification systems are positioned within the classroom, psychoeducational and psychosocial improvements occur even for children with normal hearing sensitivity (Allen 1993; Allen and Patton 1990; Benafield 1990; Berg, Bateman, and Viehweg 1989; Blair, Myrup, and Viehweg 1989; Crandell and Bess 1987; Flexer 1989; Flexer, Millin, and Brown 1990; Flexer, Richards, and Buie 1993; Gilman and Danzer 1989; Jones, Berg, and Viehweg 1989; Neuss, Blair, and Viehweg 1991; Ray, Sarff, and Glassford 1984; Rosenberg, Blake-Rahter, Allen, and Redmond 1994; Sarff 1981; Zabel and Tabor 1993). Despite this evidence, recent estimates suggest that only 4% of audiologists regularly recommend sound-field FM amplification systems (see chapter 5) for children with hearing impairment. This section will examine data on the effects of sound-field amplification on speech perception, academic achievement, behavioral characteristics, and teacher acceptance.

SOUND-FIELD FM AMPLIFICATION AND SPEECH PERCEPTION

Crandell and Bess (1987) examined the effects of sound-field amplification on the speech recognition of young children (5 to 7 years old) with normal hearing in a classroom environment (S/N ratio = +6 dB; RT = 0.45 seconds). Monosyllabic words were recorded through the KEMAR manikin at several speaker-listener distances (6, 12, and 24 feet) in amplified and unamplified conditions. Results from this investigation are presented in figure 5. The use of sound-field amplification produced significant improvements in speech recognition for the children, particularly at speaker-listener distances of 12 and 24 feet. Specifically, speech recognition scores improved 8% at 6 feet, 22% at 12 feet, and 31% at 24 feet in the aided condition.

Jones, Berg, and Viehweg (1989) compared the traditional educational strategy of improving speaker-listener distance (i.e., preferential seating) to the utilization of sound-field amplification on the speech recognition of 18 children with normal hearing and 18 children with minimal degrees of SNHL. Speech recognition was assessed by the Northwestern Children's Perception of Speech Test (NU-CHIPS) (Katz and Elliott 1978) presented at a commonly reported speaker-listener distance (12 feet), a speaker-listener distance that represented preferential seating (4 feet), and under a sound-field amplification listening condition. Results indicated that both groups of children, particularly the children with minimal degrees of SNHL, obtained

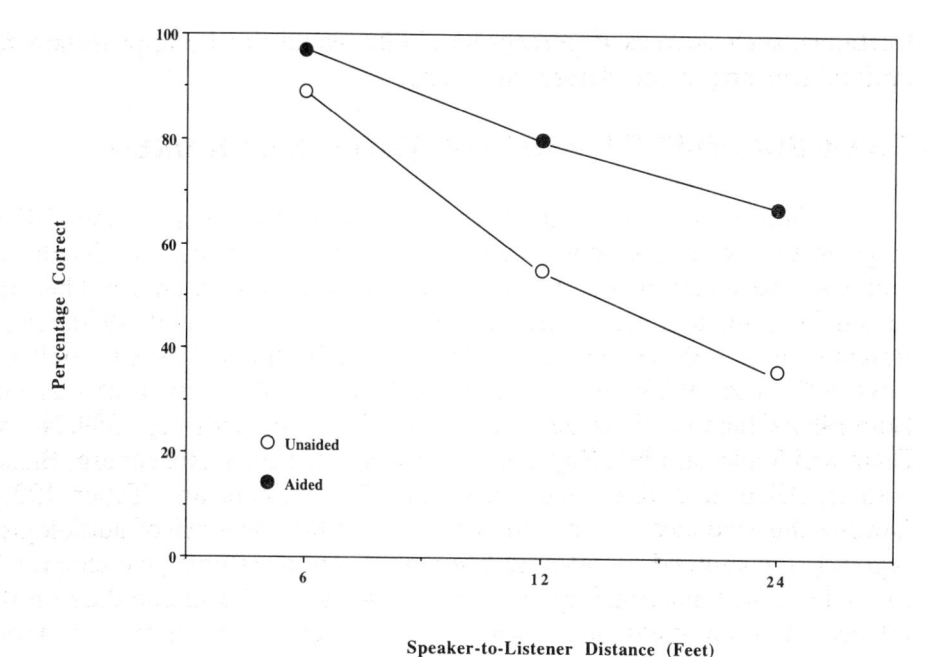

[Figure: Line graph showing Percentage Correct vs Speaker-to-Listener Distance (Feet) for Unaided (open circles) and Aided (closed circles) conditions at 6, 12, and 24 feet.]

Figure 5. Mean sentential recognition scores, in percentage correct, for children with normal hearing in an amplified (closed circles) and unamplified (open circles) listening condition. Crandell and Bess (1987).

higher speech-recognition scores under sound-field listening conditions or preferential seating than at commonly reported speaker-listener distances. For example, the children with minimal degrees of SNHL obtained recognition scores of 97%, 96%, and 81% for the sound-field, preferential seating, and traditional seating conditions, respectively. No significant differences in performance were noted between the amplified listening conditions and preferential seating. However, because of teacher movement, few children who receive preferential seating are at speaker-listener distances of 4 feet or less throughout the majority of the academic day. In fact, it appears that the only time in the classroom setting where such a speaker-listener distance is routinely obtained is during small group instruction (Crandell, Smaldino, and Flexer 1995).

Flexer, Millin, and Brown (1990) investigated whether sound-field amplification could improve monosyllabic word recognition in nine students with normal hearing who had developmental disabilities. Subjects ranged in age from 4 to 6 years and were all enrolled in a primary-level class for children with developmental disabilities. Speech perception, which was assessed in the children's classroom, was determined by the Word Intelligibility by Picture Identification (WIPI) Test (Ross and Lerman 1970).

Two conclusions were drawn from the investigation. First, each of the nine children made significantly fewer errors on a word identification task when the teacher presented the words through the sound-field amplification system (1.4 average errors) than when the words were presented without amplification (3.9 average errors). Second, an informal observational analysis showed the children to be more relaxed and to respond more quickly to the teacher's instruction in the amplified listening condition.

Zabel and Tabor (1993) investigated the influence of sound-field amplification on spelling test performance in 145 elementary school (third, fourth, and fifth grade) children with normal hearing. Spelling words were taken from the Iowa Spelling Scale (Green 1954). All words were presented in a traditional, unamplified (S/N ratio = 0 dB) and amplified (S/N ratio = +12 dB) listening condition. Data from this investigation indicated that each of the grade groups achieved significant improvements in spelling scores under the amplified listening conditions. Overall, mean average spelling scores improved from 78% to 92% correct in the amplified listening condition.

Despite the well-recognized perceptual difficulties of children with SNHL, few studies have examined the effects of sound-field amplification on children with hearing impairment. Blair, Myrup, and Viehweg (1989) assessed word-recognition ability in a classroom under three different conditions of amplification: (1) sound-field amplification in conjunction with the child's personal hearing aid; (2) personal hearing aid; and (3) personal FM system with a neckloop configuration. Subjects consisted of ten children with mild-to-moderate degrees of SNHL. Although statistical analyses were not conducted by the authors, mean data indicated that the personal FM unit provided the highest speech-recognition scores (87%). In addition, mean data indicated that the combination of the child's personal hearing aid with a sound-field FM amplification system produced higher recognition scores (82%) than just the utilization of a personal hearing aid (70%).

Neuss, Blair, and Viehweg (1991) examined the perceptual abilities of seven children with minimal degrees of SNHL under three classroom listening conditions: (1) aided with personal amplification; (2) unaided; and (3) sound-field amplification. All children exhibited pure-tone thresholds ranging from 15 to 40 dB HL. The RT of the experimental classrooms used in this investigation was 0.5 seconds, and the S/N ratio was +5 dB. Phonetically Balanced Kindergarten (PBK-50) word lists were presented to each child at a speaker-listener distance of 6 feet. Results indicated that there was a significant difference between speech-recognition scores obtained in the sound-field FM and unaided listening conditions (57% to 47%). However, no significant differences in speech-recognition performance were noted between the use of the sound-field FM amplification system (57%) and the child's personal hearing aid (55%). Individual data indicated that three of the

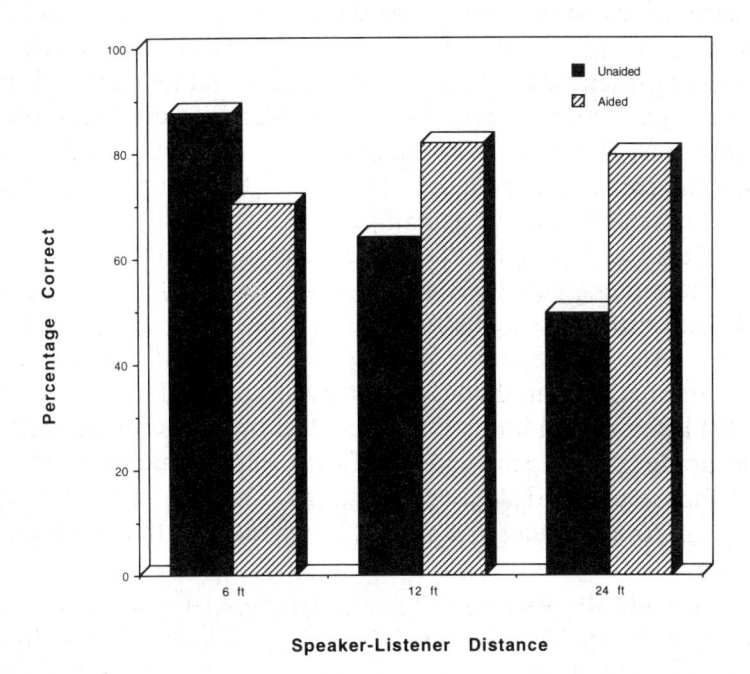

Figure 6. Mean sentential recognition sores, in percentage correct, for non-native English-speaking children in an amplified (dashed bars) and unamplified listening condition (solid bars). Reprinted with permission from Crandell, C., Smaldino, J., and Flexer, C. 1995. *Sound field FM amplification: Theory and practical applications*. San Diego: Singular Press.

subjects obtained higher recognition scores when using sound-field amplification, three performed best with their personal amplification, and one demonstrated the most improvement in the unaided listening condition.

Crandell (1995) studied the amplified and unamplified speech recognition of native and non-native English-speaking children with normal hearing at various speaker-listener distances (6, 12, and 24 feet) in a classroom environment (S/N ratio = +6 dB; RT = 0.6 seconds). PBK-50 monosyllabic word lists were recorded through the KEMAR manikin in amplified and unamplified listening conditions at several speaker-listener distances. Results from this investigation (figure 6) indicated that the speech recognition of the non-native English-speaking children was significantly improved with the utilization of sound-field amplification at speaker-listener distances of 12 and 24 feet. It is interesting to note that sound-field amplification provided consistent recognition scores of approximately 80% for the non-native children at each speaker-listener distance.

SOUND-FIELD FM AMPLIFICATION AND ACADEMIC ACHIEVEMENT

In what is often considered the original investigation on sound-field amplification, the Mainstream Amplification Resource Room Study (MARRS) examined the following educational strategies on academic achievement: (1) children in typical classrooms; (2) children receiving regular classroom instruction supplemented by resource room instruction; and (3) children educated in the regular classroom utilizing sound-field amplification (Ray, Sarff, and Glassford 1984; Sarff 1981). Students consisted of children with normal hearing and children with minimal degrees of SNHL. Results indicated that both groups of children, particularly the ones with minimal hearing impairment, demonstrated significant improvements in academic achievement, particularly in reading, when receiving amplified instruction. Younger children tended to demonstrate greater academic improvements than older children. Further, improvements in academic achievement in the amplified group were obtained at a faster rate, to a higher level, and with reduced cost when compared to the unamplified group.

In a three-year longitudinal investigation, the Putnam County (Ohio) Office of Education examined the influence of sound-field amplification on various academic areas for kindergarten and lower-grade elementary school children (Flexer 1989). The Iowa Test of Basic Skills (TBS) (1967), conducted pre- and postsound-field implementation, indicated significantly higher Iowa TBS scores in vocabulary, math concepts, math computation, math problem solving, listening, and language for children receiving amplified instruction. Data from this investigation revealed the most significant improvements in these areas within the younger (kindergarten) children. Teachers involved in this study noted that when children utilized the sound-field system to interact with other students, they displayed improved voicing skills, produced longer utterances, and displayed more confidence when speaking. Moreover, observational studies revealed that students in amplified classrooms exhibited improved on-task behaviors. Finally, school principals reported a reduction in teacher absences due to vocal fatigue and/or laryngitis when teachers used amplified instruction.

The Improving Classroom Acoustics (ICA) Project compared student behavior, listening skills, and academic achievement in amplified and unamplified classrooms for kindergarten to second grade students (Rosenberg, Blake-Rahter, Allen, and Redmond 1994). Pre- and postamplification information was obtained for 855 students in 20 experimental (amplified) classrooms and 20 control (unamplified) classrooms. Student behavior, listening skills, and academic achievement were evaluated at three time intervals (presound-field placement, 6 weeks postplacement, and 12 weeks postplacement) by materials developed by the Florida Department of Education. Results of this investigation indicated that students in the amplified classrooms demonstrated significantly greater improvements in behavior, listening, and academic achievement than students in traditional classroom teaching environments. These significant differences in performance were noted even after only 6 weeks of sound-field utilization. Moreover, 93.3% of the students responded affirmatively to the use of the sound-field systems, while 100% of the teachers wanted to keep the system in the classroom after the study was completed.

SOUND-FIELD AMPLIFICATION AND BEHAVIORAL CHARACTERISTICS

Sound-field amplification has also been shown to positively affect student classroom behavior. Gilman and Danzer (1989), for example, conducted a pre- and postassessment of classroom amplification effects on the behavioral characteristics of second and fourth grade students. Results indicated that in classrooms with sound-field amplification, students demonstrated an increased attentiveness to verbal instruction and an increased ability to hear and follow classroom instruction. Allen and Patton (1990), using observational assessments, noted that children under amplified instruction were less distractable, required fewer repetitions by the teacher, exhibited higher on-task behavior, and were generally more attentive. Benafield (1990) reported that sound-field amplification improved physical attending behaviors in 4- to 5-year-old children with speech and language delays.

Flexer, Richards, and Buie (1993) examined teacher perception of no-risk children (children with a negative history of hearing difficulties) and at-risk children (children with a history of early, recurrent hearing difficulties in amplified and unamplified classroom listening conditions). A total of 283 children were evaluated in this investigation. Teacher perception was evaluated by the Screening Instrument for Targeting Educational Risk (SIFTER) (Anderson 1989). The SIFTER includes 15 questions in the areas of attention, communication, class participation, school behavior, and academics. The SIFTERs were completed by the teachers four times during the academic year. SIFTER data indicated that both groups of children, particularly the at-risk students, achieved significantly higher teacher ratings (across all areas assessed by the SIFTER) when amplified instruction was used. The at-risk students who were receiving unamplified instruction obtained the lowest teacher appraisals on the SIFTER.

TEACHER PERCEPTION OF SOUND-FIELD AMPLIFICATION

Research suggests that teachers overwhelmingly accept sound-field amplification systems once they either receive an in-service on the instrumentation or actually utilize the equipment (Allen 1993; Berg 1993;

Crandell, Smaldino, and Flexer 1995). Crandell, Smaldino, and Flexer (1995) reported that 90% to 95% of all teachers readily accept sound-field amplification once they have been provided the opportunity to use this equipment, even on a limited basis. Allen (1993) conducted a teacher survey of the importance of instructional delivery equipment (televisions, overhead projectors, computers, VCRs, CD-ROMs, filmstrip projectors, and sound-field amplification) in three groups of teachers. The groups consisted of teachers with (1) no experience with sound-field amplification; (2) indirect experience with sound-field amplification; and (3) direct experience (at least three days) with sound-field amplification. Results of this investigation indicated that when the teachers received even minimal contact with sound-field systems, such equipment quickly became the top choice (34%) in instructional delivery equipment. Further, teachers who indicated no or indirect experience with sound-field amplification rated the overhead projector as the most beneficial instructional delivery equipment in the classroom.

COMPARATIVE ANALYSIS OF COMMERCIALLY AVAILABLE SOUND-FIELD AMPLIFICATION SYSTEMS

Although sound-field amplification systems have consistently been shown to benefit both speech recognition and academic achievement, it remains unclear which commercially available system is the most cost-effective for use in the classroom. Mills (1991) compared preschool and kindergarten teacher opinions concerning maintenance, cost-effectiveness, and sound fidelity. Three sound-field units were evaluated: (1) Comtek Omni-2001; (2) Lifeline Freefield Classroom Amplification System; and (3) Phonic Ear Easy Listener. Results indicated that the teachers felt that the Phonic Ear Easy Listener was the easiest to maintain, most cost-effective, and most maintenance free.

Crandell (1993b) examined the effectiveness of various commercially available FM sound-field amplification systems on the speech-recognition abilities of children with normal hearing sensitivity in a classroom setting. Specifically, the amplified and unamplified monosyllabic word recognition of 20 children with normal hearing was evaluated at three speaker-listener distances (6, 12, and 24 feet) in a commonly reported classroom environment (S/N ratio = +6 dB; RT = 0.64 seconds). Four FM sound-field amplification units were evaluated: (1) Comtek Omni-2001; (2) Lifeline Freefield Classroom Amplification System; (3) Phonic Ear Easy Listener; and (4) Radio Shack.[1] Two findings from this investigation are pertinent to this

---

[1] Although Radio Shack does not commercially market an FM sound-field system for the classroom, Radio Shack components are often utilized in classroom settings.

discussion. First, results revealed that each of the FM sound-field amplification systems significantly improved recognition ability in a commonly reported classroom environment. Second, two of the sound-field units (Radio Shack, Lifeline) provided significantly better speech recognition than others (Comtek, Phonic Ear). It was noted, however, that his latter finding must be interpreted with some degree of caution. Although the present investigation attempted to replicate a commonly reported classroom environment (S/N ratio = +6 dB; RT = 0.64 seconds), performance scores may differ significantly in real-world learning environments with dissimilar room volumes and/or varying levels of ambient noise and/or reverberation.

A second concern of this investigation is the speaker placement. In this investigation, a three-speaker placement paradigm (one front/two side speakers) was used for each of the sound-field systems. Several of these systems do not regularly recommend such speaker installation. For example, the Lifeline system recommends a four-speaker placement, while the Phonic Ear suggests a one- to four-speaker placement, depending on the room. Additional factors, other than improved speech recognition, must be considered prior to the recommendation and/or placement of an FM sound-field system in a classroom. These factors include (1) cost of the unit; (2) sound quality; (3) distortion characteristics; (4) durability; (5) service availability; (6) portability: and (7) ease of installation. The authors are currently examining these parameters across the individual units.

COST-EFFECTIVENESS OF SOUND-FIELD AMPLIFICATION

Sound-field amplification systems in the classroom have been shown to be extremely cost-effective for several reasons. First, such systems are typically the most inexpensive of all of the available classroom amplification systems. For example, the average price of a sound-field system is approximately $700, while personal FM systems often cost approximately $900 to $1500. Second, sound-field systems provide benefit for every child in the classroom, while personal FM systems or personal hearing aids benefit only the individual user. In addition, since sound-field systems provide amplification for all children in the classroom, these systems do not stigmatize specific children, which can be the situation with personal FMs or hearing aids. Third, sound-field systems are often the most inexpensive procedure for improving classroom acoustics. Acoustic modifications, such as acoustic ceiling tile, wall panels, or acoustically modified furniture, can cost several thousands of dollars per classroom. However, essentially all classrooms will require at least a minimal degree of acoustic modification prior to the installation of sound-field amplification. Finally, the use of sound-field amplification systems has been shown to reduce the number of children

Table 2
Average cost of a sound-field amplification system per child over a ten-year time span.

Initial cost of sound-field amplification system	$ 700.00
Cost per student (25 students)	$ 28.00
Cost per student over 10 years	$ 2.80

requiring resource room assistance (Crandell, Smaldino, and Flexer 1995; Flexer 1992).

The cost-effectiveness of sound-field amplification systems is shown in table 2. If it is estimated that the average cost of a sound-field system is $700, and the cost is divided by all of the children in the classroom (since it will benefit all children in the room), this equals approximately $28 per child (considering a class size of 25 students). If this cost per student is computed over a ten-year period (the estimated life span of a sound-field system), the unit cost per child is only $2.80. Because sound-field systems significantly improve the classroom listening environment, additional cost-effectiveness is obtained by reducing the number of children requiring resource room assistance. For instance, when the Putnam County school district in Ohio placed 60 sound-field units in regular classrooms, the number of children requiring resource room assistance for learning disabilities was reduced by 40% (Crandell, Smaldino, and Flexer 1995). Hence, if it costs approximately $2600 a year to implement special education services for these children (Berg 1993), and each child requires a minimum of five years in the resource room setting, a savings of $13,000 would occur for the school per child. If only 20 children with learning disabilities were removed from resource room services because of classroom amplification, the savings to the school would be more than $250,000.

COMPARISON OF SOUND-FIELD AMPLIFICATION WITH PERSONAL FM AMPLIFICATION

At present, limited information is available for comparing the effectiveness of sound-field FM amplification with personal FM systems (Flexer 1992; Nabelek, Donahue, and Letowski 1986). Clearly, the personal FM system offers a more favorable S/N ratio, and consequently improved speech-recognition scores, than the sound-field system. Nabelek, Donahue, and Letowski (1986) examined speech perception through a public address system and personal FM unit in elderly individuals, listeners with normal hearing sensitivity, and listeners with SNHL. While both systems provided improved speech-recognition scores over unamplified conditions, results indicated that each group obtained significantly higher recognition scores with the personal FM system.

Since sound-field systems can be expected to produce only about 10 dB of amplification, such systems would not provide sufficient gain for students with moderate-to-severe degrees of SNHL. Thus, for children with greater than mild degrees of SNHL and/or severe perceptual difficulties in noise, a personal FM system may be more appropriate amplification. Moreover, such children are more likely to require an improved classroom S/N ratio throughout their academic career (Flexer 1992). Since it is not feasible for a child to carry a sound-field amplification system to each classroom, a personal FM unit would presumably be the preferred amplification system. However, many children, particularly those in junior or senior high school, may not utilize personal FM systems due to the potential stigma associated with such devices.

CONCLUSIONS

The preceding discussion has highlighted several salient points concerning classroom acoustics and the utilization of sound-field amplification in the educational setting. First, a number of investigations have demonstrated that noise and reverberation levels in learning environments are typically higher than recommended standards (ASHA 1995). Second, commonly reported classroom acoustics may have a deleterious effect on the speech recognition of various populations of children with normal hearing sensitivity. Such findings are alarming because it is well recognized that inappropriate classroom acoustics can deleteriously affect not only speech-recognition ability but also psychoeducational and psychosocial achievement. Consequently, inappropriate classroom acoustics may place many populations of children at risk for later language, social, and academic difficulties. Finally, this discussion has addressed one strategy (sound-field amplification) that has been shown to augment speech perception and academic achievement for children with normal hearing and children with SNHL in the classroom.

In conclusion, it is important to review the benefits and potential disadvantages of sound-field amplification discussed in this chapter (Anderson 1991; Crandell, Smaldino, and Flexer 1995). First, sound-field amplification systems can be used with all of the populations of children with normal hearing who exhibit perceptual difficulties, as well as children with sensorineural hearing loss. Second, such systems can provide benefit to children with SNHL while malfunctioning hearing aids or personal FM systems are being repaired. Third, sound-field systems are often the most inexpensive method of improving classroom acoustics. Fourth, a sound-field system provides amplification for all children in the classroom; therefore, these systems do not stigmatize specific children, which can be the situation with auditory trainers or hearing aids. Fifth, 90% to 95% of all teachers willingly accept sound field-amplification systems. Sixth, teachers report lessened stress and vocal strain during teaching activities when using sound-field amplification. Seventh, students can use the system for oral report and oral reading, and for asking/answering questions, thus enhancing listening and academic performance. Finally, equipment malfunction is immediately obvious to the teacher with sound-field amplification; thus, it is easier to troubleshoot than personal amplification systems.

There are several potential disadvantages of sound-field amplification. First, sound-field amplification systems may not provide adequate benefit in excessively reverberant or noisy learning environments. Eight to 10 dB of amplification may not be enough to overcome the effects of a particularly poor acoustic environment. Second, the improper placement of speakers in a classroom could increase both the level of the desired direct sound and the undesired reflected sound energy. In addition, because of varying amounts of sound cancellation and distortion, it may make it difficult to obtain the desired uniform sound amplification throughout the classroom without proper speaker placement. For discussions on appropriate speaker placement/arrangement, the reader is directed to Berg (1993), Crandell, Smaldino, and Flexer (1995), and Flexer (1992). Third, in smaller classrooms, the amplified sound may be less than 10 dB because of feedback problems associated with the synergistic effects of reflective surfaces and speaker closeness. At present, it is not clear how much benefit limited amplification can provide. Fourth, both the teacher and the student need appropriate in-service information for the sound-field system to provide maximum benefit in the classroom.

Sound-Field FM System Manufacturers

Anchor Audio, Inc.
913 West 223rd Street
Torrance, CA 90502
(800) 262-4671

Audio Enchancement
1748 West 12600 South
Riverton, UT 84065
(800) 383-9362

Custom Audio Design
Box 597
Wenatchee, WA 98807-0598
(800) 355-7525

LightSPEED Technologies, Inc.
15812 Southwest Upper Boones Ferry Road
Lake Oswego, OR 97035
(800) 732-8999

Telex Communications, Inc.
9600 Aldrich Avenue South
Minneapolis, MN 55420
(800) 328-3102

Phonic Ear, Inc.
3880 Cypress Drive
Petaluma, CA 94954-7600
(800) 227-0735

Lifeline Amplification Systems
55 South 4th Street
Platteville, WI 53818
(800) 236-4327

Williams Sound Corporation
10399 W. 70th Street
Eden Prairie, MN 55344
(800) 328-6190

REFERENCES

Allen, L. 1993. Promoting the usefulness of classroom amplification. *Educational Audiology Monograph* 3:32-34.

Allen, L., and Patton, D. 1990. Effects of sound field amplification on students' on-task behavior. Paper presented at the American Speech-Language-Hearing Association convention, Seattle, Washington.

American Speech-Language-Hearing Association. 1995. Position statement and guidelines for acoustics in educational settings. *Asha* 37(Suppl. 14):15.

Anderson, K.L. 1989. *Screening instrument for targeting educational risk (S.I.F.T.E.R.).* Austin: Pro-Ed.

Anderson, K.L. 1991. Speech perception in children. *Educational Audiology Monograph* 1(1):15-29.

Benafield, N. 1990. The effects of sound field amplification on the attending behaviors of speech and language-delayed preschool children. Master's thesis, University of Arkansas at Little Rock.

Bench, J., Koval, A., and Bamford, J. 1979. The BKB (Bamford-Koval-Bench) sentence lists for partially-hearing children. *British Journal of Audiology* 13:108-112.

Beranek, L. 1954. *Acoustics.* New York: McGraw-Hill.

Berg, F.S. 1987. *Facilitating classroom listening.* Boston: College-Hill Press.

Berg, F.S. 1993. *Acoustics and sound systems in schools.* Boston: College-Hill Press.

Berg, F.S., Bateman, R., and Viehweg, S. 1989. Sound field FM amplification in junior high school classrooms. Paper presented at the American Speech-Language-Hearing Association convention, St. Louis, Missouri.

Bess, F.H. 1985. The minimally hearing-impaired child. *Ear and Hearing* 6:43-47.

Bess, F.H., and McConnell, F. 1981. *Audiology, education and the hearing-impaired child.* St. Louis: C.V. Mosby.

Bess, F.H., and Tharpe, A.M. 1986. An introduction to unilateral sensorineural hearing loss in children. *Ear and Hearing* 7(1):3-13.

Blair, J.C. 1977. Effects of amplification, speechreading, and classroom environment on reception of speech. *Volta Review* 79:443-449.

Blair, J.C., Myrup, C., and Viehweg, S. 1991. Comparison of the effectiveness of hard-of-hearing children using three types of amplification. *Educational Audiology Monograph* 1(1):48-55.

Blair, J.C., Peterson, M.E., and Viehweg, S. 1985. The effects of mild hearing loss on academic performance of young school-age children. *Volta Review* 87(2):87-93.

Boney, S., and Bess, F.H. 1984. Noise and reverberation effects in minimal bilateral sensorineural hearing loss. Paper presented at the American Speech-Language-Hearing Association convention, San Francisco, California.

Crandell, C. 1991. Classroom acoustics for normal-hearing children: Implications for rehabilitation. *Educational Audiology Monograph* 2(1):18-38.

Crandell, C. 1992. Classroom acoustics for hearing-impaired children. *Journal of the Acoustical Society of America* 92(4):2470.
Crandell, C. 1993a. Speech recognition in noise by children with minimal hearing loss. *Ear and Hearing* 14(3):210-216.
Crandell, C. 1993b. A comparison of commercially-available frequency modulation sound field amplification systems. *Educational Audiology Monograph* 3:15-30.
Crandell, C. 1994. Speech perception in noise by children for whom English is a second language. Paper presented at the annual American Academy of Audiology meeting, Phoenix, Arizona.
Crandell, C. 1995. The effects of sound field amplification on the speech perception of ESL children. Paper presented at the annual American Academy of Audiology meeting, Dallas, Texas.
Crandell, C., and Bess, F.H. 1986. Speech recognition in a "typical" classroom setting. *Asha* 28:82.
Crandell, C., and Bess, F.H. 1987. Sound field amplification in the classroom setting. *Asha* 29:87.
Crandell, C., and Smaldino, J. 1992. Sound field amplification in the classroom. *American Journal of Audiology* 1(4):16-18.
Crandell, C., and Smaldino, J. 1995a. An update of classroom acoustics for children with hearing impairment. *Volta Review* 96:291-306.
Crandell, C., and Smaldino, J. 1995b. The importance of room acoustics. In R.S. Tyler and D. Schum (eds.), *Assistive listening devices*. Baltimore: Williams and Wilkins.
Crandell, C., Smaldino, J., and Flexer, C. 1995. *Sound field FM amplification: Theory and practical applications.* San Diego: Singular Press.
Crum, D., and Matkin, N.D. 1976. Room acoustics: The forgotten variable. *Language, Speech, and Hearing Services in the Schools* 7:106-110.
Davis, J., Elfenbein, J., Schum, R., and Bentler, R. 1986. Effects of mild and moderate hearing impairments on language, educational, and psychosocial behavior of children. *Journal of Speech and Hearing Disorders* 51:53-62.
Elliott, L. 1979. Performance of children aged 9 to 17 years on a test of speech intelligibility in noise using sentence material with controlled word predictability. *Journal of the Acoustical Society of America* 66:651-653.
Elliott, L. 1982. Effects of noise on perception of speech by children and certain handicapped individuals. *Sound and Vibration*, December, 9-14.
Elliott, L., Connors, S., Kille, E., Levin, S., Ball, K., and Katz, D. 1979. Children's understanding of monosyllabic nouns in quiet and in noise. *Journal of the Acoustical Society of America* 66:12-21.
Finitzo-Hieber, T. 1988. Classroom acoustics. In R.J. Roeser (ed.), *Auditory disorders in school Children* (pp. 221-233). 2d ed. New York: Thieme and Stratton.
Finitzo-Hieber, T., and Tillman, T. 1978. Room acoustics effects on monosyllabic word discrimination ability for normal and hearing-impaired children. *Journal of Speech and Hearing Research* 21:440-458.
Flexer, C. 1989. Turn on sound: An odyssey of sound field amplification. *Educational Audiology Association Newsletter* 5:6-7.
Flexer, C. 1992. Classroom public address systems. In M. Ross (ed.), *FM auditory training systems: Characteristics, selection and use* (pp. 189-209). Timonium, Md.: York Press.

Flexer, C., Millin, J., and Brown, L. 1990. Children with developmental disabilities: The effects of sound field amplification in word identification. *Language, Speech, and Hearing Services in the Schools* 21:177-182.

Flexer, C., Richards, C., and Buie, C. 1993. Sound field amplification for regular kindergarten and first grade classrooms: A longitudinal study of fluctuating hearing loss and pupil performance. Paper presented at the American Academy of Audiology convention, Phoenix, Arizona.

Fourcin, A., Joy, D., Kennedy, M., Knight, J., Knowles, S., Knox, E., Matin, M., Mort, J., Penton, J., Poole, D., Powell, C., and Watson, T. 1980. Design of educational facilities for deaf children. *British Journal of Audiology* Suppl. 3:1-24.

Gengel, R. 1971. Acceptable signal-to-noise ratios for aided speech discrimination by the hearing impaired. *Journal of Auditory Research* 11:219-222.

Gilman, L., and Danzer, V. 1989. Use of FM sound field amplification in regular classrooms. Paper presented at the American Speech-Language-Hearing Association convention, St. Louis, Missouri.

Green, H. 1954. *The Iowa spelling test.* Iowa City, Iowa: State University of Iowa.

Iowa Test of Basic Skills. 1967. Boston: Houghton Mufflin Company.

Jones, J., Berg, F.S., and Viehweg, S. 1989. Close, distant, and sound field overhead listening in kindergarten classrooms. *Educational Audiology Monograph* 1:56-65.

Kalikow, D., Stevens, K.N., and Elliott, L. 1977. Development of a test of speech intelligibility in noise using sentence materials with controlled word predictability. *Journal of the Acoustical Society of America* 61:1337-1351.

Katz, D., and Elliott, L. 1978. Development of a new children's speech discrimination test. Paper presented at the annual American Speech and Hearing Association, Chicago, Illinois.

Knudsen, V., and Harris, C. 1978. *Acoustical designing in architecture.* Washington, D.C.: American Institute of Physics for the Acoustical Society of America.

Kodaras, M. 1960. Reverberation times of typical elementary school settings. *Noise Control* 6:17-19.

Leavitt, R., and Flexer, C. 1991. Speech degradation as measured by the Rapid Speech Transmission Index (RASTI). *Ear and Hearing* 12:115-118.

Markides, A. 1986. Speech levels and speech-to-noise ratios. *British Journal of Audiology* 20:115-120.

McCroskey, F., and Devens, J. 1975. Acoustic characteristics of public school classrooms constructed between 1890 and 1960. *NOISEXPO Proceedings,* 101-103.

Mills, M. 1991. A practical look at classroom amplification. *Educational Audiology Monograph* 2(1):39-42.

Nabelek, A., Donahue, A., and Letowski, T. 1986. Comparison of amplification systems in a classroom. *Journal of Rehabilitation Research and Development* 23(1):41-52.

Nabelek, A., and Nabelek, I. 1985. Room acoustics and speech perception. In J. Katz (ed.), *Handbook of clinical audiology.* 3d ed. Baltimore: Williams and Wilkins.

Nabelek, A., and Robinson, P.K. 1982. Monaural and binaural speech perception in reverberation for listeners of various ages. *Journal of the Acoustical Society of America* 71(5):1242-1248.

Neuss, D., Blair, J.C., and Viehweg, S. 1991. Sound field amplification: Does it improve word recognition in a background of noise for students with minimal hearing impairments? *Educational Audiology Monograph* 2(1):43-52.

Niemoeller, A. 1968. Acoustical design of classrooms for the deaf. *American Annals of the Deaf* 113:1040-1045.

Olsen, W.O. 1977. Acoustics and amplification in classrooms for the hearing impaired. In F.H. Bess (ed.), *Childhood deafness: Causation, assessment and management*. New York: Grune and Stratton.

Olsen, W.O. 1981. The effects of noise and reverberation on speech intelligibility. In F.H. Bess, B.A. Freeman, and J.S. Sinclair (eds.), *Amplification in education*. Washington, D.C.: Alexander Graham Bell Association for the Deaf.

Olsen, W.O. 1988. Classroom acoustics for hearing-impaired children. In F.H. Bess (ed.), *Hearing impairment in children*. Parkton, Md.: York Press.

Paul, R. 1967. An investigation of the effectiveness of hearing aid amplification in regular and special classrooms under instructional conditions. Ph.D. diss., Detroit: Wayne State University.

Pearsons, K., Bennett, R., and Fidell, S. 1977. Speech levels in various noise environments. *EPA 600/1-77-025*. Washington, D.C.: Office of Health and Ecological Effects.

Ray, H. 1987. Put a microphone on the teacher: A simple solution for the difficult problems of mild hearing loss. *Clinical Connection*, Spring, 14-15.

Ray, H., Sarff, L., and Glassford, F.E. 1984. Sound field amplification: An innovative educational intervention for mainstreamed learning disabled students. *Directive Teacher* 6(2):18-20.

Rosenberg, G., Blake-Rahter, P., Allen, L., and Redmond, B. 1994. Improving classroom acoustics: A multi-district pilot study on FM classroom amplification. Poster session presented at the American Academy of Audiology Annual convention, Richmond, Virginia.

Ross, M. 1978. Classroom acoustics and speech intelligibility. In J. Katz (ed.), *Handbook of clinical audiology*. Baltimore: Williams and Wilkins.

Ross, M., and Giolas, T.G. 1971. Effects of three classroom listening conditions on speech intelligibility. *American Annals of the Deaf,* December, 580-584.

Ross, M., and Lerman, J. 1970. A picture identification test for hearing impaired children. *Journal of Speech and Hearing Research* 13:44-53.

Sanders, D. 1965. Noise conditions in normal school classrooms. *Exceptional Child* 31:344-353.

Sarff, L. 1981. An innovative use of free field amplification in regular classrooms. In R.J. Roeser and M.P. Downs (eds.), *Auditory disorders in school children* (pp. 263-272). New York: Thieme and Stratton.

Sarff, L., Ray, H., and Bagwell, C. 1981. Why not amplification in every classroom? *Hearing Aid Journal* 11:44, 47-48, 50, 52.

Zabel, H., and Tabor, M. 1993. Effects of classroom amplification on spelling performance of elementary school children. *Educational Audiology Monograph* 3:5-9.

PART III.

New Technologies

12

Transposition Hearing Aids for Children

Judith S. Gravel and Patricia M. Chute

INTRODUCTION

The abiding goal for pediatric audiologists has been to provide audible acoustic cues to infants and children with hearing loss such that speech information could be incorporated into an auditory repertoire that would serve as the basis for aural-oral language development. For children with severe and profound hearing loss, these attempts are often frustrated by both the lack of residual hearing necessary for optimum speech intelligibility and a restricted dynamic range.

Logically, one solution to such auditory limitations has been the concept of shifting or in some other way "transposing" inaudible high-frequency speech energy into lower-frequency auditory regions where more hearing usually exists. This chapter overviews past attempts to transpose speech and to describe current commercially available, wearable transposers that provide a means of making otherwise undetectable speech cues audible to children with hearing loss.

HISTORICAL REVIEW OF FREQUENCY TRANSPOSITION

Attempts to transpose high-frequency speech information into lower-frequency spectral regions began more than 30 years ago. In Sweden, Bertol Johansson in the early 1960s reported on a transposer hearing aid he developed in both desk and body-worn models (cited in Erber 1971). The device was specifically designed to provide a means of detecting high-frequency speech phonemes. The Johansson device filtered energy in the

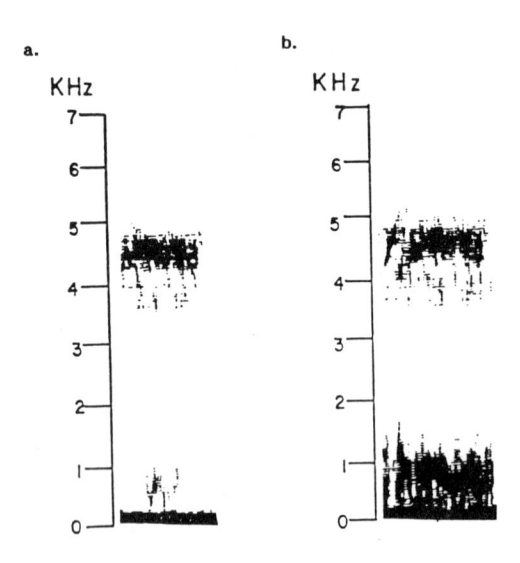

Figure 1. Spectrograms of the consonant /s/: **1A** depicts the /s/ amplified conventionally; **1B** depicts the /s/ transposed through the Johansson transposer. Note the addition of low-frequency energy (below 1500 Hz) in the transposed spectrogram. Adapted from Foust and Gengel 1973.

incoming speech signal above 4000 Hz and modulated that information with a 5000 Hz carrier frequency. The difference components (noise below 1500 Hz) created by this process were mixed with the original signal. As depicted in figure 1, the spectrogram of an /s/ is presented conventionally amplified (1A) and transposed by the Johansson device (1B). The transposed spectrum includes the normal high-frequency frication of the /s/ as well as the added noise below 1500 Hz. Phonemes without high-frequency energy above 4000 Hz were unaffected by the high-pass filtering.

Wedenberg (1961) and Johansson (1966; both cited in Erber 1971) studied the utility of the device in several children with hearing loss. In the Johansson study, the children were able to accurately discriminate /sa/ versus /Sa/ after two sessions of using the transposer. They also obtained improved recognition of the syllables /sa/, /Sa/, /ka/, and /tSa/ with the device versus conventional amplification when these stimuli were presented to the young listeners in a closed-set format.

Hirsh, Greenwald, and Erber (1967 unpublished study; cited in Erber 1971), however, found no differences for children with profound hearing loss who were trained and tested with the Johansson transposer when performance was compared to their conventional amplification. A study of the Johansson device by Ling also demonstrated no greater success in consonant and vowel discrimination with or without transposition for eight children with profound hearing loss (Ling 1968; cited in Erber 1971). This was the case even when children were provided with a ten-day auditory training period. There was, however, a learning effect demonstrated for the transposition condition. Unfortunately, an extended period of training (36 days) provided to four of the original subjects failed to corroborate the earlier finding; none of the four subjects demonstrated any consistent improvement with the device over time.

In a systematic study at Gallaudet College, Foust and Gengel (1973) examined the utility of Johansson's transposer in nine young adults with hearing losses ranging from moderate to profound. Monosyllabic word recognition (closed-set modified rhyme task) performance was studied using the transposer and conventional amplification in auditory-alone and visual-plus-auditory conditions. Training was provided with both devices. Subjects gave feedback on a regular basis. The study period lasted for six weeks; however, the device was used only in the laboratory setting.

Mean performance data failed to demonstrate differences between the transposed and conventional listening conditions in auditory-alone presentations. A significant learning effect across the six weeks of the study was evident with use of the Johansson transposer, a result not apparent with conventional amplification. In the visual-plus-auditory (combined) condition, significantly better performance was obtained with the transposed signal than with conventional amplification.

Individual performance results were mixed. One listener showed significantly better performance with the transposed than conventional signal. Though disliking the transposer initially, by the end of the six-week trial, this subject ultimately preferred the transposer over the regular hearing aid. Another subject disliked the transposer and performed poorer with it than with the conventional amplification throughout the study.

Ling and Druz (1967; Ling 1968; cited in Erber 1971) also attempted to devise a system to provide high-frequency speech cues to children with severe and profound hearing loss. This instrument coded speech energy occurring in the 2000 to 3000 Hz range by presenting a pure-tone analog of the signal in the range of 750 to 1000 Hz. In another variation, Ling and Doehring (1969; cited in Ling and Maretic 1971) transposed sounds in the 1000 to 4000 Hz regions. Ten logarithmically spread bandwidths in this range provided analogs at intervals of 100 Hz from 100 to 1000 Hz. Conventional linear amplification was also provided in the 70 to 7000 Hz range. Conventional amplification could be provided to one ear alone or mixed with the transposed signal. Essentially, studies with both devices in children with profound hearing loss showed improvement over time on various measures of syllable and word discrimination. However, control groups of children trained similarly with a conventionally amplified signal only also demonstrated improved perception with training. In no case was there a significant difference in overall performance for the transposed versus conventional signal. Ling and Maretic (1971) examined the speech production capabilities of children who were trained with the Ling and Doehring coder as well as with conventional amplification. No significant difference was made in the intelligibility of expressive speech with either device.

Other attempts at making high-frequency energy detectable for the listener with hearing loss were made in the 1960s. A vocoder developed by Guttman and Nelson (1968) and Guttman, Levitt, and Bellefleur (1970; both cited in Erber 1971) coded high-frequency speech energy through low-frequency analog pulse trains and mixed this coded speech with linear amplification. Generally, listeners' success using this vocoder was no different from conventional amplification.

These early attempts at transposition provided additional cues (noise or a pulse train) to the speech signal in order to make high-frequency information detectable. Overall, the perceptual quality of coded speech was reduced. These attempts may have interfered with the natural relationships that exist between consonants and vowels, or added energy may have masked critical speech cues.

Relevant to the discussion of current transposition devices that follows, Oeken (1963; cited in Erber 1971) devised a spectral transposition method that shifted speech one-half to one octave through use of a rotating magnetic storage drum and magnetic playback head. Oeken met with some success in children with hearing loss, but differences between the transposition device and use of conventional amplification could not be demonstrated when children received training with both. Bennett and Byers (1967) reported on the use of a "slow-play tape" spectral transposition. This process proportionally shifted speech to lower-frequency regions. The frequency transposition could not be accomplished in real time, however (AVR/Communications Ltd. 1993). The advantage of such a method would be to preserve the relationships between acoustic features of speech, thereby in theory, maintaining speech quality. Unfortunately, for all the methods previously discussed, numerous technological limitations prohibited transposition or speech coding devices from being practical for long-term daily wear.

CURRENT TRANSPOSITION INSTRUMENTS

Clinical uses of frequency transposition hearing aids were all but abandoned in the mid-1970s and 1980s as new technology (including the development of power ear-level amplification) became available to listeners with severe and profound hearing loss. In the 1990s, cochlear implants, personal FM systems, and improved wearable vibrotactile device technology provide options for clinicians seeking better methods to provide speech cues to young listeners with hearing loss. However, despite the advances, there are still children for whom instrumentation is inadequate or a surgically implanted device is contraindicated.

Two commercially available transposition hearing instruments have recently entered the marketplace. Both can be called transposers, given a broad definition of the term *transpose* (e.g., "to reverse or transfer the order or place of, interchange; to alter in form or nature; transform," *American Heritage Dictionary* 1985). These are the EMILY™ (Audiologic-Sarl) and the TranSonic™ FT-40 MKII. The EMILY, however, is described by its developers not as a transposer but as a signal processor. EMILY was developed in France, and distribution is being established at this time. On the other hand, the TranSonic was specifically designed as a frequency transposition hearing aid. The instrument was developed in Israel and is distributed in the U.S. by AVR Sonovation, Chanhassen, Minnesota. Some basics about the two instruments are provided below.

THE EMILY DEVICE

Briefly, the signal processing utilized in EMILY imposes additional harmonics that are delivered with the conventionally amplified signal. The harmonics are created by the multiplication and division of a tone representing the peak energy of the second formant (F2). Figure 2 depicts the basic EMILY processing strategy.

A bandpass filter one octave in width passes speech energy occurring between 1000 and 2000 Hz, encompassing the region of the normal occurrence of F2. The prominent or center frequency of this bandpassed energy is detected from moment to moment in time. A tone (Tn) corresponding to the spectral peak of the bandpassed signal is created. The tone is a representation of F2. This tone is subsequently divided (F2/2) and/or multiplied (F2x2). The amplitude of the harmonics created by multiplying the signal is maintained at one-half the amplitude of harmonics created by the tone's division. The signal is then mixed with the conventionally amplified speech signal and delivered to the ear. The processed portion of the signal may be adjusted differentially.

The current manufacturer's literature on the device is not specific regarding the rationale for the creation and delivery of additional harmonics to the impaired ear. Presumably, the purpose of the speech processing is to enhance detection of cues (F2) that might otherwise be inaudible. Audiogram configuration and/or the development of a "curve of auditory distortions" (termed the clarity test®) is utilized to fit the EMILY. The curve is said to be representative of the distortions inherent in an individual's hearing loss.

Presently, the EMILY device is worn on the body and interfaces with the child's personal hearing aid. It is approved by the Food and Drug

258 • NEW TECHNOLOGIES

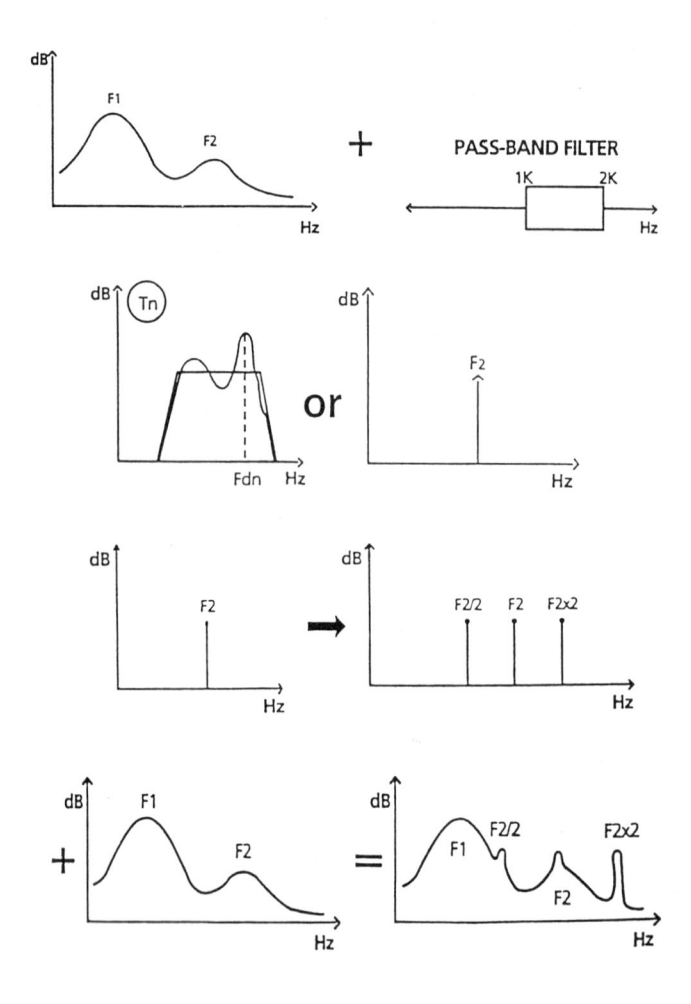

Figure 2. Schematic representation of speech processing strategy utilized by the EMILY device. Adapted from product brochure, EMILY, Audiologic-Sarl, France.

Administration (FDA) only for use in combination with Phonak hearing instruments. Currently, only two models of Phonak behind-the-ear (BTE) hearing aids can be used with the EMILY. While initially devised for severe-to-profound losses, the EMILY processor's signal enhancement schema is reported to be useful for children with even moderate degrees of hearing loss. The distributor reports that about 20 devices are currently (1994) in use by children in the U.S. Also according to the U.S. distributor, the device is worn by about 500 children in France. Reports of its use by French children and by some children attending a school for the Deaf in Texas suggest that speech recognition at the syllabic and word level can be enhanced through use of the device. However, to our knowledge, published reports (e.g., intelligibility data) on the usefulness of providing additional harmonics to the amplified speech signal are currently unavailable.

THE TRANSONIC FREQUENCY TRANSPOSITION HEARING AID

As stated previously, the TranSonic FT-40 MKII was specifically designed as a frequency transposition hearing aid. Transposition is accomplished by frequency dividing the incoming speech energy. This results in a narrowing or compressing of the speech signal and a shift of energy to

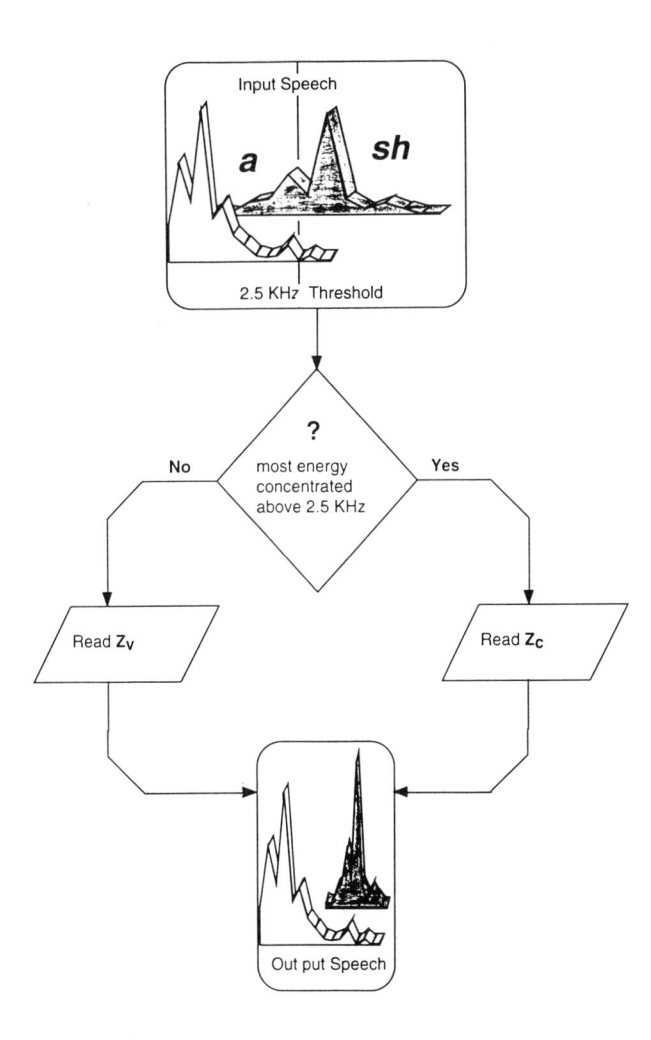

Figure 3. Schematic representation of the basic strategy of the TranSonic illustrating when the transposition coefficients (Zv and Zc) are activated by speech input. Adapted from a product brochure, AVR Sonovation, Chanhassen, Minnesota.

lower-frequency regions. The manufacturer describes the transposition as "compression in the frequency domain." The process is similar to a "slow-play tape" effect (AVR/Communications Ltd. 1993).

Two transposition coefficients may be set on the TranSonic, each activating transposition in two different frequency regions. The process is depicted schematically in figure 3. The instrument uses a spectral balance detector that analyzes the incoming speech signal. At any moment in time, if the energy concentration of incoming speech is 2500 Hz or above, the Zc (consonant) transposition coefficient is applied to the signal and all spectral information occurring at that moment in time is divided by the selected transposition coefficient and proportionally shifted to a lower-frequency region. Similarly, if the Zv (vowel) transposition coefficient has been activated, incoming spectral information with an energy concentration occurring below 2500 Hz is divided and proportionally shifted into lower-frequency regions.

The transposition is accomplished in "perceptual real time." However, there is a time delay from detection of the incoming signal to the completion of the transposition process. Indeed, even in the neutral position (Zc = 1; Zv = 1), the time delay for the transposition is approximately 9 milliseconds (ms). Depending on the setting of the two transposition coefficients, the processing delay can be as much as 13 ms.

Spectrograms of the nonsense word /isat/ are presented in figure 4 (A, B, and C). Figure 4A represents a high-fidelity recording of the nonsense

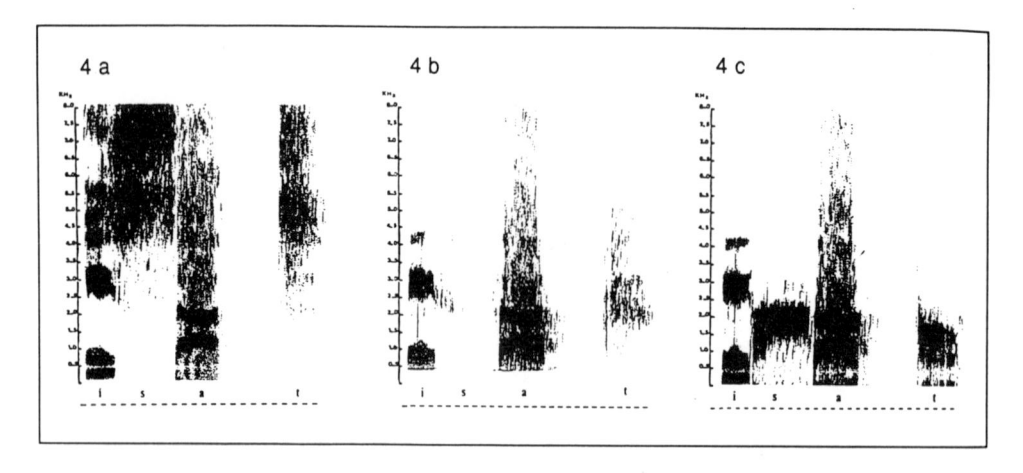

Figure 4. Spectrograms representing the nonsense word /isat/: **4A** shows the word recorded through a high-fidelity recording system; **4B** through a conventional hearing aid; and **4C** through the TranSonic with Zv = 1, Zc = 4. Note that the high-frequency speech energy in the /s/ and /t/ phonemes in **4B** that are absent or reduced in intensity (due to the response characteristics of the conventional hearing aid) are present in the transposed condition. Reprinted with permission, AVR Sonovation, Chanhassen, Minnesota.

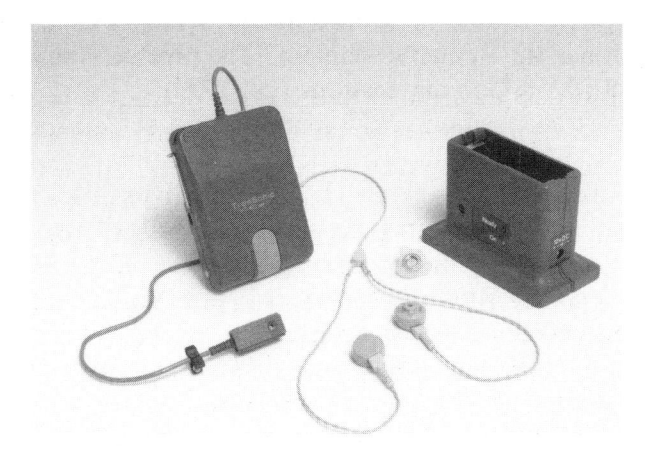

Figure 5. The TranSonic with external receiver. Reprinted with permission, AVR Sonovation, Chanhassen, Minnesota.

word. Note the energy concentrations above 2500 Hz in the /s/ and /t/. Figure 4B displays the same word transduced through a conventional hearing aid. Observe the reduction in high-frequency energy above 3000 Hz attributable to the response characteristics of the hearing aid's receiver. Figure 4C displays the same /isat/ transposed by the TranSonic device set with a Z_c = 4 and Z_v set in the neutral (Z_v = 1) position. Note that since the energy concentration occurs above 2500 Hz in the consonants /s/ and /t/, the sounds were transposed (Z_c activated) into the region of 625 Hz. The vowels have been left unaltered since their energy concentration is below 2500 Hz; thus, no transposition was imposed (as Z_v = 1).

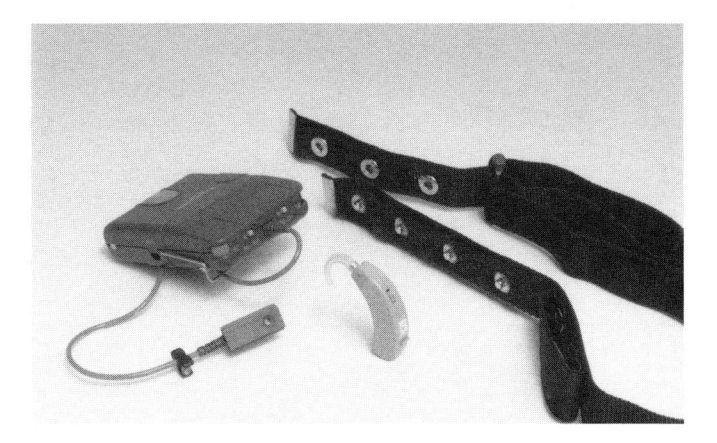

Figure 6. The TranSonic with coupling to the ear achieved by transducing the transposed signal via FM by a waist belt. Signal received by an FM receiver at ear level. Courtesy of AVR Sonovation, Chanhassen, Minnesota.

A Dynamic Consonant Boost® (DCB) circuit can be activated on the TranSonic. Activating the DCB allows the audiologist to increase the intensity of the transposed Zc signal (from 1 to 16 dB; however, exceeding 9 dB of DCB is generally not recommended by the manufacturer), thereby boosting the less-salient high-frequency cues in order to increase their potential for audibility. This also allows use of a lower Zc transposition coefficient.

The TranSonic is a body-worn hearing aid. As seen in figure 5, the transposed signal may be delivered to the ear via an external receiver (or receivers as in a Y-cord arrangement) or via an ear-level receiver (SLR) as seen in figure 6. In the latter arrangement, the body-worn unit, connected to a waist belt-antenna, converts the transposed signal to an FM signal. The FM signal is then delivered to an FM receiver worn in a BTE case. An external microphone is worn close to the mouth in both coupling arrangements.

Depicted in figure 7 is a comparison of the aided sound field responses obtained for a child fit with a conventional hearing aid and the TranSonic. Such measures demonstrate the detectability of otherwise unavailable high-frequency energy with the use of the transposer. Audibility, however, does not imply that the cues will be useful for speech perception.

Candidacy Issues

The manufacturer suggests that candidates for the TranSonic are those with hearing impairments within the moderately severe-to-profound

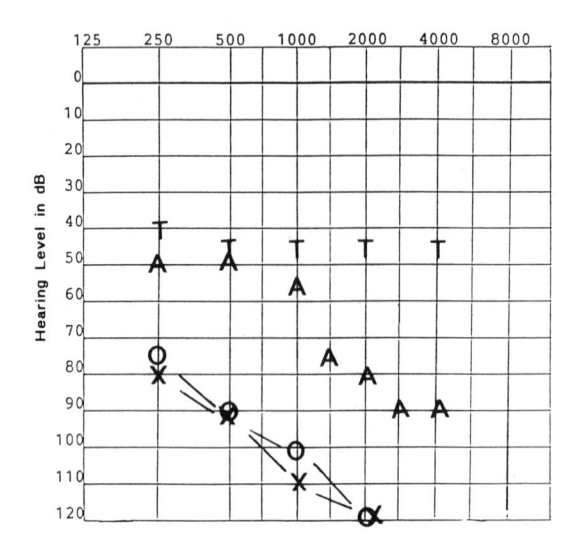

Figure 7. Sound field aided audiogram of a child utilizing a conventional power ear-level hearing aid (A) and the TranSonic (T).

hearing loss range. Thus, some children who fall into this broad audiometric range also might be considered candidates for cochlear implants. Indeed, it is somewhat unfortunate that the TranSonic has been suggested by some clinicians to be a substitute for a cochlear implant. Such a representation of the transposition device could, in our opinion, lead to unreasonable expectations for the TranSonic, on the one hand, and the elimination of some potentially good candidates for frequency transposition, on the other. Said differently, children fit with the TranSonic might be expected to perform similarly to cochlear implant recipients while others might be eliminated as candidates for the TranSonic because they were deemed to have too much hearing for a device that is considered an implant substitute.

Studies of the Benefit of Transposition

While anecdotal reports of the benefit of the TranSonic used as personal amplification are increasing, published reports that quantify outcomes (e.g., prefit and postfit speech detection, discrimination, and/or recognition scores) in both children and adults are lacking. Similarly, objective reports of the utility of the TranSonic as a specific auditory training device and/or speech therapy aid are also currently unavailable.

A report by Plant and Franklin (1994) provides an encouraging clinical case study investigation of the TranSonic. These authors quantified the benefit of frequency transposition through systematic training and testing of a woman with acquired profound hearing loss; she was a regular user of conventional binaural BTE amplification. This subject received two two-hour auditory training sessions per week for a three-month period with the TranSonic. She was encouraged to use the device for at least one hour per day on those days she was not receiving direct training. Multiple types of speech materials (based on the Analytika Auditory Training Program; Plant 1994) were utilized for training and testing.

Plant and Franklin found no significant performance difference for this listener between the hearing instruments (TranSonic versus personal hearing aids) on a 21 consonant /vCv/ syllable identification task. This was true for both an auditory-alone and a visual-plus-auditory condition. However, they found that this listener demonstrated significant benefit on auditory tasks such as detection of the consonant sounds /s/, /n/, /t/, and /d/ and closed-set identification of consonant-initial contrasts in words. Even more difficult high-frequency initial consonant contrasts were more readily recognized with the TranSonic versus her conventional hearing aids in the closed-set format. Also impressive were the results obtained on recognition of connected speech materials for the TranSonic versus conventional hearing aids condition. Ultimately, this subject did not elect to use the transposer, preferring her personal hearing aids.

As stated previously, some have suggested that the TranSonic might be used in place of, or perhaps even in addition to, a cochlear implant. We (Chute, Gravel, and Popp 1995) have begun to examine this issue in a small group of adult cochlear implant users. In a clinical trial under way at Manhattan Eye, Ear and Throat Hospital's Cochlear Implant Center, five adult volunteers who are considered successful users of a multichannel cochlear implant (use time: 2½ to 7 years) agreed to participate in a prospective six-month trial of the TranSonic. Subjects use the TranSonic alone for two hours daily in the nonimplanted ear. The remainder of the day, they use both devices together whenever possible.

All volunteers received formal testing at the time of the fitting of the TranSonic in the following conditions: (1) transposer alone, (2) cochlear implant alone, and (3) combined devices. The protocol is to evaluate all subjects at one, two, four, and six months after the initial fitting. Tests include phoneme detection, discrimination of speech features, closed- and open-set word identification, and sentence identification. No formal auditory training is provided.

Figures 8 and 9 depict the audiograms and some preliminary data displayed beneath the audiometric results. Subject 1 demonstrates comparable sound field audiograms and speech awareness thresholds with the TranSonic (T) in the right ear and cochlear implant (C) in the left. To date, this subject

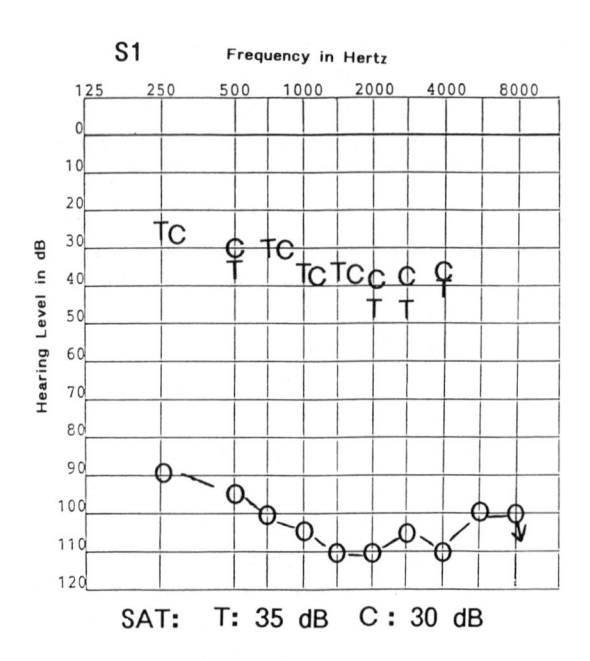

Figure 8. Audiogram (0) and responses with the TranSonic (T) for the right ear. Cochlear implant (C) responses for the left ear. SAT=Speech Awareness Threshold.

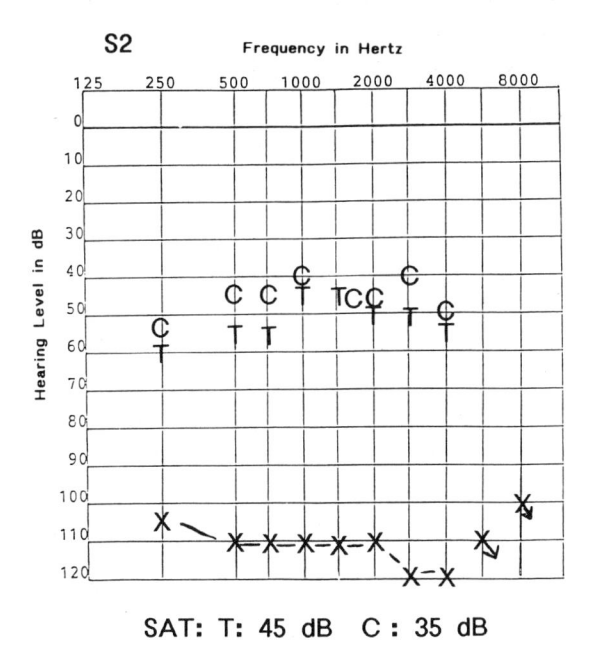

Figure 9. Audiogram (X) and responses with the TranSonic (T) for the left ear. Cochlear implant (C) responses for the right ear. SAT=Speech Awareness Threshold.

has been evaluated twice. On most measures the results show essentially comparable performance with the two devices: Performance on the GASP (Glendonald Auditory Screening Procedure, Erber 1982) words, GASP stress, and minimal pairs (combined) feature discrimination was above chance performance for both devices. On the Minimal Pairs Test (Robbins, Renshaw, Miyamoto, Osberger, and Pope 1988) one month after TranSonic fitting, this subject demonstrated above-chance performance, whereas at the initial fit, scores on this measure were below chance. At least by Subject 1's measured performance scores, there does not currently appear to be a benefit to using both devices. However, subjectively, Subject 1 stated that he felt that sounds were clearer and easier to understand when wearing both the implant and the TranSonic together.

Note Subject 2's sound field responses for the same conditions. Similar to Subject 1, this listener performs best when using his implant. His performance demonstrates well-above-chance performance on GASP words, GASP stress, and minimal pairs discrimination. However, with the TranSonic alone on these tasks, this subject's performance is currently below chance. Despite these findings on the formal measures, this subject also reported enjoying using both the cochlear implant and the TranSonic together. Both subjects desire to remain in the protocol.

OBJECTIVELY FITTING THE TRANSONIC TO YOUNG CHILDREN

Thus far, setting and evaluating the TranSonic with children have, in our opinion, been highly subjective. Indeed, the manufacturer's product literature suggests both candidacy criteria and evaluation procedures that incorporate either (1) detection and discrimination of vowels and consonants (/s/ and /S/) produced by the clinician at various physical distances from the listener, or (2) assessment of sound field aided responses to narrow bands of noise, attempting to achieve some preset aided threshold value (i.e., 40 dB HL) across audiometric speech frequencies. Based on these behavioral responses, adjustments to the transposition coefficients, volume control, and DCB are made. Moreover, loudness judgments (most comfortable levels and loudness discomfort levels) solicited from the listener are utilized in the fitting and evaluation strategy.

While the value of subjective methods for the examination of function is undisputed, in our judgment, removing some of the subjectivity associated with current recommended strategies for fitting the TranSonic device appears warranted. This is particularly important when clinicians are considering the transposer for young children. Therefore, we (Gravel, Chute, and Popp 1994) have devised a method to fit the TranSonic that utilizes the desired sensation level (DSL) prescriptive hearing aid selection and evaluation procedure developed by Seewald and his colleagues (chapter 8; Seewald 1992; Seewald and Ross 1988; Seewald, Ramji, Moodie, Sinclair, and Jamieson 1994). The DSL is a carefully devised and efficient method specifically developed for use with infants and young children. The basic components of this objective strategy for fitting and evaluating the TranSonic are described below.

First, some standard electroacoustic measurements are made with the TranSonic set in the neutral position (i.e., no transposition: $Z_c = 1$, $Z_v = 1$). These measures are utilized for determining how well the device achieves the prescribed DSL coupler targets in the neutral setting. For example, measuring the device in the test box allows the audiologist to predetermine whether the instrument achieves the DSL HA-2 gain and output targets in the range of interest; that is, below 2500 Hz. Moreover, the HA-2 coupler values are useful to the audiologist in setting the position of the volume control (VC) on the TranSonic. (Indeed, in this strategy, we suggest that once the VC has been set to achieve targets in the test box, it should remain in that position for the remainder of the transposition fitting process.) The manufacturer recommends using a linear step-by-step acoustic test procedure for electroacoustic measurements of the TranSonic (automatic test sequences should not be utilized).

When available, real-ear measures are very useful for individualizing DSL targets. Even without real-ear measurements, the DSL provides real-ear-to-coupler corrections for children across the pediatric age range. Real-ear

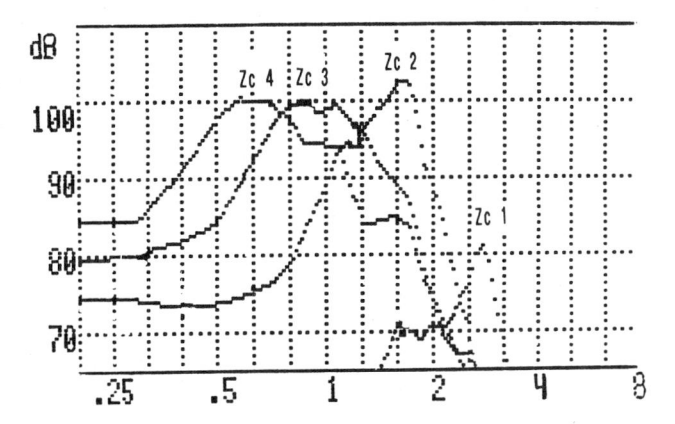

[Figure: graph showing dB vs frequency (.25 to 8 kHz) with curves labeled Zc 1, Zc 2, Zc 3, Zc 4]

Figure 10. The effects of varying the Zc transposition coefficient (from 1 to 4) on the TranSonic. Input signal was a 3000 Hz narrow band of noise. See text for details.

measurements of the TranSonic with the transposition activated are possible only when using a real-ear measurement system with an FFT analyzer (Fonix 6500, Frye Electronics) set to "spectrum mode," that is, with the regular source signal(s) turned off. In this FFT analysis mode (set to the highest noise reduction value of 16), and using narrow bands of noise generated by an audiometer as the input stimuli, the audiologist may examine the result of frequency transposition (within a 2cc coupler or the listener's ear). Figure 10 displays data obtained utilizing the preceding suggestions. The figure presents the effects of varying transposition coefficient (Zc) values. A 3000 Hz narrow band noise generated by a clinical audiometer was used as the input signal. Measurements were made with button transducer of the transposer connected to a 2cc coupler and the microphone of the TranSonic positioned in the sound field. Note the clearly observable shift of the peak of the signal as Zc was increased from the neutral (Zc = 1) to Zc = 4 position.

Our recommended TranSonic fitting strategy begins conventionally. Audiometric thresholds are entered into the DSL version 3.1 prescriptive fitting program, and the various DSL targets are generated for that child's individual hearing loss. These include the desired sensation levels for speech at each frequency, real-ear saturation response (RESR), insertion gain, aided sound field thresholds, etc. In addition, the electroacoustic parameters of gain and saturation sound pressure level (SSPL) 90 are provided for the amplification. In the case of the TranSonic, these may be measured in the acoustic test box using an HA-2 coupler with the device set at neutral (Zc = 1, Zv = 1). The DSL program also provides a verification table in which the measured responses are compared to the targets and difference values computed.

268 • *NEW TECHNOLOGIES*

The first step of the TranSonic fitting strategy is to select an initial Zc transposition coefficient for the child. This is done by first identifying an appropriate "transposition target frequency." The child's desired sensation levels for speech at each frequency below 2500 Hz are examined. Generally speaking, these values can be thought to represent the child's dynamic range as a function of frequency: A large desired sensation level value indicates a broad dynamic range and vice versa. The "transposition target frequency" is the highest nominal frequency below 2500 Hz where a reasonably large desired sensation level for speech exists. As an example, if a child's desired sensation level for speech at 500 Hz is 12 dB; 750 Hz, 11 dB; 1000 Hz, 9 dB; and at 1500 and 2000 Hz, 3 and 1 dB, respectively, the child's "transposition target frequency" is selected to be 1000 Hz. While 1500 and 2000 Hz might be considered, the desired sensation levels for speech at these frequencies are small, and thus, 1000 Hz appears to be the most appropriate value.

Next, (in all cases) the nominal value of 4000 Hz is utilized to represent high-frequency speech energy that occurs in the 3000-6000 Hz region. In our current example, the child's selected "transposition target frequency" of 1000 Hz is divided into 4000 Hz. The product (in this case, 4)

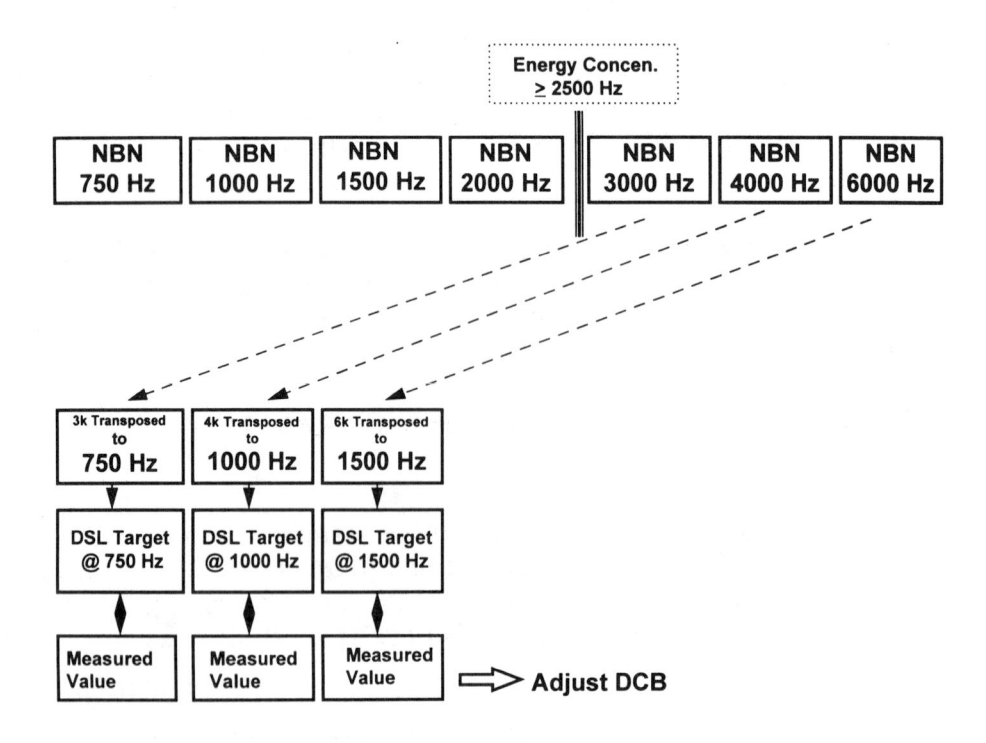

Figure 11. Schematic representation of a suggested fitting approach for the TranSonic hearing aid based on the desired sensation level (DSL) prescriptive fitting procedure. In this example, Zv =1, Zc = 4. See text for complete explanation.

becomes the Zc transposition coefficient. (Zv is maintained in the neutral 1 position.) In this example with Zc = 4 and Zv = 1, input energy concentrated below 2500 Hz is unaltered, while an energy concentration occurring at 2500 Hz and above is transposed by a factor of 4. (Note: the manufacturer cautions against setting Zc > 4.5.)

Figure 11 provides a means of conceptualizing frequency transposition and our DSL-TranSonic fitting strategy. Consistent with our current example, the values Zc = 4 and Zv = 1 have been used for display purposes in this figure. (If different Zc or Zv coefficients are selected, the values would vary from those depicted here.) Note that when input signals (narrow bands of noise) at 3000, 4000, and 6000 Hz are transposed by a factor of 4, the signals become 750, 1000, and 1500 Hz, respectively. Thus, when considering frequency transposition, the audiologist must examine the target values in the DSL program specified for the *newly transposed* frequency rather than the *original* input frequency. Therefore, verification of the achievement of DSL target values for frequencies above 2500 Hz is considered for the "transposed" rather than the nominal input frequency. Adjustments in DCB may be appropriate if measured response values are less than the specified DSL target values.

As the child gains listening experience with the transposed speech signal, the Zc value on the TranSonic may be adjusted. It is desirous to set the Zc transposition coefficient to the lowest value (that is, the least spectral compression) possible while maintaining speech perception abilities. Thus, after setting the initial Zc transposition coefficient value, any further adjustment of the setting should occur only as part of an ongoing aural habilitation process.

This procedure is offered to clinicians considering fitting the TranSonic and desiring a more objective method to initially fit the device to young children. Functional verification of the efficacy of such a fitting and evaluation approach still requires investigation.

DEVELOPING GUIDELINES FOR STUDYING TRANSPOSITION HEARING AIDS

Although reports of the benefit of current transposition devices appear encouraging, the need to adopt some guidelines for the study of these devices seems warranted. We have modeled the following suggestions for guidelines after those proffered by Erber (1971) nearly 25 years ago for the study of early systems.

1. There is a need for a clear delineation of candidacy criteria. Case reports that carefully delineate the degree and configuration of the hearing losses of individuals who use transposition hearing

aids are necessary. Moreover, the in-depth examination of the perceptual abilities of the users in quiet and noise will be necessary in order to quantify the benefits of a transposition device over conventional amplification.

2. There should be some agreement on a method by which devices will be fit particularly to young children. That is, objective protocols in addition to subjective methods should be considered and investigated. These methods should include means to select response characteristics and device parameters. Materials used for the assessment of auditory perception should be specified. Collection of data from a number of centers agreeing to use similar protocols and procedures (similar to those specified for the children's cochlear implant trials) would be beneficial. Short- and long-term efficacy of the device should be studied by examining the young listener's performance over time with the instrument.

3. Particularly with children, there is a need to provide specific auditory training as part of device provision. Only in this way will it be possible to compare and contrast how perceptual abilities may be enhanced by changes in transposition coefficient values and signal intensity variations.

4. In cases in which a cochlear implant is being considered for a child, it may be useful to examine individual performance with the transposer with the group data from the prospective study of pediatric implant recipients. In this way, performance comparisons can be made for comparable periods of use-time and decisions regarding appropriate intervention made.

With the advent of newer technology, the pediatric audiologist has an ever-expanding armamentarium of amplification devices that undoubtedly will prove useful to children with hearing loss. Our mission is to determine how best to match the device with the individual child so that the goal of maximizing a child's use of auditory input through amplification may be realized.

ACKNOWLEDGMENTS

The authors wish to thank Tad Zelski and Amy L. Popp for their valuable contributions to this chapter.

REFERENCES

American Heritage Dictionary. 1985.

Audiologic-Sarl. 1991. A new approach for auditory rehabilitation. Laboratorie d'audiologie Duprés-Lefevre, Montbeliard, France.

AVR/Communications Ltd. 1993. *TranSonic™ fitting and evaluation procedures manual.* Chanhassen, Minnesota.

Bennett, D.N., and Byers, V.W. 1967. Increased intelligibility in the hypacusic by slow-play frequency transposition. *Journal of Auditory Research* 7:107-118.

Chute, P.M., Gravel, J.S., and Popp, A.L. 1995. Speech perception abilities of adults using a multi-channel cochlear implant and frequency transposition hearing aid. *Annals of Otology, Rhinology, Laryngology* (Suppl.), September pp. 260-263.

Erber, N.P. 1971. Evaluation of special hearing aids for deaf children. *Journal of Speech and Hearing Disorders* 6:527-537.

Erber, N.P. 1982. *Auditory training.* Washington, D.C.: Alexander Graham Bell Association for the Deaf.

Foust, K.O., and Gengel, R. 1973. Speech discrimination by sensorineural hearing-impaired persons using a transposer hearing aid. *Scandinavian Audiology* 2:161-170.

Gravel, J.S., Chute, P.M., and Popp, A.L. 1994. Objective fitting of the TranSonic™ hearing aid. Paper read at the annual meeting of the American Speech-Language-Hearing Association, November, New Orleans, Louisiana.

Ling, D., and Druz, W.S. 1967. Transposition of high frequency sounds by partial vocoding of the speech spectrum: Its use by deaf children. *Journal of Auditory Research* 7:133-144.

Ling, D., and Maretic, H. 1971. Frequency transposition in the teaching of speech to deaf children. *Journal of Speech and Hearing Research* 14:37-46.

Plant, G. 1994. *Analytika* (Auditory Training Program). Somerville, Mass.: Audiological Engineering Corporation.

Plant, G., and Franklin, L. 1994. Providing high frequency speech cues to profoundly hearing-impaired listeners: Two approaches. Paper read at the International Conference on Tactile Aids, Hearing Aids and Cochlear Implants, May, Coral Gables.

Robbins, A.M., Renshaw, J.J., Miyamoto, R.T., Osberger, M.J., and Pope, M.L. 1988. *Minimal pairs test.* Indianapolis: Indiana University School of Medicine.

Seewald, R.C. 1992. The desired sensation level method for fitting children: Version 3.0. *Hearing Journal* 45(4):36-41.

Seewald, R.C., Ramji, K.V., Moodie, K.S., Sinclair, S.T., and Jamieson, D.G. 1994. *Desired sensation level method—version 3.1.* London, Ontario: Department of Communication Disorders, University of Western Ontario.

Seewald, R.C., and Ross, M. 1988. Amplification for young children. In M.C. Pollack (ed.), *Amplification for the hearing impaired* (pp. 213-271). 3d ed. Orlando, Fla.: Grune and Stratton.

13

Behind-the-Ear FM Systems: New Technology for Children

Patricia A. Chase and Fred H. Bess

INTRODUCTION

A properly fitted and functioning hearing aid is absolutely essential if a young child with hearing impairment is to realize the maximum potential for learning. Ross (1975) emphasizes the importance of amplification in the habilitation/rehabilitation process: "For most children with sensorineural hearing loss, the early, appropriate, and supervised use of hearing aid amplification is the single most effective rehabilitation tool we have. Amplification is the only therapeutic measure that focuses directly on the primary cause of the handicap, that is, the hearing loss itself. Effectively applied within the boundaries of a complete rehabilitative program, it affords the greatest possibility of minimizing the usual consequences of congenital sensorineural hearing loss."

The most commonly used amplification systems in the educational setting include the personal hearing aid and frequency modulated (FM) auditory training systems. The personal hearing aid offers several distinct advantages in the educational environment including mobility, child-to-child communication and self-monitoring, and electroacoustic characteristics that are considered appropriate for the hearing loss. One principal drawback to the personal hearing aid is the separation between the sound source and the pickup microphone. This distance factor creates variable and unfavorable signal-to-noise listening conditions as well as a signal level that may not be sufficient to overcome the hearing loss. If the hearing loss does not exceed 90 dB and the ambient noise level does not exceed 40 dB, a personal hearing aid can be used with success in the classroom (Boothroyd 1981). Unfortunately, most classrooms exceed 40 dB, prompting the need for FM systems (Bess and McConnell 1981; Bess, Sinclair, and Riggs 1984; Crandell 1993; Olsen 1988; Ross 1992a).

The most widely used system in education today is the wireless FM trainer. Introduced more than 25 years ago, these amplification devices are designed to improve the signal-to-noise relationship between the primary signal and background noise (Ross 1992b). According to Ross, FM systems are the most significant therapeutic tool developed for children with hearing impairment since the advent of personal and group amplification devices. The use of FM technology affords the child with hearing impairment a high quality signal, thus improving speech recognition by compensating for listening problems associated with background noise, distance from the speaker, and reverberation.

A number of techniques have been developed for coupling sound from the body-worn FM receiver to the child's ear. These techniques include ear button transducers, direct audio input hearing aids, and neckloops and silhouette inductors coupled with personal hearing aids. Recently, a new technology has been developed that provides the listening advantages associated with traditional FM auditory trainers while simultaneously eliminating many of the problems associated with older body-worn FM receivers. These systems, which combine an FM receiver/hearing aid worn by the listener, are manufactured by two companies and marketed as Extend-Ear® and FreeEar®. The integrated behind-the-ear (BTE) FM receiver/hearing aid eliminates coupler options and offers new choices both inside and outside the classroom for providing the FM advantage to children with hearing losses.

In this chapter, we describe the BTE FM system, discuss its apparent benefits and limitations, review the electroacoustic characteristics of these systems, offer suggestions for the appropriate evaluation of these systems, and project future needs.

COMPONENTS AND FEATURES

The BTE FM receiver and two FM transmitter/microphone options currently available in the marketplace are shown in figure 1. The lapel microphone transmitter, which can also be belt or pocket worn, has a volume control for adjusting FM gain relative to hearing aid gain and a high-frequency tone control to enhance speech understanding. A pen-shaped lavalier transmitter microphone and a small personal transmitter microphone with a retractable antenna are both compatible with most FM receivers, including wide and narrow band channels. Features of the lavalier transmitter and the personal transmitter include automatic gain control circuitry for

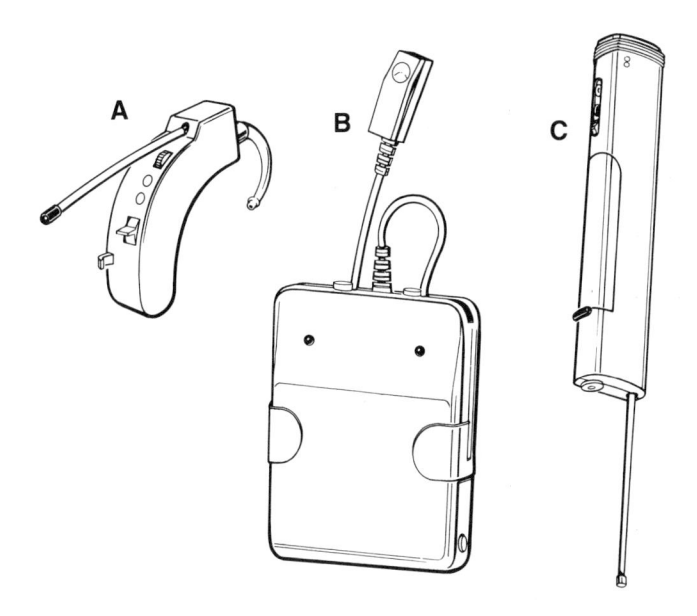

Figure 1. Schematic of BTE FM receiver (A) and two transmitter microphone (B, C) options.

adjusting audio gain relative to the loudness of the speaker's voice as well as gain control and high-frequency tone control trimmers that allow FM adjustments relative to the hearing aid part of the receiver.

An important feature of these amplification devices is wide fitting flexibility thus enabling BTE FM receivers to be used as primary amplification. Moderate, power, and superpower hearing aids are available as well as aids for precipitous losses. Similar to traditional FM systems, the BTE FM receivers have three operational modes: FM only, hearing aid only, and combined FM/hearing aid. Detachable FM antennas are available as well as squelch circuitry for eliminating white noise when the FM signal is not present. A mild gain, low output, FM only receiver with no internal microphone has been developed for children identified with central auditory processing disorders.

POTENTIAL BENEFITS AND LIMITATIONS

Because BTE FM hearing systems are relatively new, their benefits and limitations have not been clearly delineated. However, as these systems become more widely used, children, parents, teachers, and audiologists will begin to determine the various advantages and shortcomings for specific listening situations.

Indeed, the cosmetic acceptability of BTE FM systems to both children and their parents is a distinct benefit of these integrated FM receiver/hearing aid units. Similar in size to other BTE hearing aids, these units eliminate the bulky body-worn receivers associated with traditional FM systems. Moreover, the subsequent elimination of ear button transducers, cords, neckloops, and silhouette inductors enhances the wearability of BTE FM systems and improves significantly the manageability of these systems. Cosmetic appeal frequently becomes a greater issue as students approach middle school, and BTE FM systems offer another alternative for this challenging age group. The downside of cosmetic appeal may be its attraction to parents even when another FM fitting might be more appropriate for their child. Further research is needed to determine whether very young children and children with multiple disabilities benefit more from BTE FM systems or traditional body-worn fittings.

Clearly, a major benefit of BTE FM systems is the elimination of confounding variables associated with coupling body-worn FM receivers and personal hearing aids using neckloops, direct audio input, and silhouette inductors. For example, Hawkins and Schum (1985) measured frequency response curves from FM system-hearing aid combinations under four different coupling conditions and found that the high-frequency responses were reduced when hearing aids were coupled to FM systems as compared to the frequency response curve obtained for the hearing aid alone. Also, Hawkins and Schum (1985) reported considerable variability in volume control taper characteristics for FM system-hearing aid combinations using three different coupling conditions.

Lewis and colleagues (Lewis, Feigin, Karasek, and Stelmachowicz 1991) obtained a family of frequency response curves at seven volume control wheel settings from a single FM system using a 75 dB SPL pure-tone signal. Harmonic distortion was also measured for each of the seven volume control settings. The effect of adjusting the volume control wheel on output occurred primarily at only the first two (#2 and #3) settings. The specific FM system under investigation was driven beyond its linear operating range at volume control settings beyond #3, and this effect was particularly evident for the 250 to 4000 Hz frequency range. Harmonic distortion measurements at 500 Hz and 1000 Hz using these same seven volume control wheel settings revealed distortion of 20% or greater at 500 Hz for settings above #2 and at 1000 Hz for settings above #3.

Seewald and Moodie (1992) contend that successful FM system fittings provide children with a consistent amplified speech signal across listening conditions. The electroacoustic end product provided by the child's hearing aid alone and that provided by the FM system must be in close approximation. Recent studies (Lewis et al. 1991; Thibodeau, McCaffrey, and Abrahamson 1988) support the difficulty of maintaining consistent electroacoustic performance even when the FM system-hearing aid combination and coupling method are held constant; slight movements of a silhouette inductor result in significant effects on the FM output (Lewis et al. 1991), and changes in head orientation result in large frequency response variations in FM system-hearing aid combinations using a neckloop coupling method (Thibodeau et al. 1988). Seewald and Moodie (1992) offer an excellent review and summary of the FM system-related variables that can affect the signal a child receives from an FM system—many of these variables are related to coupling FM systems and personal hearing aids.

ELECTROACOUSTIC CHARACTERISTICS

Although no electroacoustic measurement standard presently exists for FM systems, the FM component and the hearing aid component require separate evaluations. Full-on gain, SSPL90, and harmonic distortion measurements should be compared to those values published by each equipment manufacturer (American Speech-Language-Hearing Association 1994). Our own electroacoustic measurements of the two systems currently available for clinical use found both units to be operating within each manufacturer's published specifications.

Because antenna length can significantly affect FM transmission ranges for traditional body-worn systems, equipment manufacturers recommend that transmitter antennas remain straight and completely extended for optimal distance transmission. We investigated the effect of receiver antenna placement on the transmission ranges of BTE FM systems using conversational speech intelligibility as the outcome measure. In a simulated classroom environment, speaker/listener distance was systematically increased and measured to determine transmission range. An adult listener qualitatively judged when conversational speech produced by a stationary adult speaker became unintelligible. BTE receiver antennas were either clipped tightly against the receiver case or unclipped and fully extended. Transmitter microphone placement was either optimal—with the antenna fully extended and the microphone located six inches from the sound source—or poor—with the antenna incompletely extended and the microphone more than six inches from the sound source. Each of the two commercially available BTE FM systems, hereafter referred to as Product A and Product B, was evaluated under the following four test conditions: (1) antenna unclipped with optimal microphone placement; (2) antenna unclipped with poor microphone placement; (3) antenna clipped with optimal microphone placement; and (4) antenna clipped with poor microphone placement. The results of this analysis are shown in figure 2. Product A demonstrated a steady decline in FM transmission range across the four test conditions with maximal transmission range (81 feet) occurring under condition 1 and minimal transmission range

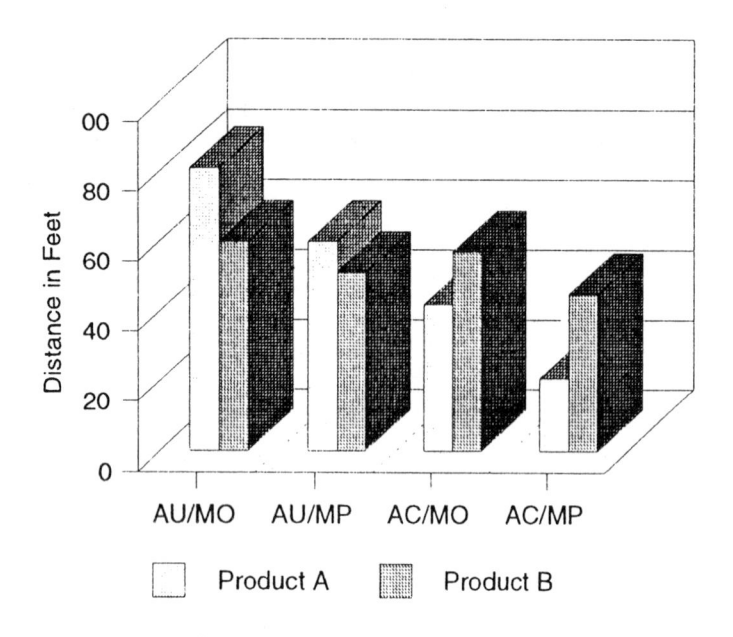

Figure 2. Transmission ranges for two different systems in the FM mode with lapel microphone transmitter. Receiver antenna was unclipped (AU) or clipped (AC), and microphone placement was optimal (MO) or poor (MP).

(21 feet) in condition 4. Product B demonstrated less variability in transmission range across conditions (condition 1—60 feet; condition 4—45 feet).

Transmission ranges were also measured for Product A under the same four test conditions using a lapel microphone transmitter with the receiver in the FM only mode and in the combined FM/hearing aid (FM/HA) mode. Again, maximal transmission range was obtained when the antenna was unclipped with optimal microphone placement (condition 1). Transmission ranges steadily decreased in test conditions 2, 3, and 4 with minimal transmission ranges occurring in both the FM only and the combined FM/HA mode when the receiver antenna was clipped and the microphone poorly placed.

Transmission ranges were again measured for Product B under test conditions 1 and 3 using a lavalier microphone transmitter with the receiver in the FM only mode and in the combined FM/HA mode. There was little difference between transmission ranges in the FM only mode and the combined FM/HA mode. Transmission ranges were only slightly better with the antenna unclipped (FM only—42 feet; FM/HA—40 feet) versus the antenna clipped condition (FM only—39 feet; FM/HA—37 feet).

These data support the following conclusions regarding the use of BTE FM systems with children. First, optimal FM transmission range requires that the receiver antenna be flexed out rather than clipped to the case and that the transmitter antenna be fully extended with microphone placement about six inches from the sound source. Second, the combined FM/HA mode, often used by children to hear the primary speaker, monitor their own voice, and receive environmental sound input is subject to the same conditions as the FM only receiver mode for maximizing transmission ranges. Third, the poor microphone placement used in this investigation is often seen in classrooms when teachers wear lapel microphones and will likely become more common as FM use increases. Because lavalier microphones are designed to be suspended about six inches from the speaker's mouth, there may be less opportunity for inadvertent poor placement. Audiologists must consider where and how BTE FM systems will be used and educate parents, caregivers, and teachers regarding the most effective FM technique.

ASHA 1994 GUIDELINES FOR FITTING AND MONITORING FM SYSTEMS

The American Speech-Language-Hearing Association (ASHA) published Guidelines for Fitting and Monitoring FM Systems (1994) to provide direction in a clinical practice area where standardized protocols are virtually nonexistent. These guidelines focus on personal and self-contained FM systems used by children and adults with hearing loss. Ear-level FM systems or BTE FM systems are considered self-contained systems within these guidelines because they couple directly to the ear as opposed to personal FM systems, which couple to an individual's own hearing aids.

The audiologist is the professional most qualified to evaluate, fit, and dispense FM systems, though other personnel may perform daily monitoring checks on the units after receiving instruction from a certified audiologist. The guidelines address preselection and management considerations including the need for daily and comprehensive monitoring as well as audiologic re-evaluation.

Though no validated measurement procedures presently exist for fitting FM systems, several current approaches are detailed in the guidelines and serve as the basis for the recommended procedures for FM system performance measurements. Performance measurements enable the audiologist to adjust FM system control settings to achieve the desired frequency response, output, and gain, and to evaluate speech recognition ability with the FM system as compared to performance with the personal hearing aids. Two approaches for fitting and adjusting FM systems are presented: electroacoustic measures in a 2-cm^3 coupler and real-ear measurements using a probe microphone.

The recommended procedure for adjusting FM systems using 2-cm^3 coupler measurements is a modified version of the protocol proffered by

Seewald and Moodie (1992). Key assumptions of this approach are that the individual's personal hearing aids have been fitted appropriately, that the hearing aids are functioning properly, and that relative differences between hearing aid performance and FM system performance measured in a 2-cm^3 coupler will hold constant in the real ear (Lewis et al. 1991; Seewald and Moodie 1992). Complete details for adjusting FM systems using 2-cm^3 coupler measurements are provided in the ASHA guidelines.

Functional gain assessments and probe-microphone measurements are the two real-ear approaches most commonly used for fitting and adjusting FM systems. The limitations of aided sound-field threshold measurements (Lewis et al. 1991; Seewald, Hudson, Gagné, and Zelisko 1992; Seewald and Moodie 1992) have resulted in increased use of probe-microphone measurements for assessing real-ear gain/frequency response and maximum output. The suggested procedure in these guidelines for fitting FM systems using probe-microphone measurements is based on the detailed work of several investigators (Hawkins 1987, 1992, 1993; Lewis 1994; Lewis et al. 1991; Seewald, Zelisko, Ramji, and Jamieson 1991; Sullivan 1987). Like the 2-cm^3 coupler measurements noted above, one of the recommended probe-microphone approaches relies on appropriately functioning personal hearing aids as the basis for matching real-ear FM system output. The other suggested approach utilizes a procedure to determine desired amplification characteristics for the FM system without regard for the variables associated with personal hearing aid performance. Detailed descriptions for the adjustment of FM systems using probe-microphone measurements are provided in the ASHA guidelines. A procedure developed by Lewis and colleagues (1991) for assessing speech recognition performance with FM systems is also included within the ASHA guidelines. Procedures are described for speech recognition testing in the following conditions: FM only mode with the environmental microphones not activated, hearing aid only mode with no FM signal present, and combined FM and hearing aid mode with the FM signal present and environmental microphones activated. Complete details for obtaining all three measurements are described in the ASHA guidelines.

SUMMARY AND CONCLUSIONS

A young child with hearing impairment must have a properly fitted and functioning hearing aid to optimize classroom learning. Personal hearing aids are appropriate for some children in the educational environment. However, many youngsters need FM systems to overcome the problems of speaker/listener distance, poor classroom acoustics, and excessive background noise. Although wireless FM auditory trainers are widely used in education today, there are many problems associated with coupling sound from traditional body-worn FM receivers to the individual child's ear. New technology integrating a BTE FM receiver and hearing aid offers solutions to some of the issues related to body-worn FM units. In this chapter we describe the BTE FM system, discuss apparent benefits and limitations, and offer suggestions for appropriate evaluation of these systems.

BTE FM systems are flexible and capable of accommodating varying degrees of hearing impairment. Cosmetic acceptability and the elimination of confounding variables associated with coupling body-worn FM receivers and personal hearing aids are major benefits of these new units. The elimination of ear button transducers, cords, neckloops, and silhouette inductors greatly enhances the manageability of BTE FM systems. Transmission range varies as a function of both antenna and microphone placement with optimal signal transmission occurring when the receiver antenna is flexed out and the transmitter antenna is fully extended with the microphone located six inches from the sound source.

Because this technology is new, benefits and limitations will be forthcoming as BTE FM systems are used in different settings with children who have varying degrees of hearing loss. Systematic research and inquiry will enable us to better determine the role of BTE FM technology in effectively maximizing a child's residual hearing. As younger and younger children are identified with hearing impairment, pediatric audiologists have more opportunities for implementing new technological solutions into the rehabilitation process. Along with these opportunities come increased responsibilities for professional consensus regarding the most appropriate strategies for fitting young children with these systems. Future research needs must also focus on the efficacy of using BTE FM systems with children who have milder forms of hearing loss as well as those who exhibit problems with higher order processing. Practical issues associated with using BTE FM systems in various listening environments merit further study. Although no standardized protocols exist for fitting FM systems, ASHA guidelines (1994) offer direction for audiologists who evaluate, dispense, and monitor BTE FM systems used by children with hearing loss.

ACKNOWLEDGMENTS

The authors express appreciation to AVR Sonovation, Carolina Hearing and Speech Services, and Phonic Ear for providing equipment for this research.

REFERENCES

American Speech-Language-Hearing Association. 1994. Guidelines for fitting and monitoring FM systems. *Asha* 36 (Suppl. 12):1-9.

Bess, F.H., and McConnell, F. 1981. *Audiology, education and the hearing impaired child.* St. Louis: C.V. Mosby.

Bess, F.H., Sinclair, J.S., and Riggs, D. 1984. Group amplification in schools for the hearing impaired. *Ear and Hearing* 5:138-144.

Boothroyd, A. 1981. Group hearing aids. In F.H. Bess, B.A. Freeman, and J.S. Sinclair (eds.), *Amplification in education.* Washington, D.C.: Alexander Graham Bell Association for the Deaf.

Crandell, C. 1993. Speech recognition in noise by children with minimal degrees of sensorineural hearing loss. *Ear and Hearing* 14:210-216.

Hawkins, D.B. 1987. Assessment of FM systems with probe tube microphone system. *Ear and Hearing* 8(5):301-303.

Hawkins, D.B. 1992. Selecting SSPL 90 using probe-microphone measurements. In H.G. Mueller, D.B. Hawkins, and J.L. Northern (eds.), *Probe microphone measurements: Hearing aid selection and assessment.* San Diego: Singular Publishing Group.

Hawkins, D.B. 1993. Assessment of hearing aid maximum output. *American Journal of Audiology* 2(1):36-37.

Hawkins, D.B., and Schum, D. 1985. Some effects of FM-system coupling on hearing aid characteristics. *Journal of Speech and Hearing Disorders* 50:132-141.

Lewis, D. 1994. Assistive devices for classroom listening: FM systems. *American Journal of Audiology* 3(1):70-83.

Lewis, D., Feigin, J.A., Karasek, A., and Stelmachowicz, P.G. 1991. Evaluation and assessment of FM systems. *Ear and Hearing* 12(4):268-280.

Olsen, W.O. 1988. Classroom acoustics for hearing impaired children. In F.H. Bess (ed.), *Hearing impairment in children.* Parkton, Md.: York Press.

Ross, M. 1975. Hearing aids for young children. *Otolaryngologic Clinics of North America* 8:125-141.

Ross, M. 1992a. Room acoustics and speech perception. In M. Ross (ed.), *FM auditory training systems: Characteristics, selection, and use.* Timonium, Md.: York Press.

Ross, M. 1992b. Preface. In M. Ross (ed.), *FM auditory training systems: Characteristics, selection, and use.* Timonium, Md.: York Press.

Seewald, R.C., Hudson, S., Gagné, J.P., and Zelisko, D.L. 1992. Comparison of two methods for estimating the sensation level of amplified speech. *Ear and Hearing* 13(3):142-149.

Seewald, R.C., and Moodie, K.S. 1992. Electroacoustic considerations. In M. Ross (ed.), *FM auditory training systems: Characteristics, selection, and use.* Timonium, Md.: York Press.

Seewald, R.C., Zelisko, D.L., Ramji, K.V., and Jamieson, D.G. 1991. *DSL 3.0 user's manual.* London, Ontario, Canada: University of Western Ontario.

Sullivan, R. 1987. Aided SSPL 90 response in the real ear: a safe estimate. *Hearing Instruments* 38:36.

Thibodeau, L.M., McCaffrey, H., and Abrahamson, J. 1988. Effects of coupling hearing aids to FM systems via neck loops. *Journal of the Academy of Rehabilitative Audiology* 21:49-56.

14

Cochlear Implants and Tactile Aids for Children with Profound Hearing Impairment

Mary Joe Osberger, Amy M. Robbins, Susan L. Todd, Allyson Riley, Karen Iler Kirk, and Arlene Earley Carney

INTRODUCTION

A research program has been under way since 1987 at the Indiana University School of Medicine that is designed to obtain a better understanding of the benefits that children with profound hearing impairments derive from different sensory aids. A series of longitudinal studies have been conducted that compare the speech perception performance of children with profound hearing impairment who use cochlear implants, tactile aids, or hearing aids. The purpose of this chapter is to provide a summary of these studies and highlight future research directions. Information is presented on (1) the speech perception materials used to evaluate device effectiveness, (2) the description of experimental and control groups, (3) comparisons of single/dual-channel and multichannel devices, (4) comparisons of multichannel devices and hearing aids, (5) additional studies with multichannel implant users, and (6) summary of major findings and directions for research.

EVALUATION MATERIALS

The outcome measures used to determine sensory aid benefit consisted of a battery of tests that assessed a range of speech perception skills. At the time that our research was initiated, relatively few tests existed that were appropriate to assess the performance of children with profound hearing impairments. Consequently, new measures were developed and evaluated to examine a range of skills in the population under study. The Change/No Change procedure (Carney, Osberger, Carney, Robbins, Renshaw, and Miyamoto 1993) assesses detection of a change in a suprasegmental or segmental feature of speech in a sequence of ten consonant-vowel (CV) syllables. All ten syllables are the same on a no-change trial, whereas the last five syllables differ from the first five on a change trial. The child is instructed to respond "same" on a no-change trial and "different" on a change trial. The Change/No Change Test is recorded and presented at 70 dB SPL in the sound field. There are seven subtests, each of which contrasts a different feature of speech. This procedure was used most often during our initial studies when the subjects' perceptual skills were limited by the use of single-channel implants or tactile aids. In the more recent investigations in which subjects have used multichannel devices, performance was reported on the following speech identification or recognition tasks.

The Minimal Pairs Test (Robbins, Renshaw, Miyamoto, Osberger, and Pope 1988) consists of pairs of pictured words, with members of a pair differing in terms of a single vowel or consonant. Vowel items are analyzed in terms of the features of vowel height and place; consonant items are analyzed in terms of the features of voicing, manner, and place. The test consists of a total of 20 word pairs, 12 with consonant contrasts and 8 with vowel contrasts. Each word in a pair is presented as a test item but in random order, totaling 40 different items. Each word is presented two times, also in random order, totaling 80 items on the entire test. Performance is expressed in terms of the percentage of total words correctly identified or as a function of vowel or consonant feature (chance level of performance = 50%).

The Common Phrases Test (Robbins, Renshaw, and Osberger 1988) was developed to assess understanding of familiar phrases used in everyday situations using a modified open-set format with pretest familiarization of item topics. The child is shown a set of ten pictured items and told that simple questions, commands, or statements will be said about the items. The card with the pictured items is removed before testing begins. There are six lists with ten items per list. Performance is scored in terms of the percentage of phrases correctly understood. That is, the child must repeat correctly all words in a phrase to receive credit for that item (if a question is asked, the child is given full credit for answering the question appropriately). Because there are no alternatives from which the subject chooses the answer, this is considered to be an "open-set" test of speech recognition (chance level of performance = 0%).

The Phonetically Balanced Kindergarten (PBK) Test (Haskins 1949) assesses recognition of monosyllabic words in an open set. Performance is scored in terms of the number of phonemes as well as the number of words correctly understood.

The Minimal Pairs, Common Phrases, and PBK Tests were administered with auditory (or tactile) cues only. In addition, the Common Phrases Test was administered with combined auditory (or tactile) cues plus visual cues. Live-voice testing was employed with the examiner seated across the table from the child in a quiet room. For tests administered without speechreading cues, the examiner held a mesh-covered screen in front of her face. A team of four examiners (one audiologist and three speech-language pathologists), who had extensive experience with live-voice testing, evaluated the children. The stimuli were articulated clearly and precisely in a manner described by Picheny, Durlach, and Braida (1986) at levels that ranged roughly from 70 to 75 dB SPL (as determined from sound-level meter readings during a pilot study). The limitations of this type of testing are recognized. However, this format was necessary due to the limited attention spans and perceptual abilities of the subjects under study. Had recorded materials been used, floor effects would have precluded meaningful assessment of the children's performance.

A major limitation with many existing evaluation procedures is the lack of data on test-retest reliability, making it difficult to isolate significant changes in performance from random variations. Therefore, a secondary aim of our research was to determine the test-retest reliability of the measures in our test battery. To address this issue, 21 subjects with profound hearing losses who used conventional hearing aids were tested on the measures on two separate occasions, with an interval of approximately two weeks between test sessions. The mean unaided better-ear pure-tone average (500 Hz, 1000 Hz, 2000 Hz) was 97 dB HL, and the mean aided threshold obtained in the sound field with warble tones while the subjects were wearing their hearing aids was 45 dB HL. The mean chronological age of the subjects was 7.4 years (range = 4.3 to 11.0 years). Table 1 shows the scores between the first and second test administration and the correlation coefficients. These data show

Table 1
Mean differences (percentage) and correlations between test and retest scores on implant test battery for 21 subjects. Time interval between tests = 2 weeks.

	Change[a]	Min Pairs[b]	CP: Aud[c]	CP + LR[d]	PBK: Words	PBK:Phone[e]
Mean Difference	2.0	2.5	1.5	2.5	0.5	2.5
r	0.97	0.90	0.91	0.97	0.94	0.89

[a] Change/No Change Test
[b] Minimal Pairs Test
[c] Common Phrases Test with auditory cues only
[d] Common Phrases Test with auditory plus lipreading cues
[e] PBK Test: phoneme score

very small differences between repeated administration of the tests and good test-retest reliability on all measures.

SUBJECTS

The subjects consisted of experimental groups of children who used either cochlear implants or tactile aids and control groups who had varying degrees of profound hearing loss and who used conventional hearing aids. There were four experimental groups who used the following devices: 3M/House single-channel implant, Tactaid II+ vibrotactile aid, Nucleus multichannel cochlear implant, or Tactaid 7 multichannel vibrotactile aid. The initial studies compared children's performance with the 3M/House single-channel implant or the Tactaid II+ vibrotactile aid. Subsequent studies compared the performance of the children who received either the Nucleus multichannel cochlear implant or the multichannel vibrotactile aid, the Tactaid 7. The experimental subjects received a cochlear implant or tactile aid because they derived negligible benefit from conventional hearing aids. All testing was performed while the subjects were wearing their implants or tactile aids only (i.e., subjects were not tested with hearing aids and implants or tactile aids). Subjects who received a cochlear implant were referred for these devices by parents and professionals. Subjects who matched the characteristics of the implanted subjects were recruited for the tactile aid groups. Many of the tactile aid subjects were recruited from the same schools attended by the subjects with cochlear implants.

EXPERIMENTAL GROUPS AND DEVICES

The 3M/House device (Fretz and Fravel 1985) consists of a single electrode implanted in the cochlea, along with a ground electrode and an internal induction coil. Microphone output is directed to a speech processor that amplifies, filters (bandpass from 340 to 2700 Hz), and amplitude modulates a 16 kHz sinusoidal carrier. The Nucleus device (Patrick and Clark 1991) is a multichannel intracochlear implant system with an electrode array of 22 platinum bands. The WSP III processor uses a feature extraction scheme that encodes fundamental frequency and first and second formant (F0/F1/F2) information. For each stimulus frame, the processor selects two electrode positions for sequential (i.e., nonsimultaneous) stimulation, one corresponding to the estimated F1 (300 to 1000 Hz) and the other to the estimated F2 (800 to 4000 Hz). The electrodes are stimulated at a rate equal to the estimated F0 during voiced sounds, and at an average of 100 pulses per second (pps) during unvoiced segments. Subjects implanted after 1989 received the next generation Nucleus processor, the Mini Speech Processor (MSP) that employs refined techniques for feature extraction for the

F0/F1/F2 strategy, presentation of pulses between 200 and 300 Hz during unvoiced sounds, enhanced resolution of amplitude encoding, and a more compressive mapping function to derive pulse amplitudes from the bandpass outputs. The MSP also can be programmed with the Multipeak (MPeak) scheme that employs a combined feature extraction and waveform representation strategy. In addition to extraction of F1 and F2, the MPeak strategy measures the energy present in three higher frequency bands: band 3: 2000 to 2800 Hz; band 4: 2800 to 4000 Hz; and band 5: 4000 to 7000 Hz. With MPeak, four pulses are delivered in each stimulus frame. During voiced sounds, the electrodes for bands 4 and 3, and for F1 and F2 are stimulated in base-to-apex order. During unvoiced sounds, electrodes for bands 5, 4, 3, and for F2 are stimulated. The newer MSP also substitutes digital for the analog hardware of the WSP (Wilson 1993).

The Tactaid II+ (Franklin 1988) is a two-channel vibrotactile device that transposes the incoming signal to frequencies around 275 Hz and splits it by low-pass (2.5 kHz cutoff) and high-pass (1.2 kHz cutoff) filtering. The filter outputs are then sent to two vibrators, which are worn on the wrist or sternum, with one vibrator responding to low frequencies and the other to high frequencies. The Tactaid 7 (Franklin 1991) is a seven-channel device that consists of seven filter bands that correspond roughly to the F1 (bands 1 to 4) and F2 (bands 4 to 7) of speech. The incoming signal is analyzed so that the highest spectral peaks in these bands are selected and then delivered to the corresponding vibrators. The vibrator array is worn on the sternum.

CONTROL GROUPS

The approach that has been used most often to evaluate tactile aid or implant benefit is a within-subjects design wherein the subject serves as his or her own control. A limitation with this type of design is that it is difficult to interpret the results relative to the performance of other children with profound hearing impairments who have not received an implant or tactile aid. Even though there might be statistically significant differences between pre- and postimplant or tactile aid scores, the clinical significance of these differences often is not clear. In our laboratory, we have compared the performance of children with implants to that of children with profound hearing impairments who use conventional hearing aids. Previous research has shown that children with profound hearing impairments demonstrate a wide range of auditory capabilities (Boothroyd 1984; Erber 1972). Using the results of these investigators as a guide, we divided hearing aid users into three groups based on the unaided better-ear pure-tone thresholds at 500, 1000, and 2000 Hz. Subjects classified as *Gold* hearing aid users demonstrated pure-tone thresholds of 90 to 100 dB HL at two of the three frequencies, with none of the three thresholds greater than 105 dB HL. *Silver* hearing aid users demonstrated thresholds of 101 to 110 dB HL at two of the three frequencies, whereas *Bronze* hearing aid users demonstrated two of three thresholds greater than 110 dB HL (the majority of Bronze hearing aid users subsequently received a tactile aid or cochlear implant).

Using this approach, we viewed the Gold hearing aid users as setting the "gold standard of performance" for children with profound hearing impairments because research has shown that children with this amount of residual hearing develop the most viable oral communication skills (e.g., Smith 1975). It was hypothesized that the Gold hearing aid users would demonstrate better speech perception skills than the implant or tactile aid subjects. At the other end of the continuum are Bronze hearing aid users who appear to respond to sound on the basis of vibrotactile rather than auditory sensation (Boothroyd and Cawkwell 1970). Subjects who received cochlear implants or tactile aids in the studies that follow were classified as Bronze hearing aid users. The performance of the Silver hearing aid users was predicted to fall intermediate to that of the Gold and Bronze hearing aid users. The performance of Silver hearing aid subjects was examined to determine if it was better or poorer than that of the multichannel implant and tactile users. A finding of poorer performance by the Silver hearing aid users than the multichannel implant or tactile aid users suggests that children with hearing levels of 100 dB HL and higher might benefit more from these devices than from continued use of only conventional acoustic amplification.

COMPARISON OF SINGLE/DUAL-CHANNEL AND MULTICHANNEL DEVICES

SINGLE- AND MULTICHANNEL COCHLEAR IMPLANTS

Most pediatric studies have reported on the performance of either single- or multichannel implant users. Several investigations in our laboratory compared the performance of matched groups of children who used either the 3M/House device or the Nucleus multichannel cochlear implant over time (Miyamoto, Osberger, Robbins, Myres, Kessler, and Pope 1992; Osberger, Robbins, Miyamoto, Berry, Myres, Kessler, and Pope 1991). The results of these studies revealed that the performance of the Nucleus users was higher than that of the 3M/House users on every speech perception measure, even on measures that assessed aspects of speech purportedly transmitted the best by the single-channel device (i.e., prosodic information). Thus, the multichannel implant not only permitted better word recognition without speechreading, but it also conveyed better information about the time-intensity cues in speech. Even though some reports have shown that a small percentage of children demonstrated open-set speech recognition with the

3M/House implant (Berliner, Tonokawa, Dye, and House 1989), the highest level of performance achieved by the *majority* of single-channel users is the perception of stress pattern and syllable number in speech.

DUAL- AND SEVEN-CHANNEL TACTILE AIDS

In another study, the speech perception skills of matched groups of subjects who used either the Tactaid II+ or the Tactaid 7 were compared. There were six subjects in each group who were matched according to chronological age and duration of tactile aid use. The mean age of the subjects at the time of testing was 8.8 years for the Tactaid II+ users and 7.6 years for the Tactaid 7 users. The mean duration of tactile aid use was 1.8 years for both groups. The mean scores obtained by each group of subjects on the battery of speech perception tests appear in table 2. The data in table 2 show similar scores for both groups of subjects on all measures, except on the Common Phrases Test when it was administered with lipreading. On this measure the score of the Tactaid II+ users was substantially higher than that of the Tactaid 7 users, which probably reflects a sampling problem and better lipreading skills of some of the Tactaid II+ subjects (note the size of the standard deviation) rather than device differences. The performance of both groups of subjects on the recognition of words based on vowel or consonant distinctions after nearly two years of device use was close to chance, and neither group showed evidence of open-set speech recognition (i.e., score greater than zero on the Common Phrases Test). Subjective feedback from the subjects and their parents suggested, however, that children wore the Tactaid 7 more consistently than was observed for the Tactaid II+ subjects.

Table 2
Mean scores (percentage correct) for Tactaid II+ (n=6) and Tactaid 7 (n=6) users on a battery of speech perception tests.

	Chng/No Chng[a]		MinPair:Vow[b]		MinPair:Con[c]		Com Phr:A/T[d]		Com Phr:+LR[e]	
	Mean	sd	Mean	sd	Mean	sd	Mean	sd	Mean	sd
TA2	64	9	51	12	58	9	0	0	56	38
TA7	71	13	54	10	50	5	0	0	25	16

[a]Change/No Change Test
[b]Minimal Pairs: vowels
[c]Minimal Pairs: consonants
[d]Common Phrases with auditory/tactile cues only
[e]Common Phrases with auditory/tactile cues plus lipreading.
Chance score on Change/No Change and Minimal Pairs= 50%.

However, unlike the results observed with implants, increasing the number of channels on a vibrotactile aid did not improve speech perception performance. Improvements might be observed if the tactile aid had more than seven channels; however, no such device is commercially available at this time.

MULTICHANNEL COCHLEAR IMPLANTS, TACTILE AIDS, OR HEARING AIDS

The purpose of the next study was to compare the performance of children in two experimental groups who used multichannel tactile aids or cochlear implants to that of control groups of children who used conventional hearing aids. The hearing aid subjects were classified as Gold or Silver hearing aid users, according to the criteria described above. Subjects in the hearing aid groups were matched to the implant and tactile aid subjects by chronological age at the time of testing. Tables 3 and 4 provide demographic information on the groups of subjects.

In the first experiment, a pre- and postdevice comparison was performed between the two experimental groups. In the preimplant or tactile

Table 3
Characteristics of the implant and tactile aid subjects at the predevice interval.

Variable	Nucleus	Tactaid 7
n	10	9
PTA (dB HL)	>110	>110
Age at Onset of Deafness (years)	1.1	.8
Chronological Age (years)	5.2	5.5

Table 4
Characteristics of the implant and tactile aid subjects at the postdevice interval compared to those of the hearing aid subjects.

Variable	Nucleus	Tactaid 7	Silver	Gold
n	10	9	10	10
PTA (dB HL)	>110	>110	103	94
Age at Onset of Deafness (years)	5.2	5.5	1.0	1.9
Chronological Age (years)	7.1	7.5	7.4	7.5

aid condition, the performance of the implant and tactile aid subjects was evaluated while they used conventional hearing aids (except that five of the tactile aid subjects were using a Tactaid I or II+). At the postdevice interval, the mean length of device use was 1.8 and 2.1 years for the Nucleus and Tactaid 7 users, respectively.

Repeated measures analysis of variance (RMANOVA) with a split-plot factorial design was used to compare pre- and postdevice performance for the two groups of subjects. The mean scores for each group of subjects on the vowel and consonant items of the Minimal Pairs Test appear in figure 1. The results of the RMANOVA on the vowel items revealed a significant group effect ($p<.001$), a significant time effect ($p<.05$), and a significant group by time interaction ($p<.01$). In the preimplant or Tactaid 7 condition, the mean score for each group was at chance level of performance. At the postdevice interval, the implant group's mean vowel recognition score was about 80%, whereas the mean score of the Tactaid 7 users remained around 50% (i.e., chance).

A similar pattern of performance was present for the consonant items of the Minimal Pairs Test. A significant effect was observed for group ($p<.05$) and time ($p<.01$), and there was a significant group by time interaction ($p<.04$). In the predevice condition, the mean score for each group was at chance. At the postdevice interval, the score of the implant group

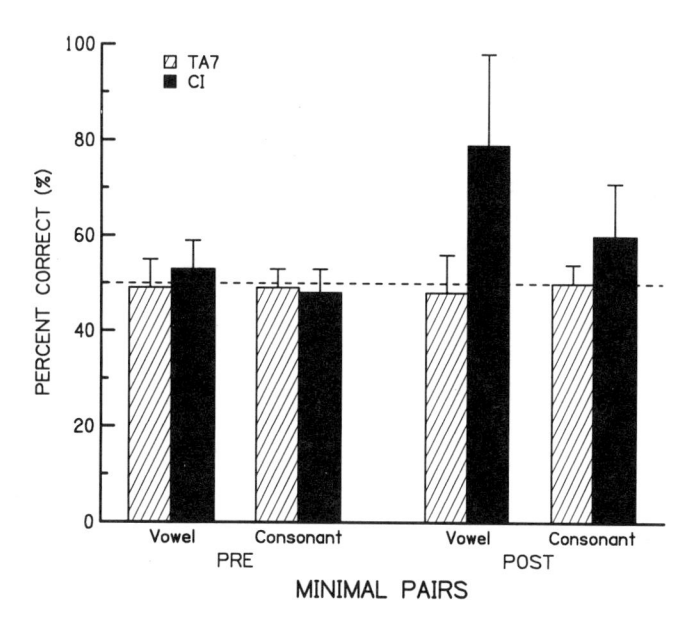

Figure 1. Mean scores (percentage) and standard deviations (vertical bars) of multichannel implant and tactile aid groups on the Minimal Pairs Test, which was administered with tactile or auditory cues only. Chance performance is marked by the dashed horizontal lines.

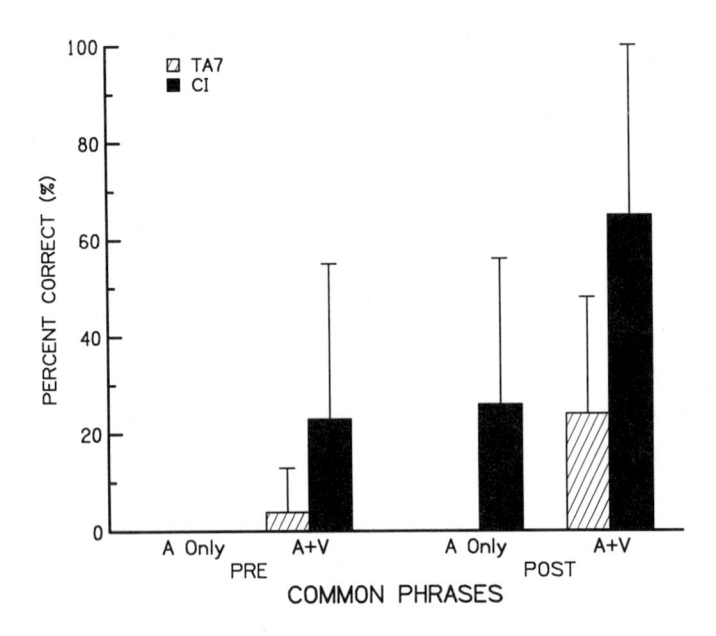

Figure 2. Mean scores (percentage) and standard deviations (vertical bars) of multichannel implant and tactile aid groups on the Common Phrases Test, which was administered with auditory or tactile cues only (A Only) or combined auditory or tactile and visual cues (A+V). Chance performance is equal to 0%.

improved to about 60%, but there was no improvement observed in the mean score of the tactile aid users. Examination of the postimplant data on the Minimal Pairs Test suggests that subjects obtained more information about vowels than consonants from the Nucleus implant.

Figure 2 shows the performance of the two groups of subjects on the open-set speech recognition measure, the Common Phrases Test, which was administered with and without lipreading. The results of the RMANOVA revealed a significant effect of group ($p<.05$) and time ($p<.05$) and a significant group by time interaction ($p<.05$) when the test was administered with auditory cues only. In this condition, both groups of subjects scored 0% at the predevice interval. At the postdevice interval, the mean score of the implant group was about 26%, whereas the score for the tactile aid group remained at zero. A RMANOVA was performed to examine the groups' performance on the Common Phrases Test when it was administered with lipreading. Significant main effects of group ($p<.01$) and time ($p<.001$) were observed, but there was no significant group by time interaction. At the predevice interval, the mean score of the implant group was higher than that of the tactile aid users. Unlike their performance on tests administered with only tactile cues, there was an improvement in the mean score of the Tactaid

7 users at the postdevice interval when testing permitted the use of visual cues (i.e., Common Phrases Test administered with auditory and visual cues). At the postdevice interval, however, the mean score of the implant group remained significantly higher than that of the tactile aid group. At this point in time, the average score of the implant group was approximately 65% compared to a mean score of 22% for the Tactaid 7 group at the postdevice interval.

In the next experiment, the mean scores of the two experimental groups at the postdevice interval were compared to those of the two control groups of hearing aid users. Figure 3 shows the mean scores for the Nucleus and Tactaid 7 subjects on the Minimal Pairs Test, along with the scores for the age-matched Gold and Silver hearing aid users. The results of the RMANOVA for vowel recognition on the Minimal Pairs Test revealed a significant group effect ($p<.0001$). The Scheffe post hoc test indicated that the performance of the Tactaid 7 subjects was significantly poorer than that of the implant, Gold, or Silver hearing aid subjects ($p<.05$). There were no significant differences between the performance of the implant group and either of the hearing aid groups.

The results of the RMANOVA for the Minimal Pairs consonant recognition items revealed a significant effect of group ($p<.01$). Post hoc

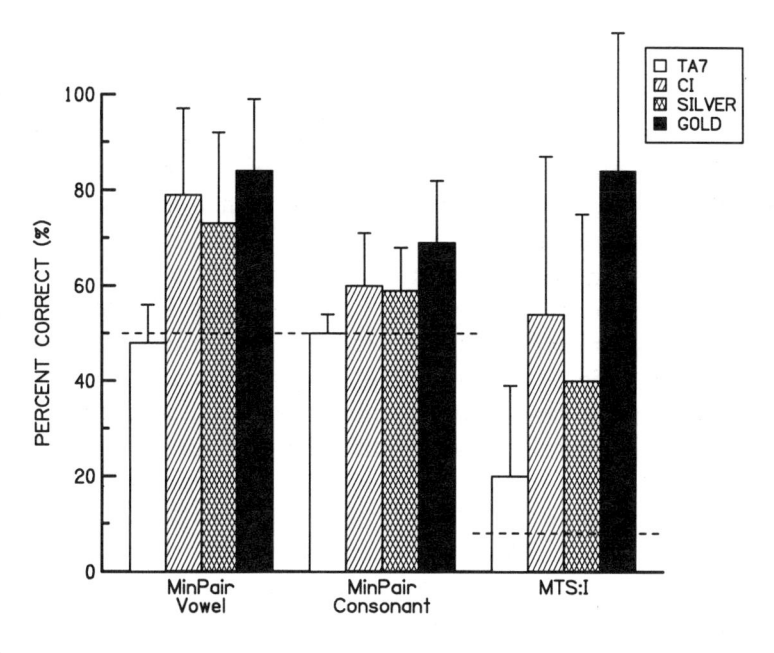

Figure 3. Mean scores (percentage) and standard deviations (vertical bars) of multichannel implant, tactile aid, Silver hearing aid (mean pure-tone average = 103 dB HL), and Gold hearing aid (mean pure-tone average = 94 dB HL) groups on the Minimal Pairs (Vowel and Consonant) and MTS:I (Monosyllable Trochee Spondee: Identification) Tests, which was administered with tactile or auditory cues only. Chance performance is marked by the dashed horizontal lines.

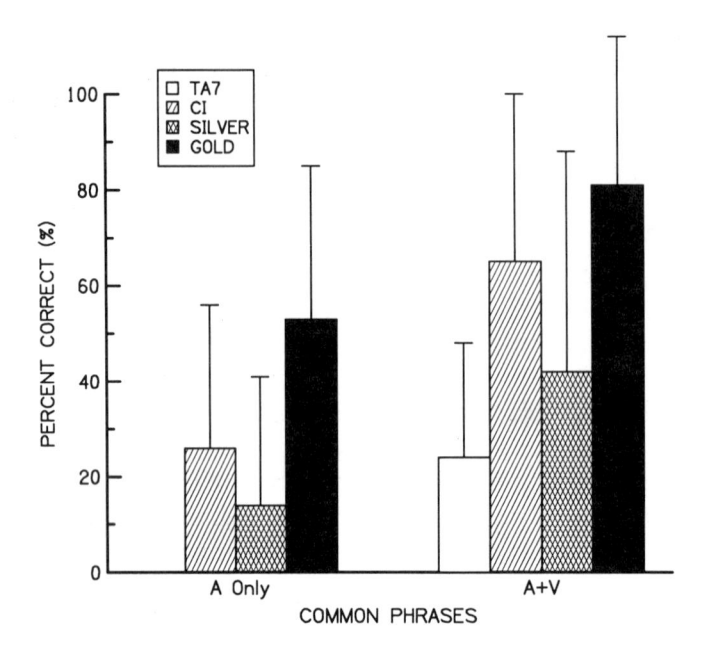

Figure 4. Mean scores (percentage) and standard deviations (vertical bars) of multichannel implant, tactile aid, Silver hearing aid (mean pure-tone average= 103 dB HL), and Gold hearing aid (mean pure-tone average= 94 dB HL) groups on the Common Phrases Test, which was administered with auditory or tactile cues only (A Only) or combined auditory or tactile and visual cues (A+V). Chance performance is equal to 0%.

testing revealed that the consonant recognition score of the tactile aid group was significantly poorer than that of the Gold hearing aid users ($p<.01$). No other group comparisons were significant.

Figure 4 shows the mean scores for the tactile aid, implant, and two hearing aid groups on the Common Phrases Test, administered with auditory or tactile cues only and with combined auditory or tactile cues and lipreading. The effect of group was significant ($p<.001$) when only auditory or tactile cues were available. Post hoc testing revealed that the scores of the tactile aid users were significantly poorer than those of the Gold hearing aid users ($p<.05$). No other group comparisons yielded significant differences. The effect of group also was significant ($p<.01$) when the test was administered with lipreading cues. Post hoc testing revealed that there was no significant difference between the scores of the implant and hearing aid groups, but the Tactaid 7 group performed more poorly than did the Gold hearing aid users ($p<.05$).

The results of this study revealed that the speech perception performance of the tactile aid and implant subjects was similar in the predevice interval when the subjects entered the study, at least on the measures administered without lipreading. After roughly two years of multichannel device use, the performance of the implant users improved significantly on all measures, whereas the scores of the Tactaid 7 users did not. The results of the Common Phrases Test, administered with only auditory or tactile cues, revealed that none of the tactile aid users demonstrated open-set speech recognition. In contrast, the mean score of the implant users on this measure was 26%, with scores ranging from 0 to 60%.

A different pattern of performance was observed on the Common Phrases Test when the subjects had access to lipreading cues. In the predevice condition, the mean score of the implant group was higher than that of the tactile aid group, suggesting that the subjects with implants entered the study with lipreading skills superior to those of the tactile aid users. At the postdevice interval, after about two years of multichannel use, both groups showed improved performance, but the mean score of the implant users remained higher than that of the tactile aid group. These data suggest that both types of multichannel devices enhance speechreading, although the implant appears to do so to a greater extent than the tactile aid. This finding, however, is confounded by the better speechreading skills of the implant subjects at the start of the study. The finding that the Tactaid 7 enhanced speechreading is in general agreement with those of Weisenberger and Kozma-Spytek (1991) and Eilers, Vergara, Oller, and Balkany (1993) who reported that the greatest benefit in speech perception performance with a tactile aid was observed when cues from the device were combined with other modalities, such as vision or audition.

A comparison of the implant and tactile aid groups with the hearing aid groups showed that the mean score of the Tactaid 7 users was significantly poorer than that of the Gold hearing aid subjects on all measures, and poorer than that of the Silver hearing aid users on open-set sentence recognition when only auditory or tactile cues were available. In contrast, there were no significant differences between the performance of the implant group and the hearing aid groups on the measures. Thus, these data suggest that the performance of children with implants are comparable to that of children with profound hearing impairments who obtain some benefit from conventional hearing aids.

STUDIES WITH MULTICHANNEL IMPLANT USERS

LONGITUDINAL EVALUATION OF MULTICHANNEL COCHLEAR IMPLANT USERS

This study employed a within-subjects design to examine changes over time in the speech perception scores of 17 prelingually deafened subjects (mean age at onset of deafness=.9 years; mean age implanted=5.6 years).

Subjects were tested preimplant (Time 1) and at .5, 1.0, and 1.5 years postimplant with the Nucleus device (Times 2, 3, and 4, respectively). Table 5 summarizes their scores on the tests described above (Change/No Change, Minimal Pairs, Common Phrases: auditory only and auditory-plus-visual cues). Data also are presented on the subjects' performance on the HAVE (Hoosier Auditory Visual Enhancement Test; Renshaw, Robbins, Miyamoto, Osberger, and Pope 1988). The HAVE is administered with both auditory and visual cues. Performance is scored on the basis of distinguishing a pair of homophenous words (*m*an *p*an) from a visually distinct word (*f*an) (HAVE:Visual), and on the basis of correct word identification (e.g., correct identification of the target word). On a given trial, only one of the homophenous words is presented; therefore, the word identification score primarily reflects perception of acoustic/phonetic distinctions (e.g., *m*an versus *p*an) because minimal visual cues distinguish the words. This test was developed to examine the integration of auditory and visual information and also to assess the speechreading skills of the subjects with single words that were maximally contrastive. The data were analyzed using RMANOVA with post hoc testing of means with Scheffe's test.

The results show that after only 6 months of implant use (Time 2), there was a significant improvement in discriminating changes between speech features (Change/No Change Test) and recognition of words in a closed set based on visual distinctions (HAVE:Visual). Significant improvements in the auditory identification of words in a closed set (HAVE:Word) or words on the basis of vowel features (height and place) or consonant voice or place features did not occur until after 1.5 years of multichannel implant use. There was no significant improvement in recognition of words based on manner distinctions or in open-set speech recognition even after 1.5 years of implant use (Common Phrases: auditory only) unless the stimuli were presented with visual as well as auditory cues (Common Phrases + lipreading). These findings suggest that improvements in the discrimination of nonsegmental speech changes and visual speech perception precede improvements in auditory word recognition. In fact, significant improvements in closed-set word recognition do not appear until after 1.5 years of use, and improvements in open-set speech recognition without lipreading occur even later than this. This finding is in general agreement with other investigators (Fryauf-Bertschy, Tyler, Kelsay, and Gantz 1992; Gantz, Tyler, Woodworth, Tye-Murray, and Fryauf-Bertschy 1994). A finding of particular interest is the *significant improvement in speechreading skills* that occurred after children received an implant. This finding is consistent with the improvements in selective visual attention reported by Quittner, Smith, Osberger, Mitchell, and Katz (1994), which preceded gains in auditory word recognition in children with cochlear implants.

Table 5
Mean scores (percentage correct) and standard deviations ( ) over time for 17 Nucleus implant users. Numbers in ***bold italics*** denote statistically significant differences (p<.05).

	Change/[a] No Chg	Vowel[b] Height	Vowel[c] Place	Cons[d] Voice	Cons[e] Manner	Cons[f] Place	HAVE: Visual	HAVE: Word	Com Ph[g] + LR	Com Ph[h] A only
T1	***52***(5)	***50***(11)	***51***(8)	***46***(9)	51(13)	***47***(9)	75(27)	***42***(13)	***18***(31)	0
T2	66(15)	63(15)	59(15)	52(10)	61(16)	55(14)	***89***(11)	48(16)	25(34)	2(10)
T3	70(15)	64(21)	65(23)	53(9)	53(15)	55(12)	94(8)	54(13)	38(42)	8(23)
T4	80(15)	72(18)	***69***(20)	***59***(16)	57(15)	***62***(14)	98(3)	***60***(9)	***48***(40)	9(23)

Table 6
Mean scores (percentage correct) and standard deviations ( ) over time for 16 hearing aid users. Numbers in ***bold italics*** denote statistically significant differences (p<.05).

	Change/[a] No Chg	Vowel[b] Height	Vowel[c] Place	Cons[d] Voice	Cons[e] Manner	Cons[f] Place	HAVE: Visual	HAVE: Word	Com Ph[g] + LR	Com Ph[h] A only
T1	***79***(17)	79(21)	69(17)	70(19)	72(18)	56(16)	96(6)	64(19)	54(41)	26(34)
T2	85(15)	84(19)	67(21)	67(21)	74(21)	56(12)	97(5)	65(19)	59(41)	29(36)
T3	86(13)	80(20)	70(21)	67(17)	72(21)	51(12)	97(3)	69(17)	59(44)	31(37)
T4	***91***(8)	86(17)	73(17)	61(20)	70(20)	54(14)	98(3)	69(18)	62(37)	28(36)

[a]Change/No Change Test
[b]Minimal Pairs: vowel height
[c]Minimal Pairs: vowel place
[d]Minimal Pairs: consonant voice
[e]Minimal Pairs: consonant manner
[f]Minimal Pairs: consonant place
[g]Common Phrases with auditory cues plus lipreading
[h]Common Phrases with auditory cues only

LONGITUDINAL EVALUATION OF HEARING AID USERS

This study, which paralleled the one above, was designed to examine changes over time in the speech perception skills of 16 hearing aid users (mean age=7.4 years at Time 1), the majority of whom were classified as Silver hearing aid users (mean unaided pure-tone average=99 dB HL; mean aided pure-tone average=43 dB HL). Subjects were tested when they entered the study (Time 1) and .5, 1.0, and 1.5 years later (Times 2, 3, and 4, respectively). The data for the hearing aid users appear in table 6. These data show very little change in performance over time, except on the Change/No Change Test, suggesting that subjects with hearing thresholds of roughly 100 dB HL, on the average, reach a plateau in the development of their auditory and visual speech perception skills by an average age of 7 to 8 years. Comparison of the data for the hearing aid users at Time 4 (table 6) with the data for the implant users at Time 4 (table 5) reveals similar scores for both groups on nearly all measures. The exception to this pattern is the higher performance of the hearing aid users on the Change/No Change Test, vowel height of the Minimal Pairs Test, and the Common Phrases Test in both conditions. However, the subjects with hearing aids received their devices at an earlier age and used them for a longer period of time than did the subjects with implants. In fact, examination of the data from the 12 subjects, who participated in the previous study and who have used their Nucleus implant for 3.5 years, revealed that these differences disappear after the subjects have had more experience with their implants, as shown in table 7. The data in table 7 reveal that the implant users eventually catch up to the hearing aid users with more extended implant experience. In fact, the scores of the implant users were actually higher than those of the hearing aid users on the features of vowel height, vowel place, consonant manner, and consonant place on the Minimal Pairs Test, and on the Common Phrases Test in both conditions when the stimuli were administered with auditory cues alone or combined with visual cues.

EFFECT OF AGE AT ONSET OF DEAFNESS ON IMPLANT PERFORMANCE

It was hypothesized that age at onset of deafness would be a significant variable in explaining performance differences among pediatric implant users. The results of Osberger, Todd, Berry, Robbins, and Miyamoto (1991) revealed that there were no significant differences in speech perception performance of children with implants (3M/House and Nucleus subjects pooled) as a function of age at onset of deafness unless the subjects lost their hearing at age 5 or later. Subjects who were postlingually deafened (i.e., onset of deafness at or after age 5) achieved significantly higher scores than subjects with congenital deafness or deafness acquired before age 3. In

Table 7

Mean scores (percentage correct) and standard deviations ( ) for 12 Nucleus subjects after 3.5 years of implant use.

Change[a] No Chg	Vowel[b] Height	Vowel[c] Place	Cons[d] Voice	Cons[e] Manner	Cons[f] Place	HAVE: Visual	HAVE: Word	Com Ph[g] + LR	Com Ph[h] A only
89(11)	94(7)	90(11)	68(18)	81(16)	66(7)	(100)(1)	(72)(13)	90(15)	48(31)

[a]Change/No Change Test
[b]Minimal Pairs: vowel height
[c]Minimal Pairs: vowel place
[d]Minimal Pairs: consonant voice
[e]Minimal Pairs: consonant manner
[f]Minimal Pairs: consonant place
[g]Common Phrases with auditory cues plus lipreading
[h]Common Phrases with auditory cues only

Table 8

Mean scores (percentage) on vowel height and consonant place features on the Minimal Pairs Test as a function of type of Nucleus processor (only significant measures considered).

		Minimal Pairs: Vowel Height				Minimal Pairs: Consonant Place			
		Mean	sd		Mean	sd		Mean	sd
WSP	T1	54	21	T2	90	12	**WSP** T1	54	12	T2	53	15
MSP	T1	83	11	T2	95	7	**MSP** T1	69	9	T2	64	15

WSP = WSP and F0/F1/F2 processing scheme
MSP = Mini speech processor with MPeak strategy
T1 = Time 1 (Early interval – 1 year postimplant use)
T2 = Time 2 (Late interval – 3 years postimplant use)

a more recent study (Miyamoto, Osberger, Robbins, Myres, and Kessler 1993), which included only multichannel implant users with prelingual deafness, the results showed no significant difference between the mean scores of a group of subjects with congenital deafness and the mean scores of a second group of subjects with deafness acquired before age 3 on 12 of the 13 speech perception tests administered in the postimplant condition. The general finding of similar performance between children with congenital and early acquired deafness is probably influenced by the secondary effects of meningitis (i.e., neurologic problems and cochlear ossification) on implant performance in the subjects with acquired deafness. That is, children who sustain deafness secondary to meningitis also might manifest other associated problems (e.g., neurologic deficits) that affect their acquisition of speech perception skills with an implant. Nevertheless, the results of the Miyamoto et al. study indicate that children who are born deaf have the potential to derive the same benefit from a multichannel cochlear implant as do children who had some exposure to spoken language before the onset of their deafness from meningitis.

VARIABLES AFFECTING IMPLANT PERFORMANCE

This study (Miyamoto, Osberger, Todd, Robbins, Stroer, Zimmermann-Phillips, and Carney 1994) examined the variables that contribute to the large individual differences in the speech perception skills of children with the Nucleus implant. Sixty-one children were tested on four measures of speech perception: two tests of closed-set word recognition, one test of open-set recognition of phrases, and one open-set monosyllabic word test, scored on the basis of the percentage of phonemes as well as words identified correctly. The mean age at onset of deafness of the 61 subjects was 1.3 years (range = birth to 10 years), the mean age implanted was 7.6 years (range = 2.8 to 14.2 years), and the mean length of implant use at the time of testing was 2 years (range .1 to 5 years). Approximately half of the subjects used oral communication and half used total communication (manually coded English plus speech). About two-thirds of the subjects used the Nucleus MSP processor and the MPeak strategy, whereas the remainder of the subjects used the WSP with the F0/F1/F2 strategy. A series of regression analyses were performed to determine the contribution of the following variables to speech recognition performance: age at onset of deafness, age implanted, length of deafness before implantation, length of implant use, and type of Nucleus processor (i.e., processing strategy). The results of the regression analyses revealed that the five variables accounted for roughly 35% of the variance on the speech perception measures. Duration of implant use accounted for the most variance on all of the measures, highlighting the need to study the performance of children with implants over an extended time.

COMPARISON OF PROCESSING SCHEMES IN CHILDREN

The speech perception abilities of six children who used the WSP and the F0/F1/F2 processing scheme (WSP group) were compared to six children who used the MSP with the MPeak strategy (MSP group). The groups were matched for age at onset of deafness (mean = 1.3 and 1.0 years for WSP and MSP users, respectively) and age implanted (mean = 5.9 years for both groups). Subjects were tested on measures described above at an *early* postimplant interval (after one year of implant use) and at a *late* interval (after three years of implant use). The data were subjected to an RMANOVA using a split-plot factorial design with processor (WSP or MSP) as the between-groups variable and interval (early or late) as the within-groups variable. Separate analyses were performed on all of the speech perception tests in the battery, as well as on the feature scores (vowel height and place, consonant voice, manner, and place) on the Minimal Pairs Test. Only the measures on which there was a significant processor or processor by interval interaction are considered (table 8). For vowel height, there was a significant processor effect ($p<.041$), a significant interval effect ($p<.001$), and a significant interaction between processor and interval ($p<.01$). As shown in table 8, the initial vowel height score of the MSP group was higher than that of the WSP group, but the scores were similar for the two groups at the later interval. For consonant place, the mean score of the MSP group was significantly higher than that of the WSP group at both intervals ($p<.05$).

The MSP group's better perception of vowel height and consonant place distinctions suggests that the MPeak strategy provides improved access to high-frequency information than the F0/F1/F2 scheme. These results indicate that advances in signal processing result in improved performance in pediatric implant users. Moreover, the results in table 8 suggest *initial* higher levels of performance with the MSP than the WSP (i.e., MSP scores higher than WSP at Time 1). This finding suggests that children show an *accelerated rate of learning with improved processing schemes*. However, recognition of vowel height was similar for both groups at the later interval, and there was no additional improvement in recognition of consonant place by the MSP group at the later interval.

SUMMARY OF RESULTS

Taken together, the findings of the above studies reveal the following information. First, the mean scores of the multichannel (Nucleus) implant users were significantly higher than those of the single-channel (3M/House) users on every speech perception test. Thus, the data suggest that increasing the number of channels on a cochlear implant results in marked improvement in speech perception performance. In contrast, there was no difference between the performance of groups of subjects who used tactile aids with a limited number of channels (Tactaid II+) and seven channels (Tactaid 7). Thus, unlike the findings observed with implants, increasing the number of channels on a tactile aid did not result in improved speech perception benefits.

Second, the mean scores of the multichannel Nucleus users were significantly higher than those of the multichannel Tactaid 7 users on all measures of word and sentence recognition administered with only auditory or tactile cues. The multichannel implant users showed significant improvement in speech recognition over time, whereas the tactile aid users did not, except on a test that assessed recognition of simple phrases with *combined* tactile and visual cues. The multichannel implant users were able to understand words in an open set without speechreading, suggesting that the information transmitted by the implant was sufficient for these children to develop underlying phonetic representations of spoken language. The results revealed no evidence of open-set speech recognition in the tactile aid users, even in subjects who used the seven-channel device.

Third, the time course over which auditory perceptual skills develop in prelingually deafened children who use multichannel implants extends over many years. In fact, duration of implant use was the factor that accounted for the most variance in subject performance on measures of open- and closed-set word recognition. Significant improvements in auditory word recognition skills did not emerge in prelingually deafened children until after 1.5 years of multichannel implant use.

Fourth, there was essentially no improvement in auditory word recognition in a group of hearing aid users who were evaluated over a period of 1.5 years. Presumably, auditory learning in these children occurred *before* they entered the study because they had used their sensory aids a number of years prior to the time of testing. In addition, there was no obvious difference between the postimplant speech perception performance of children with congenital deafness and deafness acquired before age 3 from meningitis.

Fifth, after roughly two years of multichannel device use, there was no significant difference between the speech perception performance of Nucleus users and the Silver and Gold hearing aid users. These data suggest that children with hearing levels of 90 dB HL and greater might benefit more from a multichannel cochlear implant than from continued use of only hearing aids.

Finally, preliminary data suggest that processing schemes, which have been shown to improve the performance of postlingually deafened adults (i.e., MPeak), also improve the speech perception performance of prelingually deafened children. The improvement was noted in terms of overall higher levels of performance (at least on two speech features) and a faster rate of learning. Even with the most advanced processing scheme evaluated (i.e.,

MPeak), however, consonant recognition was still relatively limited in the population studied.

FUTURE RESEARCH DIRECTIONS

Based on the above findings and the results of other investigators, the following research directions are proposed. First, there is a growing trend to implant very young children (i.e., between ages 2 and 3). Because of the increased concern in using an invasive device in this population and the difficulty in assessing their auditory perceptual skills to determine candidacy and device efficacy, it is important that this population be studied carefully. The majority of prelingually deafened children for whom long-term cochlear implant data currently are available were implanted between the ages of 4 and 9 years. Given the substantial improvements in auditory perception skills that have been realized by these children, the next logical step is to implant younger children who might demonstrate even higher levels of implant performance than have been reported for children implanted at an older age. Early auditory stimulation not only provides early experience with sound and spoken language, but it might prevent neural degeneration of the auditory system as well. For example, Leake and colleagues (Leake, Hradek, Rebscher, and Snyder 1991) found that chronic stimulation via cochlear prostheses delayed and/or prevented the otherwise progressive degeneration of spiral ganglion neurons in neonatally deafened cats. Recent data reported by Waltzman and colleagues substantiate the benefits of early implantation. In a sample of 14 children implanted between the ages of 2 and 3 years, Waltzman, Cohen, Gomolin, Shapiro, Ozdamar, and Hoffman (1994) reported open-set sentence recognition scores ranging from 57% to 100% and open-set monosyllabic word identification (PBK) scores ranging from 15% to 92% after two to four years of implant use. Although it seems intuitive that children implanted below age 5 will ultimately demonstrate higher levels of performance with the implant than children implanted at a later age, careful and systematic investigation of this issue needs to be undertaken.

Another area of change in implant work involves the audiologic criteria used to determine candidacy. The first children to be implanted were clear-cut candidates because they did not even detect sound with powerful hearing aids (i.e., unaided pure-tone thresholds >110 dB HL). Longitudinal speech perception results have shown that the performance of these children with implants is better than that of children with unaided pure-tone thresholds between 100 and 105 dB HL who use hearing aids (Miyamoto, Osberger, Todd, and Robbins 1993; Skinner 1994). These children are now considered to be implant candidates because they have poor hearing-aided thresholds above 1000 Hz (i.e., thresholds $\geq$50 dB HL) and most speech cues in the high frequencies are inaudible to them. Thus, these subjects perceive primarily vowel information but limited consonant cues through their hearing aids. This occurs because the high-frequency limit of transducers used in hearing aids for persons with profound hearing losses is seldom above 3.5 kHz (Boothroyd 1993). With electrical stimulation of individual electrodes in response to the peak frequency and amplitude of the incoming sound, the implant provides more information to the auditory system than does a hearing aid. In addition, the transformed acoustic signal is programmed into the electrical dynamic range of the implant, eliminating some of the dynamic range problems encountered with acoustic amplification. Children who demonstrate some residual hearing are being implanted at centers around the country (Skinner 1994), but few, if any, teams are investigating this issue in a systematic manner. Given that the process of implantation destroys any residual hearing, it is crucial that implant benefits derived by these children be studied carefully and systematically so that well-defined audiologic criteria are developed. The outcome of such research might indicate that a far greater number of children are implant candidates than was predicted several years ago.

A final area of important research is evaluation of children's performance with new and improved implant processing schemes. Recently, two new schemes have become available for use in the pediatric population, both of which provide a better representation of the speech waveform than the earlier feature extraction schemes. Recall that the rationale underlying the feature extraction approach is that people with limited perceptual capabilities may not be able to use all of the information in the speech signal. Therefore, the most important features of speech are extracted, while other, presumably less important, features are eliminated. In contrast, the several new processing schemes make no a priori assumption about the importance of individual speech features but rather provide a representation of the incoming acoustic waveform so that the listener can extract the relevant information needed for speech recognition. Feature extraction strategies have been used exclusively in children in the United States because the only device approved for commercial distribution by the U.S. Food and Drug Administration for use in children (i.e., Nucleus 22-Channel Cochlear Implant System) employs this type of processing scheme (i.e., the F0/F1/F2 and MPeak schemes). A recently introduced strategy from Nucleus is SPEAK (Spectral Peak), which represents the waveform using a vocoder (filterbank) strategy (McDermott, McKay, and Vandali 1992). In this strategy, the amplitudes of each of 20 bands are estimated, and on average, the 6 channels with the highest amplitudes are identified and pulses are delivered in a nonoverlapping sequence to electrodes whose positions correspond to the identified channel (the number of electrodes stimulated can vary from 1 to 10, depending on the spectral content of the incoming signal). The rate of stimulation on each channel, however, remains relatively low (i.e., 180 to 300 pps). Data reported for postlingually deafened adults (Skinner et al. 1994) revealed higher performance levels with the SPEAK than the MPeak strategy. Data comparing children's performance with the MPeak and SPEAK strategies are lacking at this time.

A state-of-the-art waveform representation scheme is the CIS (continuous interleaved sampling) strategy, developed by Wilson and colleagues (Wilson, Finley, Lawson, Wolford, Eddington, and Rabinowitz 1991). The CIS strategy is now available in the eight-channel Clarion device, manufactured by Advanced Bionics Corporation (Schindler and Kessler 1993). Key features of the CIS scheme are nonsimultaneous, pulsatile stimulation, a relatively high rate of stimulation on each channel, and channel-by-channel compression (Wilson 1993). Results obtained in postlingually deafened adults with the Clarion revealed high levels of speech recognition performance and very fast learning rates with the CIS strategy (Kessler, Loeb, and Barker 1994), with over one-half of the subjects achieving a score of 50% or better on CID sentences and over one-third of the subjects achieving a score of 75% or better on CID sentences. A clinical trial of the Clarion in the pediatric population began during the first quarter of 1995. Data reported by several investigators indicate higher levels of speech recognition performance in postlingually deafened subjects who use the Clarion than in subjects who use the Nucleus MPeak strategy (Battmer, Gnadeberg, Allum-Mecklenburg, and Lenarz 1994; Gantz, Tyler, Lowder, and Woodworth 1994). Comparison studies between SPEAK and CIS strategies are lacking in both adults and children.

ACKNOWLEDGMENTS

The authors gratefully acknowledge Wendy Myres, Kathy Kessler, and Kim Veselik of Indiana University School of Medicine and Denise Dettman, Debbie Johnson, Natalie Justice, and Ann Karasek of Boys Town National Research Hospital for their assistance in data collection. The research reported in this manuscript was conducted while the first author was on the staff of the Department of Otolaryngology, Indiana University School of Medicine, Indianapolis, Indiana and while the last author was on the staff of Boys Town National Research Hospital, Omaha, Nebraska. The work was supported by NIH-NIDCD grants DC00064 and DC00423 awarded to the Indiana University School of Medicine.

REFERENCES

Battmer, R., Gnadeberg, D., Allum-Mecklenburg, D.J., and Lenarz, T. 1994. Matched-paired comparisons for adults using the Clarion or Nucleus devices. Paper presented at the

International Cochlear Implant, Speech and Hearing Symposium, October 24-28, Melbourne, Australia.

Berliner, K.I., Tonokawa, L.L., Dye, L.L., and House, W.F. 1989. Open-set speech recognition in children with single-channel cochlear implants. *Ear and Hearing* 10:237-242.

Boothroyd, A. 1984. Auditory perception of speech contrasts by subjects with sensorineural hearing loss. *Journal of Speech and Hearing Research* 27:134-144.

Boothroyd, A. 1993. *Profound deafness.* In R.S. Tyler (ed.), *Cochlear implants.* San Diego: Singular Publishing Group.

Boothroyd, A., and Cawkwell, S. 1970. Vibrotactile thresholds in pure tone audiometry. *Acta Otolaryngologica* 69:384-387.

Carney, A.E., Osberger, M.J., Carney, E., Robbins, A.M., Renshaw, J.J., and Miyamoto, R.T. 1993. A comparison of speech discrimination with cochlear implants and tactile aids. *Journal of the Acoustical Society of America* 94:2036-2049.

Eilers, R.E., Vergara, K., Oller, D.K., and Balkany, T.J. 1993. Evaluating hearing-impaired children's usage of tactual vocoders. In *Proceedings of the Second International Conference on Tactile Aids, Hearing Aids, and Cochlear Implants.* Stockholm: Akademitryck AB.

Erber, N.P. 1972. Auditory, visual, and auditory-visual recognition of consonants by children with normal and impaired hearing. *Journal of Speech and Hearing Research* 15:413-422.

Franklin, D. 1988. *Tactaid II+ users manual.* Somerville, Mass.: Audiological Engineering Corp.

Franklin, D. 1991. *Temporary users manual for the Tactaid 7.* Somerville, Mass.: Audiological Engineering Corp.

Fretz, R.J., and Fravel, R.P. 1985. Design and function: A physical and electrical description of the 3M/House cochlear implant system. *Ear and Hearing* 6 (Suppl.):14S-19S.

Fryauf-Bertschy, H., Tyler, R.S., Kelsay, D.M., and Gantz, B.J. 1992. Performance over time of congenitally deaf and postlingually deafened children using a multichannel cochlear implant. *Journal of Speech and Hearing Research* 35:913-920.

Gantz, B.J., Tyler, R.S., Lowder, M.W., and Woodworth, G.G. 1994. Preliminary results with three different multichannel cochlear implant systems in postlingually deafened adults. Paper presented at the International Cochlear Implant, Speech and Hearing Symposium, October 24-28, Melbourne, Australia.

Gantz, B.J., Tyler, R.S., Woodworth, G., Tye-Murray, N., and Fryauf-Bertschy, H. 1994. Results of multichannel cochlear implants in congenital and acquired prelingual deafness in children: Five-year follow-up. *American Journal of Otology* 15 (Suppl. 2):1-8.

Haskins, H. 1949. A phonetically balanced test of speech discrimination for children. Master's thesis, Northwestern University, Evanston, Illinois.

Kessler, D.K., Loeb, G.M., and Barker, M.J. 1994. Distribution of speech recognition results with the Clarion cochlear prosthesis. Paper presented at the International Cochlear Implant, Speech and Hearing Symposium, October 24-28, Melbourne, Australia.

Leake, P.A., Hradek, G.T., Rebscher, S.J., and Snyder, R.L. 1991. Chronic intracochlear electrical stimulation induces selective survival of spiral ganglion neurons in neonatally deafened cats. *Hearing Research* 54:251-271.

McDermott, H.J., McKay, C.M., and Vandali, A.E. 1992. A new portable sound processor for the University of Melbourne/Nucleus Limited multielectrode cochlear implant. *Journal of the Acoustical Society of America* 91:3367-3371.

Miyamoto, R.T., Osberger, M.J., Robbins, A.M., Myres, W.A., and Kessler, K. 1993. Prelingually deafened children's performance with the Nucleus multichannel cochlear implant. *American Journal of Otology* 14:437-445.

Miyamoto, R.T., Osberger, M.J., Robbins, A.M., Myres, W.A., Kessler, K., and Pope, M.L. 1992. Longitudinal evaluation of communication skills of children with single- or multichannel cochlear implants. *American Journal of Otology* 13:215-222.

Miyamoto, R.T., Osberger, M.J., Todd, S.L., and Robbins, A.M. 1993. Speech perception skills of children with multichannel cochlear implants. In I.J. Hochmair-Desoyer and E.S. Hochmair (eds.), *Advances in cochlear implants*. Manz, Austria: Datenkonvertierung, Reproduktion und Druck.

Miyamoto, R.T., Osberger, M.J., Todd, S.L., Robbins, A.M., Stroer, B.S., Zimmermann-Phillips, S., and Carney, A.E. 1994. Variables affecting implant performance in children. *Laryngoscope* 104:1120-1124.

Osberger, M.J., Robbins, A.M., Miyamoto, R.T., Berry, S.W., Myres, W.A., Kessler, K., and Pope, M.L. 1991. Speech perception abilities of children with cochlear implants, tactile aids, or hearing aids. *American Journal of Otology* 12 (Suppl.):105-115.

Osberger, M.J., Todd, S.L., Berry, S.W., Robbins, A.M., and Miyamoto, R.T. 1991. Effect of age at onset of deafness on children's speech perception abilities with a cochlear implant. *Annals of Otology, Rhinology and Larnygology* 100:883-888.

Patrick, J.F., and Clark, G.M. 1991. The Nucleus 22-Channel Cochlear Implant System. *Ear and Hearing* 12 (Suppl.):3S-9S.

Picheny, M., Durlach, N.I., and Braida, L.D. 1986. Speaking clearly for the hard of hearing II: Acoustic characteristics of clear and conversational speech. *Journal of Speech and Hearing Research* 29:434-446.

Quittner, A.L., Smith, L.B., Osberger, M.J., Mitchell, T.V., and Katz, D. 1994. The impact of audition on the development of visual attention. *Psychological Science* 5:347-353.

Renshaw, J.J., Robbins, A.M., Miyamoto, R.T., Osberger, M.J., and Pope, M.L. 1988. *Hoosier Auditory Visual Enhancement Test (HAVE)*. Indianapolis: Indiana University School of Medicine.

Robbins, A.M., Renshaw, J.J., Miyamoto, R.T., Osberger, M.J., and Pope, M.L. 1988. *Minimal Pairs Test*. Indianapolis: Indiana University School of Medicine.

Robbins, A.M., Renshaw, J.J., and Osberger, M.J. 1988. *Common Phrases Test*. Indianapolis: Indiana University School of Medicine.

Schindler, R.A., and Kessler, D.K. 1993. Clarion cochlear implant: Phase I investigational results. *Laryngoscope* 102:1006-1013.

Skinner, M.W. 1994. The borderline child. Paper presented at the Fifth Symposium on Cochlear Implants in Children, February 5, New York.

Skinner, M.W., Clark, G.M., Whitford, L.A., Seligman, P.M., Staller, S.J., Shipp, D.B., Shallop, J.K., Everingham, C., Menapace, C.M., Arndt, P.L., Antogenelli, T., Brimacombe, J.A., Pijl, S., Daniels, P., George, C.R., McDermott, H.J., and Beiter, A.L. 1994. Evaluation of a new spectral peak (SPEAK) coding strategy for the Nucleus 22 Channel Cochlear Implant System. *American Journal of Otology* 15 (Suppl. 2):15-27.

Smith, C.R. 1975. Residual hearing and speech production in deaf children. *Journal of Speech and Hearing Research* 18:795-811.

Waltzman, S.B., Cohen, N.L., Gomolin, R., Shapiro, W.H., Ozdamar, S., and Hoffman, R. 1994. Long-term results of early cochlear implantation in congenitally and prelingually deafened children. *American Journal of Otology* 15(Suppl. 2):9-14.

Weisenberger, J.M., and Kozma-Spytek, L. 1991. Evaluating tactile aids for speech perception and production by hearing-impaired adults and children. *American Journal of Otology* 12 (Suppl.):188-200.

Wilson, B.S. 1993. Signal processing. In R.S. Tyler (ed.), *Cochlear implants*. San Diego: Singular Publishing Group.

Wilson, B.S., Finley, C.C., Lawson, D.T., Wolford, R.D., Eddington, D.K., and Rabinowitz, W.M. 1991. Better speech recognition with cochlear implants. *Nature* 52:236-238.

PART IV.

Amplification and Special Populations

15

The Potential Benefits of Amplification for Young Children with Normal Hearing

Noel D. Matkin

BACKGROUND

Including the topic of children with normal hearing in an international conference highlights how broad our scope of audiologic practice has become with respect to the use of classroom amplification. At the outset, it is worthwhile to briefly review key developments over the past 40 years. Until the early 1970s, discussion of classroom amplification primarily focused on children with severe-to-profound bilateral hearing impairments who often were educated in self-contained classrooms. Recall that in the late 1950s there was a move away from stationary hardwired systems with a bank of earphones to the use of induction loop amplification units. This advance permitted unlimited movement of children but only in classrooms with a loop installation. Wireless FM systems became increasingly popular by the late 1960s. These systems not only facilitated experiential learning for groups of children outside the school building but also made it feasible to mainstream a single child with a hearing impairment into a regular classroom that was often noisy and reverberant since there was little or no acoustic treatment.

With the 1970s came increased awareness of the linguistic, academic, and social/emotional deficits seen among children with milder degrees of bilateral sensorineural hearing loss. Davis, Berg and Fletcher, Ross and Giolas (1977, 1970, 1978), among others, documented the fact that so-called mild and moderate hearing losses often result in major obstacles to early language development and later academic achievement. At the same time, Public Law 94-142, passed in 1975, mandated a free and appropriate education for all children with developmental disabilities in the least restrictive environment. This term was viewed often as synonymous with mainstreaming. As a result, audiologists broadened considerably their scope of practice since there are six or seven children who are hard of hearing and need the support provided by classroom amplification for each child who is deaf (Elssmann, Matkin, and Sabo 1987).

Research in the past decade again required all of us to broaden our focus and consider the adverse impact of so-called minimal hearing losses, including children with unilateral impairments and children with conductive impairments related to recurrent otitis media, especially of early onset. Crandell (1993) also alerted the professional community to the adverse impact of limited high-frequency bilateral impairments among children, especially those placed in noisy learning environments.

ENVIRONMENTAL CONSIDERATIONS

With the passage of Public Law 99-457, we began to see many children, ages 3 to 5, with normal hearing but with developmental delays, placed in special needs rooms in the public schools. Many of these younger children, however, still are not being served. Valuable developmental time will be lost if we ignore the possibility of intervening before age 3. With increasing numbers of single working parents and two career couples, many toddlers and young children spend many of their waking hours during the workweek in day care. It was estimated in a recent national news broadcast that 11 million children under age 5 are placed in day care centers in the U.S.A. While there is a paucity of controlled studies relative to the noise levels in such environments, casual observations quickly confirm that they are extremely noisy much of the day.

Noisy day care centers should be of concern to the professional community since it is well documented that many of the auditory processes prerequisite to successful speech and language development and later classroom learning are developed during these early preschool years. For example, the period from 6 months to the first birthday appears to be a crucial auditory developmental period. During this time, infants move from being universal listeners to those focused on the salient acoustic features of the primary language spoken in their home (Kuhl, Williams, Lacerda, Stevens, and Lindblom 1992).

As noted many years ago, the development of key auditory skills is related to normal language acquisition, school readiness, and academic achievement (Zigmond and Cicci 1968). For this reason, early identification and intervention are crucial for children who have delayed or disordered auditory development. In this context, the hierarchy developed by Myklebust many years ago is quite relevant (1964). Recall that this hierarchy indicates that receptive language development precedes expressive language acquisition. In other words, input precedes output during the early preschool years. Once a child is of school age, reception of the printed form of language (reading) precedes expression (writing).

Aram and Nation (1982) discuss five basic auditory operations that they view as interdependent and basic to the processing of speech through the auditory channel. These include attention, rate, sequencing, discrimination, and memory. Two of these processes, auditory attention and auditory discrimination, can be observed and measured with relative ease in the child's learning environment.

Auditory attention is a process of primary interest in that attention is not only a precursor, but a prerequisite, to efficient learning. Although it is a complex auditory process, attention can be analyzed relative to three components: focusing on the primary signal, maintaining such attention, and then shifting attention to an alternate auditory signal or to another sensory modality such as vision. There is good evidence that the quality of all three components are age related and, thus, are developmental in nature. Feagans, Sanyal, Henderson, Collier, and Appelbaum (1987) observed that children with early otitis media histories had deficits not only in language processing but also in attention when studied in the classroom at age 5 and at age 7. A later study (Feagans, McGhee, Kipp, and Blood 1990) found similar attention deficits among toddlers even during story time. Fortunately, there also is growing evidence that such attending behaviors can be enhanced by increasing the intensity of the primary signal, thereby improving the signal-to-noise ratio (Rosenberg and Blake-Rahter 1995).

For a number of years, a comparison of the speech recognition performance of children with normal hearing and children with hearing impairments in noisy and reverberant listening situations has been made using the Finitzo dissertation data (Finitzo-Hieber and Tillman 1978). Relevant to this topic, it is revealing to compare the speech recognition scores for monosyllabic words of adults with normal hearing as collected by Crum (1974) with the scores of children with normal hearing. Even at age 10, children with normal hearing still experience more difficulty on speech recognition tasks than adults with normal hearing in adverse listening situations. In fact, Elliott (1979) found children up to age 13 with normal hearing have poorer speech perception in background noise than do young adults. Data from Keith's SCAN-A (1986) also suggested there are positive changes in auditory performance up to age 13. Such auditory growth was seen on the low pass filtered word test, the auditory figure-ground task, and the competing word tests. Further, Nabelek and Robinson (1982) reported an increase of 10 dB in the speech signal was required for young children to perform at an equivalent level with young adults. Thus, it is reasonable to speculate that if Finitzo's study was replicated with 3-, 4-, and 5-year-old children, an even greater difference in scores would be noted. Gravel and Wallace (1992) found that at age 4, children with histories of early and recurrent otitis media required a more positive signal-to-noise ratio to perform at the same level as their otitis negative peers. In other words, learning to listen in noise appears to be developmental and, thus, is a much more difficult auditory task for young children with normal hearing than one might suspect.

It is imperative that audiologists consider noise levels of day care centers as well as developmental preschool classrooms in attempting to provide and to maintain optimal amplification for preschoolers with normal hearing who are at developmental risk.

CLASSROOM AMPLIFICATION

As we consider utilization of classroom amplification with school-age children with normal hearing, it is beneficial first to consider what ages should be targeted. School-age children of any age may benefit from amplification, especially those in untreated, noisy classrooms. However, we need to keep in mind that until children develop good reading comprehension skills, typically by grade four, they largely depend on comprehending the verbal instruction of their teacher through listening. Therefore, the first four years of formal schooling merit our primary focus. During this time many basic academic skills, which are prerequisite to later academic success, are acquired. If we are conservative and use 3% as an estimate of children at risk for communication disorders, and then consider that there are 15 million children across this country in grades one through four, there are at least 450,000 children in this country who could benefit from classroom amplification.

A review of the literature suggests that there are at least five types of children who may well benefit from improving the signal-to-noise ratio in the educational listening environment. First, a significant number of youngsters now have normal hearing but had early onset otitis media with fluctuating conductive hearing loss due to retained middle ear effusion. The prevalence of such children may approach 8 in 1,000 (Teele, Klein, Rosner, and the Greater Boston Otitis Media Study Group 1984). A second type is the child with significant speech-language delay whose problems may or may not be related to early onset otitis media. Even with comprehensive evaluation, the cause of such delays often is unknown. This group undoubtedly includes a variety of children with special needs. Another group includes youngsters with attention deficits coupled with difficulties listening in compromised environments. These children may later be identified as having specific learning disabilities. Some investigators include children with central auditory processing disorders in this former group while others view such youngsters

Table 1
Potential Benefits of Classroom Amplification

Increased
    Attending skills
    Eye contact
    On-task behavior
    Rate of response
    Awareness of verbal cues
    Auditory memory
    Verbal comprehension: noise academic performance

Decreased
    Distractibility
    Body movement
    Extraneous verbalizations

as comprising a distinct category. Of additional concern is the estimate that by the turn of the century, many children with special needs will come from culturally and linguistically different populations where standard English is a second language (Kayser 1994). Finally, we need always to keep in mind those preschoolers who have relatively weak auditory skills. High noise levels in many day care centers may well limit their range of opportunities for auditory learning.

The primary objective in using amplification with children with normal hearing, regardless of their ages, is to improve receptive communication by making speech the most audible signal, thereby accelerating learning. Table 1 highlights the behaviors cited one or more times by a variety of investigators when discussing the benefits of amplification. Attention, on-task behavior, eye contact with the speaker, and increased awareness of verbal cues have all been noted to improve. One study of particular interest by Flexer and Savage (1993) indicated that with mild gain amplification, children's test-taking time was shortened significantly. If both time on task and rate of response are improved with classroom amplification, then the findings from this study intuitively make good sense. Other authors report that auditory memory, verbal comprehension in noise and, subsequently, academic performance also improve with classroom amplification (Rosenberg and Blake-Rahter 1995). Of equal importance is the observation that distractibility, extraneous body movement, and verbalizing out of turn have been noted to decrease among children classified as language/learning disabled upon using FM amplification systems (Blake, Field, Foster, Platt, and Wertz 1991).

Recall that the classic MARRS study (Mainstream Amplification Resource Room Study) was implemented in 1977 with two stated objectives.

First, the investigators wanted to determine whether or not students with minimal hearing loss experienced educational deficits. Second, they attempted to determine if such educational deficits, found on standardized tests, could be remediated within the mainstream classroom setting (Sarff 1981). Two intervention strategies were used in testing the second objective. The first involved the use of a resource room setting in the instruction of standard curriculum. The second employed the use of a sound field amplification system in a regular classroom. Children in grades four, five, and six were selected to participate in this two-year study.

A significantly greater academic improvement at a faster rate and lower cost was noted for the students receiving amplified instruction as compared to those receiving resource room instruction. Findings also suggested amplified teacher instruction may be more beneficial in the earlier grades where language skills so critical to academic success are established (Ray, Sarff, and Glassford 1984; Sarff 1981). It was with the success of the MARRS project that the importance of sound field amplification gained recognition in this country.

As we move toward national education of parents, caregivers, and educators relative to use of amplification with children with normal hearing, there are three important questions regarding such treatment efficacy (Carney and Moeller 1994). First, does the treatment work? The evidence to date, while limited with certain age groups and types of disability, is most encouraging in this respect. The second question, which is more difficult at this time to answer, is: Does one treatment work better than another? Whether a mild gain/low maximum output (MPO) wireless personal FM system or a free field classroom amplification system is most beneficial with different types of children remains to be definitively answered. Finally, how does a treatment alter behaviors? This third question needs a more solid database before one can answer it with assurance. As we consider the need for future research, it should be noted that any one of these three questions can be answered in any one of three ways: with group experimental designs, with single subject designs, or with case studies.

The ASHA Committee on Amplification for the Hearing Impaired published its report in 1991 (American Speech-Language-Hearing Association 1991). It addresses several concerns relative to selection of instrumentation and monitoring of hearing status. The issues of consumer safety, professional liability, and the potential for noise-induced hearing loss must be considered when one uses any type of amplification with children having normal peripheral hearing.

When we were discussing classroom amplification for children with normal hearing, one major decision to be made is whether to provide treatment for a single child in the form of a personal wireless FM unit or whether a sound field classroom system is more suitable. The obvious advantages of a sound field system include the following:

1. The child benefits from treatment without active cooperation required. Thus, the issue of rejection becomes a moot point.
2. No one child is singled out for treatment. Thus, the potential stigma of using amplification is eliminated.
3. Equipment malfunction is readily obvious to everyone in the classroom. This is a major concern when one considers the rate of malfunction seen among pediatric hearing aid users.
4. There is a major financial advantage in that the cost of amplifying a classroom is roughly equivalent to the cost of providing only one child with a single FM unit.

These advantages are appealing, but several concerns must be addressed. At present, there is no national standardization with respect to quality of the sound system or its installation. A number of school systems have reported assembling their own units by purchasing inexpensive electronic components. They have further attempted to save money by only installing one loudspeaker per classroom. This defeats the purpose of the system in that the signal-to-noise ratio will not be consistently advantageous throughout the classroom unless multiple loudspeakers are used.

While the use of sound field amplification in educational environments is gaining popularity, there are distinct advantages of individual low gain/low MPO FM units that should be considered as decisions about the preferable type of amplification are made. First, with stable placement of the teacher microphone and the use of Walkman-type earphones or ear buds, there is greater consistency of the signal-to-noise ratio regardless of the child's physical location in the classroom. A second advantage is that there is a good deal more use gain than the 12 dB or so typically measured with sound field systems. Another major advantage relates to mobility. If the school system requires the child to change classrooms for different academic subjects, the advantage of the self-contained FM system is readily seen.

Finally, in some instances, school personnel are reluctant to invest in amplification for a specific child without evidence of its benefit. By using an instrument such as the SIFTER, it is often possible to demonstrate the benefit of amplification through a single subject study by comparing pre- and post-treatment scores (Anderson 1989). Since the SIFTER is completed by the classroom teacher, positive differences in scores take on a face validity to administrators and to parents that is advantageous to the child.

CONCLUSION

This chapter has reviewed a number of positive reports relative to the use of amplification with a variety of children with normal hearing in different age categories. However, many of the studies cited, especially those with preschoolers, are descriptive in nature. It is now time to move toward well-designed, longitudinal empirical studies in which the characteristics of pediatric research subjects are well defined. In other words, it is now time to develop a solid research base if, as a profession, we are to justify recommendations for wide-scale use of classroom amplification with children having normal hearing. This is an excellent opportunity for school audiologists and research centers to initiate collaborative investigations. It is important to elicit input from teachers who spend much of the day with these children. The SIFTER has been invaluable in collecting pre- and post-treatment data from teachers so that the benefits of a particular management, such as use of classroom amplification, can be more objectively delineated.

With the implementation of P.L. 99-457, increasing numbers of young children are being considered for placement in special needs preschools. At present, a preschool version of the SIFTER is being field tested as a screening instrument for use with children considered for placement in such special programs. Screening is only the first step. Once a child is identified as being at risk, there is a pressing research need to identify a battery of psychometric instruments designed to detect both changes in auditory and communication behaviors and improvements in academic achievement. A national study committee needs to generate a position paper in which a preferred test battery and test protocol are delineated. Such a battery would facilitate collaborative efforts making it possible to develop a national data bank and compare data across test sites with different groups of children.

After a decade or more, it is now time to move away from descriptive studies and anecdotal reports. Recommendations for using amplification with children having normal peripheral hearing sensitivity should now be supported with data from well-designed research investigations. One important goal is for each of us to become more proactive in early identification of children in need. We must avoid the continued use of a failure-based model when recommending amplification for young children, even those with normal hearing. This is our challenge in the nineties!

ACKNOWLEDGMENTS

I want to acknowledge gratefully the time and effort expended by Kate Peters, B.A., University of Arizona, in researching this topic and in preparing this manuscript.

REFERENCES

American Speech-Language-Hearing Association. 1991. Amplification as a remediation technique for children with normal peripheral hearing. *Asha* (Suppl). 5:22-24.

Anderson, K.L. 1989. *Screening instrument for targeting educational risk.* Austin: Pro-Ed.

Aram, D.M., and Nation, J.E. 1982. *Child language disorders.* St. Louis: C.V. Mosby.

Berg, F.S., and Fletcher, S.G. 1970. *The hard of hearing child.* New York: Grune and Stratton.

Blake, R., Field, B., Foster, C., Platt, F., and Wertz, P. 1991. Effect of FM auditory trainers on attending behaviors of learning-disabled Children. *Language, Speech, and Hearing Services in Schools* 22:111-114.

Carney, A.E., and Moeller, M.P. 1994. Treatment efficacy: Hearing loss in children. *Asha Technical Paper.*

Crandell, C. 1993. Speech recognition in noise by children with minimal degrees of sensorineural hearing loss. *Ear and Hearing* 14(31):210-216.

Crum, M.A. 1974. The effects of noise reverberation and speaker-to-listener distance on speech understanding. Ph.D. diss., Northwestern University, Evanston, Illinois.

Davis, J. (ed.). 1977. Our forgotten children: Hard-of-hearing pupils in the regular classroom. National Support Systems Project. Washington, D.C.: Department of Health, Education, and Welfare.

Elliott, L. 1979. Performance of children aged 9 to 17 years on a test of speech intelligibility in noise using sentence material with controlled word predictability. *Journal of the Acoustical Society of America* 66:651-653.

Elssman, S.F., Matkin, N.D., and Sabo, M.P. 1987. Early identification and habilitation of hearing impaired children: fact or fiction. *Proceeding of a Symposium in Audiology* (1):1-33.

Feagans, L., Sanyal, M., Henderson, F., Collier, A., and Appelbaum, M. 1987. Relationship of middle ear disease in early childhood to later narrative and attentional skills. *Journal of Pediatric Psychology* 12:581-594.

Feagans, L.V., McGhee, S., Kipp, E., and Blood, I. 1990. Attention to language in day-care attending children: A mediating factor in the developmental effects of otitis media. Paper presented at the Meeting of the International Conference of Infancy Studies, Montreal, Canada.

Finitzo-Hieber, T., and Tillman, T. 1978. Room acoustic effects on monosyllabic word discrimination ability for normal and hearing-impaired children. *Journal of Speech and Hearing Research* 21:440-458.

Flexer, C., and Savage, H. 1993. Use of a mild gain amplifier with preschoolers with language delay. *Language, Speech, and Hearing Services in Schools* 24:151-155.

Gravel, J.S., and Wallace, I.F. 1992. Listening and language at 4 years of age: Effects of early otitis media. *Journal of Speech and Hearing Research* 35:588-595.

Kayser, H. 1994. Service delivery issues for multicultural populations. In R. Lubinski and C. Frattali (eds.), *Professional Issues in Speech-Language Pathology and Audiology* (pp. 282-292). San Diego: Singular Publishing Group.

Keith, R.L. 1986. A test for auditory processing disorders in adolescents and adults (SCAN-A). San Antonio: The Psychological Corporation, Harcourt Brace and Company.

Kuhl, P.K., Williams, K.A., Lacerda, F., Stevens, K.N., and Lindblom, B. 1992. Linguistic experience alters phonetic perception in infants by 6 months of age. *Science* 255(1):606-608.

Myklebust, H.R. 1964. *Auditory disorders in children.* New York: Grune and Stratton.

Nabelek, A., and Robinson, P.K. 1982. Monaural and binaural speech perception in reverberation for listeners of various ages. *Journal of the Acoustical Society of America* 71:1242-1248.

Ray, H., Sarff, L., and Glassford, F.E. 1984. Sound field Amplification: An innovative educational intervention for mainstreamed learning-disabled children. *Directive Teacher*, Summer-Fall, 18-20.

Rosenberg, G. and Blake-Rahter, P. 1995. Sound field amplification: A review of the literature. In C.C. Crandell, J. Smaldino, and C. Flexer (eds.), *Sound field FM amplification* (pp. 107-123). San Diego: Singular Publishing Group, Inc.

Ross, M. and Giolas, T.G. 1978. *Auditory management of hearing impaired children.* Baltimore: University Park Press.

Sarff, L. 1981. An innovative use of free field amplification in regular classrooms. In R.J. Roeser and M.P. Downs (eds.), *Auditory disorders in children* (pp. 263-272). New York: Thieme and Stratton.

Teele, D.W., Klein, J.O., Rosner, B.A., and the Greater Boston Otitis Media Study Group 1984. Otitis media with effusion during the first three years of life and development of speech and language. *Pediatrics* 74(2):282-287.

Zigmond, N.K., and Cicci, R. 1968. *Auditory learning.* Belmont, Calif.: Fearon Publishers.

16

Amplification for Children with Minimal Hearing Loss

Carol Flexer

INTRODUCTION

Minimal is defined as "the least possible degree or quantity" (Webster's 1992). The term implies without consequence—insignificant. Because a minimal hearing loss is the least measurable hearing loss, also implicit in the term is permission to provide the least possible intervention and the fewest management strategies. Traditionally, parents have been advised that minimal hearing loss will pose little, if any, academic or communicative difficulties for their child. Contrary to that belief, minimal hearing loss in children can have negative consequences (Northern and Downs 1991).

Children with minimal hearing loss are often behind in school (Davis 1990), may have subtle language problems and reading difficulties (Ross 1991), and may have behavior problems (Cargill and Flexer 1991). Intervention needs to be as thoughtful and rigorous for children with minimal hearing loss as for children who experience any other degree of hearing loss. The purpose of this chapter is to discuss why minimal hearing impairments are problematic for children, and to identify the technology that can be used to overcome the barrier of hearing poorly, especially in classrooms.

DEFINITION AND DESCRIPTION OF MINIMAL HEARING IMPAIRMENTS

There are about 39½ million schoolchildren in the United States with 8 million having some type and degree of hearing loss. This makes children with hearing problems the largest population of children who require special services in the schools (Berg 1986; Hull and Dilka 1984; Ross, Brackett, and Maxon 1991). There are approximately 700 audiologists employed within school settings to manage these 8 million children (Berg 1987; Wilson-Vlotman and Blair 1986). It is reasonable to assume that these overburdened audiologists will focus their attention on children with the most severe degrees of hearing loss.

NORMAL HEARING

Normal hearing for children is defined as thresholds of 15 dB HL or better at all frequencies in both ears. Thresholds greater than 15 dB HL are considered abnormal and place a child at risk for academic failure.

MINIMAL HEARING IMPAIRMENT

A *minimal* or *slight* hearing impairment is defined as thresholds from 16 to 25 dB HL for children. A child with a minimal hearing impairment could experience problems hearing faint or distant speech, hearing subtle conversational cues, tracking fast-paced communicative interactions, and hearing word-sound distinctions that form morphological markers for plurality, tense, possessives, and so on (Davis 1990; Roeser and Downs 1995). Furthermore, a child with a minimal hearing impairment may appear immature and be more fatigued than peers with normal hearing due to the increased level of effort needed to hear (Anderson 1991). A minimal hearing loss could have a major negative impact on a child who needs to be able to hear a clear, complete, and consistent speech signal.

Otitis media is the primary cause of hearing loss in children. Most hearing losses caused by otitis media are in the minimal-to-mild hearing loss range (Paradise 1980). The audiologic/educational intervention for the hearing loss caused by ear infections should not vary from interventions used for other hearing impairments because it is the hearing impairment, and not the disease, that is at issue. Audiologic interventions are used in addition to, not instead of, medical interventions. See chapter 17 for more information about managing children with fluctuating hearing impairment.

MILD HEARING IMPAIRMENT

Mild hearing impairments also have been described erroneously as insignificant. A mild hearing impairment is defined as thresholds from 26 to 40 dB HL. If unmanaged, a child who experiences a 30 dB hearing loss can miss 25% to 40% of the speech signal depending on the noise level in the environment, the distance from the speaker, and the configuration of the hearing loss (Mueller and Killion 1990; Olsen, Hawkins, and Van Tasell

1987). Furthermore, the child probably will not benefit from incidental learning because he or she will be unable to overhear conversational transactions.

UNILATERAL HEARING IMPAIRMENT

Professionals in audiology, education, and medicine typically have considered unilateral hearing loss to be a mild hearing impairment and of minimal consequence to communicative and academic performance. However, recent research has revealed that children with unilateral hearing loss are ten times more likely than the general population of schoolchildren to experience academic failure, and five times more likely to need academic support services (Bess 1985; Bess and Tharpe 1986; Oyler, Oyler, and Matkin 1988).

The incidence of monaural hearing impairment ranges from 2 per 1000 to 13 per 1000 with nearly 50% of these children experiencing educational difficulties (Bess 1986; Oyler et al. 1988). The auditory skills that are crucial for academic performance, including understanding speech in noise, identifying morphological markers, and localizing sound sources, are confusing for the monaural listener, especially in noisy conditions or when speech is directed toward the poorer ear (Bess 1986; Giolas and Wark 1967; Moncur and Dirks 1967). Additionally, Sarff (1981) has shown evidence of academic deficits, specifically in reading comprehension, reading vocabulary, spelling, and mathematics, in children with unilateral hearing loss.

Stein (1983) and Culbertson and Gilbert (1986) found that children with unilateral hearing impairment tend to have interpersonal and social adjustment problems and are often described as more distractible, frustrated, dependent, and less confident than their peers who have normal hearing sensitivity. Behavioral difficulties may be more obvious than hearing problems in the child who has a unilateral hearing impairment (Cargill and Flexer 1991). Unfortunately, negative behaviors rarely are linked to the unilateral hearing impairment because the child has one perfectly good ear and, thus, is believed to be able to hear what and when he or she wants to.

Children with unilateral hearing losses are at risk for educational and behavioral difficulties. A child with a unilateral hearing impairment who also experiences repeated ear infections is at risk for the educational delays and behavioral problems that result from unmanaged hearing impairment (Cargill and Flexer 1991).

WHY AND HOW DOES MINIMAL HEARING LOSS NEGATIVELY IMPACT LEARNING?

Childhood hearing loss of *any* degree places a child at risk for educational difficulties because mainstream classrooms are auditory-verbal environments, "data input" is insufficient, and distance hearing is compromised (Bess 1985; Davis 1990; Downs 1988; Flexer 1994).

MAINSTREAM CLASSROOMS ARE AUDITORY-VERBAL ENVIRONMENTS

Auditory discrimination has primary importance for the development of basic academic competencies that provide the framework for school success (Elliott, Hammer, and Scholl 1989). Mainstream classrooms are auditory-verbal settings with information presented through the speech of the teacher (Simon 1985). To the extent that a child cannot clearly and consistently hear the teacher, the entire premise of the educational system is undermined. Academic achievement, therefore, is based largely on the pupil's ability to listen and to discriminate word-sound differences (Berg 1987; Elliott et al. 1989).

Speech-to-noise ratio (S/N ratio) is a critical concept relative to the reception of intelligible speech in a classroom environment. S/N ratio is the relationship between the primary speech or input signal and background sounds. Background noise includes all sounds that interfere with the reception of the auditory signal of choice such as other talkers, heating or cooling systems, classroom sounds, traffic noise, televisions, computer hums, playground noise, gym sounds, internal biological noise, wind, and so on. The more favorable the S/N ratio—the louder the primary auditory signal relative to background sounds—the more intelligible that speech signal will be for a child.

Adults with normal hearing sensitivity typically require an S/N ratio of +6 dB for the reception of intelligible speech. Persons with hearing impairment are believed to need a more favorable S/N ratio of at least +20 dB even when they are wearing hearing aids (Finitzo-Hieber and Tillman 1978). Because of noise, reverberation, and changes in teacher and pupil locations, the average classroom S/N ratio is only +4 dB, and it may be worse than 0 dB. This is less than ideal even for children with normal hearing sensitivity (Berg 1993).

COMPUTER ANALOGY

Hearing impairment has been described as an invisible acoustic filter (Davis 1990; Ling 1989). One negative effect of the invisible acoustic filter of hearing impairment is its detrimental impact on spoken language development. If a child cannot hear clear, consistent, and intelligible sounds because of minimal, mild, fluctuating, or unilateral hearing impairment, then that child's spoken language skills probably will not be clear either unless deliberate intervention occurs (Ling 1989).

Another negative consequence of the invisible acoustic filter effect of hearing loss is its destructive impact on the higher-level linguistic skills of reading and writing. That is, if verbal language skills are deficient, then reading skills likely will be deficient also because reading is a secondary linguistic function built on speaking (Simon 1985). If a child has poor reading skills, then academic options likely also will be limited because literacy certainly is linked to academics (Wallach and Butler 1984). The core problem of hearing loss needs to be recognized, and hearing must be accessed before intervention at the secondary levels of spoken language, reading, and academics can be effective (Ling 1989; Ross, Brackett, and Maxon 1991).

As a result of the acoustic filter effect, speech might be audible but not intelligible to someone with a hearing loss (Bess 1985; Dobie and Berlin 1979). That is, a child with a hearing loss might hear *show, showing, shows, shown, showed,* all as __ow. That child "heard" the teacher but did not intelligibly discern all of the morphological markers, causing the teacher to be misled into believing that deficient language and academic skills are independent problems rather than the effects of hearing loss. Furthermore, when a child mishears even a single speech sound, inappropriate behaviors may result that could be interpreted, by an uninformed teacher, as student noncompliance. Until that hearing loss is directly managed to allow maximum intelligibility of speech, success from language and academic intervention could be limited.

A computer analogy can be used to illustrate the potentially negative effects of any type and degree of hearing problem on spoken language development and on academic performance. A child must have information (data) in order to learn. A primary way that information is entered into the brain is through hearing (Berg 1987; Lennenberg 1967; Leonard 1991). If data are entered incompletely or inconsistently, analogous to using a malfunctioning computer keyboard or to having one's fingers on the wrong keys of a computer keyboard, the child will have faulty information to process. Logically, a child's learning will be compromised when the information that reaches the brain is deficient. Is the computer program in error if the entered data are incomplete? Unfortunately, children who have inaccurate data entry may be labeled learning disabled, hyperactive, attention disordered, or noncompliant even though their behavior is the result of faulty data entry caused by hearing loss.

Once the keyboard is repaired or the fingers are placed consistently on the correct keys, analogous to using amplification technology that enables a child to detect word-sound distinctions, what happens to all of the previously entered inaccurate and incomplete information? Do the inaccurate data automatically convert to correct and complete information? Unfortunately, faulty data need to be identified, and correct data need to be reentered. Consequently, the longer a child's hearing problem remains unrecognized and unmanaged, the more damaging are the preventable sequelae of that hearing impairment.

Hearing is the first step in the scheme of intervention. As soon as hearing is accessed through appropriate speech-to-noise enhancing technology, the child will have an opportunity to discriminate word-sound distinctions, learn and expand spoken language, which then provides an opportunity to acquire knowledge. All levels of the acoustic filter effect of hearing impairment need to be identified, understood, and managed. The longer a child has inaccurate data entry, the more destructive the acoustic filter effect will be on the child's overall development. On the other hand, the more intelligible the entered data are, the better opportunity the child will have to learn language, to acquire reading skills, and to develop academic competencies.

DISTANCE HEARING AND PASSIVE LEARNING

Distance hearing, or earshot, is a critical concept that needs to be understood relative to managing the hearing of children with minimal, mild, unilateral, or fluctuating hearing losses. Distance hearing is the distance over which speech sounds are intelligible and not just audible (Ling 1989). Hearing loss of any type and degree (even minimal) reduces the distance over which speech sounds are intelligible, even with amplification. Typically, the greater the hearing impairment, the greater the reduction in earshot. This reduction in earshot has tremendous consequences for classroom performance. Distance hearing is linked to passive/casual/incidental listening and learning (Ramsdell 1978; Ross, Brackett, and Maxon 1991).

Children who experience a hearing loss, even a minimal or unilateral hearing loss, cannot casually overhear what people are saying or the events that are occurring around them. Most children with normal hearing seem to absorb information from their surroundings without expending much effort. Hearing impairment presents a barrier to the casual acquisition of information, so children who have hearing problems often seem oblivious to environmental events that are not directed actively to them (Pollack 1985). Therefore, due to this reduction in earshot and the elimination of casual listening and learning caused by hearing impairments, children with even a minimal hearing loss may need to be taught directly many skills and concepts that other children learn incidentally (Erber 1982).

The reduction of distance hearing has additional implications for a child with hearing problems, including lack of redundancy of instructional information, lack of access to social cues (Conway 1990), and the need for a remote microphone to expand earshot (Leavitt 1991). Listening is necessarily an active and not a passive process for children with hearing impairment.

Another area that is affected by reduction in distance hearing is the learning of appropriate social skills. Much of what a child understands about how other children behave is learned through casual observation of communicative interactions—also known as eavesdropping. Children with hearing impairments, even minimal ones, have a very difficult time overhearing conversations that are not directed to them (Ling 1989). Consequently, auditory rehabilitation goals often need to include planned teaching of social skills, especially to young children.

RATIONALE FOR THE USE OF SIGNAL-TO-NOISE RATIO ENHANCING TECHNOLOGY

It is well known that sound is degraded as it is propagated across a physical space. The magnitude of the degradation probably has been underestimated because of the difficulty of relating the physical components of high-fidelity sound—dynamic range, frequency, intensity, reverberation, and S/N ratio—to speech perception. Therefore, Leavitt and Flexer (1991) used the Bruel and Kjaer's Rapid Speech Transmission Index (RASTI) to measure the effect of a listening environment on a speechlike signal. The RASTI score is a measure of the integrity of the acoustic signal as it is propagated across the classroom; a perfect reproduction of the RASTI signal at the receiver is depicted by a score of 1.0.

RASTI measurements were made at 17 different seating locations in an occupied classroom. Results showed that significant sound degradation occurred as the RASTI receiver was moved away from the RASTI transmitter. Even in the front-row center seat—preferential seating—the RASTI score dropped to 0.83. In the back row, the RASTI score was only 0.55, showing a loss of 45% of equivalent speech intelligibility in a quiet, occupied classroom. Note that a perfect RASTI score of 1.0 could be attained only at the six-inch reference position.

The RASTI study demonstrated the importance of being close to the speaker (within six inches), physically or through the use of a remote location microphone for the purpose of obtaining a complete speech signal. That is, as soon as a pupil moves farther away than six inches from the teacher's mouth, the speech signal begins to degrade. If a student does not receive a complete speech signal, that student is being denied access to instructional information.

Certainly, we want to use the best available hearing aid technology when amplifying children. However, hearing aids alone in a classroom may not be enough to allow the reception of intelligible sound. The best current hearing aids can amplify only the sounds that reach the microphone port. A remote microphone placed close to the source of the sound (the teacher's mouth) may be needed to enhance the speech signal.

SPEECH-ENHANCING TECHNOLOGY

Historically, the recommendation of preferential seating was thought to address the classroom listening needs of children with minimal hearing losses. Recent research, however, shows that an intact signal is not received from the teacher even when a child is seated in the front-row center seat (Leavitt and Flexer 1991).

Hearing aids are not necessarily the first choice for amplifying children with minimal, mild, unilateral, or fluctuating hearing impairments. These children could receive the most immediate benefit in the classroom from an initial fitting of a mild gain personal FM unit. These same children might also benefit from sound field amplification units instead of personal FM systems. If functional audiometric testing and teacher, parent, and child report show that the child is having the greatest difficulty when listening and attending in the classroom, then amplification should initially address the areas of greatest need.

Updike (1994) compared FM auditory trainers, CROS hearing aids, and personal amplification for six children with unilateral hearing losses. She found that all six children in her study experienced significantly better performance with the FM auditory trainer than with hearing aids. The children with the greatest hearing losses received the greatest benefit from the FM systems.

Cargill and Flexer (1991) found, after evaluating numerous coupling options (Walkman headphones, earbud, standard earmold), that a custom standard earmold designed to accommodate the FM button receiver, with a short canal, belled bore, and IROS venting, appeared to be the most effective and comfortable way of coupling the FM unit to the better ear of children with unilateral hearing impairments. Such coupling allowed the children to hear the teacher at a favorable S/N ratio while not occluding their ears to their own and classmates' voices. The use of sound field amplification was not evaluated for these children, but it is a recommended direction for future research.

PERSONAL FM SYSTEMS

For children with minimal hearing impairments, an FM system is not intended to function as a hearing aid. Rather, the FM unit is fit to enhance acoustic accessibility of intelligible speech and to provide instructional redundancy in a classroom environment. The S/N ratio is improved because the teacher wears the (remote) wireless microphone transmitter, and the child wears the receiver. The situation is comparable to the teacher speaking within six inches of the child's ear at all times no matter where the teacher or the child is located within the classroom.

AMPLIFICATION AND MINIMAL HEARING LOSS • 329

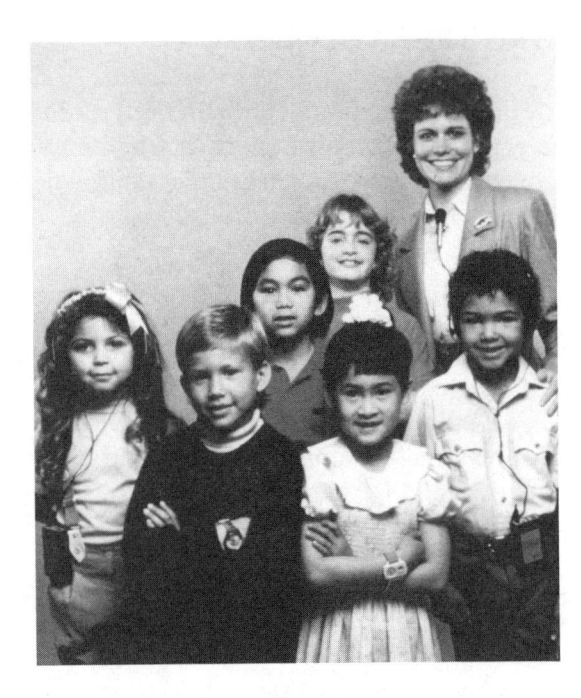

Figure 1. A child with a minimal, mild, fluctuating, or unilateral hearing loss can be fit with a low-power-output FM unit to improve the S/N ratio in a classroom; the signal can be delivered to a child's ears through lightweight Walkman earphones. (Photo Courtesy of Phonic Ear Inc.)

Children with minimal hearing losses require a low-power-output FM unit that also has low gain. The output and gain must be specified, measured, and controlled by an audiologist. Coupling arrangements may include lightweight Walkman earphones (figure 1), earbuds, stetoclips, or button earphones attached to special custom earmolds. See chapter 13 for a thorough discussion of FM systems.

SOUND FIELD AMPLIFICATION

A sound field FM system is an exciting educational tool that allows control of the acoustic environment in a classroom, thereby facilitating acoustic accessibility of teacher instruction for all children in the room. Sound field units are small wireless high-fidelity public address systems that are self-contained in a classroom (Crandell, Smaldino, and Flexer 1995). The classroom is amplified through the use of one to five wall- or ceiling-mounted loudspeakers (figure 2). A wireless FM microphone transmitter, just like the one used for a personal FM unit, is worn by the teacher. The radio signal is sent to an amplifier that is connected to the loudspeakers. See chapter 11 for detailed information about sound field amplification.

330 • AMPLIFICATION AND SPECIAL POPULATIONS

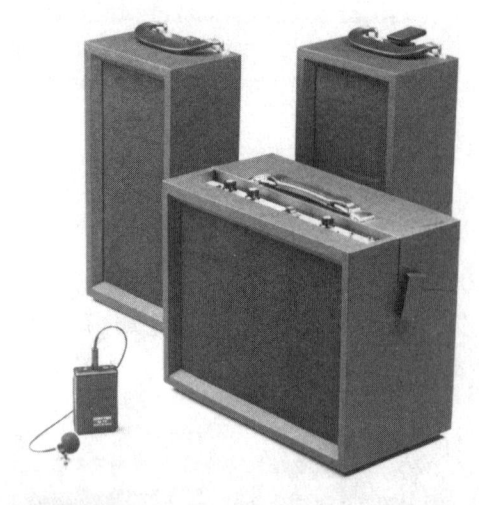

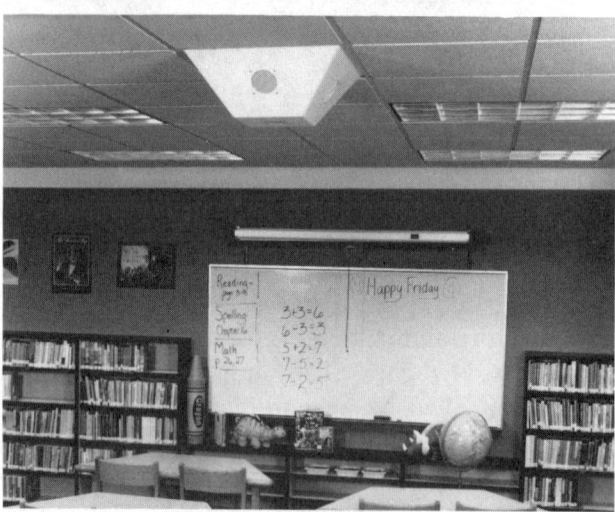

Figure 2. Sound field FM systems amplify an entire classroom through the use of one to five wall- or ceiling-mounted loudspeakers. (**2A** Photo Courtesy of Audio Enhancement; **2B** Photo Courtesy of Custom Audio Design.)

A major difference between sound field FM units and personal FM systems is that the personal FM, if fit appropriately, can provide the most favorable S/N ratio: +20 to +30 dB (Hawkins 1984). With a personal FM unit, the speech signal travels directly from the microphone transmitter that is located about six inches from the teacher's mouth to the ear of the child who is wearing the FM receiver. With a sound field unit, the teacher's speech is transmitted from the microphone worn six inches from his or her mouth to the amplifier/loudspeakers that are located at some distance from the child. The child can be closer to loudspeakers than to the teacher, but not as close as the child could be to the headphones of a personal FM receiver. Sound field FM units typically improve the classroom's S/N ratio by about 10 dB (Berg 1993).

Evidence is accumulating that pupil performance improves significantly in regular and in special education classrooms where sound field amplification is employed (Flexer 1989; Ray, Sarff, and Glassford 1984). In a three-year study, the Putnam County Project evaluated the effectiveness of 47 sound field units and found (1) the number of students receiving special services or requiring special placement decreased from 945 students prior to amplified classrooms to 850 students, even though the overall pupil count in the county had increased, (2) amplified kindergarten classes showed the most dramatic results on the Iowa TBS achievement tests with significantly higher scores on listening, language, and word analysis than scores obtained by children in unamplified classrooms, and (3) better student production and on-task behaviors were noted in amplified classrooms.

Flexer, Millin, and Brown (1990) found that the nine students in a primary-level classroom for children with developmental disabilities scored significantly fewer errors on a word identification task when the classroom was amplified. Flexer et al. (1990) found that only one child in that classroom had normal hearing sensitivity as defined by thresholds being 15 dB or better at all frequencies bilaterally. That is, all but one child had minimal hearing impairment. None of the children were recognized by school personnel as having hearing impairment.

EVALUATING THE EFFICACY OF FM USE: SIFTER

There is a need for a measurement tool that can be used in a repeated fashion, over time, to monitor the effectiveness of FM use for children who experience minimal hearing impairments. The SIFTER (Screening Instrument for Targeting Educational Risk) can be used in this fashion (Anderson 1989). The SIFTER is the only instrument currently available that specifically screens the classroom performance of children with hearing problems. The SIFTER is a brief checklist filled out by the classroom teacher that asks questions about student performance in five different areas: academic, attention, communication, class participation, and school behavior. There are 3 questions in each area for a total of 15 questions. The questions ask the teacher to compare the student's performance (in this case the student with a minimal hearing loss who is using an FM system, personal or sound field) to that of his or her classmates by rating the student from 1 to 5. The teacher's ratings are then plotted on a scoring grid that shows if the student in question passes, fails, or has marginal performance in each of the five areas.

Matkin (1990) reported that the SIFTER was effective for screening the classroom performance over time of children with minimal hearing losses. Note that the SIFTER is a screening and not a diagnostic tool. Nevertheless, it is easy and fast, and it adds the important facet of involving the classroom teacher, in a collaborative fashion, in the management of the child with a minimal hearing loss.

FUNCTIONAL AUDIOMETRIC INFORMATION

Children cannot be fit for amplification using the same decision-making paradigm used for fitting adults. Again, referring to the computer analogy, children are still receiving new auditory-linguistic data. They do not have the sophisticated linguistic systems, speech perceptual abilities, or concentration skills that adults have (Davis 1990). In addition, the complexity and multiplicity of children's listening and learning environments must be considered when selecting amplification options. A child needs to be able to hear teacher instruction and peer response during interaction in the classroom including large group and small group dynamics, instruction in gym class, and on the playground and playing field, all environments where the teacher is not close to the child. Further, peer interaction in the cafeteria, conversation on the school bus, conversation while riding in the car with parents in the front seat and the child restrained in the backseat, and family interactions at home are but a few of the diverse listening/learning domains. In addition, children tend to be very active, which means that they often run and jump, fall down, and sweat. There is a tremendous variety of listening demands on a child who must function in dynamic and often unpredictable environments. All of these factors must be considered when selecting amplification systems for children.

One way to demonstrate the impact of a minimal, mild, unilateral, or fluctuating hearing impairment on a child's classroom listening is to present phonetically balanced (PB) words at 45 dB HL in quiet and noise (+5 dB S/N) in the sound field. Forty-five dB HL was selected because that is the average loudness level at which speech is received by a child in a favorable classroom listening environment (Berg 1987). A child might appear to hear all of the PB words in quiet but have a great deal of difficulty hearing those words in noise. Noise is always present in classrooms. Therefore, it is not logical to test a child in an acoustically perfect (quiet) sound room and then make inferences about listening in a noisy classroom.

Obtaining functional audiometric data is important for evaluating children with unilateral hearing losses. When performing sound field testing at 45 dB HL with a +5 dB S/N ratio, two different conditions should be utilized. First, present the PB words from the loudspeaker that is directed to the good ear, with the speech noise or multitalker speech babble directed to the poor ear. Next, present the PB words directed toward the poor ear, with the noise directed toward the good ear. Then compare the scores.

There will be many times in class when the desired speech signal is directed toward the poor ear. Preferential seating is not possible because of constant changes in teacher and pupil position, background noise, and reverberation. Speech-enhancing technology must be employed.

ACOUSTIC ACCESSIBILITY AND SECTION 504

Special services for children with hearing problems in schools are mandated by three federal laws (DuBow, Geer, and Strauss 1992). These include Education of All Handicapped Children Act of 1975 (Public Law 94-142), Education of All Handicapped Children Act Amendments of 1986 (Public Law 99-457), and the Rehabilitation Act of 1973, specifically, Section 504. In 1990, Public Law 99-457 was amended and its name was changed to the Individuals with Disabilities Education Act, commonly referred to as IDEA. In addition, the Rehabilitation Act of 1973 was amended twice, in 1978 and again in 1992 (Rehabilitation, Comprehensive Services and Developmental Disabilities Amendments of 1978; Rehabilitation Act Amendments of 1992).

IDEA accesses special education funds by developing an Individualized Education Plan (IEP) to identify necessary accommodations for a child with a disability. Most students who experience minimal, mild, or unilateral hearing impairments do not qualify for special school services through IDEA because their hearing impairments are not severe enough. Consequently, Section 504 of the Rehabilitation Act of 1973 probably will be the most relevant legislation for them. This act assures accessibility to educational programs for individuals with disabilities. Audiologists should recommend speech-enhancing technology for children with minimal hearing losses to ensure *acoustic accessibility*.

Audiologists can advocate, proactively, that a child's hearing problem interferes with her or his opportunity to have access to spoken instruction. By not having acoustic accessibility, the child is being denied an appropriate education. By performing the speech-in-noise testing in a sound room that was discussed earlier in this chapter, an audiologist can furnish evidence that a child cannot hear clearly in a typical classroom.

CONCLUSION

The following ideas were emphasized in this chapter:

1. There is no such thing as an insignificant hearing impairment in children. Hearing is a first-order event for learning spoken language and for developing academic competencies.

2. A child with a minimal hearing impairment experiences problems hearing faint or distant speech, hearing subtle conversational cues that could cause a child to react inappropriately, tracking fast-paced communicative interactions, and hearing word-sound distinctions.
3. Children with unilateral hearing losses are ten times more likely than the general population of schoolchildren to experience academic failure, and they tend to have interpersonal and social adjustment problems.
4. As a result of their reduction in earshot and the elimination of casual listening, children with minimal, unilateral, or fluctuating hearing impairments need to be taught directly many skills and concepts that other children learn incidentally.
5. To obtain functional audiometric information the audiologist should perform word identification testing at 45 dB HL in quiet and in noise in the sound field.
6. If a child does not hear clearly in the presence of typical classroom noise, then that child does not have acoustic accessibility to classroom instruction.
7. Speech-to-noise ratio is a critical concept relative to the reception of intelligible speech. Hearing aids alone in a classroom, therefore, may not be enough. A remote microphone placed within six inches of the sound source may be necessary.
8. The audiologist should fit FM technology first, before hearing aids, to facilitate classroom listening for children with minimal hearing impairments.
9. Children with unilateral hearing impairments may perform better in the classroom with FM units than they do with personal amplification or with CROS hearing aids.
10. The SIFTER is a measurement tool that can be used to monitor the effectiveness of FM use in the classroom.
11. Most children with minimal hearing impairments will not qualify for special school services through IDEA because their hearing impairments are not severe enough. Section 504 of the Rehabilitation Act of 1973 probably will be the most relevant legislation for them.

Audiologists, by providing information about hearing and by advocating for and accessing the critically important auditory modality, are the primary professionals who can promote service for this neglected population of children with minimal hearing impairments. It's time to take a more active role!

REFERENCES

Anderson, K.L. 1989. *Screening instrument for targeting educational risk.* Austin: Pro-Ed.

Anderson, K.L. 1991. Hearing conservation in the public schools revisited. In C. Flexer (ed.), Current audiologic issues in the educational management of children with hearing loss. *Seminars in Hearing* 12:340-364.

Berg, F.S. 1986. Characteristics of the target population. In F.S. Berg, J.C. Blair, S. Viehweg, and A. Wilson-Vlotman (eds.), *Educational audiology for the hard of hearing child* (pp. 1-24). New York: Grune and Stratton.

Berg, F.S. 1987. *Facilitating classroom listening: A handbook for teachers of normal and hard of hearing students.* Boston: College-Hill Press/Little, Brown.

Berg, F.S. 1993. *Acoustics and sound systems in schools.* San Diego: Singular Publishing Group.

Bess, F.H. 1985. The minimally hearing-impaired child. *Ear and Hearing* 6:43-47.

Bess, F.H. 1986. The unilaterally hearing-impaired child: A final comment. *Ear and Hearing* 7:52-54.

Bess, F.H., and Tharpe, A.M. 1986. An introduction to unilateral sensorineural hearing loss in children. *Ear and Hearing* 7:3-13.

Cargill, S., and Flexer, C. 1991. Strategies for fitting FM units to children with unilateral hearing losses. *Hearing Instruments* 42:26-27.

Conway, L.C. 1990. Issues relating to classroom management. In M. Ross (ed.), *Hearing-impaired children in the mainstream.* Parkton, Md.: York Press.

Crandell, C., Smaldino, J., and Flexer, C. 1995. *Sound field amplification: A practical user's guide.* San Diego: Singular Publishing Group.

Culbertson, J.L., and Gilbert, L.E. 1986. Children with unilateral sensorineural hearing loss: Cognitive, academic and social development. *Ear and Hearing* 7:38-42.

Davis, J. (ed.). 1990. *Our forgotten children: Hard-of-hearing pupils in the schools.* Bethesda, Md.: Self Help for Hard of Hearing People.

Dobie, R.A., and Berlin, C.I. 1979. Influence of otitis media on hearing and development. *Annals of Otology, Rhinology, and Laryngology* 88:46-53.

Downs, M.P. 1988. Contribution of mild hearing loss to auditory language learning problems. In R.J. Roeser and M.P. Downs (eds.), *Auditory disorders in school children* (pp. 186-199). 2d ed. New York: Thieme Medical Publishers.

DuBow, S., Geer, S., and Strauss, K.P. 1992. *Legal rights: The guide for deaf and hard of hearing people.* 4th ed. Washington, D.C.: Gallaudet University Press.

Elliott, L., Hammer, M.A., and Scholl, M.E. 1989. Fine-grained auditory discrimination in normal children and children with language-learning problems. *Journal of Speech and Hearing Research* 32:112-119.

Erber, N. 1982. *Auditory training.* Washington, D.C.: Alexander Graham Bell Association for the Deaf.

Finitzo-Hieber, T., and Tillman, T. 1978. Room acoustics effects on monosyllabic word discrimination ability for normal and hearing-impaired children. *Journal of Speech and Hearing Research* 21:440-458.

Flexer, C. 1989. Turn on sound: An odyssey of sound field amplification. *Educational Audiology Association Newsletter* 5:6-7.

Flexer, C. 1994. *Facilitating hearing and listening in young children.* San Diego: Singular Publishing Group.

Flexer, C., Millin, J., and Brown, L. 1990. Children with developmental disabilities: The effect of sound field amplification on word identification. *Language, Speech, and Hearing Services in Schools* 21:177-182.

Giolas, T.G., and Wark, D.J. 1967. Communication disorders associated with unilateral hearing loss. *Journal of Speech and Hearing Disorders* 41:336-343.

Hawkins, D.B. 1984. Comparisons of speech recognition in noise by mildly-to-moderately hearing-impaired children using hearing aids and FM systems. *Journal of Speech and Hearing Disorders* 49:409-418.

Hull, R., and Dilka, K. 1984. *The hearing impaired child in school.* New York: Grune and Stratton.

Leavitt, R. 1991. Group amplification systems for students with hearing impairment. In C. Flexer (ed.), Current audiologic issues in the educational management of children with hearing loss. *Seminars in Hearing* 12:380-388.

Leavitt, R., and Flexer, C. 1991. Speech degradation as measured by the rapid speech transmission index (RASTI). *Ear and Hearing* 12:115-118.

Lennenberg, E.H. 1967. *Biological foundations of language.* New York: John Wiley and Sons.

Leonard, L.B. 1991. New trends in the study of early language acquisition. *Asha* 33:43-44.

Ling, D. 1989. *Foundations of spoken language for hearing impaired children.* Washington, D.C.: Alexander Graham Bell Association for the Deaf.

Matkin, N.D. 1990. Recognizing cultural diversity when counseling families of children with hearing impairment. Presentation at Pediatric Audiology Update Conference, June, Providence, Rhode Island.

Moncur, J.P., and Dirks, D.D. 1967. Binaural and monaural speech intelligibility in reverberation. *Journal of Speech and Hearing Research* 10:186-195.

Mueller, H.G., and Killion, M.C. 1990. An easy method for calculating the articulation index. *Hearing Journal* 43:14-22.

Northern, J.L., and Downs, M.P. 1991. *Hearing in children.* 4th ed. Baltimore: Williams and Wilkins.

Olsen, W.O., Hawkins, D.B., and Van Tasell, D.J. 1987. Representation of the longterm spectra of speech. *Ear and Hearing* 8 (Suppl. 5):100-108.

Oyler, R.F., Oyler, A.L., and Matkin, N.D. 1988. Unilateral hearing loss: Demographics and educational impact. *Language, Speech, and Hearing Services in School* 19:201-210.

Paradise, J.L. 1980. Otitis media in infants and children (review article). *Pediatrics* 65:917-943.

Pollack, D. 1985. *Educational audiology for the limited hearing infant and preschooler.* 2d ed. Springfield, Ill.: Charles C. Thomas.

Ramsdell, D.A. 1978. The psychology of the hard-of-hearing and deafened adult. In H. Davis and S.R. Silverman (eds.), *Hearing and deafness.* 4th ed. New York: Holt, Rinehart and Winston.

Ray, H., Sarff, L., and Glassford, F.E. 1984. Sound field amplification: An innovative educational intervention for mainstreamed learning disabled students. *Directive Teacher*, Summer-Fall, 18-20.

Rehabilitation Act of 1973, P.L. 93-112. September 26, 1973. *United States Statutes at Large* 87:355-394.

Roeser, R.J., and Downs, M.P. 1995. *Auditory disorders in school children.* 3d ed. New York: Thieme Medical Publishers.

Ross, M. 1991. A future challenge: Educating the educators and public about hearing loss. In C. Flexer (ed.), Current audiologic issues in the educational management of children with hearing loss. *Seminars in Hearing* 12:402-413.

Ross, M., Brackett, D., and Maxon, A.B. 1991. *Assessment and management of mainstreamed hearing impaired children.* Austin: Pro-Ed.

Sarff, L. 1981. An innovative use of sound field amplification in the classroom. In R.J. Roeser and M.P. Downs (eds.), *Auditory disorders in school children: The law, identification, remediation* (pp. 263-272). New York: Thieme Medical Publishers.

Simon, C.S. 1985. *Communication skills and classroom success.* San Diego, Calif.: College-Hill Press.

Stein, D.M. 1983. Psychosocial characteristics of school-age children with unilateral hearing loss. *Journal of the Academy of Rehabilitative Audiology* 16:12-22.

Updike, C.D. 1994. Comparison of FM auditory trainers, CROS aids, and personal amplification in unilaterally hearing impaired children. *Journal of the American Academy of Audiology* 5:204-209.

Wallach, G.P., and Butler, K.G. (eds.). 1984. *Language learning disabilities in school age children.* Baltimore: Williams and Wilkins.

Webster's II New Riverside Dictionary. 1992. New York: Berkley Books.

Wilson-Vlotman, A.L., and Blair, J.C. 1986. A survey of audiologists working full-time in school systems. *Asha* 27:33-38.

17

Special Considerations for Children with Fluctuating/Progressive Hearing Loss

Anne Marie Tharpe

INTRODUCTION

Hearing loss that fluctuates and/or progresses poses a unique challenge to a child's audiologic, otologic, and educational management. An additional complication, particularly with younger children, is that audiologists may assume that changes in audiometric results reflect attention, or nonsensory factors, as opposed to true changes in hearing sensitivity. Such assumptions may result in delayed adjustments to hearing aid settings and delayed referrals for otologic management. Further, many young children, with or without hearing impairment, do not have the requisite language skills for informing their care providers of a change in hearing status. Not identifying audiologic changes in a timely manner can have far-reaching medical, linguistic, and educational implications for a child. It is the role of audiologists to monitor a child's hearing and provide this information to parents, otologists, and other appropriate professionals such as speech/language pathologists and school personnel.

This chapter attempts to raise the reader's level of suspicion for fluctuating/progressive hearing loss in children by reviewing several causes and patterns of such changes. Although this review is by no means exhaustive, it covers the most likely causes of progressive/fluctuating hearing loss in children. In addition, recommendations for audiologic management of children with fluctuating or progressive hearing loss will be suggested.

PREVALENCE OF FLUCTUATING/PROGRESSIVE HEARING LOSS

The likelihood of a child with sensorineural hearing loss (SNHL) demonstrating a progressive loss of auditory sensitivity is reported to be between 2% and 33% (Barr and Wedenberg 1965; Brookhouser, Worthington, and Kelly 1991; Newton and Rowson 1988; Parving 1988; Ruben and Fishmann 1981). It is assumed that these wide variations in prevalence reports are due to differences in study populations (i.e., varying etiologies) and study methodologies, specifically, audiologic criteria used to document progression and length of follow-up. Brookhouser and Worthington (1994), in examining children with fluctuating and/or progressive hearing losses in the absence of middle ear dysfunction, found that 21% of their study population of children with SNHL demonstrated threshold variations of 10 dB or greater for at least one frequency between 250 and 8000 Hz. The majority (57%) of the study ears with threshold variations demonstrated progressive losses with intermittent upward fluctuations at one or more test frequencies. Only 6% had purely progressive hearing loss with no intermittent upward fluctuation while 37% had intermittent threshold fluctuation without a permanent decrease in hearing sensitivity. One must interpret these findings with caution, however, because a 10 dB change in auditory response is considered by many to represent normal clinical variance depending on the step size used to obtain threshold.

CAUSES OF FLUCTUATING/PROGRESSIVE HEARING LOSS IN CHILDREN

GENETIC HEARING LOSS WITHOUT ASSOCIATED ABNORMALITIES

Autosomal Dominant Progressive SNHL

This progressive hearing loss is characterized by early or late onset bilateral progressive SNHL. Much is unknown about the genes involved in nonsyndromic deafness, although differences in age of onset of hearing loss, degree of loss, and rate of progression suggest defects in different genes (Konigsmark and Gorlin 1976; Meyerhoff, Cass, Schwaber, Sculerati, and Slattery 1994). Several genes for dominant SNHL have been localized (Chen, Ni, Fukushima, Marietta, O'Neill, Coucke, Willems, and Smith 1995; Coucke et al. 1994; Leon, Raventos, Lynch, Morrow, and King 1992). For example, Leon and colleagues have located a gene on chromosome 5 causing Monge deafness, one form of dominantly inherited progressive hearing loss, in a large Costa Rican kindred (Leon, Raventos, Lynch, Morrow, and King 1992) while Coucke et al. (1994) have mapped a gene in some families with early onset autosomal dominant hearing loss to chromosome 1.

Autosomal Recessive Progressive SNHL

Recessive hearing loss without associated anomalies is considered to be the most common cause of deafness in early childhood. Genes causing recessive nonsyndromic deafness are difficult to locate due to genetic heterogeneity. Meyerhoff et al. (1994) have described a nonsyndromic hearing loss with onset between approximately 1 and 6 years of age rapidly progressing to the severe-to-profound loss range by 6 years of age. Such losses have been reported in offspring of consanguineous marriages.

X-Linked Progressive Hearing Loss

Nonsyndromic recessive X-linked hearing loss is a clinically variable condition between and among pedigrees. It accounts for approximately 5% to 6% of all male genetic hearing loss. X-linked hearing impairment has been classified according to age of onset of hearing loss and audiometric characteristics. These include (1) congenital sensorineural loss; (2) early onset sensorineural loss; (3) progressive sensorineural loss; and (4) mixed loss with stapes footplate fixation (Gusher's syndrome) (Reardon, Bellman, Phelps, Pembrey, and Luxon 1993). Progression of the hearing loss has also been reported in this latter classification (Glasscock 1973).

Otosclerosis

Although otosclerosis usually begins in early adulthood, it can manifest itself in childhood. The hearing loss associated with this disorder is usually conductive or mixed; however, a progressive SNHL can occur. The cause of the conductive component in most cases is the result of stapedial footplate fixation (Meyerhoff et al. 1994). The process can, however, surround the cochlea resulting in a sensorineural component (Linthicum 1993). The causative agent of otosclerosis is unknown, and the mode of genetic transmission also remains unclear (Konigsmark and Gorlin 1976; Linthicum 1993). Surgical and medical intervention is considered highly effective in most cases (Colletti and Fiorino 1994; Farrior 1994; Shea 1994).

GENETIC HEARING LOSS WITH ASSOCIATED ABNORMALITIES

Albers-Schonberg Disease

Also known as marble bone disease or osteosclerosis fragilis generalisata, this syndrome is characterized by osteopetrosis and may have associated progressive, mixed hearing loss, optic atrophy, and facial paralysis. The pattern of inheritance is autosomal recessive for the infantile severe form while a benign adult form of this disorder has an autosomal dominant expression. Incidence of osteopetrosis is between 1 in 100,000 and 1 in 500,000 (Manusov, Douville, Page, and Trivedi 1993). The etiology of osteopetrosis is unknown, although we do know that the disease results from congenital alteration of mesenchyma, with excessive deposit of calcium at the level of bones, cartilages, tendons, viscera, and vessels (Filip, Golu, Filip, Scavera, and Ciuchi 1994). Although osteopetrosis can be treated with bone marrow transplantation, splenectomy, blood replacement, and systemic corticosteroids, results are variable and prognosis is poor (Gerritsen, Vossen, van Loo, Hermans, Helfrich, Griscelli, and Fischer 1994; Manusov et al. 1993).

Alport's Syndrome

This syndrome is associated with hereditary nephritis, ocular lesions, and progressive SNHL. The mode of inheritance of this syndrome is X-linked or autosomal dominant, and occurrence has been reported at a rate of 1 in 200,000 (Brown, Meyerhoff, and Ginsburg 1986; Buyse 1990). The cause of the X-linked form of this disorder has been identified as mutations in the collagen alpha 5 (IV) gene (Coucke et al. 1994); however, the etiology of the hearing loss remains unclear. This is the first genetic basement disease whose gene has been cloned, thus enabling the development of antibodies and DNA probes for accurate diagnosis.

Approximately 40% to 50% of persons with Alport's syndrome will demonstrate a slowly progressive SNHL. The hearing loss begins in the second decade of life and generally ranges from mild to moderately severe in the mid to high frequencies, being more severe in males than females (Flinter, Cameron, Chantler, Houston, and Bobrow 1988). Variants of Alport's syndrome (i.e., Epstein's and Fleckner syndromes) consist of nephritis, macrothrombocytopenia, and progressive SNHL (Konigsmark 1969).

Branchio-Oto-Renal (BOR) Syndrome

An autosomal dominant inherited disorder, BOR syndrome is associated with external, middle, and inner ear malformations, branchial cleft sinuses, cervical fistulas, mixed hearing loss, and renal anomalies (Gutierrez, Bardaji, Bento, Martinez, and Conde 1993; Kumar, Kimberling, Connolly, Tinley, Marres, and Cremers 1994). Notable external ear anomalies include malformation of the antihelix, severe microtia, preauricular cartilaginous appendages, and preauricular pits (Fraser, Ling, Clogg, and Nogrady 1978). Although approximately 1% of the general newborn population has preauricular pits, 1 in 500 with pits is diagnosed with BOR syndrome (Fraser,

Sproule, and Halal 1980). Hearing loss is the most common characteristic of BOR syndrome affecting approximately 80% of the carriers (Fraser et al. 1978). Although the loss is most often mixed in nature, it may also be conductive or sensorineural, may range in degree from mild to profound, and may be progressive or nonprogressive (Fraser et al. 1980). The gene for BOR syndrome has been mapped to the long arm of chromosome 8 (Kumar et al. 1994).

CHARGE Syndrome

The acronym CHARGE was proposed to describe a recurring association of defects that include colobomata of the eyes, heart disease, choanal atresia, retarded growth and development and/or central nervous system anomalies, genital hypoplasia, and ear anomalies/hearing loss (Guyot, Gacek, and DiRaddo 1987; Pagon, Graham, Zonana, and Yong 1981). CHARGE syndrome is considered to be one of the most common multiple-anomaly conditions (Hall 1979). Although it is generally regarded as a group of anomalies and not as a specific syndrome, researchers have described kindreds in which the transmission of the disease is consistent with dominant or recessive inheritance. Both X-linked and autosomal patterns of inheritance have been noted, and these findings have been interpreted as suggesting that CHARGE is a syndrome (Davenport, Hefner, and Mitchell 1986; Davenport, Hefner, and Thelin 1986; Mitchell, Giangiacomo, Hefner, Thelin, and Pickens 1985; Pagon et al. 1981; Thelin, Mitchell, Hefner, and Davenport 1986).

Approximately 90% of those with CHARGE association demonstrate ear abnormalities and/or hearing loss. External, middle, and inner ear anomalies have been noted. The hearing loss is typically sensorineural in nature, although conductive or mixed losses are not uncommon. The degree of hearing loss ranges from mild to severe. Asymmetry between ears is a frequent finding (Brown and Israel 1991), and progression has been reported in some cases (Thelin et al. 1986).

Mucopolysaccharidoses Syndrome (MPS)

This metabolic disorder is caused by congenital lack of a lysosomal enzyme for degradation of a glycosaminoglycan molecule (Meyerhoff et al. 1994). Children with MPS exhibit no abnormality at birth; however, a progressive buildup of the glycosaminoglycan molecules within cells results in progression of the disorder. The MPS disorders are characterized by skeletal deformity, dwarfism, coarse facial features, mental retardation, and cardiovascular disease. Hearing loss associated with MPS is progressive and usually mixed. The more common varieties of MPS include (1) Hurler's syndrome: an autosomal recessive disorder associated with growth failure early in infancy (Meyerhoff and Liston 1991); (2) Hunter's syndrome: an X-linked recessive disorder similar to but less severe than Hurler's syndrome; and (3) Maroteaux-Lamy syndrome: an autosomal recessive disorder that is less severe than both Hurler's and Hunter's syndromes (Meyerhoff et al. 1994). Bone marrow transplantation has been advocated as a possible therapy for MPS (Bekassy and Ringden 1992).

Neurofibromatoses Type 1 and Type 2 (NF1 and NF2)

NF1 is a relatively common inherited disease that usually manifests in early childhood as a multisystem progressive disorder. It is usually characterized by pigmentary lesions (café-au-lait spots) present at, or soon after, birth. Increased growth of neurofibromas and multisystem symptomatology generally occur at puberty (Bolande 1981). Audiologic findings are highly variable and can range from normal hearing sensitivity to profound hearing loss. The NF1 gene has been identified and many different mutations have been reported (Xu, O'Connell, Viskochil, Cawthon, Robertson, Culver, Dunn, Stevens, Gesteland, White, and Weiss 1990). NF2 is an inherited tumor syndrome. It is characterized by an insidious or rapidly progressive SNHL, beginning in childhood, secondary to bilateral acoustic neuromas (Young, Eldridge, and Gardner 1970). However, pure-tone sensitivity may be well within normal limits even in advanced cases of NF2 (Pikus 1990). The defective gene has been identified, and its structure and function suggest that it may be involved in multiple tumor types in addition to brain neoplasms (Trofatter et al. 1994). Both of these genetically distinct disorders have an autosomal dominant pattern of transmission; NF1 is on chromosome 17 and NF2 is on chromosome 22. Surgery is the only treatment available to prevent total deafness.

Osteogenesis Imperfecta (Van Der Hoeve's Syndrome)

This syndrome exhibits an autosomal dominant mode of transmission with associated multiple fractures, weak joints, blue sclera, and skeletal deformities. The progressive hearing loss is usually conductive (60% of cases) or sensorineural in the higher frequencies (Riedner, Levin, and Holliday 1980) and results from osteoclast activation in the temporal bone (Chole 1993). The rate of occurrence is approximately 2 to 4 per 100,000 births (Buyse 1990).

Retinitis Pigmentosa

Several inherited disorders are associated with retinitis pigmentosa and progressive hearing loss. Usher syndromes (USH) are autosomal recessive disorders characterized by retinitis pigmentosa and congenital SNHL. USH1 is associated with profound SNHL and vestibular involvement while USH2 is associated with mild-to-severe SNHL; the hearing loss in USH3 is progressive (Moller et al. 1989; Sankila et al. 1995; Smith et al. 1994). Prevalence ranges from 3 to 4 per 100,000 (Boughman, Vernon, and Shaver 1983; Nuutila 1970). At least five distinct genes are known to cause the Usher syndrome, one of which has been identified as myosin VIIA (Weil et al. 1995). Refsum syndrome is characterized by progressive SNHL beginning in the second decade of life, retinitis pigmentosa, icthyosis, and hypertrophic peripheral neuropathy (Konigsmark 1969). Other syndromes associated with progressive SNHL and ocular disease include Alstrom syndrome (Alter and Moshang 1993), Norrie syndrome (Holmes 1971), and Cockayne's syndrome (Shemen, Mitchell, and Farkashidy 1984).

Stickler Syndrome (Hereditary Arthro-Ophthalmopathy)

Stickler syndrome is an autosomal dominant disorder of the connective tissue, which includes ocular and systemic manifestations. It is characterized by progressive and severe myopia, vitreal degeneration, retinal detachment, progressive sensorineural deafness, cleft palate, and mandibular hypoplasia. The disorder may be caused by mutations in type II collagen, which is the most abundant protein of cartilage (Ahmad, McDonald-McGinn, Zackai, Knowlton, LaRossa, DiMascio, and Prockop 1993; Brunner, van Beersum, Warman, Olsen, Ropers, and Mariman 1994). Sensorineural deafness could be related to the observation that type II collagen is also present in the inner ear (Rai, Wordsworth, Coppock, Zaphiropoulos, and Struthers 1994). It is one of the more common inherited disorders of connective tissue with an incidence of between 1 per 10,000 and 1 per 20,000 (Buyse 1990; Pyeritz 1993).

Waardenburg's Syndrome

This autosomal dominant disorder has variable penetrance and is characterized by pigmentary abnormalities that include a white forelock and nonpigmented skin, heterochromia irides, hyperplasia of medial portion of eyebrows, and lateral displacement of medial canthi. Sensorineural hearing loss occurs in 50% of cases, may be unilateral or bilateral, mild to profound, and may or may not be progressive (Meyerhoff et al. 1994; Pantke and Cohen 1971). In about 60% of cases, the cause of this disorder is a mutation in the PAX3 gene, which is involved in embryonic development (Coucke et al. 1994).

ACQUIRED HEARING LOSS

PRENATAL CAUSES

Infections

The most common cause of congenital viral-induced hearing impairment, *cytomegalovirus* (CMV) is presumed to infect 0.5% to 2.4% of all live births (Pass, Stagno, Myers, and Alford 1980; Schildroth 1994). The infection is usually asymptomatic in the mother; therefore, it is difficult to determine which stage of intrauterine development is most vulnerable to CMV. CMV can also be contracted in the perinatal period during delivery through the birth canal. Approximately 10% to 15% of children with congenital CMV demonstrate mental retardation or hearing loss. The hearing loss associated with congenital or prenatally acquired CMV is sensorineural in nature with variable configuration, can be unilateral or bilateral, mild to profound, and is frequently progressive (Dahle, McCollister, Stagno, Reynolds, and Hoffman 1979). Onset may occur as late as 7 years of age (Stagno et al. 1977). When CMV is acquired perinatally, it is believed that there is no associated hearing loss at least through 3 years of age (Johnson, Hosford-Dunn, Paryani, Younger, and Malachowski 1986). Serologic titers must be obtained within the first 3 weeks of life in order to reliably diagnose CMV (Meyerhoff et al. 1994). Currently, there is no vaccine to prevent the CMV infection nor is there any effective treatment for individuals infected with the virus (Koszinowski, Del Val, and Reddehase 1990; Stagno 1990).

Although immunization is available, *congenital rubella* remains a cause of severe-to-profound sensorineural hearing loss in some children and congenital conductive loss in others. Hearing loss occurs in 50% of surviving infants affected in the first trimester, making it the most common of rubella defects (Davis and Johnson 1983). The sensorineural losses have been reported with delayed onset, progression, and/or fluctuation (Bergstrom 1988; Newton and Rowson 1988). A few cases of SNHL following rubella immunization have been reported (Stewart and Prabhu 1993).

The advent of prenatal serology and penicillin in the 1950s led to a marked decline in cases of congenital *syphilis* through the mid-1980s. The number of cases, however, increased by 34% in the U.S. between 1981 and 1989 (Dehner and Gersell 1994; Starling 1994). Congenital syphilis is characterized as early, *infantile,* or late, *tardive*. Onset in infancy is usually associated with sensorineural hearing loss that is sudden, bilateral, progresses rapidly, and may fluctuate. Hearing loss with later onset (early childhood as opposed to infancy) presents as a bilaterally symmetrical, sensorineural deficit with a sudden onset and slow progression (Dennis and Neely 1991; Schuknecht 1974). Identification is made through Venereal Disease Research

Laboratory (VDRL) or fluorescent treponemal antibody absorption (FTA) screening and is treated with penicillin and corticosteroid therapy. Hearing levels can be stabilized and/or improved in early onset cases with prompt treatment.

Other prenatal infections associated with progressive or fluctuating hearing loss include *herpes simplex virus, varicella* (chicken pox), and *rubeola* (measles) (Meyerhoff et al. 1994).

Inner Ear Malformations

Several inner ear malformations are associated with progressive/fluctuating hearing losses. These include *Mondini's dysplasia*, which is a developmental disorder of the inner ear involving the bony capsule and the membranous labyrinth and is associated with large vestibular aqueduct, endolymphatic sac, and endolymphatic hydrops (Triglia, Nicollas, Ternier, and Cannoni 1993). Hearing loss is reported as fluctuating and progressive supposedly due to the presence of the hydrops. Endolymphatic shunt operations have been recommended to halt the progression of the loss (House 1964; Mangabeira-Albernaz, Fukaka, Chammas, and Gananca 1981).

Another inner ear malformation associated with progressive hearing loss is *Scheibe dysplasia*. The most common of inner ear dysplasias, Scheibe is characterized by involvement of the membranous labyrinth of the cochlea and saccule (cochleosaccular dysgenesis). Although it most commonly results in profound, bilateral sensory hearing loss, Scheibe dysplasia may present with early onset, progressive hearing loss (Konigsmark and Gorlin 1976).

Large vestibular aqueduct syndrome (LVAS) may be an isolated finding or may accompany other congenital malformations of the inner ear such as aplasia and hypoplasia as well as malformations of the semicircular canals and vestibule (Jackler and De La Cruz 1989; Levenson, Parisier, Jacobs, and Edelstein 1989). The hearing loss associated with LVAS is characterized as being bilateral, sensory, ranging in degree from mild to profound, and progressive (without fluctuations) in nature with onset in early childhood. The cause of the progression is unknown. Jackler and De La Cruz (1989) believe that LVAS is relatively common in children and is underdiagnosed due to a lack of radiographic evaluations in children with SNHL and interpretive expertise.

PERINATAL CAUSES

Hyperbilirubinemia

Also called jaundice, hyperbilirubinemia is the result of excessive bilirubin in the blood (blood concentration levels >6 to 8 mg/dl).

Hyperbilirubinemia can progress to kernicterus, a condition that is usually fatal; 80% of surviving infants demonstrate some degree of sensorineural hearing loss among other severe neurologic symptoms. The hearing loss is caused by accumulation of bilirubin in the striatum and cranial nerves (Roger, Koziel, Vert, and Nehlig 1993). The hearing loss is usually sensorineural and characterized by a saucer-shaped audiometric configuration. Cases of improvement in auditory thresholds over time have been reported (Schwartz and Costello 1988). Phototherapy and photochemotherapy are the most common effective treatments for neonatal hyperbilirubinemia while exchange transfusions are reserved for severe cases (Lazar, Litwin, and Merlob 1993).

Persistent Pulmonary Hypertension of the Newborn (PPHN)

Also known as persistent fetal circulation, PPHN is a cardiac abnormality exhibiting persistence of the fetal vessel joining the pulmonary artery to the aorta resulting in severe hypoxemia. Approximately 20% to 40% of infants diagnosed with PPHN demonstrate sensorineural hearing loss (Leavitt, Watchko, Bennett, and Folsom 1987; Sell, Gaines, Gluckman, and Williams 1985; Walton and Hendricks-Munoz 1991). The synergistic effect of aminoglycosides, furosemide, and use of hyperventilation in treatment is believed to contribute to the onset of hearing loss (Hendricks-Munoz and Walton 1988; Walton and Hendricks-Munoz 1991). The hearing loss associated with PPHN has been described as bilateral, progressive, sensorineural, with variability in degree and the possibility of delayed onset (Hendricks-Munoz and Walton 1988; Naulty, Weiss, and Herer 1986).

POSTNATAL CAUSES

Autoimmune Inner Ear Disease

Autoimmune disease can present as a systemic or localized otologic immune disorder affecting the auditory and vestibular mechanisms (McCabe 1979). Although it is most common for this disease to appear in middle age, it can also begin in childhood (Hughes, Barna, Kinney, Calabrese, and Nalepa 1988). The pathogenesis of autoimmune disease is believed to be multifactorial (cellular and humoral) (Hughes, Kinney, Barna, and Calabrese 1984). It is assumed that the hearing loss is the result of vasculitis (inflammation) of vessels supplying the inner ear, autoantibodies directed against inner ear antigenic epitopes, or cross-reacting antibodies (Harris and Sharp 1990; McKusick 1992). Tissue destruction may occur involving the tympanic membrane, the entire middle ear, the middle ear and mastoid, and/or facial nerve. The hearing loss is characterized by unilateral or bilateral involvement, fluctuating progression over weeks or months, and sudden onset

(Hughes et al. 1984). Unsteadiness and ataxia in darkness are common complaints with autoimmune disease (McCabe 1979). At least one researcher has reported that the vertiginous spells associated with autoimmune disease differ from those of Ménière's in that one may experience several in one day as opposed to one or two per week or month (McCabe 1989). Autoimmune disease is one of the few forms of SNHL for which there is treatment. Not only may progression of hearing loss be halted, but improvement in hearing sensitivity has been reported (Hughes et al. 1984). However, therapeutic recommendations in autoimmune disease remain controversial.

Ménière's Disease

Estimates are that only 3% of all patients with Ménière's disease are children while occurrence is most frequent between 40 and 50 years of age (Meyerhoff, Paparella, and Shea 1978). Early reports of childhood Ménière's first appeared in the late 1930s and early 1940s with children as young as 4 years of age demonstrating symptoms (Crowe 1938; Simonton 1940). Hearing loss associated with Ménière's disease is typically unilateral (80%), fluctuating, and primarily in the lower frequencies in the early stages of disease. Vertigo and tinnitus commonly accompany the hearing loss. Progression of the disease usually results in a moderate or moderately-severe sensory hearing loss. Because Ménière's disease is most often associated with endolymphatic hydrops, it is usually responsive to low-sodium diet, diuretics, and antivertiginous medications.

Meningitis

The incidence of neonatal meningitis varies across reports between 2 and 10 cases per 10,000 live births (Saez-Llorens and McCracken 1990). Over 80% of bacterial meningitis cases are the result of three pathogens: *Haemophilus influenzae* Type B (Hib), *Neisseria meningitidis,* and *streptococcus pneumoniae* with Hib being the most common cause among these (Lieberman, Greenberg, and Ward 1990). The peak age of incidence of invasive Hib disease is 6- to 12-month-old infants when antibody levels are the lowest. Approximately 1 in 250 children under the age of 5 develops invasive Hib disease with about half of these being meningitis (Lieberman et al. 1990).

Approximately 15% of meningitis survivors have neurologic sequelae that may include hearing loss, seizures, paresis, and learning or developmental disabilities (Kallio, Kilpi, Anttila, and Peltola 1994). Pneumococcal meningitis (*streptococcus pneumoniae*) is associated with a higher mortality and more serious morbidity rate than Hib meningitis (Lieberman et al. 1990). Typically, the hearing loss resulting from meningitis is bilateral, sensorineural, symmetrical, mild to profound in range, and permanent. Dodge et al. (1984) reported an incidence of hearing loss of 5% to 30% following bacterial meningitis in infants and children. Reports of recovery of meningitis-induced hearing loss have appeared sporadically in the literature (Brookhouser, Auslander, and Meskan 1988; Guiscafre, Benitez-Diaz, Martinez, and Muroz 1984; Liebman, Ronis, Lovrinic, and Katinsky 1969; Ozdamar, Kraus, and Stein 1983; Roeser, Campbell, and Daly 1975; Rosenhall and Kankkunen 1980; Wolff and Brown 1987). Even in those cases, few authors actually documented behavioral threshold improvement while others either did not report assessment technique or relied solely on auditory brainstem evoked responses (ABR).

Two ways that meningitis can affect the auditory system include a perineuritis of the eighth nerve and/or involvement of central auditory pathways in the brainstem. Since ABR results reflect the integrity of the auditory brainstem and not hearing sensitivity per se, it is possible that ABR results could initially be abnormal, suggesting hearing loss, while hearing sensitivity actually is normal. An "improvement" in hearing based on ABR alone could, in fact, be an improvement in auditory brainstem function. Documentation of hearing status following meningitis based on ABR findings alone, therefore, should be interpreted with caution.

It is anticipated that with the recent release of a preventive vaccine against *Haemophilus influenzae* Type B (Hib), hearing loss secondary to meningitis will decline markedly (Klein 1994; Stein and Boyer 1994). The Hib-protein conjugate vaccine (Hboc) was recommended by the U.S. FDA in 1990 for use in infants at 2, 4, and 6 months of age with a booster dose at 15 to 18 months (Lieberman et al. 1990). Although pneumococcal and meningococcal vaccines are also available, they are not sufficiently immunogenic to protect young children.

Otitis Media

Otitis media is the most frequent cause of auditory threshold shift in young children. Approximately one-third of children in the U.S. have recurrent and severe middle ear disease by age 3 (Klein 1992). Hearing loss associated with otitis media with effusion (OME) is conductive, unilateral or bilateral, and fluctuates. The mean threshold shift caused by otitis media is between approximately 25 and 30 dB (Brookhouser, Worthington, and Kelly 1993; Fria, Cantekin, and Eichler 1985). The peak age of acute otitis media is 7 to 12 months (Klein 1992). The insertion of tympanostomy tubes for treatment of OME is the most common operation for children in the U.S. (Kleinman, Kosecoff, DuBois, and Brook 1994). Antibiotic therapy remains the most common form of treatment for OME. The American Academy of

Pediatrics has recently published guidelines for the medical management of OME in young children (1994).

Perilymphatic Fistula (PLF)

A perilymphatic fistula is a leakage of perilymph fluid through a hole in the round window membrane or the oval window annular ligament as the result of an inner or middle ear anomaly or trauma (Grundfast and Bluestone 1978; Weissman, Weber, and Bluestone 1994). PLF, therefore, can be present at birth or caused by trauma at any age. Weber, Perez, and Bluestone (1993) reported a retrospective analysis of PLF and found that middle ear malformation, usually a malformed stapes, was responsible for 81% of cases. The associated hearing loss can be progressive, fluctuating, sudden onset SNHL with or without vertigo. Considerable controversy continues to surround the diagnosis and treatment of PLF primarily because there are no definitive laboratory, radiographic, or audiologic tests to confirm the presence of PLF. Direct viewing of the middle ear during exploratory surgery is the ultimate confirmation of PLF. Tympanotomy with repair of the fistula does not assure improvement in hearing (Seltzer and McCabe 1986).

DISCUSSION

Several questions arise when considering the significant number of children who may demonstrate a fluctuating or progressive hearing loss. How often do children with sensorineural hearing impairments need audiologic monitoring? Certainly, it is reasonable to closely monitor children whose etiologies are known to predispose them to progression or fluctuation and who are unable to report such changes to parents, perhaps every two to three months. But what about the approximately 50% of children with SNHL whose etiologies are unknown? Are we not responsible for ensuring that too much time does not lapse between audiologic visits for these children as well? It is understandable and appropriate that cost containment is at the forefront of health care concerns at this time. Excessive diagnostic testing can be costly and time consuming. The consequences of not identifying hearing sensitivity changes in a timely manner, however, cannot be ignored.

As discussed earlier, although most SNHLs are not treatable, several (such as autoimmune disease, Ménière's disease, and PLF) are. Prompt identification and treatment may result in a halt or reversal of the progression. In addition, identification of progressive or fluctuating loss may assist in determining the causative agent, which may have profound medical implications for other body systems (e.g., syphilis, autoimmune disease, neurofibromatosis). With that in mind, it is recommended that families of all children with SNHL of unknown etiology receive extensive counseling regarding the signs and symptoms of changes in auditory sensitivity. They should be encouraged to keep in close contact with their child's care providers or teachers in order to monitor potential changes in behavior or development. Audiologic monitoring should be conducted every three months or sooner if any concerns arise. This frequent monitoring schedule should continue until such time that children are considered reliable reporters of their hearing status.

Another question raised by this discussion is whether or not children with a high likelihood of progressive hearing loss resulting in severe-to-profound degree should be introduced to alternative communication approaches or strategies early in the course of progression in order to prepare them for the expected changes. If so, is a school system obligated to provide such intervention in anticipation of future difficulties? Obviously, there are many complex issues to be considered in making such a difficult decision. The first step is to discuss the prognosis with the child's otologist so that the family and all interested professionals are informed and knowledgeable about what to expect. If requested by the child's family, a multidisciplinary team meeting should be held to discuss the various educational and communicative options available.

Finally, given the evidence that some postmeningitic SNHLs improve over time, should we withhold consideration of cochlear implantation surgery for eligible children for a period of time while hearing levels are monitored? Contributing to the controversy surrounding this issue is that a consequence of surgical delay may be the development of labyrinthitis ossificans (ossification of the labyrinth). Ossification of the inner ear is a well-known sequela of meningitis (DeSouza, Paparella, Schachern, and Yoon 1991). The presence of ossification in the basal turn of the cochlea requires alteration of the introduction of an electrode in this area. Such alterations may result in partial insertion of the electrode array, which may result in reduced auditory performance (Balkany, Gantz, and Nadol 1988; Beiter, Brimacombe, Fowler-Brehm, Sinopoli, and Segel 1994; Cohen and Waltzman 1993).

It appears, therefore, that several questions remain that need to be answered in order to make a reasonable decision regarding when to implant children with postmeningitic hearing loss: What is the incidence of children with profound hearing loss secondary to meningitis who demonstrate auditory improvement, and when does such improvement occur? What are the consequences of repeated X rays used for monitoring purposes? What are the temporal characteristics of the ossification process? Until these issues are investigated, we are left with the question of how long cochlear implant surgery should be withheld while monitoring hearing levels. Brookhouser and colleagues (1988) have recommended a one-year waiting period after meningitis-induced hearing loss. Certainly during that time, hearing levels can be monitored for stability, and other amplification devices can be evaluated.

In addition, one can monitor the cochlea for initial signs of ossification, although computerized tomography may not always be a reliable indicator of the extent of ossification (Allen, Singh, McGowan, and Smith 1994). It is reasonable to assume that once the ossification process begins, no improvement in auditory sensitivity will occur and there is no longer any reason to delay cochlear implantation of suitable candidates.

CASE REPORTS

The following cases are representative of those that are the focus of this chapter. Each poses audiologic challenges and presents possible management strategies.

PATIENT 1 (E.K.)

This male presented at 4 years of age with cleft lip and palate, and a history of recurrent otitis media requiring placement of myringotomy tubes. His audiogram at that time confirmed a profound SNHL for the right ear and normal hearing sensitivity for the left ear. He was next evaluated nine months later when the hearing for his left ear was found to have dropped to a mild-to-severe SNHL. The results of a CT scan obtained two months later disclosed Mondini deformity for the right ear and large vestibular aqueduct (possible Mondini deformity) for the left ear. Figure 1 reveals the range of hearing fluctuation for E.K.'s left ear. His hearing periodically improved and declined within this range.

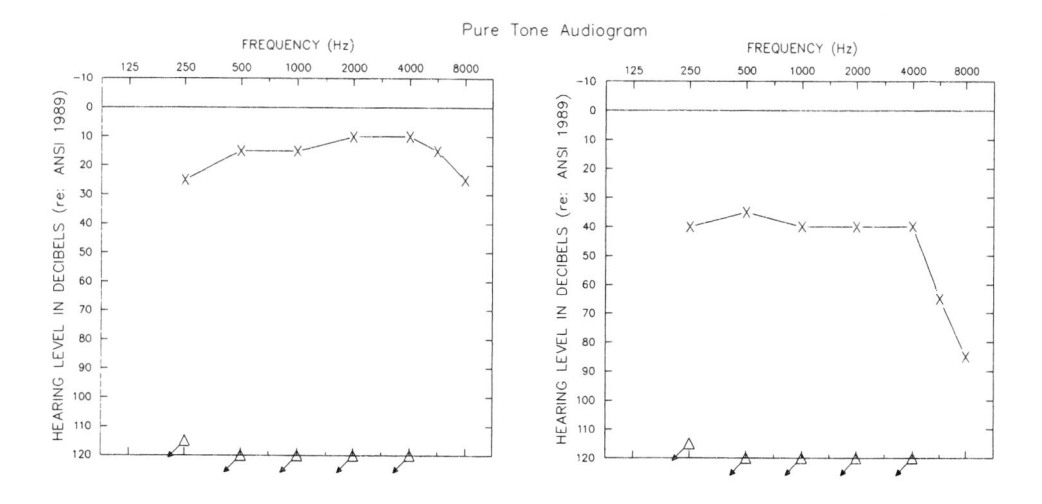

Figure 1. Representative audiograms demonstrating the range of hearing fluctuation as a result of Mondini's dysplasia (Patient 1).

The fluctuating nature of E.K.'s hearing loss created obvious audiologic challenges. You will recall that he initially demonstrated a unilateral hearing loss of the right ear with normal hearing sensitivity for the left ear. The amplification recommendation at that time was for the use of a mild gain personal FM system (with Walkman type earphones) for classroom use. When the hearing loss in his left ear began to progress, however, the FM no longer provided sufficient amplification. He was then fit with an ear-level hearing aid for the left ear. His right ear was considered unaidable due to the degree of hearing loss.

E.K. was enrolled in a rural public school that did not have on-site audiologic services. It was a minimum of an hour's drive to the nearest audiologist; therefore, frequent audiologic monitoring was impractical. In an attempt to overcome this problem, it was recommended that E.K.'s parents obtain an AudioScope manufactured by Welch Allyn in order to monitor his hearing in the left ear every morning before school (figure 2). This easy-to-use hearing screening device, which also serves as an otoscope, emits pure-tone signals at .5, 1, 2, and 4 kHz. For this child, a 30 dB signal level was requested; however, the standard device comes with 20 dB, 25 dB, and 40 dB screening levels. If E.K. failed the screening with the AudioScope™, he wore his left hearing aid to school. If he passed the screening, he wore his personal FM at school. This arrangement, though not perfect, allowed for a reasonable approximation of optimal amplification between audiologic evaluations. Another option that is available today is sound field FM amplification. The use of a sound field FM system in E.K.'s classroom would eliminate the need for his personal FM system and would benefit him even on days when wearing his hearing aid.

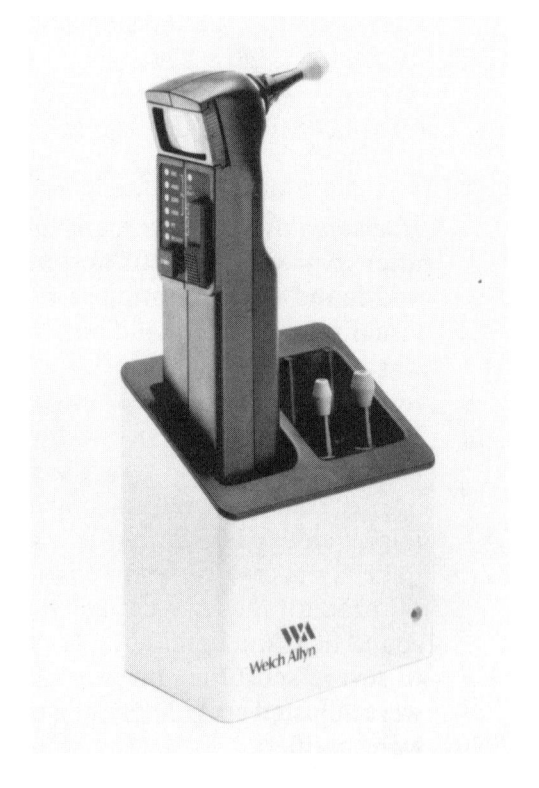

Figure 2. Welch Allyn AudioScope™ for screening hearing.

In addition to audiologic monitoring, E.K.'s academic progress was monitored with the Screening Instrument for Targeting Educational Risk (SIFTER; Anderson 1989). Briefly, the SIFTER is an easy-to-complete 15-item questionnaire designed to identify students who are educationally at risk as a result of hearing difficulties. It can serve as a reminder to teachers that a student has a hearing loss that may be educationally significant and may require special attention. In this case, the SIFTER was a conduit between the teacher and the audiologist, thus improving communication and their ability to assist E.K. with his educational and audiologic needs.

Finally, the Family Needs Survey (Bailey and Simeonsson 1990) was completed by E.K.'s parents at every audiologic visit (approximately every three months). This survey assists in identifying family concerns in the areas of family/social support, information, finances, explaining to others, child care, and community support and services. At one of their regular visits, the survey revealed that E.K. had been very concerned about his ability to have a meaningful career and adulthood because of his hearing loss. As a result of receiving that information, his audiologist was able to arrange a meeting between E.K. and a local prominent businessman who had a significant hearing impairment. This information may not have been discovered by the audiologist through routine questioning without the use of the Family Needs Survey.

PATIENT 2 (L.B.)

This 11-month-old female (L.B.) was diagnosed and hospitalized with *Haemophilus influenzae* meningitis and was treated with ampicillin. Nine days after admission while still hospitalized, she was seen for audiologic assessment and found to demonstrate a profound hearing loss in sound field utilizing visual reinforcement audiometry (VRA). ABR testing utilizing click stimuli was conducted the same day as behavioral testing. Results of the ABR and immittance testing were consistent with a profound sensorineural hearing loss bilaterally. The process of acquiring binaural amplification and enrolling in an early intervention program was begun at that time.

At two months postmeningitis, parental report indicated a possible improvement in hearing. A second ABR was conducted utilizing air- and bone-conducted click stimuli. A verifiable wave V was observed down to 70 dB nHL for the right ear and 80 dB nHL for the left ear. Results of VRA in sound field and immittance testing were consistent with a moderately-severe to severe sensorineural hearing loss for at least one ear. Her hearing aids were adjusted accordingly, and her teachers and speech/language pathologists were notified.

Another behavioral hearing test at three months postmeningitis found L.B.'s hearing to be unchanged. At five months postmeningitis, however, her

356 • *AMPLIFICATION AND SPECIAL POPULATIONS*

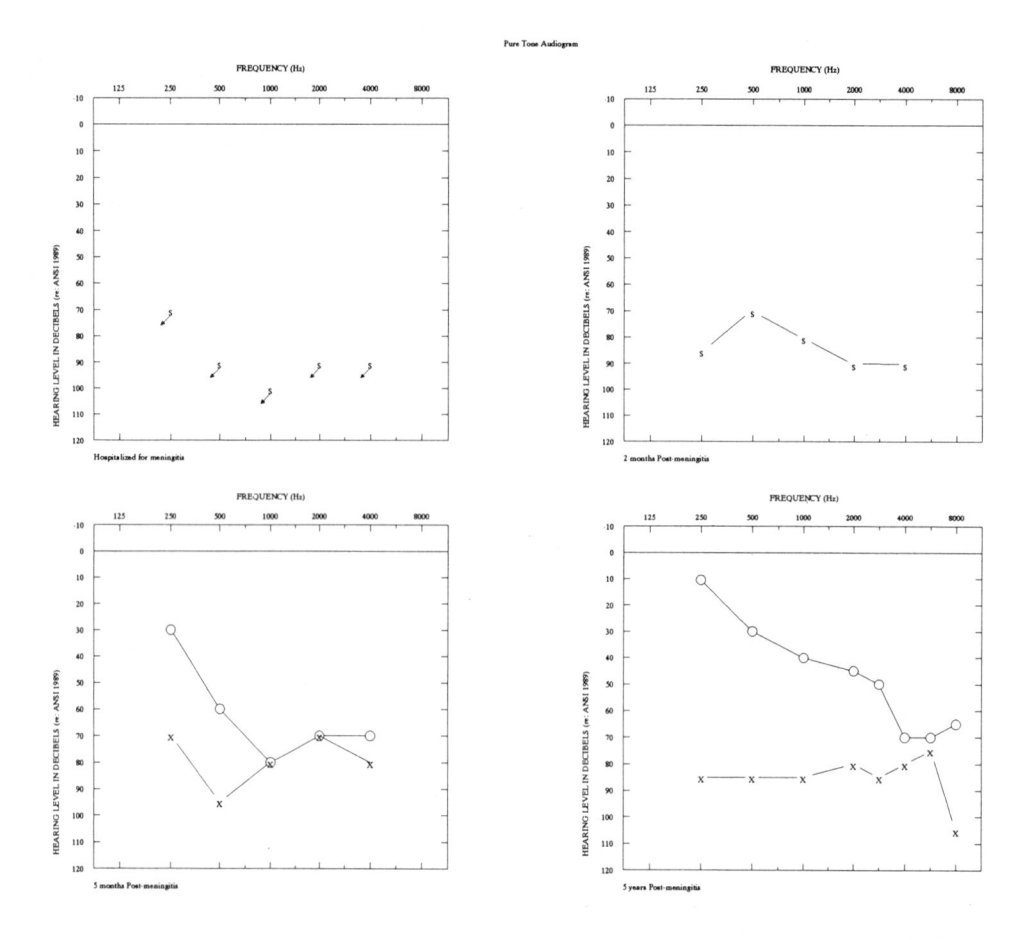

Figure 3. Serial audiograms demonstrating improvement in hearing sensitivity following H-flu meningitis (Patient 2).

hearing was found to have changed again with her right ear demonstrating a significant improvement in sensitivity between .25 and 1 kHz. L.B.'s hearing was monitored every two to three months and more often if her parents noted any change. While her left ear fluctuated slightly, her right ear continued to improve for approximately 2½ years postmeningitis before stabilizing. Figure 3 documents the changes in L.B.'s hearing over time.

L.B. was fit with binaural behind-the-ear hearing aids that provided flexibility in terms of frequency response, gain, and maximum output limiting. Due to her young age, they were ordered with tamperproof battery doors and direct-auditory input (DAI) capability. She used an FM system when in classroom/group settings. Adjustments to the hearing aid and earmold modifications were sufficient for maintaining optimal amplification. Her aided performance was monitored via probe microphone measures whenever there were changes in the hearing aid settings or earmolds. Because of reduced speech recognition ability in L.B.'s right ear (12%) and resistance to wearing a hearing aid in that ear, hearing aid use was discontinued for the right ear. Her parents, teachers, and speech/language pathologists received extensive counseling regarding functional signs of hearing fluctuation and were encouraged to return to their audiologist if any signs were noted. The SIFTER was used to facilitate communication between L.B.'s teacher and audiologist.

PATIENT 3 (R.H.)

At 5 years of age, R.H. was first seen for an audiologic evaluation in conjunction with a speech/language evaluation. Her mother's primary concern was an apparent language delay and articulation disorder. The results of that hearing test can be seen in figure 4. Utilizing play audiometric techniques, R.H. reliably demonstrated a moderate to moderately-severe mixed hearing loss for the right ear and a mild to moderate mixed loss for the left ear. Otoscopic examination revealed middle ear effusion for both ears. Immittance testing revealed reduced middle ear mobility (Type B tympanograms) bilaterally with absent ipsi- and contralateral acoustic reflexes. R.H. was referred to an otologist for medical intervention and was enrolled in speech/language therapy.

Following antibiotic therapy for otitis media, R.H.'s hearing was reevaluated with results seen in figure 4. Although the air/bone gap was closed, R.H. continued to demonstrate a minimal sensorineural hearing loss.

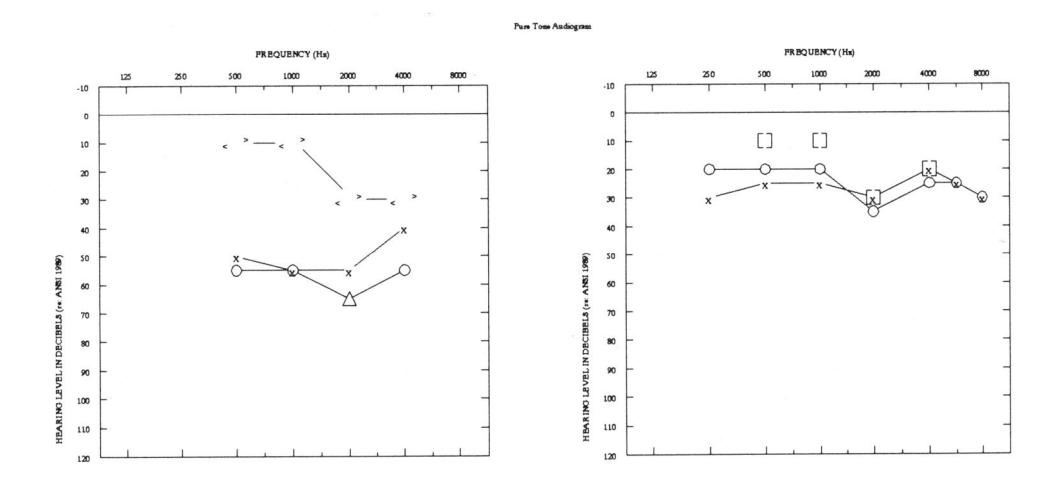

Figure 4. Audiograms reflecting the range of hearing sensitivity fluctuation with a conductive overlay secondary to otitis media with effusion (Patient 3).

In addition, R.H.'s hearing fluctuated periodically due to the intermittent presence of middle ear effusion. Audiologic management for R.H. was threefold. First, counseling included R.H. and her mother. Both were educated with regard to the cause of the fluctuations in R.H.'s hearing. R.H. was encouraged to notify her mother whenever a change was noticed, and her mother was alerted to the signs of reduced hearing sensitivity. Second, R.H.'s teacher was notified of the minimal hearing loss and the possibility of fluctuations. Her teacher was able to provide input to the managing audiologist regarding R.H.'s academic progress by completing a SIFTER approximately every two to three months. Third, because R.H. was enrolled in a public school classroom with the usual large classroom size, acoustic measurements were made revealing poor signal-to-noise (S/N) ratios that could interfere with speech recognition ability (i.e., < + 15 S/N). As a result of the classroom noise levels and teacher concerns revealed by the SIFTER, a sound field FM system was recommended. Such systems can improve the S/N ratio in the classroom, thus potentially enhancing the speech recognition ability of the students in the class. A sound field FM system has the added advantages of not singling out the child with the hearing impairment in the classroom as being "different" and, additionally, providing a listening advantage to all the children in the room.

CONCLUSIONS

This chapter has reviewed evidence that a considerable number of children with hearing loss will experience hearing fluctuation, progression, or both. Identifying these audiologic changes in a timely manner and alerting caregivers to this possibility are important roles of the audiologist. I would summarize with three practical points. First, children with hearing loss who cannot, due to developmental or linguistic limitations, relate changes in hearing sensitivity to caregivers should receive audiologic monitoring every three months or more often if indicated. Second, families of children with etiologies known to result in progressive sensorineural hearing losses should seek medical advice regarding prognosis and request multidisciplinary team meetings to plan for future educational, emotional, and communicative needs. Finally, although a waiting period used to monitor the stability of auditory thresholds prior to cochlear implantation of children with postmeningitic hearing loss appears justified, cochlear implant teams must weigh the possibility of waiting too long and risking labyrinthitis ossificans against the possibility of recovery.

REFERENCES

Ahmad, N.N., McDonald-McGinn, D.M., Zackai, E.H., Knowlton, R.G., LaRossa, D., DiMascio, J., and Prockop, D.J. 1993. A second mutation in the type II procollagen gene (COL2AI) causing Stickler syndrome (arthro-ophthalmopathy) is also a premature termination codon. *American Journal of Human Genetics* 52(1):39-45.

Allen, A.A., Singh, R.S., McGowan, K., and Smith, J. 1994. Results from patients with cochlear ossification. *Advances in Cochlear Implants: Proceedings of the Third International Cochlear Implant Conference*, 478-482.

Alter, C.A., and Moshang, T., Jr. 1993. Growth hormone deficiency in 2 siblings with Alstrom syndrome. *American Journal of Disabled Children* 147(1):97-99.

American Academy of Pediatrics. 1994. Managing otitis media with effusion in young children. *Pediatrics* 94(5):766-773.

Anderson, K.L. 1989. *Screening Instrument for Targeting Educational Risk (SIFTER)*. Austin: Pro-Ed.

Bailey, D.B., and Simeonsson, R.J. 1990. *Family needs survey*. Carolina Institute for Research on Infant Personnel Preparation, Frank Porter Graham Child Development Center. Chapel Hill: University of North Carolina.

Balkany, T.J., Gantz, B.J., and Nadol, J.B. 1988. Multichannel cochlear implants in partially ossified cochleas. *Annals of Otology, Rhinology, and Laryngology* 97 (Suppl. 135): 3-7.

Barr, B., and Wedenberg, E. 1965. Perceptive hearing loss in children with respect to genesis and the use of hearing aid. *Acta Otolaryngology Rhinology* 59:462-474.

Beiter, A.L., Brimacombe, J.A., Fowler-Brehm, N., Sinopoli, T.A., and Segel, P.A. 1994. Results with a multichannel cochlear implant in individuals with ossified cochleae. *Advances in Cochlear Implants: Proceedings of the Third International Cochlear Implant Conference*, 462-466.

Bekassy, A.N., and Ringden, O. 1992. Bone marrow transplantation and organ transplantation can cure hereditary metabolic diseases. *Lakartidningen* 89 (34):2658-2660.

Bergstrom, L. 1988. Infectious agents that deafen. In F.H. Bess (ed.), *Hearing impairment in children*. Parkton, Md.: York Press.

Bolande, R.P. 1981. Neurofibromatosis—the quintessential neurocristopathy: pathogenetic concepts and relationships. In V.M. Riccardi and J.J. Mulvihill (eds.), *Advances in neurology*, vol. 29. New York: Raven.

Boughman, J.A., Vernon, M., and Shaver, K.A. 1983. Usher syndrome: Definition and estimate of prevalence from two high risk populations. *Journal of Chronic Disease* 36:595-603.

Brookhouser, P.E., Auslander, M.C., and Meskan, M.E. 1988. The pattern and stability of postmeningitic hearing loss in children. *Laryngoscope* 98(9):940-948.

Brookhouser, P.E., and Worthington, D.W. 1994. Fluctuating and/or progressive sensorineural hearing loss in children. *Laryngoscope* 104(8 part 1):958-964.

Brookhouser, P.E., Worthington, D.W., and Kelly, W.J. 1991. Unilateral hearing loss in children. *Laryngoscope* 101(12 part 1):1264-1272.

Brookhouser, P.E., Worthington, D.W., and Kelly, W.J. 1993. Middle ear disease in young children with SNHL. *Laryngoscope* 103(4):371-378.

Brown, D.P., and Israel, S.M. 1991. Audiologic findings in a set of fraternal twins with CHARGE association. *Journal of the American Academy of Audiology* 2:183-188.

Brown, O.E., Meyerhoff, W.L., and Ginsburg, C.M. 1986. Ear, nose, throat manifestations of systemic disease. In T.J. Balkany and N.T. Pashley (eds.), *Clinical pediatric otolaryngology*. St. Louis: C.V. Mosby.

Brunner, H.G., van Beersum, S.E., Warman, M.L., Olsen, B.R., Ropers, H., and Mariman, E.C.M. 1994. A Stickler syndrome gene is linked to chromosome 6 near the COL11A2 gene. *Human Molecular Genetics* 3(9):1561-1564.

Buyse, M.L. (ed.). 1990. *The birth defects encyclopedia*. Cambridge: Blackwell Scientific Publications.

Chen, A.H., Ni, L., Fukushima, K., Marietta, J., O'Neill, M., Coucke, P., Willems, P., and Smith, R.J. 1995. Linkage of a gene for dominant non-syndromic deafness to chromosome 19. *Human Molecular Genetics* 4(6):1073-1076.

Chole, R.A. 1993. Differential osteoclast activation in endochondral and intramembranous bone. *Annals of Otology Rhinology and Laryngology* 102(8 part 1):616-619.

Cohen, N.L., and Waltzman, S.B. 1993. Partial insertion of the nucleus multichannel cochlear implant: Technique and results. *American Journal of Otology* 14(4):357-361.

Colletti, V., and Fiorino, F.G. 1994. Stapedectomy with stapedius tendon preservation: Technical and long-term results. *Otolaryngology Head and Neck Surgery* 111:181-188.

Coucke, P., Van Camp, G.V., Djoyodiharjo, B., Smith, S.D., Frants, R.R., Padberg, G.W., Darby, J.K., Huizing, E.H., Cremers, C.W., Kimberling, W.J., Oostra, B.A., Van de Heyning, P.H., and Willems, P.J. 1994. Linkage of autosomal dominant hearing loss to the short arm of chromosome 1 in two families. *New England Journal of Medicine* 331(7):425-431.

Crowe, S.J. 1938. Ménière's disease: Study based on examinations made before and after intracranial division of vestibular nerve. *Medicine* 17:1.

Dahle, A.J., McCollister, F.P., Stagno, S., Reynolds, D.W., and Hoffman, H.E. 1979. Progressive hearing impairment in children with congenital cytomegalovirus infection. *Journal of Speech and Hearing Disorders* 44:220-229.

Davenport, S.L., Hefner, M.A., and Mitchell, J.A. 1986. The spectrum of clinical features in CHARGE syndrome. *Clinical Genetics* 29:298-310.

Davenport, S.L., Hefner, M.A., and Thelin, J.W. 1986. CHARGE syndrome: Part I — External ear anomalies. *International Journal of Pediatric Otorhinolaryngology* 12:37-143.

Davis, L.E., and Johnson, L.G. 1983. Viral infections of the inner ear: Clinical virologic and pathologic studies in humans and animals. *American Journal of Otolaryngology* 4:347-362.

Dehner, L.P., and Gersell, D.J. 1994. Congenital syphilis: A reminder about the return of an old scourge. *Missouri Medicine* 91(10):630-635.

Dennis, J.M., and Neely, J.G. 1991. Otoneurologic diseases and associated audiologic profiles. In J.T. Jacobson and J.L. Northern (eds.), *Diagnostic audiology*. Austin: Pro-Ed.

DeSouza, C., Paparella, M.M., Schachern, P., and Yoon, T.H. 1991. Pathology of labyrinthine ossification. *Journal of Laryngology and Otology* 105:621-624.

Dodge, P.R., Davis, H., Feigin, R.D., Holmes, S.J., Kaplan, S.L., Jubelirer, D.P., Stechenberg, B.W., and Hirsh, S.K. 1984. Prospective evaluation of hearing impairment as a sequela of acute bacterial meningitis. *New England Journal of Medicine* 311(14):869-874.

Farrior, J.B. 1994. Small fenestra stapedectomy for management of progressive conductive hearing loss. *Southern Medical Journal* 87(1):17-22.

Filip, O., Golu, T., Filip, I., Scavera, N., and Ciuchi, V. 1994. Keratoconus in Albers-Schonberg disease. *Oftalmologia* 38(3):247-251.

Flinter, F.A., Cameron, J.S., Chantler, C., Houston, I., and Bobrow, M. 1988. Genetics of classic Alport's syndrome. *Lancet*, October, 1005-1007.

Fraser, F.C., Ling, D., Clogg, D., and Nogrady, B. 1978. Genetic aspects of the BOR syndrome—branchial fistulas, ear pits, hearing loss, and renal anomalies. *American Journal of Medical Genetics* 2:241-252.

Fraser, F.C., Sproule, J.R., and Halal, F. 1980. Frequency of the branchio-oto-renal (BOR) syndrome in children with profound hearing loss. *American Journal of Medical Genetics* 7:341-349.

Fria, T.J., Cantekin, E.I., and Eichler, J.A. 1985. Hearing acuity of children with otitis media with effusion. *Archives of Otolaryngology* 111:10-16.

Gerritsen, E.J., Vossen, J.M., van Loo, I.H., Hermans, J., Helfrich, M.H., Griscelli, C., and Fischer, A. 1994. Autosomal recessive osteopetrosis: Variability of findings at diagnosis and during the natural course. *Pediatrics* 93(2):247-253.

Glasscock, M.E. III. 1973. The stapes gusher. *Archives of Otolaryngology* 98:82-91.

Grundfast, K.M., and Bluestone, C.D. 1978. Sudden or fluctuating hearing loss and vertigo in children due to perilymph fistula. *Annals of Otology* 87(6):761-771.

Guiscafre, H., Benitez-Diaz, L., Martinez, M.C., and Munoz, O. 1984. Reversible hearing loss after meningitis: Prospective assessment using auditory evoked responses. *Annals of Otology Rhinology and Laryngology* 93:229-232.

Gutierrez, C., Bardaji, C., Bento, L., Martinez, M.A., and Conde, J. 1993. Branchio-oto-renal syndrome: Incidence in three generations of a family. *Journal of Pediatric Surgery* 28(12):1527-1529.

Guyot, J.P., Gacek, R.R., and DiRaddo, P. 1987. The temporal bone anomaly in CHARGE association. *Archives of Otolaryngology Head and Neck Surgery* 113:321-324.

Hall, B.D. 1979. Choanal atresia and associated multiple anomalies. *Journal of Pediatrics* 95:395-398.

Harris, J.P., and Sharp, P.A. 1990. Inner ear autoantibodies in patients with rapidly progressive sensorineural hearing loss. *Laryngoscope* 100:516-524.

Hendricks-Munoz, K.D., and Walton, J.P. 1988. Hearing loss in infants with persistent fetal circulation. *Pediatrics* 81:650-656.

Holmes, L.B. 1971. Norrie's disease: An X-linked syndrome of retinal malformation, mental retardation, and deafness. *Journal of Pediatrics* 70:89-92.

House, W.F. 1964. Subarachnoid shunt for drainage of hydrops: A report of 63 cases. *Archives of Otolaryngology* 79:338-354.

Hughes, G.B., Barna, B.P., Kinney, S.E., Calabrese, L.H., and Nalepa, N.J. 1988. Clinical diagnosis of immune inner-ear disease. *Laryngoscope* 98:251-253.

Hughes, G.B., Kinney, S.E., Barna, B.P., and Calabrese, L.H. 1984. Practical versus theoretical management of autoimmune inner ear disease. *Laryngoscope* 94(6):758-767.

Jackler, R.K., and De La Cruz, A. 1989. The large vestibular aqueduct syndrome. *Laryngoscope* 99(12):1238-1243.

Johnson, S., Hosford-Dunn, H., Paryani, S., Younger, A., and Malachowski, N. 1986. Prevalence of sensorineural hearing loss in premature and sick term infants with perinatally acquired cytomegalovirus infection. *Ear and Hearing* 7:325-327.

Kallio, M.J.T., Kilpi, T., Anttila, M., and Peltola, H. 1994. The effect of a recent previous visit to a physician on outcome after childhood bacterial meningitis. *Journal of the American Medical Association* 272(10):787-791.

Klein, J.O. 1992. Epidemiology and natural history of otitis media. In F.H. Bess and J.W. Hall III (eds.), *Screening children for auditory function*. Nashville, Tenn.: Bill Wilkerson Center Press.

Klein, J.O. 1994. Antimicrobial therapy and prevention of meningitis. *Pediatric Annals* 23(2):76-81.

Kleinman, L.C., Kosecoff, J., DuBois, R.W., and Brook, R.H. 1994. The medical appropriateness of tympanostomy tubes proposed for children younger than 16 years in the United States. *Journal of the American Medical Association* 271(16):1250-1255.

Konigsmark, B.W. 1969. Hereditary deafness in man. *New England Journal of Medicine* 281:713-720.

Konigsmark, B.W., and Gorlin, R.J. 1976. *Genetic and metabolic deafness*. Philadelphia: W.B. Saunders Co.

Koszinowski, U.H., Del Val, M., and Reddehase, M.J. 1990. Cellular and molecular basis of the protective immune response to cytomegalovirus infection. In J.K. McDougall (ed.), *Cytomegaloviruses*. Berlin: Springer-Verlag.

Kumar, S., Kimberling, W.J., Connolly, C.J., Tinley, S., Marres, H.A., and Cremers, C.W. 1994. Refining the region of branchio-oto-renal syndrome and defining the flanking markers on chromosome 8q by genetic mapping. *American Journal of Human Genetics* 55(6):1188-1194.

Lazar, L., Litwin, A., and Merlob, P. 1993. Phototherapy for neonatal nonhemolytic hyperbilirubinemia: Analysis of rebound and indications for discontinuing therapy. *Clinical Pediatrics* 32(5):264-267.

Leavitt, A.M., Watchko, J.F., Bennett, F.C., and Folsom, R.C. 1987. Neurodevelopmental outcome following persistent pulmonary hypertension of the neonate. *Journal of Perinatology* 7(4):288-291.

Leon, P.E., Raventos, H., Lynch, E., Morrow, J., and King, M.C. 1992. The gene for an inherited form of deafness maps to chromosome 5q31. *Proceedings of the National Academy of Science* 89:5181-5184.

Levenson, M.J., Parisier, S.C., Jacobs, M., and Edelstein, D.R. 1989. The large vestibular aqueduct syndrome. *Archives of Otolaryngology Head and Neck Surgery* 115:54-58.

Liebman, E.P., Ronis, M.L., Lovrinic, J.H., and Katinsky, S.E. 1969. Hearing improvement following meningitis deafness. *Archives of Otolaryngology* 90:92-95.

Lieberman, J.M., Greenberg, D.P., and Ward, J.I. 1990. Prevention of bacterial meningitis: Vaccines and chemoprophylaxis. In W.M. Scheld and B. Wispelwey (eds.), *Infectious Disease Clinics of North America* 4(4):703-729.

Linthicum, F.H. 1993. Histopathology of otosclerosis. *Otolaryngologic Clinics of North America* 26(3):335-352.

Mangabeira-Albernaz, P.L., Fukaka, J., Chammas, F., and Gananca, M.M. 1981. The Mondini dysplasia—A clinical study. *ORL: Journal of Oto-Rhino-Laryngology and Its Related Specialties* 43:131-152.

Manusov, E.G., Douville, D.R., Page, L.V., and Trivedi, D.V. 1993. Osteopetrosis (marble bone disease). *American Family Physician* 47(1):175-180.

McCabe, B.F. 1979. Autoimmune sensorineural hearing loss. *Annals of Otology* 88(5):585-589.

McCabe, B.F. 1989. Autoimmune inner ear disease: Therapy. *American Journal of Otology* 10(3):196-197.

McKusick, V.A. 1992. *Mendelian inheritance in man, catalogs of autosomal dominant, autosomal recessive and X-linked phenotypes.* 10th ed. Vols. 1 and 2. Baltimore: Johns Hopkins Press.

Meyerhoff, W.L., Cass, S., Schwaber, M.K., Sculerati, N., and Slattery, W.H. III. 1994. Progressive sensorineural hearing loss in children. *Otolaryngology Head and Neck Surgery* 110(6):569-579.

Meyerhoff, W.L., and Liston, S.L. 1991. Metabolic hearing loss. In M.M. Paparella, D. Shumrick, J. Gluckman, and W.L. Meyerhoff (eds.), *Otolaryngology.* 3d ed. Philadelphia: W.B. Saunders Co.

Meyerhoff, W.L., Paparella, M.M., and Shea, D. 1978. Ménière's disease in children. *Laryngoscope* 8:1504-1511.

Mitchell, J.A., Giangiacomo, J., Hefner, M.A., Thelin, J.W., and Pickens, J.M. 1985. Dominant CHARGE association. *Ophthalmological Pediatric Genetics* 6:31-36.

Moller, C.G., Kimberling, W.J., Davenport, S.L., Priluck, I., White, V., Biscone-Halterman, K., Odkvist, L.M., Brookhouser, P.E., Lund, G., and Grissom, T.J. 1989. Usher's syndrome: an otoneurologic study. *Laryngoscope* 99:73-79.

Naulty, C.M., Weiss, I.P., and Herer, G. 1986. Progressive sensorineural hearing loss in survivors of persistent fetal circulation. *Ear and Hearing* 7:74-77.

Newton, V.E., and Rowson, V.J. 1988. Progressive hearing loss in childhood. *British Journal of Audiology* 22(4):287-295.

Nuutila, A. 1970. Dystrophia retinae pigmentosa-dysacusis syndrome (DRD): A study of the Usher of Hallgren syndrome. *Journal of Genetique Humaine* 18:57-58.

Ozdamar, O., Kraus, N., and Stein, L. 1983. Auditory brainstem responses in infants recovering from bacterial meningitis. *Archives of Otolaryngology* 109:13-18.

Pagon, R.A., Graham, J.M., Zonana, J., and Yong, S.L. 1981. Coloboma, congenital heart disease, and choanal atresia with multiple anomalies: CHARGE association. *Journal of Pediatrics* 99(2):223-227.

Pantke, O.A., and Cohen, M.M., Jr. 1971. The Waardenburg syndrome. *Birth Defects* 7(7):147-152.

Parving, A. 1988. Longitudinal study of hearing-disabled children: A follow-up investigation. *International Journal of Pediatric Otorhinolaryngology* 15:233-244.

Pass, R.F., Stagno, S., Myers, G.J., and Alford, C.A. 1980. Outcome of symptomatic congenital cytomegalovirus infection: Results of long-term longitudinal follow-up. *Pediatrics* 66:758-762.

Pikus, A.T. 1990. Audiologic manifestations. In J.J. Mulvihill (ed.), Neurofibromatosis 1 (Recklinghausen Disease) and Neurofibromatosis 2 (Bilateral Acoustic Neurofibromatosis). *Annals of Internal Medicine* 113:44-47.

Pyeritz, R. 1993. Hereditable and developmental disorders of connective tissue and bone. In D.J. McCarty (ed.), *Arthritis and allied conditions: A textbook of rheumatology.* Philadelphia: Lea and Febiger.

Rai, A., Wordsworth, P., Coppock, J.S., Zaphiropoulos, G.C., and Struthers, G.R. 1994. Hereditary arthro-ophthalmopathy (Stickler syndrome): A diagnosis to consider in familial premature osteoarthritis. *British Journal of Rheumatology* 33(12):1175-1180.

Reardon, W., Bellman, S., Phelps, P., Pembrey, M., and Luxon, L.M. 1993. Neuro-otologic function in x-linked hearing loss: A multipedigree assessment and correlation with other clinical parameters. *Acta Otolaryngology* 113:706-714.

Riedner, E.D., Levin, S., and Holliday, M.J. 1980. Hearing patterns in dominant osteogenesis imperfecta. *Otolaryngology Head and Neck Surgery* 106:737-740.

Roeser, R.J., Campbell, J.C., and Daly, D.D. 1975. Recovery of auditory function following meningitic deafness. *Journal of Speech and Hearing Disorders* 40:405-411.

Roger, C., Koziel, V., Vert, P., and Nehlig, A. 1993. Effects of bilirubin infusion on local cerebral glucose utilization in the immature rat. *Brain Research Developments* 76(1):115-130.

Rosenhall, U., and Kankkunen, A. 1980. Hearing alterations following meningitis: 1. Hearing improvement. *Ear and Hearing* 1(4):185-190.

Ruben, R.J., and Fishmann, G. 1981. Otological care of the hearing impaired child. In S.E. Gerber and G.T. Mencher (eds.), *Early management of hearing loss*. San Francisco: Grune and Stratton.

Saez-Llorens, X., and McCracken, G.H., Jr. 1990. Bacterial meningitis in neonates and children. In W.M. Scheld and B. Wispelwey (eds.), *Infectious disease clinics of North America*. Vol. 4. Philadelphia: W.B. Saunders.

Sankila, E.M., Pakarinen, L., Kaariainen, H., Aittomaki, K., Karjalainen, S., Sistonen, P., and de la Chapelle, A. 1995. Assignment of an Usher syndrome type III (USH3) gene to chromosome 3q. *Human Molecular Genetics* 4(1):93-98.

Schildroth, A.N. 1994. Congenital cytomegalovirus and deafness. *American Journal of Audiology* 3(2):27-38.

Schuknecht, H.F. 1974. *Pathology of the ear*. Cambridge, Mass.: Harvard University Press.

Schwartz, D.M., and Costello, J.A. 1988. Audiologic application of auditory evoked potentials in children. In F.H. Bess (ed.), *Hearing impairment in children*. Parkton, Md.: York Press.

Sell, E., Gaines, J., Gluckman, C., and Williams, E. 1985. Persistent fetal circulation. *Archives of the Journal of Disorders of Children* 139:25-28.

Seltzer, S., and McCabe, B.F. 1986. Perilymph fistula: The Iowa experience. *Laryngoscope* 96(1):37-49.

Shea, J.J., Jr. 1994. How I do primary and revision stapedectomy. *American Journal of Otology* 15(1):71-73.

Shemen, L.J., Mitchell, D.P., and Farkashidy, J. 1984. Cockayne syndrome—An audiologic and temporal bone analysis. *American Journal of Otology* 5:300-307.

Simonton, K.M. 1940. Ménière's symptom complex: Review of the literature. *Annals of Otolaryngology* 49:80.

Smith, R.J., Berlin, C.I., Hejtmancik, J.F., Keats, B.J., Kimberling, W.J., Lewis, R.A., Moller, C.G., Pelias, M.Z., and Tranebjaerg, L. 1994. Clinical diagnosis of the Usher syndromes: Usher syndrome consortium. *American Journal of Medical Genetics* 50(1):32-38.

Stagno, S. 1990. Cytomegalovirus. In J.S. Remington and J.O. Klein (eds.), *Infectious diseases of the fetus and newborn infant*. 3d ed. Philadelphia: W.B. Saunders.

Stagno, S., Reynolds, D.W., Amos, C.S., Dahle, A.J., McCollister, F.P., Hohindra, I., Ermocilla, R., and Alford, C.A. 1977. Auditory and visual defects resulting from symptomatic and subclinical congenital cytomegaloviral and toxoplasma infections. *Pediatrics* 59:669-678.

Starling, S.P. 1994. Syphilis in infants and young children. *Pediatric Annals* 23(7):334-340.

Stein, L.K., and Boyer, K.M. 1994. Progress in the prevention of hearing loss in infants. *Ear and Hearing* 15(2):116-125.

Stewart, B.J., and Prabhu, P.U. 1993. Reports of sensorineural deafness after measles, mumps, and rubella immunization. *Archives of Diseases in Children* 69(1):153-154.

Thelin, J.W., Mitchell, J.A., Hefner, M.A., and Davenport, S.L. 1986. CHARGE syndrome: Part II—Hearing loss. *International Journal of Pediatric Otorhinolaryngology* 12(2):145-163.

Trofatter, J.A., MacCollin, M.M., Rutter, J.L., Murrell, J.R., Duyao, M.P., Parry, D.M., Eldridge, R., Kley, N., Menon, A.G., Pulaski, K., Haase, V.H., Ambrose, C.M., Munroe, D., Bove, C., Haines, J.L., Martuza, R.L., MacDonald, M.E., Seizinger, B.R., Short, M.P., Buckler, A.J., and Gusella, J.F. 1993. A novel moesin-, ezrin-, radixin-like gene is a candidate for the neurofibromatosis 2 tumor suppressor. *Cell* 72(5):791-800.

Triglia, J.M., Nicollas, R., Ternier, F., and Cannoni, M. 1993. Deafness caused by malformation of the inner ear: Current contribution of x-ray computed tomography. *Annales D Oto-Laryngologie et de Chirurgie Cervico-Faciale* 110(5):241-246.

Walton, J.P., and Hendricks-Munoz, K. 1991. Profile and stability of sensorineural hearing loss in persistent pulmonary hypertension of the newborn. *Journal of Speech and Hearing Research* 34:1362-1370.

Weber, P.C., Perez, B.A., and Bluestone, C.D. 1993. Congenital perilymphatic fistula and associated middle ear abnormalities. *Laryngoscope* 103:160-164.

Weil, D., Blanchard, S., Kaplan, J., Guilford, P., Gibson, F., Walsh, J., Mburu, P., Varela, A., Levilliers, J., Weston, M.D., Kelley, P.M., Kimberling, W.J., Wagenaar, M., Levi-Acobas, F., Larget-Piet, D., Munnich, A., Steel, K.P., Brown, S.D.M., and Petit, C. 1995. Defective myosin VIIA gene responsible for Usher syndrome type 1B. *Nature* 374 (2):60-61.

Weissman, J.L., Weber, P.C., and Bluestone, C.D. 1994. Congenital perilymphatic fistula: Computed tomography appearance of middle ear and inner ear anomalies. *Otolaryngology Head and Neck Surgery* 111(3 part 1):243-249.

Wolff, A.B., and Brown, S.C. 1987. Demographics of meningitis-induced hearing impairment: Implications for immunization of children against hemophilus influenzae Type B. *American Annals of the Deaf* 132(1):26-30.

Xu, G., O'Connell, P., Viskochil, D., Cawthon, R., Robertson, M., Culver, M., Dunn, D., Stevens, J., Gesteland, R., White, R., and Weiss, R. 1990. The neurofibromatosis gene encodes a protein related to GAP. *Cell* 62:599-608.

Young, D.F., Eldridge, R., and Gardner, W.J. 1970. Bilateral acoustic neuroma in a large kindred. *Journal of the American Medical Association* 214:347-353.

PART V.

Management of Children with Auditory Deficits

18

Developing Auditory Capabilities in Children with Severe and Profound Hearing Loss

Diane Brackett

INTRODUCTION

For the past twenty years, there has been a dwindling interest in enhancing the hearing of children with severe and profound hearing loss. Instead, more emphasis has been placed on circumventing the hearing loss by using visual communication systems. Cochlear implants, which were approved by the Food and Drug Administration (FDA) in 1990 for use in children, have provided clinicians with the opportunity to review their procedures and techniques for training auditory skills in children with profound hearing impairment. These children with cochlear implants require extensive training to obtain maximum benefit from the surgically inserted device.

As cochlear implantation emerged as a viable alternative for children with profound hearing loss, the lack of appropriate services became critical. There were only a few isolated areas of the country where auditory training services were readily available. Typically, a private therapist was engaged to provide the desired services. The combination of access to conversational speech and rapidly changing auditory skills in these children with cochlear implants convinced many professionals to include auditory skill development in their intervention protocols. This reexamination of auditory management has rekindled interest in incorporating auditory-based spoken language skills into preschool and school-age programs for children with all degrees of hearing loss.

Professionals involved with cochlear implants, specifically in documenting progress over time, were soon frustrated by the lack of evaluation tools and procedures. It seemed impossible to determine primary benefit (access to conversational level speech) and secondary benefit (speech production and language development) of cochlear implants, since the available tests were not developmentally appropriate. The tests focused on the final outcome of word recognition rather than the incremental steps that indicated growth toward the final goal. Therefore, with the renewed interest in auditory skill development, we have witnessed simultaneous development of test protocols for assessing auditory skills from their embryonic stage of alerting to sound to the birth of full speech perception of words and sentences. This emphasis on audition applies not only to children with cochlear implants but also to children with severe and profound hearing losses who, with amplification, can hear most of the intensity, time, and frequency characteristics of speech.

PROGRAM DESIGN

Designing a rehabilitation program for a child with severe-to-profound hearing impairment requires conscious attention to the following factors:

1. The acoustic cues *potentially* available through amplification—not just at the threshold, but at a level that is useful given the variable intensity of conversational speech. Consideration should be given not just to frequency-specific cues that allow recognition of phonemes, but to time and intensity cues as well. Features such as duration, intonation contour, stress, and rhythm should be considered relative to aided hearing.
2. The acoustic cues used by the child during speech perception. Skill sampling of both suprasegmental and segmental features can take place during structured evaluations or during more natural interactions as long as the stimuli are presented auditorially (without visual cues) with speech used as the response mode.
3. The discrepancy between the potential to perceive speech (according to aided results) and actual use of these acoustic cues for perceiving speech. This discrepancy becomes the focus of the rehabilitation sessions. The targets are selected according to degree of acoustic accessibility, developmental sequence, frequency of use in communication, and indicators of emergence.

Zara and Brackett (1994), in their tutorial on similarities between rehabilitation approaches for children using conventional amplification and those with cochlear implants, urge professionals to use their present knowledge of language acquisition and techniques as they plan rehabilitation sessions for children with cochlear implants. Regardless of whether the child uses electrical (cochlear implant) or acoustic (hearing aids) amplification, certain components need to be in place. These include monitoring amplification (minimally daily listening check), controlling the listening/learning environment (noise, reverberation, speaker-listener distance), and establishing the auditory-speech link (self-monitoring of speech). Device-specific issues such as the need for frequent adjustments to the cochlear implant speech processor and sensitivity to high-frequency speech energy are unique to children using cochlear implants.

Maximizing auditory capabilities includes the ability to receive the speech of others as well as to monitor one's own speech production. Boothroyd (1993) has determined that individuals with hearing loss of 100 to 110 dB can hear themselves sufficiently well to develop an auditory feedback system for monitoring their own speech production. This assumes appropriate amplification and the fact that individuals hear their own speech without the interference of distance and background noise. Reception of others is somewhat diminished at 110 dB levels due to the drop in intensity of the signal when presented at conversational distances (three to six feet). Audible features include rhythm and rate, with partial accessibility to intonation, vowels, and consonants.

Individuals with hearing loss of 90 to 100 dB can have full access to their own speech and the speech of others with appropriate amplification. Most suprasegmental and segmental features of speech, with the exception of place of articulation, can potentially be audible. Multichannel cochlear implants have the potential of increasing access to speech for children in the 110 dB range to levels similar to those of children with 90 dB losses (Osberger, Robbins, Miyamoto, Berry, Myres, Kessler, and Pope 1991).

Given the intensity of therapy required to develop spoken language in children with lesser degrees of hearing loss, it only follows that a well-designed training program is needed if a child with severe-to-profound hearing impairment is going to develop the auditory skills that are the framework for speech. A dual approach to training comprised of reception of speech from others and self immediately connects the auditory and speech channels.

SPEECH PERCEPTION TRAINING

There are two aspects to improving perception of speech addressed to a listener: (1) increasing dependence on and confidence in information received through amplification, and (2) fully utilizing available acoustic cues.

Amplification Dependence and Confidence

During training, the child uses linguistic and situational context to gain meaning from what has been said. The goal of training activities is not for precise perception of a particular target. Instead, the child is asked to concentrate on the global message, to comprehend and respond to the meaning of the message. The young child can easily learn new material through the auditory channel, resulting in a strong auditory representation of the word to use during reception and production. The older child may achieve auditory dependence only for familiar words and phrases.

General techniques for improving dependence on acoustic information include the following:

— Use familiar phrases, questions, and commands to establish a response during auditory-only practice.
— Use a natural conversational approach during which some or all of the utterances are presented without visual cues.
— Start with heavy context and reduce it over time as the child becomes more confident in his or her ability.

Optimizing Acoustic Cues

Through analytic activities, the child is made aware of acoustic cues by example, that is, by providing many stimuli to perceive and produce that exemplify the target cue (voiced/voiceless, plosive/fricative, bilabial/alveolar, question/statement, high pitch/low pitch). By hearing and producing the contrasts, the child should be able to discover the difference between them. Recognition of speech can be achieved by the following acoustic cues:

— Frequency specific information indicates formants of the vowels, and bands and spread of energy for consonants.
— Duration of vowel indicates voicing of final consonants.
— Transition of vowel to final consonant indicates place of articulation.
— Nasal murmur indicates nasality.
— Burst of noise of short duration indicates plosion.

Analytic training may lead to task-bound performance as evidenced in children with cochlear implants who are able to perform on structured tasks but still do not use sound for speech reception or for self-monitoring of speech outside the therapy setting. This task-bound behavior is especially prevalent when older children are implanted or when parents decide to implement an auditory training program for children who have already established a visually based spoken language system. Clearly, incorporating sound into communication is best accomplished at an early age when communication development is in its infancy.

When both analytic and synthetic (global) approaches are used, full carryover into spontaneous use may not be accomplished even if the child demonstrates the potential to employ the contrast during perception and production tasks. Often, this is the result of discontinuing the emphasis on the target before the job is completed. With children who have hearing loss, it is not surprising that this happens since they often have so many areas of need that one feels compelled to move at a rapid pace to fully accomplish the goal of communicative competence within the time constraints.

SPEECH PERCEPTION TRAINING TECHNIQUES

Reducing Visual Information

During a variety of activities, some or all of the spoken input can be presented without the benefit of speechreading cues. It is expected that the child will extract salient cues from the auditory signal, which will assist in

Table 1
Reduction of Visual Cues

BARRIER	
Hand covering mouth	Seated opposite; hand as barrier; high frequencies reduced; eyes visible
Fingers in front of mouth (partial)	Seated opposite; fingers as barrier; high frequencies reduced; eyes visible
Paper covering mouth (eyes exposed)	Seated opposite; paper as barrier; high frequencies reduced; eyes visible
Embroidery hoop with loosely woven cloth	Seated opposite; cloth as barrier; minimal sound interference; eyes visible
SEATING ARRANGEMENTS	
Seated behind	Seated behind; no barrier; directional microphones; face not visible
Seated beside and behind	Seated offside and behind; no barrier; unilateral reception; face not visible
Seated beside	Seated offside; no barrier; unilateral reception; face not visible

receiving and understanding the spoken message. This approach can be used during auditory dependence activities (synthetic) as well as those optimizing cues (analytic).

There are two primary ways of reducing visual reception of speech (table 1). The first uses a barrier to obscure the mouth area. The second reduces visibility through seating arrangements.

Some problems are inherent in each permutation of this technique. When the clinician is seated opposite the child, his or her face is visible, making a more natural communication situation. However, each of the methods for obscuring the mouth and cheeks causes a change in the acoustic information received by the child. Specifically, the high frequencies are reduced due to the effects of the barriers. The use of loosely woven cloth as a barrier has the least effect on the acoustic characteristics of the signal.

Alternative strategies for reducing visual cues focus on seating arrangements. When the clinician is seated directly behind the child, speech is received equally by the two microphones, which are typically front mounted and may, in addition, be directional. High frequency energy is reduced in this condition. When the adult is seated to the side of the child, primarily one ear is being stimulated. When employing this technique, the clinician must be aware of these signal variations in order to appropriately analyze the child's response. For children who are monaurally aided due to one nonfunctional ear or who use a cochlear implant (one microphone), seating should be carefully arranged so that the single microphone is receiving uncompromised speech.

For children who have learned to communicate via nonauditory means, it will be necessary to gradually decrease reliance on visual input to avoid frustration and refusal. Two approaches are useful for this population: the top-down and key word approaches. The top-down approach begins with the assumption that the child has the capability of using context to gain meaning from an utterance. The utterance is initially presented with no visual access to the mouth of the speaker. If no response is given, the presenter selects part of the utterance to present with full visual and auditory cues, quickly obscuring the lower face for the remaining portion of the utterance. The child should be able to narrow the semantic/syntactic possibilities for the obscured portion of the utterance by applying his or her linguistic knowledge. With practice, the child requires less of the utterance presented with combined auditory-visual input. For example,

Adult: "The man walked down the street."
[............Listen Alone..............]

Child: No response.

Adult:	"The man walked	down the street."
	[Look + Listen]	[Listen Alone]
Child:	"The man walked down the street."	

The second approach, key word, preselects the target word that will be presented without any speechreading cues. If the child is unable to perceive the target, then he or she is given choices of the possibilities and asked to listen to the original sentence again. Closing the set of possibilities may make this task achievable. Readers are cautioned, however, to regularly attempt higher level auditory-only activities if their ultimate goal is auditory dependence and confidence.

Adult:	"The man sat on the	bench."
	[Look + Listen]	[Listen Alone]
Child:	No response.	
Adult:	"The man sat on a chair, a bench, a rock, or a couch. Which one?"	
	[...............Look + Listen...............]	
	"The man sat on a bench."	
	[.......Listen Alone......]	
Child:	"The man sat on a bench."	

Response Analysis

When direct intervention is viewed as partially diagnostic in nature, it logically follows that each of the child's responses has diagnostic value. By determining the extent of acoustic information the child is able to glean from the stimulus, the professional can recognize emerging percepts and capitalize on them within the sessions. Further, when early developing skills are slow to emerge, it is possible to overcome inertia by loading the input with many examples of the target. Fine-tuning the rehabilitation program requires constant evaluation of the child's performance.

Selection of Stimuli

An end result of this diagnostic approach to rehabilitation is the need to carefully select stimuli according to acoustic features. To understand the reason behind specific confusions, one must determine the commonalities between the stimulus and error. For example, when the stimulus is *ship* and the error production is *shell*, the child has successfully perceived the voicing, manner, and place features for /sh/, selected a vowel that is adjacent to the stimulus /I/, but substituted a voiced glide for an unvoiced plosive. Based on these errors, practice in recognizing voicing and manner contrasts should be included in the child's rehabilitation program. If the stimulus was *Washington* and the child's response was *ton,* the most basic suprasegmental feature has not been recognized, that is, one versus three syllables.

Typically, initial contrasts should be widely different from each other (example: /sh/ versus /m/; ball [one syllable] versus birthday cake [three syllables]; "stop!" [short duration] versus "Where is Mommy?" [long duration]). As the discrepancy between the potential acoustic cues available and functional use of those cues decreases, the contrasts become less varied. Movement should be toward phonemes that differ according to only one distinctive feature (example: /p/ versus /t/ [same voicing and manner of articulation]; Neptune versus Saturn [same syllables]; "He has juice" versus "I want milk" [same sentence pattern/duration]).

Loading

Loading describes the process of artificially increasing the frequency with which a particular target occurs during spoken interactions. The selected target can be in the semantic, syntactic, pragmatic, or phonologic domains. This principle is based on the fact that children with severe-to-profound hearing impairment have reduced access to the speech of others, especially when it is not directly addressed to them. Therefore, it is difficult to gain sufficient exposure to a particular aspect of spoken language in order to learn and retain it. By loading each verbal interaction, we are increasing the opportunities for learning to occur. That is, we are compensating for the children's inability to efficiently hear or overhear the speech of others.

Integrating Speech-Language-Listening

Effective auditory training takes place within the framework of spoken language. Linking auditory perception and speech production into functional communication is the goal. Carryover of these newly developed speech perception/speech production skills occurs best when a meaningful context exists. For example, it is possible to train a child to perceive and produce the voiced/voiceless cognates /s/ and /z/ within a structured task. Using this same skill to comprehend and mark plurality or possession moves this task to a meaningful level.

RELATIONSHIP OF SPEECH PERCEPTION AND SPEECH PRODUCTION

Novelli-Olmstead and Ling (1984) document the positive effect that speech production training has on both speech production and speech perception. They divided matched pairs of students with severe and profound hearing losses into two groups: One group, discrimination only, responded to a speech perception task by pointing to the word that was said. The other group, speaking only, had to produce the word with assistance from a variety of speech correction techniques. Both groups received identical input during the training sessions. At the end of the training sessions, the speech perception and production skills of both groups were sampled. Only the speaking group showed any positive change in speech discrimination and speech production.

The authors speculate that motor speech practice rather than more precise auditory discrimination could account for the superior posttraining scores of the speaking group. Children with hearing impairment may benefit from the practice of encoding the incomplete auditory information they receive. For children with cochlear implants, the act of producing the stimuli that they are expected to perceive can solidify the auditory representation of the word.

SPEECH PERCEPTION AND PRODUCTION TRAINING

By using speech as the response in all auditory training activities and insisting on correct production, a natural joining of this auditory input and speech output develops. It also allows children to acoustically compare their own production with the prior production of the adult. The following example demonstrates using speech as the response mode for all speech perception tasks.

Adult: "Which one is it . . . shoe   chew?"
(*Show printed word or picture.*)

(*Cover pictures or print.*)
"Listen . . . shoe."

Child: "Shoe."
(*Then points to the word.*)

To further solidify the auditory-speech link, immediately reverse the task so that the child becomes the presenter (make sure he or she can produce the contrast).

Child: "shhhoe."
Adult: "Shoe." *(Then points to the picture.)*

or

Child: "shhhhToe."
Adult: "What?" *(with quizzical face)*
Child: "shhhoe."
Adult: *(Points to correct picture.)*

Erber (1982) describes effective techniques for acoustic correction of speech: repetition, exaggeration, verbal instruction, and gesture. These techniques can be applied to the child's imitated responses following an adult model in an effort to solidify a correct production. If, as Novelli-Olmstead and Ling (1984) suggest, speech production facilitates speech discrimination, then these techniques can also be considered as facilitative of speech discrimination. A description of each of these techniques follows.

Repetition

An incorrect or absent response may be the result of inattention or interference from noise, or the stimulus may have been too soft. Merely repeating the stimulus may result in a correct imitation.

Exaggeration

Abnormal stress on the misperceived element may increase its saliency for the child. Emphasis can be placed on syntactic, semantic, pragmatic, or phonologic elements. Once the correct production has been achieved, it is important to return the stimulus to its natural state.

Syntactic Stress:	"The frog IS jumping; he jumpED(t) from lily pad to lily pad."
Semantic Stress:	"He EVACUATED the rocket. He left . . . evacuated."
Pragmatic Stress:	"CAN I play?"
Phonologic Stress:	(target /-f/) "Take it oFF."

Verbal Cuing

The adult gives the child information regarding production through a variety of verbal prompts. These prompts vary in the amount of direct information they contain about the child's production. Each prompt, however, focuses on how the child's production sounds to the listener. Use of verbal cues conveys the message that it is the child's responsibility to "repair" his or her production so that it sounds acceptable to the listener. (These same prompts or requests for clarification can be used by the child when he or she has not understood what the adult has said.)

"What did you say?"
"I didn't understand you."
"You went WHERE?"
"You forgot the last sound in hat."
"Ha_?" *(error imitated)*

Gestural Prompting

Gestures or movements can highlight the acoustic event. For example, to convey the manner of production contained within the acoustic signal, the adult might use a gliding movement for the glides /r, l/, or a forward, sudden explosive movement for the plosives /p, t/. Voiced/voiceless contrasts can be portrayed by heavy (voiced) and light (voiceless) movements. These gestural assists should be used only in the phonologic acquisition phase when acoustic modifications alone are not sufficient to establish the correct production and perception of the phoneme. When used, these gestures should be dropped as soon as the target feature has been acquired to allow the child to recognize and rely on the auditory percept.

EARLY IDENTIFICATION/MANAGEMENT

For children with severe and profound hearing loss, generic language stimulation programs emphasizing exposure to language in context and to speech as a vehicle for transmitting language are insufficient for developing auditory skills. The examples do not occur frequently enough for the child to deduce the rules or figure out use patterns of language. Ling concurs that "the more severe the hearing loss, the greater need for specific training" (1989).

Intervention during this birth to age 3 period often focuses on educating the parents in the following areas: enhancing the language learning potential of daily home routines; adapting the acoustic environment; observing auditory responses with hearing aids; observing changes in speech and language. Direct service to the child may be delayed until the magical age of 3.

Since children with normal hearing make enormous changes in their communication skills between 0 and 3 years, it is unfortunate that hearing professionals assume a waiting attitude before providing direct intervention

(Cole 1991). Instead of closing the gap between the chronological age and language age, often the gap is magnified during the period from birth to age 3 before direct service is provided. Perhaps the problem lies in our definition of direct service. If we approach early intervention from a teaching perspective, then waiting until the child can benefit from group learning (approximately age 3) and can comply with the curriculum is appropriate.

Instead of our teaching infants, we should view ourselves as facilitating communication, that is, assisting the process of normal language acquisition by increasing the frequency with which a particular event (i.e., phoneme, word, phrase) occurs at an audible level. By the conscious loading of speech directed to the infant with a designated target, the probability is increased that the child will receive sufficient exposure to the target to enable incorporation into his or her spoken language system. As communication facilitators, we help what would naturally occur in the near future to occur sooner due to increased purposeful or targeted exposure. Through aggressive, early intervention, we can alter the rate of acquisition to decrease the gap between chronological age and communicative age.

PREREQUISITES FOR AUDITORY DEVELOPMENT

Boothroyd (1993) describes the full achievement of auditory performance through the multiplicative effect of auditory capability (as measured by hearing loss, aided hearing, and functional use) and listening experience (home and school listening/learning environment). The following prerequisite conditions must be in place for maximum auditory performance to result.

AMPLIFICATION

Children with severe and profound hearing loss come to intervention fitted with a variety of acoustic amplification (traditional hearing aids, transposition aids, ear-level FM units, traditional FM units), vibrotactile amplification (single and multichannel), and electrical stimulation (single and multichannel cochlear implants). Regardless of the type of listening system used, performance outcomes are influenced by amplification use pattern, appropriateness of fitting, family commitment and involvement, maintenance, and functioning.

To begin the process of auditory skill development, parents and professionals must be confident that they have exploited all available hearing through amplification. The audiologist must endeavor to maximize the child's residual hearing. Capitalizing on every decibel, every increase in sound, becomes the rehabilitation professional's responsibility. Attempting to enhance the remaining hearing through appropriate amplification and training assumes that the clinician is approaching this challenge from what the child is capable of hearing rather than what is missing (Boothroyd 1984). If training auditory skills in children with severe and profound hearing loss is the goal, then an audible signal is essential. The amount of audibility across the speech frequencies will affect the expected outcome of the training. From a rehabilitation standpoint, providing a young child with profound hearing impairment with low-frequency information at an audible level is vital for the competent development of spoken language. As with children with normal hearing, access to and use of intonation occur early in communication development. These intonation cues become the vehicle by which the infant learns the rules of conversational exchange, vocal characteristics of anger, joy, and the pragmatic requesting, questioning, and directing. To ignore the importance of this low-frequency information for children with profound hearing impairment is to set up poor speech production habits. As the child emerges from the babbling and jargon stage, many of the suprasegmental aspects of speech are already established, resulting in a lessened need for this low-frequency emphasis.

PARENTS

Parents are critical to the success of an auditory training/learning program for children with severe and profound hearing loss (Brackett 1992; Cole 1991; Maxon and Brackett 1992). The hours the child spends in the home environment can be effective for training auditory/speech skills. The preschooler spends a minimum of eight hours a day in the presence of parents and siblings (three hours in early education setting); the school-age child spends approximately five hours a day. Without varying their routines, parents can reinforce goals and objectives by consciously increasing the number of times the targets occur during conversational input and appear in the child's response.

Often parents are the force behind choosing an auditory approach or increased auditory emphasis in their child's school program. As initiators of the process, many parents are fully committed to its implementation at home and at school. This commitment can, with direction, be channeled into effective home auditory management.

EXPECTATIONS

Expecting a response to an auditory-only stimuli is the essential first step in training auditory skills. If the parents and/or professionals are ambivalent about this goal, then little forward movement will occur. An optimal situation exists when all adults in home and school environments agree with the decision to optimize residual hearing through appropriate amplification and aggressive auditory management.

CONCLUSION

The possibility of developing the auditory capabilities of children with severe-to-profound hearing loss has never been as attainable as it is now. Through technological advancements, it is possible to make most components of the speech signal audible to children with hearing loss as great as 120 dB. Stimulation by other than acoustic means may be necessary to accomplish this goal, but it is achievable. With an audible signal, the potential is there; aggressive rehabilitation is the means by which it is accomplished.

REFERENCES

Boothroyd, A. 1984. Auditory perception of speech contrasts by subjects with sensorineural hearing loss. *Journal of Speech and Hearing Research* 27:34-144.

Boothroyd, A. 1993. Profound deafness. In R.S. Tyler (ed.), *Cochlear implants.* San Diego: Singular Publishing Group.

Brackett, D. 1992. Home involvement for children with cochlear implants. *Hearing Rehabilitation Quarterly (Special Issue on Children with Cochlear Implants).* New York: New York League for the Hard of Hearing.

Cole, E. 1991. *Listening and talking.* Washington, D.C.: Alexander Graham Bell Association for the Deaf.

Erber, N. 1982. *Auditory training.* Washington, D.C.: Alexander Graham Bell Association for the Deaf.

Ling, D. 1989. *Foundations of spoken language for hearing impaired children.* Washington, D.C.: Alexander Graham Bell Association for the Deaf.

Maxon, A.B., and Brackett, D. 1992. *The hearing impaired child: Infancy through high school years.* Boston: Andover Medical Publishers.

Novelli-Olmstead, T., and Ling, D. 1984. Speech production and speech discrimination by hearing impaired children. *Volta Review* 86:72-80.

Osberger, M.J., Robbins, A.M., Miyamoto, R.T., Berry, S.W., Myres, W.A., Kessler, K.S., and Pope, M.L. 1991. Speech perception abilities of children with cochlear implants, tactile aids, or hearing aids. *American Journal of Otology* 12:105-115.

Zara, C., and Brackett, D. 1994. Cochlear implant rehabilitation: No need to reinvent the wheel. Presented at Alexander Graham Bell Association convention, July, Rochester, New York.

19

Auditory Intervention for Children with Mild Auditory Deficits

Carolyn Edwards

INTRODUCTION

To address the needs of children with mild auditory deficits, we must consider new approaches to auditory intervention. In the sixties and seventies, educational services and auditory curricula focused primarily on children with severe-to-profound sensorineural hearing loss. In the last ten to fifteen years, however, several changes have occurred. Integration of children with hearing loss into regular schools and mainstream programs is now common. The auditory difficulties of children with minimal and mild sensorineural hearing loss, unilateral sensorineural hearing loss, and recurrent otitis media are now being acknowledged in the research literature (Bess 1982, 1986; Boney and Bess 1984; Crandell 1993; Gravel and Ellis 1995; Jerger, Jerger, Alford, and Abrams 1983; Johnson and Stein 1995; Oyler, Oyler, and Matkin 1988). Children with mild auditory deficits, who were previously unamplified, are now commonly fitted with personal and/or classroom amplification devices.

The recognition of the need for intervention for children with mild degrees of hearing loss, of a fluctuating or permanent nature, must be reflected in changes in service delivery models for educational services. Therefore, service providers are now asking, What is different about auditory intervention for children with mild auditory deficits? To address the question, this chapter will consider the nature of listening and auditory intervention in its broadest scope. Based on the auditory issues presented by children with lesser degrees of hearing loss, an approach for the creation of optimal listening environments through consideration of room acoustics, amplification technology, and strategy teaching in the classroom will be described.

A MODEL FOR AUDITORY INTERVENTION

THE NATURE OF LISTENING

Listening is the ability to respond to, organize, interpret, and evaluate sounds in order to create meaning (Early Childhood Curriculum Committee 1978). The classroom is a complex listening environment. In the classroom, for example, children are expected to respond to the teacher's voice by paying attention under a variety of listening conditions. They are expected to know what to listen for and what sounds to ignore. That is, children are expected to recognize relevant instructions and conversations even when a number of activities are occurring simultaneously in the room.

The characteristics of children's listening environments are constantly changing throughout the day. For example, the sensation level of the primary signal, the speech-to-noise (S/N) ratio, and the reverberation time vary as children move from a teacher-directed activity to classroom discussion, from a quiet to a noisy activity, or from the classroom to the gymnasium. There is no single measure of listening ability that can be used to describe children's listening skills in the classroom. It is important to paint a number of pictures of children's listening skills, based on a range of listening environments encountered during the day.

Listening occurs for various purposes: to comprehend suprasegmental and segmental information, to monitor one's own speech, and to auditorily monitor the surrounding environment (Edwards 1991). All three aspects are critical within the classroom environment and need to be addressed within a comprehensive model of auditory intervention.

For children with hearing loss, the ability to interpret the incoming auditory signal is affected by a number of factors, outlined in table 1. The quality of the speech signal received at the microphone of a hearing aid is dependent on the clarity of articulation of the speaker and the room acoustics through which the signal is sent. Children's auditory potential to respond to and organize sound, and their cognitive and linguistic skills to interpret and evaluate sound, will determine the extent of the message received. In most

Table 1
Factors Affecting Comprehension of Speech

Quality of speaker signal
Transmission of signal
Reception of signal
Children's ability to utilize the auditory information
Children's ability to effect better reception of the auditory signal
School's and family's acknowledgment of children's communication needs

---

cases, the incoming signal will be somewhat distorted by the presence of background noise or long reverberation times. Although the use of assistive listening technologies will improve the quality of signal received, children will usually require some use of clarification strategies in difficult listening conditions. Children's confidence to utilize various strategies will only develop when their communication needs are recognized by school staff, classmates, and family members. Thus, children's ability to use assistive listening technologies and clarification strategies will enhance reception of the speech signal.

LISTENING FOR CHILDREN WITH MILD AUDITORY DEFICITS

Intervention can focus on enhancing comprehension of suprasegmental and segmental information, monitoring speech production, and/or monitoring the surrounding environment. Speech recognition in quiet for children with mild degrees of hearing loss is generally excellent if the vocabulary is within their language levels. Therefore, there is typically no need to focus on auditory recognition or comprehension of suprasegmentals or segmentals in quiet for school-age children. Of course, preschool children at the outset of amplification will benefit from enriched language experience and incidental work on phoneme contrasts as confusions arise. Speech intelligibility is also generally good for children with minimal-to-mild hearing loss, so formal work on auditory monitoring of speech production is usually not indicated. When speech errors arise, the clinician can check to ensure that the speech production errors are not the result of auditory recognition errors.

Monitoring the surrounding environment, however, is vital for children with mild degrees of hearing loss, since their ability to recognize speech is compromised by the presence of background noise and reverberation. Crandell (1993) showed a 58% deterioration in sentence recognition scores for children with minimal hearing loss, as compared to a 28% drop in scores for children with normal hearing when the listening condition changed from quiet to an S/N ratio of -6 dB. Similarly, children with moderate hearing loss in Finitzo-Hieber and Tillman's classic 1978 study showed a decrease of 59% in word recognition scores under adverse noise and reverberation conditions. Bess (1982, 1986) and Oyler, Oyler, and Matkin (1988) found that children with unilateral hearing loss exhibit greater difficulty understanding speech in the presence of competing background noise than do children with normal hearing, even under a monaural direct condition (i.e., speech signal directed to the ear with normal hearing and noise directed to the poorer ear). Children with histories of otitis media have demonstrated poorer performance for word or sentence recognition in a competing noise background than do peers without a history of otitis media

(Brown 1994; Gravel and Wallace 1992; Jerger, Jerger, Alford, and Abrams 1983; Schilder, Snik, Straatman, and van den Broek 1994).

Children with minimal and mild hearing loss may appear to be progressing adequately in school and, in fact, doing better than some of the other students in the classroom with normal hearing. Articulation in school-age children with mild auditory deficits is usually completely intelligible, so speech patterns do not attract attention. Alerting to the teacher's voice is also generally good, as is speech recognition in quiet environments. Thus, the lack of visibility of the effects of the hearing loss leads others to doubt the need for any intervention. Unrecognized needs can lead to children feeling less capable instead of recognizing their inability to hear as well as others (Stanley 1992). The effects of hearing loss may be reflected in social interactions with classmates. In a study reported by Davis, Shepard, Stelmachowicz, and Gorga (1981), children with mild and moderate hearing losses were perceived by parents as having more problems interacting with others or establishing friendships. In addition, 50% of the children expressed concerns about making friends or being accepted socially, as compared to 15.5% of the children with normal hearing.

The first step in intervention must, therefore, be the demonstration of the effects of mild auditory deficits. One effective in-service tool is a simulation of hearing loss where the teachers or parents wear earplugs in one or both ears during a speech recognition exercise presented in background noise. The in-service is described in detail in Edwards (1995). After the simulation experience, most teachers or caregivers are ready to commit to an auditory intervention approach for children with hearing loss.

Children with hearing loss often are unaware that others with normal hearing also may experience listening difficulties. One student with a moderate hearing loss observed a peer with normal hearing asking the teacher for repetition. She commented to the author that she did not understand why the student needed the repetition, since the student had normal hearing. The importance of sharing listening difficulties with children who have normal hearing cannot be overemphasized for children with minimal and mild loss.

Speech and hearing professionals should also be aware that our terminology may also undermine intervention efforts for children with lesser degrees of hearing loss. The terms *minimal* and *mild* suggest to school staff that a mild issue exists that may or may not need to be addressed. It is therefore recommended that audiologists add the following statement to any definition of minimal, mild, or unilateral hearing loss: This child is at risk for delays in academic and/or social/emotional development.

AUDITORY PROGRAMMING

The obvious prerequisites for auditory programming are consistent hearing aid usage and good hearing aid care and maintenance. It is notable that within the SKI-HI preschool auditory curriculum, one part of a comprehensive home intervention program originally developed in the state of Utah for infants with hearing loss and their families, no other auditory skills are trained until hearing aid usage is 100% of waking hours (Clark and Watkins 1993). This area deserves more attention than it often receives, particularly for children with minimal-to-mild hearing loss wearing hearing aids.

Programming itself can be divided into three areas of focus: listening skills training, strategies and metastrategies, and consumer information about hearing loss (table 2). The presumed outcome of programming is the development of confidence in the use of audition by children with hearing loss. Listening skills training may focus on detection, identification, or comprehension skills through activities selected from auditory curricula or implementation of auditory activities using academic curricular materials. Specific skill training must be followed by activities that reinforce use of the listening skill in the classroom. The development of communication strategies and metastrategies is the second vital area of auditory programming. In the past, most of the listening skills training for children with severe-to-profound sensorineural hearing loss focused on content, language skills, and mastery of academic content for assignments and tests rather than strategy training. Since strategies are a powerful tool to obtain information lost in the noise

Table 2
Components of Auditory Programming

Prerequisites
    Consistent hearing aid usage
    Good hearing aid care and maintenance

Components
    Listening skills training
    • Acuity
    • Identification
    • Comprehension
      through use of auditory or academic curricula

    Generalization/Carryover to Classroom
    • Strategies
    • Metastrategies

    Consumer information about hearing loss

Table 3
Auditory Goals by Age Groupings

Preschool
    Detection
    Comprehension
    Auditory attitude within home environment

Elementary School
    Comprehension
    Identification
    Teacher strategies, followed by development of child strategies
    Auditory attitude within school environment

Secondary School
    Metastrategies
    Strategies: Determination of technological support and support personnel needs
    Auditory attitude of student
    Consumer information about hearing loss

Postsecondary Years and Beyond
    Self-advocacy and possibly advocacy for others

barrage of the classroom, strategies are an important area of focus for children with mild auditory deficits. The third area of focus, consumer information about hearing loss, is equally important for children with all degrees of hearing loss in their teenage years.

Auditory programming goals change with each age group (table 3). Although the focus of this chapter is school-age children, it is important to note the differences in approach with respect to age. As previously discussed, children with mild auditory deficits require little work in detection, recognition, or comprehension of speech; the focus in auditory programming is primarily in the areas of strategy development and auditory attitude. Development of appropriate teacher strategies is followed by the development of child strategies, metastrategies and, finally, determination of technology and support needs, and consumer information about hearing loss.

CREATION OF OPTIMAL LISTENING ENVIRONMENTS

Children with mild degrees of hearing loss can benefit from a multifaceted approach to auditory management. Such an approach would address the physical listening environment, technological options, staff and students' awareness of sound and particularly noise, and use of communication strategies by teachers and students. Although these comments will be directed to school-age children, the reader can apply some of the principles of intervention to preschool children in the home, nursery school, or day care setting.

THE PHYSICAL LISTENING ENVIRONMENT

Awareness of the Effects of Noise on Listening

Before changes to the physical listening environment can be made, the classroom teacher must understand the purpose of making such changes. Increasing the teacher's awareness of noise, the interference of noise with communication, and ways to improve reception of speech in the classroom is essential. Tape-recording the classroom for short segments of the day can help the teacher become aware of problematic noise sources. As discussed earlier, simulation of hearing loss with earplugs is another in-service tool for staff and/or students. Presentation of some of the literature cited earlier showing the devastating effect of noise on the listening of children with normal hearing and children with mild degrees of hearing loss may also be useful (Crandell 1993; Finitzo-Hieber and Tillman 1978).

Changing the Acoustics within the Classroom

Use of personal and/or sound field FM technology and accessories such as a pass-around microphone increases the intensity of the speaker signal and decreases the effects of reverberation. However, during small group activities where FM systems are often not used, ability to communicate effectively is constrained by the noise levels and reverberation within the classroom. The degree of acoustic interference is determined by the number of children in the classroom and the acoustic treatment of the classroom (Melancon, Truchon-Gagnon, and Hodgson 1990).

Although significant noise sources external to the classroom ultimately need to be addressed, the initial focus for the classroom teacher is simple and inexpensive changes that will improve acoustics in the classroom. Socks or tennis balls attached to the bottom of chair and desk legs in uncarpeted classrooms can significantly decrease noise from scraping chairs. Padded table covers reduce impact noise from activities occurring at various centers around the room. The creative use of corkboard, mobile bulletin boards, and storage areas can increase absorption of noise generated within the classroom. More expensive options can include installation of carpeting with underpadding and suspended acoustic tile on the ceiling. Corkboard placed in checkerboard pattern along the rear wall of the classroom and carpeting on the floor can be particularly beneficial (Berg 1993).

DEVELOPMENT OF A CLASS APPROACH TO LISTENING SKILLS

Rationale

The purpose of involving the entire class in the development of listening skills is fivefold: (1) to address the communication needs of listeners with normal hearing and children with mild auditory deficits that are compromised by poor acoustic conditions in the classroom; (2) to provide opportunities for children with hearing loss to experience some of the similarities between their listening experiences and those of children with normal hearing, hence providing opportunities for enhancement of self-esteem; (3) to develop the transition from the teacher's use of communication strategies to the students' use of strategies among themselves; (4) for children with hearing loss to develop effective "communication partners" among their classmates rather than with the teacher only; and (5) to create an atmosphere of environmental support for the development of good listening skills.

To make lasting changes in the listening environment, one must create attitudinal changes in the teacher and students. The first step is creating awareness. Once the teacher and students have opportunities to experience different aspects of sound, and noise in particular, they are able to make choices about what type of listening environment they want.

Areas of Listening Activities

The following areas have been selected for the development of listening skills using a whole class approach. Activities from each of these areas can be introduced one at a time, perhaps one per week. The advantage of spreading listening programs out over the school year is that it keeps listening visible and a vital part of the curriculum throughout the year.

Exploring Sound

The purpose of these activities is to heighten the teacher's and children's awareness and enjoyment of sound in their activities. Use of storytelling, poetry, and singing places attention on oral listening activities. The children can create a listening logbook where they note the sounds heard that day in the home, the classroom, and the school. Onomatopoeic words are reinforced as children describe in their logbook the sounds they hear. Children can create their own onomatopoeic sounds as accompaniment to stories read by the teacher or other children. A favorite children's activity is creating and taping sound effects for ghost stories.

Self-Exploration—The Affective Side of Listening

Children need some reflective time to think about how they listen—to themselves and to others. A listening journal is often a useful tool to record children's thoughts about when they listen best, what they are listening for, when they stop listening, or what interferes with listening, as a few examples. Opportunities to share these thoughts with others in small groups and as a class will give children with hearing loss an opportunity to experience the diversity of listening experiences and possibly to experience some similarities with peers who have normal hearing.

Listening Readiness Skills

The focus of these activities is to create teacher strategies to prepare the children to listen and student strategies to obtain their classmates' attention. Some teachers create a specific space in the classroom where instructions are given so that merely walking into that area is the preparatory set for the students. Creating signals that indicate time to listen, such as clapping the hands or using a familiar phrase, is beneficial prior to instruction giving. Introduction of the concept of the talking stick, a Native American tradition, in student discussion teaches talker-listener etiquette. The children learn that the only person who can speak is the person holding the talking stick, and everyone must wait until that person is finished. Passing of the talking stick clearly indicates the next speaker. Passing of the FM transmitter in classrooms using sound field FM amplification also creates a similar readiness to listen. As good listening habits become established within the classroom, children with minimal-to-moderate hearing loss benefit from the increased ease of listening.

Choosing or Changing the Listening Environment

Noise is such a prevalent part of the classroom environment that it is often taken for granted. Therefore, a listening skills program must first focus on highlighting noise in the classroom. Experiencing differences in the classroom listening environment, such as a silent day without talking, is important so that children can make informed choices about the desired level of noise in their environment. Taping classroom activities to determine the noise levels and using a sound level meter to learn to accurately estimate loudness levels increase students' awareness of current noise levels. Students can then experiment with consciously altering the noise levels in the class and obtaining classmates' feedback regarding most desirable levels. A trial period with a sound field FM system is another effective way to demonstrate changes in S/N ratio. As the class becomes more aware of noise and its interference with communication, there is more potential for students to modify the noise levels, with resulting benefits for children with mild auditory deficits.

Clarification Strategies

In this module, children are given opportunities to experiment with various clarification strategies. Role-playing is a very effective tool to demonstrate good and poor speaking strategies, and good and poor listening strategies. Of course, the children love to play the bad listener. The teacher can model "unclear" messages and ask the children to discover the error. Simulation of telephone communication also explores communication breakdown and repair. Following directions, question games, classification games, and barrier game activities are other activities that can be used to experiment with various clarification strategies. There are many materials available within language curricula to develop these skills. Two examples of available resources are *Listening: A Basic Connection* (Micallef 1984) and *125 Ways to Become a Better Listener* (Graser 1992).

The age of the children will determine the sophistication of strategies. In kindergarten or first grade, children can make choices about the most appropriate strategy from a closed set of two or three responses. By third grade, children are able to consider a larger number of choices and formulate their own decisions. As children move into the senior grades, they are able to develop metastrategies (information about strategies), where they consider the background information necessary for selection and formulation of strategies.

SPECIFIC STRATEGY TEACHING

The class approach to development of listening skills fills in some of the gaps in listening skills for children with hearing loss and children with normal hearing, encourages the children to recognize some of the factors that interfere with communication, and creates an environment that supports clarification of communication. Some children may require more specific work on particular clarification strategies or may require a longer time to practice a strategy than is possible within the general class format. Thus, another aspect of auditory intervention for children with mild auditory deficits is specific strategy teaching in small groups. This can be done by the educational audiologist, the speech-language pathologist, or the special education teacher during small group activities within the class or outside the class.

It is important to evaluate children's current use of strategies in order to determine which strategies to select for more in-depth work. For example, when children are puzzled, what strategy do they use? Do they look quizzical?

Do they say *what*? Do they ask for repetition? Do they ask for repetition of the part of the sentence not heard? Do they paraphrase the content? One can design a teacher questionnaire such as the Evaluation of Children with Suspected Listening Difficulties (Edwards 1991) or the Observational Profile of Classroom Communication (Sanger 1988) that guides teachers in the collection of detailed observations about children's listening skills and strategies. Table 4 describes the general areas of evaluation useful for

Table 4
Evaluation of Children with Suspected Listening Difficulties

1. Overall Concerns about Listening
   - Doesn't understand appropriate listening expectations of the classroom
   - Doesn't seem to listen
   - Appears to be a good listener but work suggests misunderstanding
   - Has difficulty following directions
   - Follows single step commands but has difficulty with multistage commands
   - Frequently asks for repetition
   - Tends to quit easily when frustrated
   - Impulsive—often acts before thinking
   - Slow at beginning new tasks
   - Doesn't complete assignments
   - Has difficulty sustaining attention during oral presentations
   - Watches the speaker's face for more information

2. Current Strengths and Weaknesses
   - The child shows appropriate listening skills:

   In a Large Group Activity:
   - When activity is directed
   - When activity is independent
   - In the gymnasium
   - The noise level has impact on the student's performance

   In a Small Group Activity:
   - When activity is directed
   - When activity is independent
   - The noise level has impact on the student's performance

3. Child's Level of Awareness of Strengths and Weakness
   - Generally unaware of errors in processing information and doesn't attempt to clarify
   - Recognizes difficult listening situations
   - Recognizes that it is difficult to understand when people talk too quickly
   - Has developed preferences for certain speakers

Table 4 (continued)
Evaluation of Children with Suspected Listening Difficulties

4. Child's Current Strategies
   - Maintains eye contact with speaker
   - Will choose/request seating
     — close to speaker
     — away from noise sources
   - Will ask for repetition
     — in large group
     — with classmates
     — privately with teacher
   - Will rehearse information to retain it better
   - Will clarify by asking questions or paraphrasing
   - Will close the classroom door
   - Other strategies: list _____
   - Comments: _____

5. Current Modifications by the Teacher

   Environmental Modifications that Improve Listening Performance
   - Seating close to teacher
   - Seating away from constant noise sources (pencil sharpener, hallway, windows, etc.)
   - Seating in special areas of classroom: _____
   - Use of library/hallways for projects
   - Use of headphones by the child (for noise reduction during individual work periods)

   Teaching Strategies that Improve Listening Performance
   - Use of buddy system
   - Writing instructions on blackboard
   - Calling child's name before initiating instructions
   - Touching child on shoulder to get his/her attention
   - Simplifying instructions to single steps
   - Comprehension checks:
     — ask child to indicate when didn't understand
     — ask child to repeat the instructions heard
     — ask child to summarize instructions before work initiated
   - Slowing rate of speech
   - Use of breaks or rest periods from listening

6. Other Factors of Note (fluid build-up in the middle ear [otitis media], emotional difficulties, attention deficit disorder)

Reprinted with the permission from Edwards. 1991. *Seminars in Hearing*, 12:399-401, Thieme Medical Publishers., Inc.

program planning. When using teacher reporting forms, the clinician should ensure that teachers have a few weeks after receipt of the questionnaire to study and complete the information requested.

Questions from the SIFTER (Screening Instrument for Targeting Educational Risk; Anderson 1989) or the Preschool SIFTER (Anderson and Matkin in development) also provide observations about general aspects of the child's listening performance. Results of the Hearing Performance Inventory for Children (HPIC) (Maxon 1988) provide examples of situations where children experience listening difficulty. It is also important to interview the teacher in order to understand the listening expectations of the classroom and the strategies that would make the most impact on children's classroom performance. Information about children's degree of risk taking in the classroom, their relationships with peers, and their overall social skills will also indicate directions for strategy intervention programs.

The classroom teacher can select other students who also require work on similar listening strategies to join the child with hearing loss in a small group. This continues to affirm to children with hearing loss that some of their listening experiences are similar to those of children with normal hearing.

The design of the small group strategy sessions is experiential. Based on input from the teacher and the children, a particular situation is selected, the clinician or older students design an experiment to evaluate various strategies, and then they decide which strategy worked for them. The clinician assigns some carryover activities for the classroom to ensure that the strategy is generalized. The clinician or students may choose to focus on strategies that are implemented prior to communication and/or those that are implemented during a communication breakdown. Examples of the strategies

Table 5
Technological Strategies to Enhance Communication

Hearing aid features
- Client adjustable tone control
- Programmable options
- Hearing aid microphone off switch (for use with FM)

FM features
- Type of accessory microphone used with FM transmitter
  - Directional
  - Boom
  - Pass-around
  - Conference
- Patch cords for audio-visual equipment

selected in advance occur when the student determines that the room acoustics, such as those in the gymnasium, already indicate a potential problem for communication, and so the student institutes a buddy system for the gym. The metastrategy approach deepens the specific strategy approach for older students. For a detailed approach to communication breakdown and repair strategies used with children with moderately severe-to-profound hearing loss, see Elfenbein (1992).

Work on use of technological strategies is best completed by the student with hearing loss and the clinician. The purpose of the individual sessions is to provide the student with an opportunity to experiment with various amplification options, and then test the benefits in the classroom. Table 5 lists some of the technological strategies that the student may use with personal or FM amplification.

SUMMARY

A multifaceted approach to auditory intervention for children with mild auditory deficits focuses on the factors affecting communication in the home and classroom: room acoustics, potential amplification technologies, and listening strategies. Because the ultimate goal of auditory intervention is the development of children's self-worth, inherent in the approach described in this chapter is the message to children with hearing loss that we are all unique and we all share universal needs to communicate.

ACKNOWLEDGMENTS

The author would like to acknowledge the collaboration of her colleague, Kim Wyllie, in the development of the listening skills program described in this chapter.

REFERENCES

Anderson, K.L.. 1989. *Screening Instrument for Targeting Educational Risk (SIFTER)*. Austin: Pro-Ed.

Anderson, K.L., and Matkin, N.D. In development. *Preschool Screening Instrument for Targeting Educational Risk* (age 3-kindergarten).

Berg, F.S. 1993. *Acoustics and sound systems in schools*. San Diego: Singular Publishing Group.

Bess, F.H. 1982. Children with unilateral hearing loss. *Journal of Rehabilitative Audiology* 15:131-144.

Bess, F.H. 1986. The unilaterally hearing impaired child: A final comment. *Ear and Hearing* 7(1):52-54.

Boney, S., and Bess, F.H. 1984. Noise and reverberation effects in minimal bilateral sensorineural hearing loss. Paper presented at the American Speech-Language-Hearing Association convention, San Francisco, California.

Brown, D. 1994. Speech recognition in recurrent otitis media: Results in a set of identical twins. *Journal of American Academy of Audiology* 5:1-6.

Clark, T., and Watkins, S. 1993. The Ski-Hi Model: A comprehensive model for identification, language facilitation, and family support for hearing handicapped children through home management, ages birth to six. 5th ed. Project Ski-Hi.

Crandell, C. 1993. Speech recognition in noise by children with minimal degrees of sensorineural hearing loss. *Ear and Hearing* 14(3):211-216.

Davis, J., Shepard, N., Stelmachowicz, P.G., and Gorga, M.P. 1981. Characteristics of hearing impaired children in the public schools: Part II—Psychoeducational data. *Journal of Speech and Hearing Disorders* 46:30-137.

Early Childhood Curriculum Committee. 1978. *Listening and speaking.* Adelaide: Publications Branch, Education Department of South Australia.

Edwards, C. 1991. Assessment and management of listening skills in school-aged children. *Seminars in Hearing* 12(4):389-401.

Edwards, C. 1995. Listening strategies for teachers and students. In C. Crandell, J. Smaldino, and C. Flexer (eds.), *Sound field FM amplification: Theoretical foundations and practical applications.* San Diego: Singular Press.

Elfenbein, J. 1992. Coping with communication breakdown: A program of strategy development for children who have hearing losses. *American Journal of Audiology* 1(3):25-29.

Finitzo-Hieber, T., and Tillman, T. 1978. Room acoustics effects on monosyllabic word discrimination ability for normal and hearing impaired children. *Journal of Speech and Hearing Research* 21:440-458.

Graser, N.S. 1992. *125 ways to be a better listener.* East Moline, Ill.: Linguisystems, Inc.

Gravel, J.S., and Ellis, M. 1995. The auditory consequences of otitis media with effusion: The audiogram and beyond. *Seminars in Hearing* 16(1):44-59.

Gravel, J.S., and Wallace, I.F. 1992. Listening and language at four years of age: Effects of early otitis media. *Journal of Speech and Hearing Research* 35:588-595.

Jerger, S., Jerger, J., Alford, B.R., and Abrams, S. 1983. Development of speech intelligibility in children with recurrent otitis media. *Ear and Hearing* 4:138-145.

Johnson, C., and Stein, R. 1995. High risk listeners in the classroom. Paper presented at the American Academy of Audiology convention, Dallas, Texas.

Maxon, A.B. 1988. Hearing Performance Inventory for Children (HPIC). Paper presented at the American Speech-Language-Hearing Association convention, November, Boston, Massachusetts.

Micallef, M. 1984. *Listening: A basic connection.* Carthage, Ill.: Good Apple, Inc.

Melancon, L., Truchon-Gagnon, C., and Hodgson, M. 1990. *Architectural strategies to avoid noise problems in child care centres.* Montreal, Canada: Groupe d'Acoustique de l'Universite de Montreal.

Oyler, R.F., Oyler, A.L., and Matkin, N.D. 1988. Unilateral hearing loss: Demographics and educational impact. *Language, Speech, and Hearing Services in the Schools* 19:201-210.

Sanger, D. 1988. Observational profile of classroom communication. *Clinical Connection* 2(2):11-13.

Schilder, A., Snik, A.F.M., Straatman, H., and van den Broek, P. 1994. The effect of otitis media with effusion at preschool age on some aspects of auditory perception at school age. *Ear and Hearing* 15(3):224-231.

Stanley, S. 1992. Children with otitis media: A qualitative study. Master's thesis, York University, Toronto, Canada.

Appendix 1

Amplification for Infants and Children
with Hearing Loss

The Pediatric Working Group
Conference on Amplification for Children with Auditory Deficits

---

In October 1994, Vanderbilt University, Bill Wilkerson Center, and the Academy of Dispensing Audiologists cosponsored a conference designed to address various contemporary issues associated with hearing aids in children. The proceedings of this conference, Amplification for Children with Auditory Deficits *(Bess, Gravel, and Tharpe 1996) is available through the Bill Wilkerson Center Press, Nashville, Tennessee. Following the conference, a small working group was assembled from the conference faculty to develop a Position Statement on amplification for infants and children with hearing loss. The members of the committee who prepared the following statement include: Fred H. Bess, Chair, Vanderbilt University School of Medicine/Bill Wilkerson Center, Nashville, Tennessee; Patricia A. Chase, Vanderbilt University School of Medicine, Nashville, Tennessee; Judith S. Gravel, Albert Einstein College of Medicine, Bronx, New York; Richard C. Seewald, The University of Western Ontario, London-Ontario, Canada; Patricia G. Stelmachowicz, Boys Town National Research Hospital, Omaha, Nebraska; Anne Marie Tharpe, Louisiana State University Medical Center, New Orleans, Louisiana; and Andrea Hedley-Williams, Bill Wilkerson Center, Nashville, Tennessee.*

INTRODUCTION

The timely fitting of appropriate amplification to infants and children with hearing loss is one of the more important responsibilities of the pediatric audiologist. Although the importance of providing an audible signal for the development and maintenance of aural/oral communication for formal and informal learning is undisputed, the methods used to select and evaluate personal amplification for infants and children with hearing loss vary widely among facilities. Few audiologists use any systematic approach for selecting and fitting amplification for young children and many do not use current technologies in the fitting process (Hedley-Williams, Tharpe, and Bess 1996). Because of the improvement in early identification of hearing loss in children (Bess and Paradise 1994: Stein 1995), continued changes in technology, and a new array of amplification options available for application to infants and children, there is a critical need for a systematic, quantifiable, and evidence-based approach to providing amplification for the pediatric population. The goal is to ensure that children will receive full-time and consistent audibility of the speech signal at safe and comfortable listening levels.

The audiologist is the professional singularly qualified to select and fit all forms of amplification for children, including personal hearing aids, FM systems, and other assistive listening devices. To perform this function capably, an audiologist must have experience with the assessment and management of infants and children with hearing loss and the commensurate knowledge and test equipment necessary for use with current pediatric hearing assessment methods and hearing aid selection and evaluation procedures. Facilities that lack the expertise or equipment should establish consortial arrangements with those that do.

This statement sets forth guidelines and recommendations associated with the fitting of personal amplification to infants and children with hearing loss. The approach stresses an objective, timely strategy and discourages the traditional comparative approach. We envision the provision of appropriate, reliable, and undistorted amplification as a four-stage process involving assessment, selection, verification, and validation. We herein present a discussion on need, audiologic assessment, preselection of the physical characteristics of hearing aids, selection and verification of the electroacoustic characteristics of hearing aids, and validation of aided auditory function. Because the focus of this position statement is on the fitting process, the topics of counseling and follow-up are discussed but not treated in detail. Readers are referred elsewhere for comprehensive coverage of these important topics (Brackett 1996; Diefendorf, Reitz, Escobar, and Wynne 1996; Edwards 1996). Finally, we include a question/answer section regarding issues frequently raised by pediatric audiologists.

CRITERIA FOR PROVISION OF PERSONAL AMPLIFICATION

A child needs hearing aids when there is a significant, permanent, bilateral peripheral hearing loss. Some children with variable and/or unilateral losses may also need hearing aids. There are no empirical studies that delineate the specific degree of hearing loss at which need for amplification begins. However, if one considers the acoustic spectrum of speech at normal conversational levels in the 1000-4000 Hz range, hearing thresholds of 25 dB

HL or greater can be assumed to impede a child's ability to perceive the acoustic features of speech necessary for optimum aural/oral language development. Hence, thresholds equal to or poorer than 25 dB HL would indicate candidacy for amplification in some form. For children with unilateral hearing loss, rising or high-frequency hearing loss above 2000 Hz, and/or milder degrees of hearing loss (<25 dB HL), need should be based on the audiogram plus additional information including cognitive function, the existence of other disabilities, and the child's performance within the home and classroom environment.

THE AUDIOLOGIC ASSESSMENT

The efficacy of the hearing aid fitting is predicated on the validity of the audiologic assessment. The ultimate goal of the audiometric evaluation is to obtain ear- and frequency-specific threshold data from the child at the earliest opportunity.

When testing very young children, however, complete audiologic data are seldom obtained. In the absence of a complete audiogram, and even with one, consistencies among several audiometric measures—behavioral findings, click-evoked and/or tone evoked ABR threshold recordings, aural acoustic immittance measures (reflexes and tympanometry), evoked otoacoustic emissions, and bone-conduction responses (behavioral and/or ABR)—are essential.

For children with a developmental age at or under 6 months, behavioral responses should be confirmed with ABR threshold assessment. When behavioral results are unreliable, such as in the case of children with multiple disabilities, behavioral and ABR assessments should be completed and the findings for both measures should be examined for agreement. However, in the absence of reliable behavioral thresholds, hearing aid fitting should proceed based on frequency-specific ABR results unless neurologic status contraindicates such action.

It is not sufficient to base binaural hearing aid fitting only on soundfield thresholds, nor is it acceptable to fit hearing aids to infants and young children based solely on a click-ABR threshold. In both such cases, critical information is lacking that could affect the efficacy of the fit, or in the worst-case scenario, be detrimental to the child's performance. With regard to soundfield audiometric assessment, it is inadvisable to assume that both ears have equal hearing loss or hearing loss of the same configuration based on behavioral soundfield results alone. Therefore, it is preferable to obtain thresholds using earphones. Insert earphones are recommended because the child's real-ear-to-coupler difference (RECD) (described in the *Selection and Verification*, page 403) can then be used to convert threshold measures to real-ear SPL. Other behavioral measures such as speech detection and speech recognition may be useful in determining amplification need. The click-ABR provides insufficient information regarding both the degree and configuration of hearing loss—information that is critical for use with today's prescriptive selection and evaluation procedures. At a minimum, click and 500-Hz tone ABR thresholds should be obtained in order to reflect low- and high-frequency hearing sensitivity (ASHA 1991). Finally, auditory behaviors should be consistent with parental reports of auditory function as well as more formal, systematic observations of behavioral responses to calibrated acoustic stimuli.

PRESELECTION—PHYSICAL CHARACTERISTICS

Even at a very young age, consideration should be given to the availability of appropriate coupling options on hearing aids, so that the child will have maximum flexibility for accessing the various forms of current assistive device technology. Consequently, hearing aids for most children should include the following features: Direct Audio Input (DAI), telecoil (T), and microphone-telecoil (M-T) switching options. Hearing aids used with young children also require more flexibility in electroacoustic parameters (e.g., tone, gain, output limiting) than for adults, as well as more safety-related features such as safety-related features such as battery and volume controls that are tamper resistant.

The physical fit of the hearing aids (in most cases worn behind the pinnae) and the earmolds is important for both comfort and retention. Color of the hearing aids and earmolds needs to be considered across ages, and size of the hearing aids is an especially important cosmetic concern for older children. Earmolds should be constructed of a soft material.

While consideration needs to be given to the aforementioned physical factors, the ultimate goal is the consistency and integrity of the amplified signal that the child receives. Providing the best possible amplified speech signal should not be compromised for cosmetic purposes, particularly in the early years of life when speech-language learning is occurring at a rapid pace.

Binaural amplification should always be provided to young children unless there is a clear contraindication. Even if there is audiometric asymmetry between ears as evidenced by pure tones or speech perception, hearing aids should be fit binaurally until it is apparent from behavioral evidence that a hearing aid fitted to the poorer ear is detrimental to performance.

In general, behind-the-ear (BTE) hearing aids are the style of choice for most children. However, for children with profound hearing loss, body aids or FM systems may be more appropriate because of acoustic feedback problems limiting sufficient gain to provide full audibility of the speech signal in BTE arrangements. Other circumstances that may indicate the need for body-worn amplification include children with restricted motor capacities and those confined by a head restraint. In-the-ear (ITE) hearing aids may be considered appropriate when ear growth has stabilized—at about 8-10 years of age—as long as the flexibility and options available are not markedly restricted by concha and ear-canal size.

SELECTION AND VERIFICATION OF ELECTROACOUSTIC CHARACTERISTICS

The use of a systematic approach when selecting the electroacoustic characteristics of hearing aids for children is considered of utmost importance. Sound pressure levels measured in infants' and young children's ears typically exceed adult values (Bratt 1980; Feigin, Kopun, Stelmachowicz, and Gorga 1989; Nelson Barlow, Auslander, Rines, and Stelmachowicz 1988) and external ear resonance characteristics vary as a function of age (Bentler 1989; Kruger 1987; Kruger and Ruben 1987). In addition, children may be unable to provide subjective feedback regarding their hearing aid fittings (i.e., comfortable and uncomfortable listening levels). Therefore, probe microphone measurements of real-ear hearing aid performance should be obtained with children whenever possible (Stelmachowicz and Seewald 1991). If probe measures are used, target values for frequency/gain and frequency/output limiting characteristics should be selected via a systematic approach that seeks to optimize the audibility of speech (e.g., Byrne and Dillon 1986; Byrne, Parkinson, and Newall 1991; McCandless and Lyregaard 1983; Schwartz, Lyregaard, and Lundh 1988; Seewald 1992; see Section A for details). For selecting maximum hearing aid output, similar approaches exist (e.g., McCandless and Lyregaard 1983; Seewald 1992; Skinner 1988; see Section A for details). Many of these prescriptive approaches were developed for adults and may not be appropriate for children in the process of developing speech and language without some modification. However, such approaches do provide a starting point after which modifications can be made in the verification and validation stages of the process. Some procedures for calculating target gain and output limiting characteristics for children are available in computer-assisted formats (Seewald, Ramji, Sinclair, Moodie, and Jamieson 1993) although such values can also be calculated manually (Moodie, Seewald, and Sinclair 1994; see Section A for details).

Once the preselected hearing aid frequency-gain and output characteristics have been determined theoretically, verification of the selected electroacoustic parameters should be completed. Because large variability in RECDs are expected in young children, custom earmolds should be available at the time hearing aid performance is verified. Prior to the direct evaluation of the hearing aid on the child, the hearing aid gain and maximum output characteristics should be preset in a hearing aid test box using published or preferably measured RECD values (Feigin et al. 1989; Seewald et al. 1993; see Section A, table A-7).

Probe microphone measurements are preferable for use in the verification stage. When probe microphone measures of real-ear hearing aid performance are not possible, however, real-ear hearing aid performance can be predicted by applying average RECD values to coupler measures. Average RECD values from adults, however, are not appropriate for use with children due to the differences in adult and child ear-canal characteristics (Bentler and Pavlovic 1989; Hawkins, Cooper, and Thompson 1990). Thus, transforms designed for use with infants and children should be used to predict hearing aid performance (Moodie et al. 1994; Seewald, Sinclair, and Moodie 1994; Sinclair et al. 1994). Examples of how to use age-appropriate correction factors for determining target gain and maximum output values for children are shown in Section A: worksheets 1 and 2. No facility should fit hearing aids to children if it lacks the equipment for electroacoustic evaluation.

VERIFICATION OF OUTPUT LIMITING

The primary purposes of output limiting are to protect the child from loudness discomfort and to avoid potential damage to the ear from amplified sound. Setting the output-limiting characteristics of hearing aids for children is considered of equal, if not greater, importance as other amplification selection considerations. To this end, the audiologist must know what output levels exist in the ear canal of the child. Coupler-based SSPL targets are insufficient for use with infants and young children in particular unless RECDs are applied (Seewald 1991; Snik and Stollman 1995). Recommended options for determining output-limiting levels include direct measurement of the real-ear saturation response (RESR) for each ear or the use of measured or average age-related RECD values added to the tabled response (see Section A, table A-7B for HA-2/RECD values). It is recommended that swept pure tones or swept warble tones should be used when measuring hearing aid output (Revit 1991; Stelmachowicz 1991; Stelmachowicz, Lewis, Seewald, and Hawkins 1990).

Clearly, these approaches are predicated on the availability of frequency-specific threshold data. Thus, in cases where full audiometric information is not available, the clinician must make a "best estimate" of the residual hearing across the frequency range important for speech. The use of formulae may necessitate some extrapolation and interpolation of audiometric information from limited audiometric data, taking into account additional clinical and/or familial information that may be available. In such cases, continued observation and assessment of the child are mandatory.

Although none of the threshold-based selection procedures is guaranteed to ensure that a child will not experience loudness discomfort or that output levels are safe, the use of a systematic objective approach that incorporates age-dependent variables into the computations is preferred. Finally, frequency-specific loudness discomfort levels should be obtained when children are old enough to provide reliable responses (Gagné, Seewald, Zelisko, and Hudson 1991; Kawell, Kopun, and Stelmachowicz 1988; Macpherson, Elfenbein, Schum, and Bentler 1991; Stuart, Durieux-Smith, and Stenstrom 1991).

VERIFICATION OF GAIN/FREQUENCY RESPONSE

The hearing aid should be adjusted to approximate the previously determined target gain values for each ear. Aided soundfield threshold measurements are not the preferred procedure for verifying the frequency-gain characteristics of hearing aids in children for several reasons: (a) prolonged cooperation from the child is required, (b) time needed for such testing can be excessive, (c) frequency resolution is poor, and (d) test-retest reliability is frequently poor (Seewald, Moodie, Sinclair, and Cornelisse 1996). In addition, misleading information may be obtained in cases of severe to profound hearing loss, minimal/mild loss, or when nonlinear signal processing is used (Macrae 1982; Schwartz and Larson 1977; Seewald, Hudson, Gagné, and Zelisko 1992; Snik, van den Borne, Brokx, and Hoekstra 1995; Stelmachowicz and Lewis 1988).

Gain should be verified using probe-microphone measures or 2cc coupler and RECD (individually measured or age-related average) values. A 60-dB SPL input using swept pure tones or speech-weighted noise should be used with linear hearing aid systems (Stelmachowicz 1991; Stelmachowicz et al. 1990). When using nonlinear instruments with children, audiologists should be using advanced verification technology such as the use of multiple signal levels and types to obtain a family of response characteristics (Revit 1994).

VALIDATION OF AIDED AUDITORY FUNCTION

Once the prescriptive procedure is complete and the settings of the hearing aids have been verified, the validation process begins. Validation of aided auditory function is a critical, yet often overlooked, component of the pediatric amplification provision process. The purpose of validating aided auditory function is to demonstrate the benefits/limitations of a child's aided listening abilities for perceiving the speech of others as well as his or her own speech. Validation is accomplished, over time, using information derived through the aural habilitation process, as well as the direct measurement of the child's aided auditory performance.

With input provided by parents, teachers, and speech-language pathologists, the pediatric audiologist determines whether the ultimate goals of the hearing aid fitting process have been achieved. These goals are that the speech signal is audible, comfortable, and clear, and that the child is resistant to noise interference in the vast majority of communication environments in which formal and informal learning takes place. Measurements of aided performance quantify the child's auditory abilities at the time of the initial hearing aid fitting, and, as importantly, serve as a baseline for monitoring the child's incorporation of audible speech cues into his or her communication repertoire. Examples of measures of aided auditory performance include aided soundfield responses to various stimuli, including speech measures (see Section B, table A-1 for examples of speech materials to be used with children). Other functional performance measures include the SIFTER (Anderson 1989), the Pre-school SIFTER (Anderson and Matkin in development), and the Meaningful Auditory Integration Scale (MAIS; Robbins, Renshaw, and Berry 1991). Measures of aided performance are not to be used for the purpose of changing hearing aid settings unless there is an obvious behavioral indicator to the contrary. These include loudness tolerance problems or an inability to perceive particular speech cues that should be audible in the aided condition. It is recommended that performance measures be obtained in a binaural presentation mode unless one's intent is to document asymmetry in aided auditory performance.

It is stressed that the contributions provided by all members of the habilitation team promote an atmosphere of mutual cooperation and respect that ultimately results in more effective management for the child with hearing impairment (Edwards 1996).

INFORMATIONAL COUNSELING AND FOLLOW-UP

In order to ensure that hearing aids will be used successfully, proper counseling, monitoring, and follow-up are essential. Hearing aid orientation programs should include all family members who will be assisting the child with the hearing aid and any professionals working directly with the child and his or her family (e.g., teachers and therapists). The need for parents, teachers, and therapists to receive in-service training on the routine troubleshooting of the child's hearing instruments and the child's performance using amplification cannot be overemphasized. When appropriate, children should be assisted in understanding the details of their hearing loss; instructed in the use, care, and monitoring of their personal hearing aids; and given information on communication strategies under different listening conditions (Edwards 1996; Elfenbein 1994; Seewald and Ross 1988).

It is recommended that young children be seen by an audiologist every 3 months during the first 2 years of using amplification; thereafter children should be seen at least every 6 months if there are no concerns. Reasons for more aggressive monitoring include fluctuating and/or progressive hearing loss (Tharpe 1996). The follow-up examinations should include audiometric evaluation, electroacoustic evaluation and listening checks of the hearing aid(s), and re-evaluation of the RECD and other probe-microphone measures as appropriate. In addition, the RECD should be measured whenever earmolds are replaced.

Functional measures, as discussed above, should be obtained on a periodic basis to document the development of auditory skills. These measures should include input from family, educators, and other interested professionals regarding communication and educational abilities, and social and behavioral development (Diefendorf et al. 1996). Finally, the audiologist should routinely assess the acoustic conditions in which children use amplification and offer suggestions on ways to optimize the listening environments (Crandell 1993).

QUESTIONS AND ANSWERS

The following section has been developed to provide information about questions commonly asked by audiologists working with the pediatric population.

1. Can an FM system be used in lieu of traditional hearing aids for an infant or young child?

Theoretically, an FM system (in the FM mode of operation) should provide an improved signal-to-noise (S/N) ratio for any user. A number of investigators have suggested that use of FM systems as primary amplification can be advantageous for children with severe to profound hearing loss (Benoit 1989; Brackett 1992; Kramlinger 1985; Madell 1992). In addition, Moeller, Donaghy, Beauchaine, Lewis, and Stelmachowicz (1996) monitored language acquisition in a small group of young children with mild to moderate hearing loss fitted with FM systems in the home setting over a 2-year period. In this study, practical problems such as system bulkiness, signal interference, multiple talkers, the need for extensive parent/caregiver training, and the complications associated with inappropriate mode of operation (e.g., FM transmission of irrelevant conversations and communication at great distances) limited and/or complicated FM system use in many situations. At the end of the 2-year study, the parents reported that they preferred to use the FM system as an assistive device rather than as primary amplification. Although manufacturers have attempted to address some of these practical problems with recent technological advances (e.g., BTE FM systems, voice-activated microphones), currently no single system can be expected to solve all of these problems. If an FM system is recommended for a young child, the practical issues cited above should be considered in the context of the child's degree of hearing loss, environment, and family structure.

2. What assistive devices, if any, are appropriate for young children?

Assistive devices are often overlooked in the management of young children with hearing loss. Assistive devices can help ensure safety, foster independence, and maintain privacy for older children with hearing loss. FM systems can be used as assistive devices even for very young children in situations where noise, reverberation, and/or distance are a concern. Normal-hearing children learn the meaning of various environmental sounds in an incidental fashion. If a child cannot be expected to hear environmental sounds such as the telephone, doorbell, smoke alarm, or alarm clock when he or she is unaided, the use of appropriate alerting devices should be considered. There will be many situations (e.g., bath time, sleeping) when hearing aids will not be worn, yet the children with hearing loss should be able to identify and respond to familiar environmental and alerting signals. Normal-hearing children begin to attend to television programs by 2-4 years of age. A TV amplifier can provide access to television for children with varying degrees of hearing loss. In addition, for children with severe to profound hearing loss, closed captioning can be introduced at this early age to foster preliteracy skills, such as print awareness. Children with normal hearing are often introduced to the concept of telephone conversations shortly after their first birthday; something as simple as a telephone amplifier may enable the child with hearing loss to talk to friends, grandparents, or other relatives. Children with more severe hearing loss may require a telephone device for the deaf (TDD). TDDs can be used once the child can read and write. See Compton (1989) for a more thorough discussion of assistive devices in general and Lewis (1991) for a discussion of the application of these devices with young children.

3. Is there a minimum age at which hearing aids should be fitted? And what factors need to be considered when fitting hearing aids to children under 6 months of age?

If the clinical picture clearly suggests that a permanent, educationally significant hearing loss exists and the family is motivated to proceed with habilitation, then the child is a candidate for amplification regardless of age. Consider, for example, a child who is screened at birth because of a family history of hearing loss (two older siblings with severe bilateral sensorineural hearing loss). If the ABR shows elevated click-evoked and/or tone-burst thresholds, an absence of otoacoustic emissions, and normal middle ear function, there is little reason to delay the hearing aid fitting once the infant is awake sufficient lengths of time to introduce the device effectively. If the clinical picture is less straightforward, then additional testing is warranted before the hearing aid fitting.

Under 6 months of age, a successful hearing-aid fitting can often be compromised by practical issues. The complicating factors include: parental acceptance of the hearing loss, ear canal and concha size, financial considerations, additional handicapping conditions or health concerns, conductive component to the hearing loss, problems with retention of the earmold/hearing aid, and acoustic feedback. Some of these problems can be circumvented by the use of loaner hearing aids, body-worn hearing aids, specialized devices to assist with device retention (kiddie tone hooks, double-sided tape, headbands, bonnets, Huggie Aids™) and feedback control via use of a remote microphone. In cases where the hearing aid fitting must be delayed, it is still important to proceed with counseling, parent education, and habilitative services.

4. What about a young child with a conductive hearing loss or a conductive overlay?

In these cases, the first goal is to determine if the hearing loss is entirely conductive or mixed in nature. If it is entirely conductive and cannot be treated medically or surgically (e.g., congenital ossicular anomalies), then it should be viewed in the same way as a sensorineural hearing loss. An air-conduction hearing aid, if it can be used, is preferable to a bone-conduction aid. Bone-conducted amplification is limited by several factors, including low fidelity, the complexity and number of components, the difficulty of keeping the bone vibrator against the mastoid, and, in some cases, malformation of the skull.

If the hearing loss is caused by otitis media, then the child should be followed closely in lieu of amplification. In cases where the conductive component is substantial, ossicular anomalies and/or a cholesteatoma should be ruled out by the managing physician.

When a child has a mixed hearing loss, a bone-conduction hearing aid may or may not be appropriate, depending on the degree and configuration of the sensorineural component and the reason for the conductive component. (Again, air-conduction hearing aid fittings are most appropriate.) In these cases, it is important to work closely with the managing physician.

When a conductive component exists, concern for overamplification is minimized, since the SPL actually reaching the cochlea will be reduced by the amount of the conductive component.

5. How should children with progressive or fluctuating hearing loss be managed?

Progressive hearing loss is known to be associated with certain etiologies (e.g., cytomegalovirus, branchio-oto-renal syndrome, Stickler syndrome, family history of progressive hearing loss). In addition, it has been reported that as many as 21% of children with sensorineural hearing loss showed evidence of fluctuating and/or progressive hearing loss that is not related to middle ear disease (Brookhouser, Worthington, and Kelly 1994). Accordingly, parents, caregivers, and teachers should be counseled to be aggressive if changes in auditory awareness are suspected in a young child. Obviously, in some cases (e.g., fistula), early medical intervention may halt or actually reverse the progression of hearing loss. When progressive or fluctuating hearing loss has been identified, close follow-up by both the audiologist and the managing otolaryngologist is essential, and a referral to a geneticist may be warranted. Professional counseling should be considered for older children with progressive hearing loss to help them cope with potential changes in their communication abilities. Hearing aids should have flexible frequency response and maximum output characteristics. It may be necessary to recommend more than one volume control setting and/or changes in the internal settings as hearing changes. In some instances, programmable or multi-memory hearing aids may be the best choice.

6. What about amplification for young children with minimal hearing loss, unilateral hearing loss, rising or unusual configuration, or hearing loss only above 2000 Hz?

Minimal, unilateral, rising, and high-frequency hearing losses are not often identified at an early age (Bess and Tharpe 1986; Mace, Wallace, Whan, and Stelmachowicz 1991). When identified, however, they pose a special challenge for the pediatric audiologist. These losses should be monitored closely for progression, and middle-ear problems should be treated aggressively. Parents, caregivers, and teachers should be counseled to watch for changes in auditory awareness. Safety issues should be discussed for children with unilateral hearing loss, and the topic of hearing protection should be addressed. Hearing aids and other assistive devices should be considered on a case-by-case basis. Factors such as speech and language development, additional handicapping conditions, academic performance, and communication needs should be considered in conjunction with the audiological data when making decisions about amplification.

7. What additional factors need to be considered when fitting hearing aids/assistive devices to children with multiple handicapping conditions?

Estimates suggest that as many as 30% of children with permanent sensorineural hearing loss have at least one additional handicapping condition (Karchmer 1985). For many of these children, the accurate determination of hearing status may be difficult. Developmental delays often preclude behavioral audiological testing, and neurological problems often complicate the interpretation of ABR measures. In cases where the existence of educationally significant hearing loss can be established, however, a multidisciplinary approach is mandatory. Parents, physicians, audiologists, teachers, speech-language pathologists, physical and/or occupational therapists, and social workers need to be involved in the decision to proceed with amplification. Because these children often have atypical early life experiences, a primary goal should be to meet the needs of both the child and his or her family. It is important to recognize that for many of these children, hearing per se may not be a priority for the family. In many cases, it may be appropriate to delay the hearing aid fitting or to use some type of assistive device instead of conventional amplification. (A child on a ventilator, for example, may benefit from a hearing aid with a remote microphone.)

When a decision is made to proceed with amplification, it is essential to evaluate its impact in relation to the child's physical challenges, environment, and communication needs.

FUTURE DIRECTIONS

The selection and evaluation of properly fitted and functioning hearing aids for children with hearing loss is one of the major challenges facing today's pediatric audiologist. This challenge is compounded by a continued decrease in the average age of identification of hearing loss in children, as well as the ever-changing technology in hearing aids and the associated instrumentation used in the selection and evaluation of hearing aids. Hence, it is critical for the pediatric audiologist to stay abreast of the trends, practices, and technologies used in the hearing assessment and hearing aid fitting of very young children. To this end, the pediatric working group recognizes the need for systematic research and encourages controlled studies in all areas of pediatric amplification. Examples of important directions for future research include:

- Develop/validate audiometric assessment protocols for fitting amplification in infants.
- Examine the relationship between aided performance and auditory/communicative function.
- Develop additional psychoacoustic data from children with hearing loss, and consider the implications of such data on amplification selection and evaluation.
- Validate various prescriptive procedures for this population.
- Evaluate current technologies designed to enhance signal-to-noise ratio.
- Develop procedures and guidelines for fitting advanced-technology hearing aids to children.

- Determine the efficacy of amplification for children with minimal hearing loss, unilateral hearing loss, or unusual audiometric configurations.
- Develop better models for predicting performance and establishing safety and efficacy.

REFERENCES

American Speech-Language-Hearing Association. 1991. Guidelines for the audiologic assessment of children from birth through 36 months of age. *Asha* 33(Suppl. 5):37-43.

Anderson, K.L. 1989. *Screening Instrument for Targeting Educational Risk (SIFTER)*. Austin: Pro-Ed.

Anderson, K., and Matkin, N.D. in development. *Preschool S.I.F.T.E.R. Screening Instrument for Targeting Educational Risk in Preschool Children (age 3-kindergarten)*.

Benoit, R. 1989. Home use of FM amplification systems during the early childhood years. *Hearing Instruments* 40(3):8-12.

Bentler, R. 1989. External ear resonance characteristics in children. *Journal of Speech and Hearing Disorders* 54:264-268.

Bentler, R., and Pavlovic, C.V. 1989. Transfer functions and correction factors used in hearing aid evaluation and research. *Ear and Hearing* 10:58-63.

Bess, F.H., Gravel, J.S., and Tharpe, A.M. (eds.). 1996. *Amplification for children with auditory deficits*. Nashville, Tenn.: Bill Wilkerson Center Press.

Bess, F.H., and Paradise, J.L. 1994. Universal screening for infant hearing impairment: A reply. *Pediatrics* 94(6):959-963.

Bess, F.H., and Tharpe, A.M. 1986. Case history data on unilaterally hearing-impaired children. *Ear and Hearing* 7(1):14-19.

Brackett, D. 1992. Effects of early FM use on speech perception. In M. Ross (ed.), *FM auditory training systems—Characteristics, selection and use*. Timonium, Md.: York Press.

Brackett, D. 1996. Developing auditory capabilities in children with severe and profound hearing loss. In F.H. Bess, J.S. Gravel, and A.M. Tharpe (eds.), *Amplification for children with auditory deficits*. Nashville, Tenn.: Bill Wilkerson Center Press.

Bratt, G. 1980. *Hearing and receiver output in occluded ear canals in children*. Unpublished doctoral dissertation. Nashville, Tenn.: Vanderbilt University.

Brookhouser, P.E., Worthington, D.W., and Kelly, W.J. 1994. Fluctuating and/or progressive sensorineural hearing loss in children. *Laryngoscope* 104:958-964.

Byrne, D., and Dillon, H. 1986. The National Acoustic Laboratories' (NAL) new procedure for selecting the gain and frequency response of a hearing aid. *Ear and Hearing* 7:257-265.

Byrne, D., Parkinson, A., and Newall, P. 1991. Modified hearing aid selection procedure to severe profound hearing losses. In G.A. Studebaker, F.H. Bess, and L.B. Beck (eds.), *The Vanderbilt hearing-aid report II*. Parkton, Md.: York Press.

Compton, C. 1989. *Assistive devices: Doorways to independence*. Washington, D.C.: Gallaudet University.

Crandell, C.C. 1993. Speech recognition in noise by children with minimal degrees of sensorineural hearing loss. *Ear and Hearing* 14:210-216.

Diefendorf, A.O., Reitz, P.S., Escobar, M.W., and Wynne, M.K. 1996. Initiating early amplification: *TIPS* for success. In F.H. Bess, J.S. Gravel, and A.M. Tharpe (eds.), *Amplification for children with auditory deficits*. Nashville, Tenn.: Bill Wilkerson Center Press.

Edwards, C. 1996. Auditory intervention for children with mild auditory deficits. In F.H. Bess, J.S. Gravel, and A.M. Tharpe (eds.), *Amplification for children with auditory deficits*. Nashville, Tenn.: Bill Wilkerson Center Press.

Elfenbein, J. 1994. Monitoring preschoolers' hearing aids: Issues in program design and implementation. *American Journal of Audiology* 3(2):65-70.

Feigin, J.A., Kopun, J.G., Stelmachowicz, P.G., and Gorga, M.P. 1989. Probe-tube microphone measures of ear canal sound pressure levels in infants and children. *Ear and Hearing* 10(4):254-258.

Gagné, J.P., Seewald, R.C., Zelisko, D.L., and Hudson, S.P. 1991. Procedure for defining the auditory area of hearing-impaired adolescents with a severe/profound hearing loss II: Loudness discomfort levels. *Journal of Speech-Language Pathology and Audiology* 15(4):27-32.

Hawkins, D.B., Cooper, W.A., and Thompson, D.J. 1990. Comparison among SPL's in real ears, 2CM^3 and 6CM^3 couplers. *Journal of the American Academy of Audiology* 1:154-161.

Hedley-Williams, A., Tharpe, A.M., and Bess, F.H. 1996. Fitting hearing aids in children: A survey of practice procedures. In F.H. Bess, J.S. Gravel, and A.M. Tharpe (eds.), *Amplification for children with auditory deficits*. Nashville, Tenn.: Bill Wilkerson Center Press.

Karchmer, M.A. 1985. A demographic perspective. In E. Cherow (ed.), *Hearing impaired children and youth with developmental disabilities*. (pp. 37-56) Washington, D.C.: Gallaudet Press.

Kawell, M.E., Kopun, J.G., and Stelmachowicz, P.G. 1988. Loudness discomfort levels in children. *Ear and Hearing* 9(33):133-136.

Kramlinger, M. 1985. How I helped my children communicate: Adapting an auditory trainer for everyday use. *Exceptional Parent* 15:19-25.

Kruger, B. 1987. An update on the external ear resonance in infants and young children. *Ear and Hearing* 8(16):333-336.

Kruger, B., and Ruben, J.A. 1987. The acoustic properties of the infant ear. *Acta Oto-Laryngologica* (Stockholm) 103:578-585.

Lewis, D. 1991. FM systems and assistive devices: Selection and evaluation. In J.A. Feigin and P.G. Stelmachowicz (eds.), *Pediatric amplification: Proceedings of the 1991 national conference*. Omaha: Boys Town National Research Hospital.

Mace, A.L., Wallace, K.L., Whan, M.A., and Stelmachowicz, P.G. 1991. Relevant factors in the identification of hearing loss. *Ear and Hearing* 12:287-293.

Macpherson, B.J., Elfenbein, J.L., Schum, R.L., and Bentler, R. 1991. Thresholds of discomfort in young children. *Ear and Hearing* 12(3):184-190.

Macrae, J. 1982. Invalid aided thresholds. *Hearing Instruments* 33(9):20, 22.

Madell, J.R. 1992. FM systems for children birth to age five. In M. Ross (ed.), *FM auditory training systems—Characteristics, selection and use*. Timonium, Md.: York Press.

McCandless, G.A., and Lyregaard, P.E. 1983. Prescription of gain/output (POGO) for hearing aids. *Hearing Instruments* 34:16-21.

Moeller, M.P., Donaghy, K., Beauchaine, K., Lewis, D.E., and Stelmachowicz, P.G. 1996. Longitudinal study of FM system use in non-academic settings: Effects an language development. *Ear and Hearing* 17:28-41.

Moodie, K.S., Seewald, R.C., and Sinclair, S.T. 1994. Procedure for predicting real-ear hearing aid performance in young children. *American Journal of Audiology* 3(1):23-31.

Nelson Barlow, N., Auslander, M.C., Rines, D., and Stelmachowicz, P.G. 1988. Probe-tube microphone measures in hearing-impaired children and adults. *Ear and Hearing* 9:243-247.

Revit, L.J. 1991. New tests for signal-processing and multi-channel hearing instruments. *Hearing Journal* 44:20-23.

Revit, L.J. 1994. Using coupler tests in the fitting of hearing aids. In M. Valente (ed.), *Strategies for selecting and verifying hearing aid fittings*. New York: Thieme Medical Publishers.

Robbins, A.M., Renshaw, J.J., and Berry, S.W. 1991. Evaluating meaningful auditory integration in profoundly hearing impaired children. *American Journal of Otology* 12:144-150.

Schwartz, D.M., and Larson, V.D. 1977. A comparison of three hearing aid evaluation procedures for young children. *Archives of Otolaryngology* 103:401-406.

Schwartz, D., Lyregaard, P., and Lundh, P. 1988. Hearing aid selection for severe-to-profound hearing loss. *Hearing Journal* 41:13-17.

Seewald, R.C. 1991. Hearing aid output limiting considerations for children. In J. Feigin and P.G. Stelmachowicz (eds.), *Pediatric amplification: Proceedings of the 1991 national conference*. Omaha: Boys Town National Research Hospital.

Seewald, R.C. 1992. The desired sensation level method for fitting children: Version 3.0. *The Hearing Journal* 45(4):36-41.

Seewald, R.C., Hudson, S.P., Gagné, J.P., and Zelisko, D.L. 1992. Comparison of two procedures for estimating the sensation level of amplified speech. *Ear and Hearing* 13(3):142-149.

Seewald, R.C., Moodie, K.S., Sinclair, S.T., and Cornelisse, L.E. 1996. Traditional and theoretical approaches to selecting amplification for infants and young children. In F.H. Bess, J.S. Gravel, and A.M. Tharpe (eds.), *Amplification for children with auditory deficits*. Nashville, Tenn.: Bill Wilkerson Center Press.

Seewald, R.C., Ramji, K.V., Sinclair, S.T., Moodie, K.S., and Jamieson, D.G. 1993. *Computer-assisted implementation of the desired sensation level method for electroacoustic selection and fitting in children: User's manual*. London, ON: University of Western Ontario.

Seewald, R., and Ross, M. 1988. Amplification for young hearing-impaired children. In M. Pollack (ed.), *Amplification for the hearing impaired*. New York: Grune and Stratton.

Seewald, R.C., Sinclair, S.T., and Moodie, K.S. 1994. Predictive accuracy of a procedure for electroacoustic fitting in young children. Presented at the XXII International Congress of Audiology, July, Halifax.

Sinclair, S.T., Beauchaine, K.L., Moodie, K.S., Feigin, J.A., Seewald, R.C., and Stelmachowicz, P.G. 1994. Repeatability of a real-ear to coupler difference measurement as a function of age. Presented at the American Academy of Audiology Sixth Annual Convention, April, Richmond.

Skinner, M. 1988. *Hearing aid evaluation*. Englewood Cliffs, NJ: Prentice Hall.

Snik, A.F.M., and Stollman, M.H.P. 1995. Measured and calculated insertion gains in young children. *British Journal of Audiology* 29:7-11.

Snik, A.F.M., van den Borne, S., Brokx, J.P.L., and Hoekstra, C. 1995. Hearing aid fitting in profoundly hearing impaired children; comparison of prescription rules. *Scandinavian Audiology*.

Stein, L.K. 1995. On the real age of identification of congenital hearing loss. *Audiology Today* 7(1):10-11.

Stelmachowicz, P.G. 1991. Clinical issues related to hearing aid maximum output. In G.A. Studebaker, F.H. Bess, and L.B. Beck (eds.), *The Vanderbilt hearing-aid report* (pp. 141-148). Parkton: York Press.

Stelmachowicz, P.G., and Lewis, D.E. 1988. Some theoretical considerations concerning the relation between functional gain and insertion gain. *Journal of Speech and Hearing Research* 31:491-496.

Stelmachowicz, P.G., Lewis, D.E., Seewald, R.C., and Hawkins, D.B. 1990. Complex vs. pure-tone stimuli in the evaluation of hearing aid characteristics. *Journal of Speech and Hearing Research* 33:380-385.

Stelmachowicz, P.G., and Seewald, R.C. 1991. Probe-tube microphone measures in children. *Seminars in Hearing* 12:62-72.

Stuart, A., Durieux-Smith, A., and Stenstrom, R. 1991. Probe-tube microphone measures of loudness discomfort levels in children. *Ear and Hearing* 12:140-143.

Tharpe, A.M. 1996. Special considerations for children with fluctuating/progressive hearing loss. In F.H. Bess, J.S. Gravel, and A.M. Tharpe (eds.), *Amplification for children with auditory deficits*. Nashville, Tenn.: Bill Wilkerson Center Press.

Section A
Procedures for calculating target gain and output limiting characteristics for children

A.1 PRESCRIPTION OF GAIN AND OUTPUT (POGO)

POGO was introduced in 1983 by McCandless and Lyregaard. It is based on the following assumptions: (a) frequency-gain response and maximum output limiting are essential characteristics in a basic prescriptive fitting, and (b) a valid prescriptive fitting can be derived based on audiometric information obtained with pure-tone or other stationary signals that will ensure an amplified signal that is audible and delivered at a comfortable listening level.

Required insertion gain is calculated using the formula in table A-1.

Table A-1. POGO formula for calculating required insertion gain.

Frequency (Hz)	Insertion Gain (dB) Formula
250	1/2 HTL - 10
500	1/2 HTL - 5
1000	1/2 HTL
2000	1/2 HTL
3000	1/2 HTL
4000	1/2 HTL

POGO II was introduced in 1987 to prescribe the additional gain required for individuals with severe-to-profound hearing losses. Therefore, for losses greater than 65 dB, the formula shown in table A-2 is used.

Table A-2. POGO II formula for losses greater than 65 dB.

Frequency (Hz)	Insertion Gain (dB) Formula
250	1/2 HTL + 1/2 (HL-65) - 10
500	1/2 HTL + 1/2 (HL-65) - 5
1000	1/2 HTL + 1/2 (HL-65)
2000	1/2 HTL + 1/2 (HL-65)
3000	1/2 HTL + 1/2 (HL-65)
4000	1/2 HTL + 1/2 (HL-65)

RESERVE GAIN

The POGO formula includes a 10-dB reserve gain.

CONDUCTIVE AND/OR MIXED HEARING LOSSES

The POGO formula does not provide recommendations regarding the gain requirements of those with conductive or mixed hearing loss.

MAXIMUM OUTPUT CALCULATIONS

The calculation of hearing aid maximum output characteristics requires the measurement of UCLs at .5, 1, and 2 kHz, and is made using the equation shown in table A-3.

Table A-3. Formula for maximum power output (MPO) calculations (in dB SPL re: 2cc coupler).

$$MPO = \left(\frac{UCL_{500} + UCL_{1000} + UCL_{2000}}{3}\right) + 4$$

DEFINING 2cc COUPLER CRITERIA

Table A-4 provides transformation values to convert the prescribed insertion gain for ITE or BTE hearing aids to 2cc coupler gain. The values shown in this table are subtracted from the POGO desired insertion gain values. To assist in the selection of hearing aids from manufacturer's published specification books, one must add the desired reserve gain across frequencies.

Table A-4. Correction values (in dB) to be subtracted from the POGO insertion gain values to estimate the corresponding 2cc coupler gain as a function of frequency.

	\multicolumn{6}{c}{Frequency (Hz)}
	250	500	1000	2000	3000	4000
ITE	3	1	2	-6	-6	5
BTE	3	1	0	-2	-11	-9

A.2. NATIONAL ACOUSTIC LABORATORIES (NAL) PROCEDURE

The first version of the NAL procedure was introduced in 1976 (Byrne and Tonnison). The rationale of this procedure is to amplify all frequency bands of speech to MCL. In 1986, Byrne and Dillon published a revised version of the NAL procedure (NAL-R). In the revised version, the prescribed real-ear gain is dependent on both degree of hearing loss and slope of hearing thresholds across frequencies. In 1991, the NAL-R procedure was further modified to provide more overall gain for individuals with severe-to-profound hearing losses. The calculation of X has been modified (see line 1, table A-5) to provide more overall gain for mean thresholds over 60 dB HL. In addition, when the threshold at 2 kHz is 95 dB HL or greater, more gain is prescribed in the low frequencies and less gain in the high frequencies.

Required insertion gain is calculated as a function of frequency using the formulas shown in table A-5.

RESERVE GAIN

The NAL formula includes a 15-dB reserve gain to be added to the desired insertion gain values.

Table A-5. NAL-R formulas for calculating required real-ear gain (REG) as a function of frequency modified for severe/profound hearing losses.

1. Calculate $X_{dB} = 0.05 \times (HTL_{500} + HTL_{1000} + HTL_{2000}$ up to 180 dB$) + 0.116 \times$ combined HTL in excess of 180 dB.

2. Calculate the prescribed real-ear gain (REG) at each frequency:

REG_{250} (dB) = $X + 0.31\, HTL_{250} - 17$ REG_{2000} (dB) = $X + 0.31\, HTL_{2000} - 1$
REG_{500} (dB) = $X + 0.31\, HTL_{500} - 8$ REG_{3000} (dB) = $X + 0.31\, HTL_{3000} - 2$
REG_{750} (dB) = $X + 0.31\, HTL_{750} - 3$ REG_{4000} (dB) = $X + 0.31\, HTL_{4000} - 2$
REG_{1000} (dB) = $X + 0.31\, HTL_{1000} + 1$ REG_{6000} (dB) = $X + 0.31\, HTL_{6000} - 2$
REG_{1500} (dB) = $X + 0.31\, HTL_{1500} + 1$

3. When the 2000-Hz HTL is 95-dB or greater, add the following gain (dB) values.

HTL 2 kHz	250	500	750	1000	1500	2000	3000	4000	6000
95	4	3	1	0	-1	-2	-2	-2	-2
100	6	4	2	0	-2	-3	-3	-3	-3
105	8	5	2	0	-3	-5	-5	-5	-5
110	11	7	3	0	-3	-6	-6	-6	-6
115	13	8	4	0	-4	-8	-8	-8	-8
120	15	9	4	0	-5	-9	-9	-9	-9

CONDUCTIVE AND/OR MIXED HEARING LOSSES

For these individuals, additional gain is needed at each frequency, equal to one-fourth of the difference between air- and bone-conduction thresholds.

A.3. DESIRED SENSATION LEVEL (DSL) METHOD

The general rationale of the DSL method is to use a systematic procedure to provide children with hearing loss with an amplified speech signal that is audible, comfortable, and undistorted across the broadest relevant frequency range possible. This method applies age-appropriate individual or average values for relevant acoustic characteristics that are known to vary as a function of

Table A-6. The desired real-ear aided response values (in dB gain)[a] as a function of threshold (dB HL) and audiometric frequency for the DSL method.

Threshold (dB HL)	250	500	750	1000	1500	2000	3000	4000	6000
0	1	2	3	1	4	11	14	13	6
5	1	2	3	2	5	12	16	15	8
10	1	3	4	4	7	15	18	18	10
15	2	4	5	6	10	17	21	20	13
20	3	5	7	9	12	20	24	23	16
25	5	7	9	12	15	23	27	26	19
30	7	9	11	15	18	26	30	30	23
35	10	12	14	18	22	29	34	33	27
40	13	15	17	21	25	32	38	37	31
45	17	18	20	25	29	36	41	40	35
50	20	21	24	28	32	40	45	44	39
55	24	25	28	32	36	43	49	48	43
60	28	28	31	36	40	47	53	52	47
65	32	32	35	39	44	50	57	55	51
70	36	36	39	43	48	54	60	59	55
75	41	40	42	47	51	57	64	63	59
80	44	43	46	50	55	61	67	66	62
85	48	47	50	54	58	64	71	70	66
90	52	50	53	57	62	67	74	73	69
95	55	54	56	60	65	70	76	76	71
100	58	57	59	62	67	72	79	79	73
105	-	60	62	65	70	75	81	81	-
110	-	62	64	67	72	77	83	85	-

[a] The values presented in this table assume a real-ear unaided response (REUR) approximating published average adult values (Shaw and Vaillancourt 1985). Furthermore, if audiometric data have been collected using 3A insert earphones (in dB HL), the above values assume an average adult real-ear-to-coupler difference.

age—specifically, external ear resonance characteristics and real-ear-to-2cc coupler differences (RECD). A computer-assisted implementation of the DSL method is available.

DESIRED REAL-EAR AIDED RESPONSE VALUES (in dB gain) AS A FUNCTION OF THRESHOLD (dB HL)

The real-ear aided response values, in dB gain, required to amplify the long-term speech spectrum to the desired sensation levels as a function of threshold (dB HL) and audiometric frequency are shown in table A-6.

Estimated real-ear-to-2cc coupler difference (RECD) values as a function of age are shown in table A-7. These age-appropriate estimated RECD values can be used when individual RECD measures cannot be obtained. The use of these values to derive corresponding 2cc coupler targets enables hearing aid electroacoustic response shaping to occur in the hearing aid test chamber.

Table A-7. Estimated real-ear-to-2cc coupler difference (RECD) transformations as a function of age and audiometric frequency.

A. HA-1 coupler

Frequency (Hz)

	250	500	750	1000	1500	2000	3000	4000	6000
0-12 months	5.4	9.8	10.0	13.0	14.4	14.5	18.5	21.6	22.4
13-24 months	7.3	10.2	9.9	12.6	13.7	14.2	16.1	18.5	15.5
25-48 months	4.0	8.5	8.7	11.8	13.2	13.2	15.5	16.2	15.4
49-60 months	2.8	8.0	8.5	9.8	11.9	12.7	14.0	15.0	14.8
> 60 months[a]	2.2	4.6	4.3	6.3	7.7	8.8	11.2	13.1	13.7

B. HA-2 coupler

Frequency (Hz)

	250	500	750	1000	1500	2000	3000	4000	6000
0-12 months	5.5	9.7	9.6	11.9	11.6	10.5	16.2	19.4	17.8
13-24 months	7.4	10.1	9.5	11.5	10.9	10.2	13.8	16.3	10.9
25-48 months	4.1	8.4	8.3	10.7	10.4	9.2	13.2	14.0	10.8
49-60 months	2.9	7.9	8.1	8.7	9.1	8.7	11.7	12.8	10.2
> 60 months	2.3	4.5	3.9	5.2	4.9	4.8	8.9	10.9	9.1

[a]Values for individuals > 60 months were derived by Seewald, Ramji, Sinclair, Moodie, and Jamieson (1993), at the University of Western Ontario. Values for individuals < 60 months were derived by applying age group data reported by Feigin, Kopun, Stelmachowicz, and Gorga (1989) to the values of Seewald and colleagues. HA-2 coupler values were derived by applying an HA-1 to HA-2 coupler transformation (Seewald et al. 1993) to the HA-1 coupler values.

Table A-8. The one-third octave band levels (dB SPL) of the University of Western Ontario long-term average speech spectrum for hearing aid fitting in children.

	Frequency (Hz)								
	250	500	750	1000	1500	2000	3000	4000	6000
dB SPL	62.8	64.3	60.1	56.4	52.1	51.0	45.0	42.3	42.1

THE DSL UNAMPLIFIED LONG-TERM AVERAGE SPEECH SPECTRUM

The DSL unamplified speech spectrum attempts to strike a compromise between the average speech levels of potential conversational partners and the average speech levels of a child's own speech productions at the ear-level position. The overall level of the DSL long-term average speech spectrum (LTASS) is 70 dB SPL. The DSL unamplified LTASS levels are shown in table A-8 as a function of frequency.

RESERVE GAIN

The DSL method currently applies 12 dB or reserve gain.

CONDUCTIVE AND/OR MIXED HEARING LOSSES

The DSL method does not currently provide recommendations regarding additional gain requirements for individuals with conductive or mixed hearing loss.

DESIRED REAL-EAR MAXIMUM SOUND-PRESSURE LEVEL (SPL) VALUES (in dB) AS A FUNCTION OF THRESHOLD (dB HL).

The desired real-ear maximum SPL values as a function of threshold (dB HL) and audiometric frequency are shown in table A-9.

DEFINING 2cc COUPLER CRITERIA

The DSL worksheets on pages 426 and 427 provide information on how to calculate 2cc coupler gain criteria for the purposes of electroacoustic selection and fitting.

Table A-9. The desired real-ear maximum sound-pressure level (SPL) values (in dB)[a] as a function of threshold (dB HL) and audiometric frequency for the DSL method.

Threshold (dB HL)	250	500	750	1000	1500	2000	3000	4000	6000
0	94	102	101	99	99	100	100	98	97
5	94	102	101	99	99	101	100	99	97
10	94	102	101	100	100	102	101	100	98
15	95	103	102	101	100	103	102	101	98
20	95	103	102	101	101	104	103	102	99
25	96	104	103	103	102	105	105	103	100
30	97	105	104	104	104	106	106	104	101
35	99	106	106	105	105	108	108	106	103
40	100	107	107	107	107	110	110	108	105
45	102	109	109	109	109	112	112	109	106
50	104	111	110	110	111	114	114	111	108
55	106	113	112	112	113	116	116	113	111
60	109	115	114	114	115	118	118	115	113
65	111	117	117	117	117	120	120	118	115
70	114	119	119	119	119	122	123	120	117
75	117	121	121	121	121	124	125	122	120
80	120	123	123	123	123	126	127	124	122
85	123	126	125	125	125	128	129	126	124
90	126	128	127	127	127	130	130	128	125
95	129	130	129	129	129	131	132	130	127
100	132	131	131	130	131	133	133	132	128
105	-	133	132	131	132	134	135	133	-
110	-	134	134	133	133	135	136	135	-

[a] See note at end of table A-6.

A.4 REFERENCES

POGO

McCandless, G.A. 1994. Overview and rationale of threshold-based hearing aid selection procedures. In M. Valente (ed.), *Strategies for selecting and verifying hearing aid fittings*. New York: Thieme Medical Publishers.

McCandless, G.A., and Lyregaard, P.E. 1983. Prescription of gain and output (POGO) for hearing aids. *Hearing Instruments* 3:16-21.

Schwartz, D., Lyregaard, P.E., and Lundh, P. 1988. Hearing aid selection for severe-to-profound hearing loss. *Hearing Journal* 41(2):13-17.

NAL

Battaglia, D., Dillon, H., and Byrne, D. 1991. *HASP: Version 2 user's manual.* Chatswood, Australia: The National Acoustics Laboratories.

Byrne, D., and Dillon, H. 1986. The National Acoustic Laboratories' (NAL) research for hearing aid gain and frequency response selection strategies. In G.A. Studebaker and I. Hochberg (eds.), *Acoustical factors affecting hearing aid performance* (2d ed.). Boston: Allyn and Bacon.

Byrne, D., Parkinson, A., and Newall, P. 1991. Modified hearing aid selection procedure for severe-profound hearing losses. In G.A. Studebaker, F.H. Bess, and L.B. Beck (eds.), *The Vanderbilt hearing-aid report II.* Parkton, Md.: York Press.

Byrne, D., and Tonisson, W. 1976. Selecting the gain of hearing aids for persons with sensorineural hearing impairments. *Scandinavian Audiology* 5:51-59.

DSL

Feigin, J.A., Kopun, J.G., Stelmachowicz, P.G., and Gorga, M.P. 1989. Probe-tube microphone measures of ear-canal sound pressure levels in infants and children. *Ear and Hearing* 10(4):254-258.

Seewald, R.C. 1992. The desired sensation level method for fitting children: Version 3.0. *Hearing Journal* 45(4):36-41.

Seewald, R.C., Ramji, K.V., Sinclair, S.T., Moodie, K.S., and Jamieson, D.G. 1993. *Computer-assisted implementation of the desired sensation level method for electroacoustic selection and fitting in children: User's manual.* London, ON: University of Western Ontario.

Seewald, R.C., Ross, M., and Spiro, M.K. 1985. Selecting amplification characteristics for young hearing-impaired children. *Ear and Hearing* 6(1):48-53.

Shaw, E.A., and Vaillancourt, M.M. 1985. Transformation of sownd-pressure level from the free field to the eardrum presented in numerical form. *Journal of the Acoustical Society of America* 78(3):1120-1123.

424 • APPENDIX 1

Worksheet #1: Calculating target 2cc coupler gain values as a function of frequency.

	250	500	750	1000	1500	2000	3000	4000	6000
Threshold (dB HL)									
Desired real-ear aided response									
RECD values									
Mic effects*									
Target coupler gain (row 2-3-4)									
Measured coupler gain									
Difference (row 5-6)									

* **Mic location effect values** as a function of hearing aid type and audiometric frequency.

Frequency (Hz)

	250	500	750	1000	1500	2000	3000	4000	6000
BTE	0.5	1.2	0.9	0.3	2.5	4.1	2.8	3.7	1.6
ITE	0.5	1.8	2.0	1.5	-0.3	3.8	3.3	4.3	0.4
ITC	0.3	0	0.4	1.2	-1.9	2.1	3.5	6.4	-1.8
BODY AID	3.0	4.0	2.0	0	-4	-4	0	0	0

1. Enter the individual's hearing threshold measures as a function of frequency.
2. Using table A-6, determine the desired real-ear aided response as a function of frequency and hearing threshold level. For example, if the audiometric threshold at 250 Hz is 30 dB HL, the desired real-ear aided response (in gain) is 7 dB.
3. Enter the individual's measured RECD values. If measured values cannot be obtained, use estimated age-appropriate RECD values as a function of frequency from table A-7A for ITE fittings and table A-7B for BTE fittings.
4. Enter the appropriate mic location effect values as a function of hearing aid style.
5. To determine the target 2cc coupler gain values across frequencies, subtract the RECD and mic location effect values from the desired real-ear aided response values (row 2-3-4).
6. Using the frequency-specific University of Western Ontario (UWO) LTASS values from table A-8 as a guideline for test signal input levels, adjust the electroacoustic characteristics of the hearing aid in the hearing aid test chamber to approximate the target 2cc coupler values as a function of frequency. For example, using a 50-dB stimulus level, adjust the volume control wheel to approximate the target 2cc gain at 2000 Hz. Using a 65-dB stimulus level, adjust the hearing aid tone control to approximate the target 2cc gain at 500 Hz. (Note: for linear and output compression hearing aids, set maximum output characteristics before setting the hearing aid gain/frequency response characteristics.)

Worksheet #2: Calculating target saturation SPL (SSPL) values as a function of frequency.

	250	500	750	1000	1500	2000	3000	4000	6000
Threshold (dB HL)									
Desired real-ear maximum SPL									
RECD values									
Target coupler SSPL (row 2-3)									
Measured coupler gain									
Difference (row 3-4)									

1. Enter the individual's hearing threshold measures as a function of frequency.
2. Using table A-9, determine the desired real-ear maximum SPL (dB) as a function of frequency and hearing threshold level. For example, if the audiometric threshold at 250 Hz is 30 dB HL, the desired maximum SPL (dB) is 97.
3. Enter the individual's measured RECD values. If measured values cannot be obtained, use estimated age-appropriate RECD values as a function of frequency from table A-7.
4. To determine the target SSPL values across frequencies, subtract the RECD values from the desired real-ear maximum SPL values (row 2-3).
5. With the hearing aid volume control wheel adjusted to a full-on position, place the hearing aid in the hearing aid test chamber. Using a 90-dB stimulus level, look for the primary peak in the hearing aid response. Adjust the hearing aid maximum output control so that it does not exceed the target coupler SSPL value for that frequency.
6. Using a 90-dB pure-tone stimulus level, enter the measured coupler SSPL values as a function of frequency.
7. Determine the difference between the target and measured SSPL values.
8. Once the hearing aid maximum output characteristics have been adjusted to approximate the 2cc target values, the frequency gain characteristics should be quickly re-evaluated to ensure that adjustments are not necessary. In addition, if the hearing aid being fitted is a compression instrument, an evaluation of the compression characteristics at user's settings should be conducted.

Section B
Common Speech Recognition Materials Used with Children

Table 1. Common speech recognition materials used with children. Children's lists.

Test name	Investigator(s)	Material	Number of lists	Items per list	Response format	Response task	Age range	Degree of HL
1. PBK-50	Haskins (1949)	Monosyllables	4	50	Open set	Verbal	6-9 years	Mild to moderate
2. Word Intelligibility by Picture Identification (WIPI)	Ross & Lerman (1970)	Monosyllables	4	25	Closed set (6 picture matrix)	Psycho-motor	3-6 years	Mild to severe
3. Sound Effects Recognition Test (SERT)	Finitzo-Hieber, Gerlin, Matkin, Cherow-Skalka (1980)	Environmental Sounds	3	10	Closed set (4 picture matrix)	Psycho-motor	≥3 years	Severe to profound
4. Spondee Recognition Test	Erber (1974)	Spondees	1	25	Closed set	Written	8-16 years	Severe to profound
5. Six Sound Test	Ling (1978, 1989)	Vowels /u/, /a/, /I/, /ʃ/, /s/, /m/	1	6	Open set	Psycho-motor	Infant/children	Moderate to profound
6. Glendonald Auditory Screening Procedure (GASP)	Erber (1982)	Phonemes Words Sentences	1 1 1	10 12 10	Closed set	Psycho-motor and verbal	6-13 years	Moderate to profound
7. Children's Perception of Speech (NUCHIPS)	Katz & Elliott (1978)	Monosyllables	4 randomizations	50	Closed set	Psycho-motor	≥3 years	Mild to moderate
8. Discrimination by the Identification of Pictures (DIP)	Siegenthaler & Haspiel (1966)	Monosyllables	3	48	Closed set (2 picture matrix)	Psycho-motor	3-8 years	Mild to severe
9. BKB sentences	Bench, Koval, & Bamford (1979)	Sentences	21 11	16 16	Open set	Verbal	8-15 years	Mild to moderate

Table 1 (continued). Common speech recognition materials used with children. Children's lists.

Test name	Investigator(s)	Material	Number of lists	Items per list	Response format	Response task	Age range	Degree of HL
10. Auditory Numbers Test (ANT)	Erber (1980)	Numbers	1	5	Closed set	Psycho-motor	3-8 years	Severe to profound
11. Pediatric Speech Intelligibility Test (PSI)	Jerger, Lewis, Hawkins, & Jerger (1980)	Monosyllables Sentences	1 2	20 10	Closed set	Verbal	3-10 years	Mild to moderate
12. Hoosier Auditory Visual Enhancement Test (HAVE)	Renshaw, Robbins, Miyamoto, Osberger, & Pope (1988)	Monosyllables	1	40	Closed set	Verbal/ Sign	≥2 years	Mild to profound
13. Minimal Pairs Test	Robbins, Renshaw, Miyamoto, Osberger, & Pope (1988)	Monosyllables	2	80	Closed set	Psycho-motor	≥5 years	Mild to profound
14. Imitative tests of Speech Pattern Contrast Perception (IMSPAC)	Boothroyd, Eran, & Hanin (1996)	Syllables	4 (plus random-izations)	40	Auditors: Closed set	Child: Imitation	≥3 years	Mild to profound
15. Three Interval Force Choice Test of Speech Pattern Contrast Perception (THRIFT)	Boothroyd (in press)	Syllables	1 (plus random-izations)	54 or 108	Choose odd one of 3	Pointing, Button-press, or verbal	≥7 years	Mild to profound
16. Arthur Boothroyd Lists (AB lists)	Boothroyd (1968)	Phonemes in CVC words	15	30 phonemes	Open set	Verbal/ Written	≥4 years	Mild to profound

Table 1 (continued). Common speech recognition materials used with children. Adult lists.

Test name	Investigator(s)	Material	Number of lists	Items per list	Response format	Response task	Age range	Degree of HL
1. Northwestern University Auditory Test No. 6 (NU-6)	Tillman & Carhart (1966)	Monosyllables	4	50	Open set	Verbal/Written	≥9 years	Mild to moderate
2. Central Institute for the Deaf W-22 (CID W-22)	Hirsh et al. (1952)	Monosyllables	20	50	Open set	Verbal/Written	≥7 years	Mild to moderate
3. Nonsense Syllable Test (NST)	Levitt & Resnick (1978)	Syllables	16 (7 subtests within a list)	62	Closed set	Written	≥6 years	Mild to moderate

REFERENCES

Bench, J., Koval, A., and Bamford, J. 1979. The BKB (Bamford-Koval-Bench) sentence lists for partially-hearing children. *British Journal of Audiology* 13:108-112.

Boothroyd, A. 1968. Developments of speech audiometry. *Sound* 2:3-10.

Boothroyd, A., Eran, O., and Hanin, L. 1996. Speech perception and production in children with hearing impairment. In F.H. Bess, J.S. Gravel, and A.M. Tharpe (eds.), *Amplification for children with auditory deficits*. Nashville, Tenn.: Bill Wilkerson Center Press.

Boothroyd, A. In press. Speech perception tests and hearing-impaired children. In G. Plant and C.E. Spens (eds.), *Speech communication and profound deafness*. London: Whurr Publishers.

Erber, N.P. 1974. Pure-tone thresholds and word-recognition abilities of hearing-impaired children. *Journal of Speech and Hearing Research* 17:194-202.

Erber, N.P. 1980. Use of the auditory numbers test to evaluate speech perception abilities of hearing-impaired children. *Journal of Speech and Hearing Disorders* 45:527-532.

Erber, N.P. 1982. *Auditory training*. Washington, D.C.: Alexander Graham Bell Association for the Deaf.

Finitzo-Hieber, T., Gerlin, I.J., Matkin, N.D., and Cherow-Skalka, E. 1980. A sound effects recognition test for the pediatric evaluation. *Ear and Hearing* 1:271-276.

Haskins, H.A. 1949. A phonetically balanced test of speech discrimination for children. Master's thesis, Northwestern University: Evanston, Illinois.

Hirsh, I.J., Davis, H., Silverman, S.R., Reynolds, E.G., Eldert, E., and Bensen, R.W. 1952. Development of materials for speech audiometry. *Journal of Speech and Hearing Disorders* 17:321-337.

Jerger, S., Lewis, S., Hawkins, J., and Jerger, J. 1980. Pediatric speech intelligibility test: I. Generation of test materials. *International Journal of Pediatric Otorhinolaryngology* 2: 217-230.

Katz, D.R., and Elliott, L.L. 1978. Development of a new children's speech discrimination test. Paper presented at the convention of the American Speech and Hearing Association, November 18-21, Chicago.

Levitt, H., and Resnick, S.B. 1978. Speech reception by the hearing impaired: Methods of testing and the development of new tests. *Scandinavian Audiology* 6 (Suppl.):107-130.

Ling, D. 1978. Auditory coding and reading—an analysis of training procedures for hearing impaired children. In M. Ross and T.G. Giolas (eds.), *Auditory management of hearing-impaired children* (pp. 181-218). Baltimore, Md.: University Park Press.

Ling, D. 1989. *Foundations of spoken language for hearing-impaired children*. Washington, D.C.: Alexander Graham Bell Association for the Deaf.

Renshaw, J., Robbins, A.M., Miyamoto, R., Osberger, M.J., and Pope, M. 1988. *Hoosier Auditory Visual Enhancement Test (HAVE)*. Indianapolis: Indiana University School of Medicine, Department of Otolaryngology—Head and Neck Surgery.

Robbins, A.M., Renshaw, J., Miyamoto, R., Osberger, M.J., and Pope, M. 1988. *Minimal Pairs Test*. Indianapolis: Indiana University School of Medicine, Department of Otolaryngology—Head and Neck Surgery.

Ross, M., and Lerman, J. 1970. A picture identification test for hearing impaired children. *Journal of Speech and Hearing Research* 13:44-53.

Siegenthaler, B., and Haspiel, G. 1966. Development of two standardized measures of hearing for speech by children. Project no. OE-5-10-003. Washington, D.C.: U.S. Department of Health, Education, and Welfare.

Tillman, T.W., and Carhart, R. 1966. An expanded test for speech discrimination utilizing CNC monosyllabic words. Northwestern University Auditory Test no. 6. Technical Report no. SAM-TR-66-55. Brooks Air Force Base, Tex.: USAF School of Aerospace Medicine.

Appendix 2

Case Study: Amplification in Children

Sheila T. Sinclair, K. Shane Moodie, and Richard C. Seewald

BACKGROUND

  The specific approach used at the University of Western Ontario (UWO) hearing clinic for hearing aid fitting in infants and young children applies the desired sensation level (DSL) method (Seewald 1992, 1994). Clinical implementation of this method is facilitated by the DSL version 3.1 software system (Seewald, Ramji, Sinclair, Moodie, and Jamieson 1993). The method specifies frequency specific desired sensation levels for amplified speech for all degrees of sensorineural hearing loss. Hearing aid gain characteristics are chosen to amplify the average long-term speech spectrum to the DSLs across frequencies. The method also provides clinicians with desired hearing aid maximum output target values that are derived from the child's hearing threshold levels.

  One primary advantage of this method is that acoustic factors unique to each child can be accounted for in the amplification selection and fitting process. These factors include the real-ear unaided response (REUR) and the real-ear-to-2cc-coupler difference (RECD). The RECD can be defined as the difference in dB between the level of sound measured in a real ear versus a 2cc coupler across frequencies. In young children, the difference between the absolute sound pressure levels (SPLs) measured in the real ear and the coupler will be greater than average values for adults and have been shown to vary as a function of age (Feigin, Kopun, Stelmachowicz, and Gorga 1989). The RECD measurement procedure implemented at the UWO hearing clinic is described by Moodie, Seewald, and Sinclair (1994).

  A hearing aid prescription is generated by the DSL software system on the basis of the audiometric and acoustic test results entered for a given child. This prescription is developed in the following manner. First, the audiometric data are applied in deriving a set of real-ear hearing aid performance criteria for gain and output limiting across frequencies. Second, the child's RECD values are applied in transforming the real-ear performance criteria to the 2cc coupler. In this way, the child's own real-ear-to-2cc-coupler transfer function, which includes the acoustic effects of his or her earmold coupling, is accounted for in developing performance criteria for 2cc coupler-based measures.

With the DSL software system, verification of hearing aid performance can be performed using a variety of procedures by comparing the measured electroacoustic performance with the recommended set of electroacoustic performance criteria for each child. In addition to probe microphone measures of real-ear hearing aid performance, the DSL software system provides the clinician with the option to verify hearing aid performance in the 2cc coupler. This verification option can be used to predict real-ear hearing aid performance and has been shown to be valid when it incorporates an individual measurement of the child's RECD (Seewald, Sinclair, and Moodie 1994). The primary advantage of this approach to verification with young children is that they are not required to cooperate for extended periods of time.

CASE STUDY

L.C. was initially referred to the UWO hearing clinic for an audiologic assessment at 14 months of age. Test results revealed a severe sensorineural hearing loss bilaterally. L.C. returned to our clinic within ten days of the initial assessment to allow time for fabrication of custom earmolds. The hearing aid selection and fitting process was initiated at this second visit by obtaining a measurement of L.C.'s RECD with her new earmolds. The RECD values obtained for L.C.'s right ear are shown in figure 1. In this figure, all positive values indicate the extent to which the SPL, in dB, measured in the real ear exceed the SPL measured in an HA-2/2cc coupler. The RECD values that were measured for L.C. at 14 months ranged from 5 dB at 250 Hz to 18 dB at 4000 Hz.

L.C.'s audiologic test results and RECD values were entered into the DSL: version 3.1 software system. Desired 2cc coupler frequency/gain and maximum output characteristics were derived for a behind-the-ear (BTE) hearing aid fitting. Hearing aids were selected for L.C. after several hearing aids were evaluated in an electroacoustic analyzer to determine which instrument provided the best approximation to the performance criteria for both gain and output limiting. The final results of this electroacoustic shaping process were subsequently entered into the DSL software system.

Figure 2 shows the aided SPL-O-GRAM with the hearing aid adjusted to the recommended settings. The electroacoustic verification results plotted

APPENDIX 2 • 433

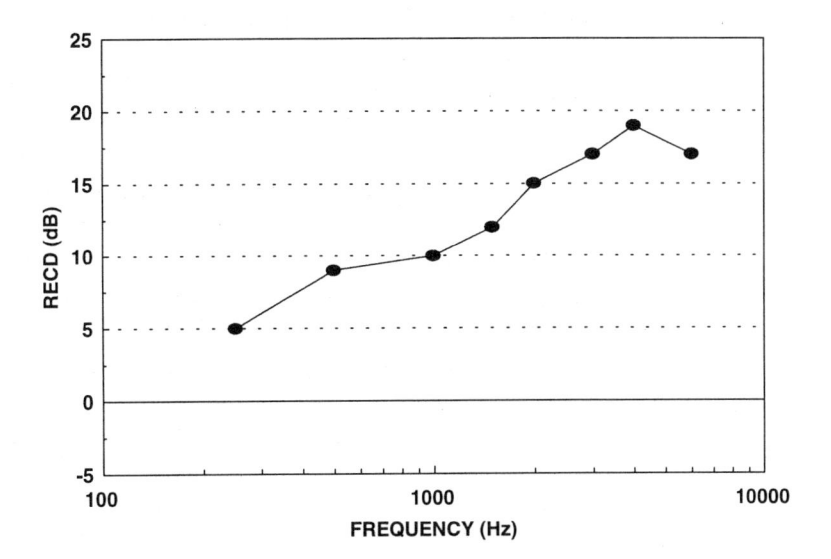

Figure 1. The real-ear-to-coupler difference (RECD) values measured, in dB, at 14 months of age using the procedure described in Moodie, Seewald, and Sinclair (1994). All positive values indicate the extent to which the SPLs measured in the child's ear canal exceeded those that were measured in an HA-2/2cc coupler.

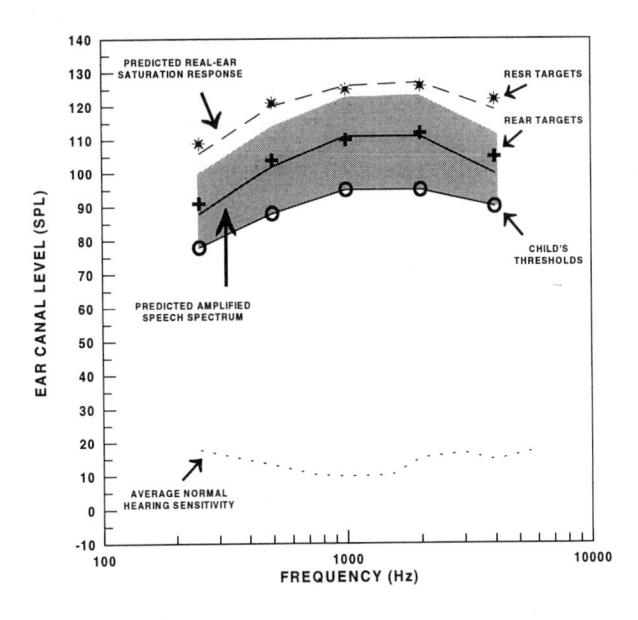

Figure 2. Predicted real-ear hearing aid performance at 14 months of age illustrated in an aided SPL-O-GRAM format. All variables including average normal hearing sensitivity, L.C.'s thresholds, target and predicted amplified speech spectrum, and target and predicted saturation response values are plotted in dB SPL (ear canal level).

in this format illustrate that a reasonable approximation has been achieved between the target values for the real-ear aided response (REAR) and real-ear saturation response (RESR) and the predicted real-ear performance of the selected instrument.

This family lived a substantial distance from our facility. Therefore, it was recommended that L.C. be followed by an audiologist in her home community. Conventional unaided and sound field aided threshold testing was conducted by the local audiologist at 15 months of age. Results obtained for the right ear are shown in figure 3 and were generally consistent with our own test findings and with the performance we would have predicted for the recommended hearing aid.

L.C. obtained new earmolds at 20 and 29 months of age. When L.C. was approximately 32 months of age, her parents expressed concern to the local audiologist that she was not performing as well as she had been with amplification. An audiologic assessment was conducted within one week and indicated that no significant change in L.C.'s unaided hearing threshold levels had occurred. Figure 4A shows a comparison of the unaided test results obtained for the right ear at 15 and 32 months of age. Impedance test findings were within normal limits for both ears. Also, an electroacoustic analysis of L.C.'s hearing aids indicated that they were operating within manufacturer's specifications. In addition, the audiologist ensured that both

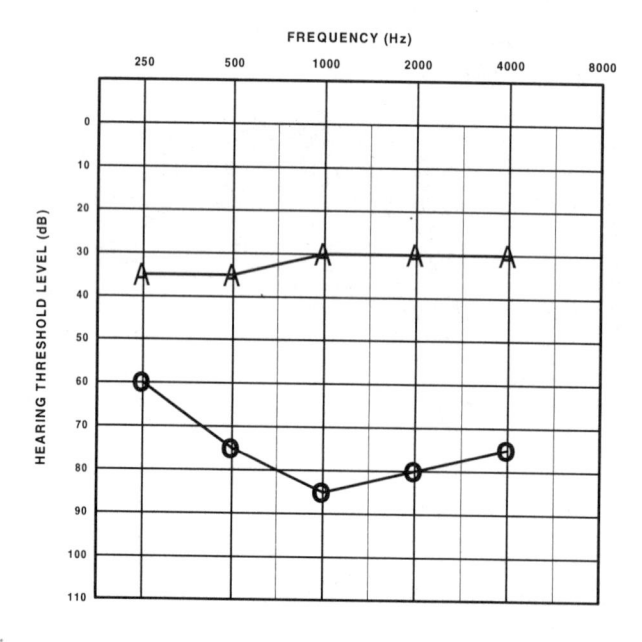

Figure 3. Monaural unaided (o) and sound field aided (A) thresholds, in dB HL, measured at 15 months of age.

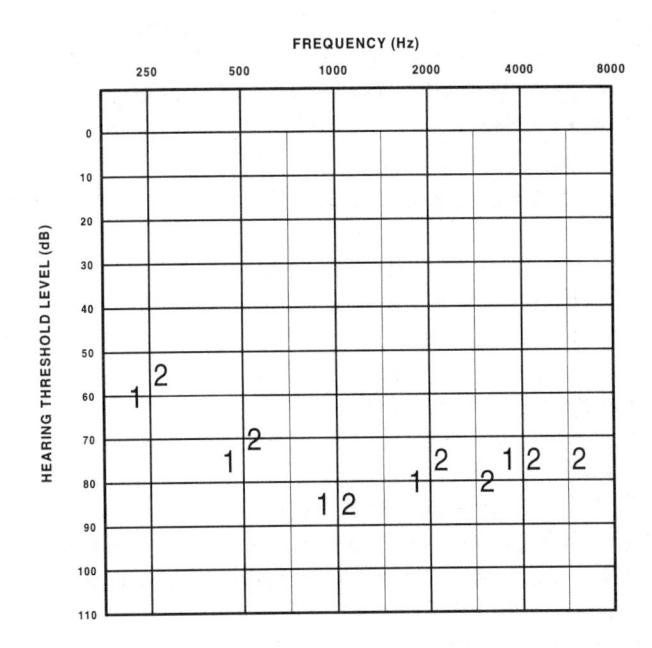

Figure 4A. Monaural unaided hearing threshold levels, in dB HL, obtained at 15 months (1) and 32 months (2) of age.

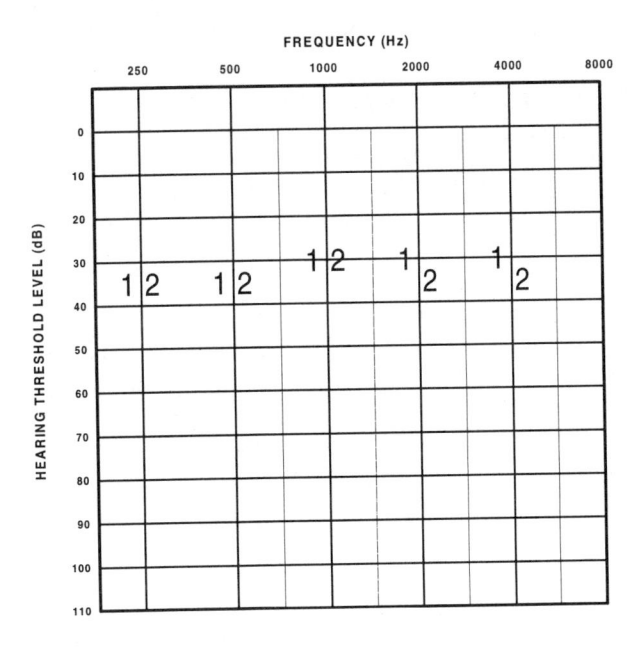

Figure 4B. Sound field aided threshold test results, in dB HL, obtained at 15 months (1) and 32 months (2) of age.

hearing aids were adjusted properly to the recommended settings. Finally, to evaluate her aided performance, sound field aided threshold testing was conducted. Figure 4B compares the sound field aided test results obtained at 15 and 32 months for the right ear. On the basis of the sound field aided threshold test results, the audiologist concluded that "there is no indication of significant change in L.C.'s aided performance with her current hearing aids."

Due to their continued concern regarding L.C.'s auditory performance with amplification, the parents requested a reevaluation at the UWO hearing clinic. A reevaluation was scheduled for L.C. at 33 months of age. The audiologic assessment performed at the UWO hearing clinic indicated no significant change had occurred in L.C.'s unaided hearing threshold levels for either ear. Electroacoustic impedance test findings were again within normal limits. Similar to her previous visit at 14 months of age, a measurement of L.C.'s RECD was obtained for both ears. Results of this measurement obtained for the right ear are shown in figure 5. As shown in this figure, L.C.'s RECD values at 33 months of age ranged from -1 dB at 250 Hz to 9 dB at 4000 Hz. For comparative purposes, the RECD values that were measured for L.C.'s right ear at 14 months of age have also been included in this figure. A substantial difference between these two sets of RECD values can be observed. Overall, the average difference between these two sets of RECD values is 9 dB. These differences can be attributed primarily to changes in the acoustic properties of the earmold coupling and growth of the external ear canal.

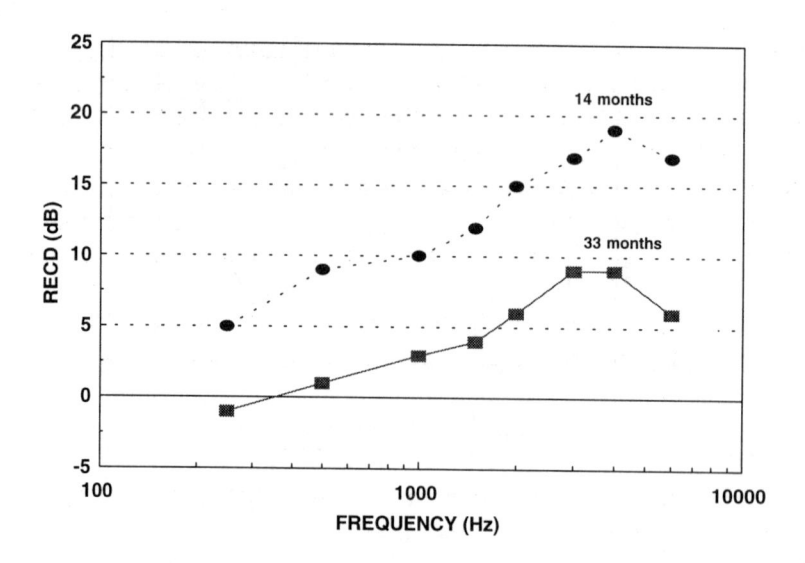

Figure 5. The RECD values, in dB, measured at 33 months of age (■). The RECD values measured at 14 months of age (●) are also shown.

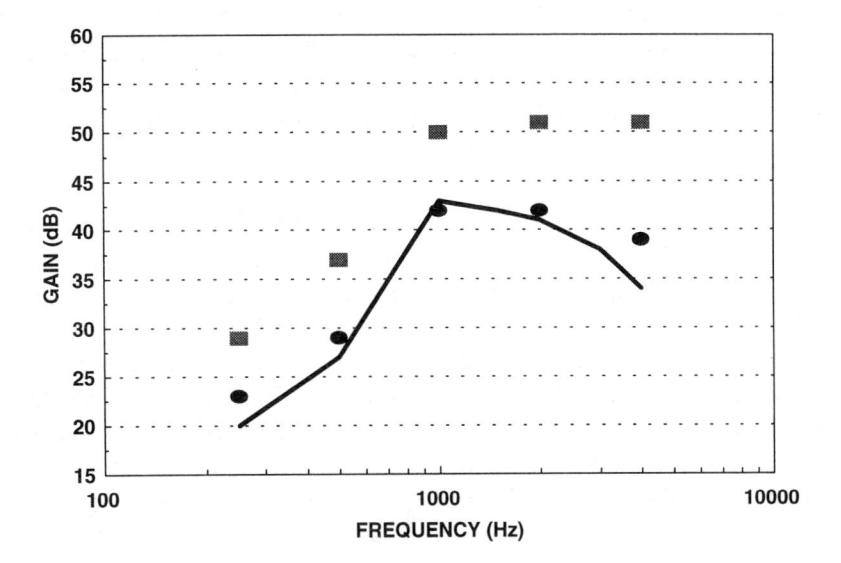

Figure 6. Target (●) and measured (■) 2cc coupler gain values obtained at 14 months of age as a function of frequency. Target (■) 2cc coupler gain values derived for 33 months of age as a function of frequency.

Recall that the DSL software system derives a set of individualized target 2cc coupler gain values as a function of frequency. The 2cc coupler gain target values and the measured frequency/gain characteristics obtained for L.C. at 14 months of age are shown in figure 6. The target 2cc coupler gain characteristics derived for L.C. at 33 months of age have also been plotted in this figure. Note that the target 2cc coupler gain values that are prescribed for L.C. at 33 months of age are significantly higher at all frequencies. For example, the target gain value at 4000 Hz is approximately 10 dB higher at 33 months of age than it was for 14 months of age. The difference in desired 2cc coupler gain characteristics can be attributed to the decrease in L.C.'s RECD values that occurred during the intervening 19 months. Consequently, as illustrated in figure 6, the gain measured in a 2cc coupler must be increased to maintain the same real-ear output that had been achieved at the time of the initial fitting. *Thus, while L.C.'s unaided hearing threshold levels had remained stable, her amplification needs had changed over time.*

Similarly, the real-ear maximum output characteristics of L.C.'s hearing aid also changed over time because of the decrease in the RECD values. The solid circles in figure 7 are the target 2cc coupler SSPL characteristics prescribed for L.C. at 14 months. The SSPL curve obtained at that time is shown by the solid line. The SSPL targets derived for L.C. at 33

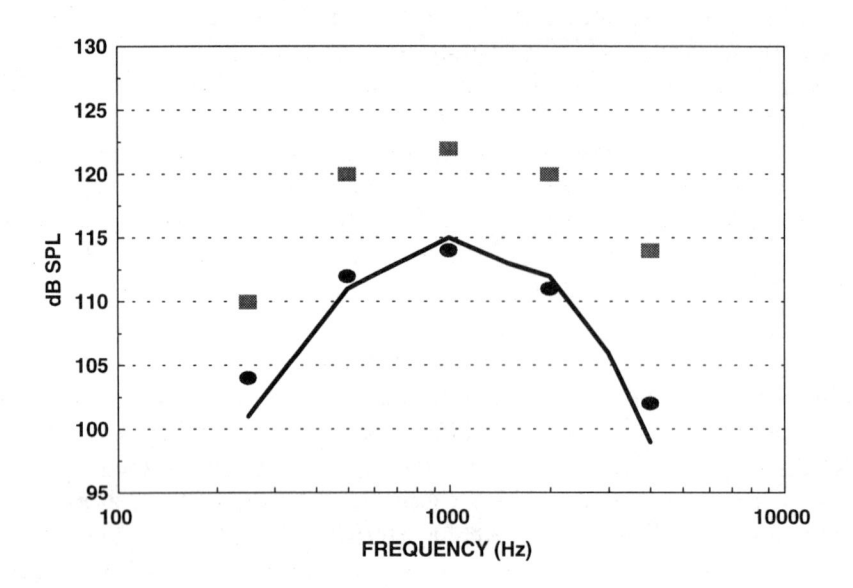

Figure 7. Target (●) and measured (■) 2cc coupler saturation response (SSPL) values obtained at 14 months of age as a function of frequency. Target (■) 2cc coupler saturation response (SSPL) values derived for 33 months of age as a function of frequency.

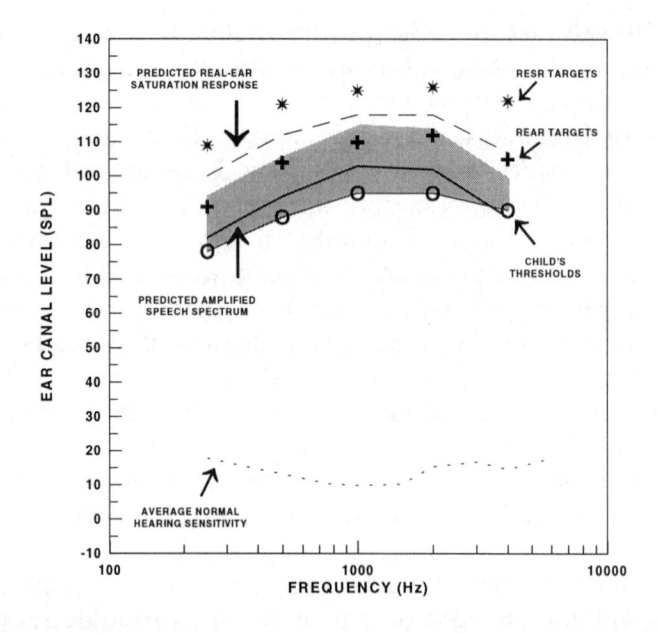

Figure 8. Predicted real-ear hearing aid performance at 33 months of age illustrated in an aided SPL-O-GRAM format. All variables including average normal hearing sensitivity, L.C.'s thresholds, target and predicted amplified speech spectrum, and target and predicted real-ear saturation response values are plotted in dB SPL (ear canal level).

months of age are shown in figure 7 as shaded squares. It can be seen that an increase in the SSPLs, measured in a 2cc coupler, is required at 33 months to match the real-ear saturation response that was obtained with L.C. at 14 months of age.

The implications of the change that had taken place, in terms of real-ear hearing aid performance, are best illustrated in the SPL-O-GRAM format. The results obtained with L.C. at 33 months were entered into the DSL software system including her unaided thresholds, RECD values, and the results of 2cc coupler-based measures of gain and output limiting. Figure 8 shows the real-ear hearing aid performance in terms of the predicted levels of amplified speech and the predicted RESR. The results shown on this SPL-O-GRAM can be compared to those shown in figure 2. Note that the predicted levels at which amplified speech will be received as well as the RESR of L.C.'s hearing aid are lower overall relative to the predicted real-ear performance obtained at the time of the initial fitting. The differences that can be observed in the real-ear performance of L.C.'s hearing aid at 14 and at 33 months are entirely consistent with the parental observation of a reduction in auditory performance. Consequently, appropriate adjustments were made to the hearing aids.

SUMMARY

1. Conventional measures of auditory and electroacoustic performance were insensitive to a change in the amplification condition that had occurred for this child.
2. Parental concern regarding a decrease in auditory performance over time can be attributed to a change in the earmold and growth of the external auditory canal.
3. In amplification-related work with preschool children, it can be assumed that the basic electroacoustic characteristics of their hearing aids, as measured in a 2cc coupler, will need to be modified to maintain consistent real-ear hearing aid performance over the first years of life.

REFERENCES

Feigin, J.A., Kopun, J.G., Stelmachowicz, P.G., and Gorga, M.P. 1989. Probe-tube microphone measures of ear-canal sound pressure levels in infants and children. *Ear and Hearing* 10:254-258.

Moodie, K.S., Seewald, R.C., and Sinclair, S.T. 1994. Procedure for predicting real-ear hearing aid performance in young children. *American Journal of Audiology* 3(1):23-31.

Seewald, R.C. 1992. The desired sensation level method for fitting children: Version 3.0. *Hearing Journal* 45(4):36-41.

Seewald, R.C. 1994. Fitting children with the DSL method. *Hearing Journal* 47(9):10, 48-51.
Seewald, R.C., Ramji, K.V., Sinclair, S.T., Moodie, K.S., and Jamieson, D.G. 1993. *Computer-assisted implementation of the desired sensation level method for electroacoustic selection and fitting in children: User's manual.* London, Ontario: University of Western Ontario.
Seewald, R.C., Sinclair, S.T., and Moodie, K.S. 1994. Predictive accuracy of a procedure for electroacoustic fitting in young children. Presented at American Academy of Audiology Sixth Annual convention, April, Richmond.

Appendix 3

Clinical Grand Rounds

At the conclusion of the Symposium, a panel composed of six of the conference speakers was convened for the purpose of presenting and discussing four cases of children with hearing loss. Each was selected from the presenter's own practice and was chosen by the speaker to highlight and make clinically relevant many of the issues and concepts that had been presented over the course of the Symposium. The four speakers were Richard Seewald, Ph.D., Jackson Roush, Ph.D., Anne Marie Tharpe, Ph.D., and Carol Flexer, Ph.D., Carolyn Edwards, M.Cl.Sc., and Judith Gravel, Ph.D. (who served as moderator), were also panel discussants. Each case is presented in its entirety (Case 1 is found in Appendix 2), followed by the exchange that occurred among the panel and the audience participants.

Discussion for CASE 1 (Case 1 is described in Appendix 2.)

Richard Seewald, Ph.D., Discussant
Panel and Participant Exchange

Ms. Edwards: The two comments I have really speak to intervention; first, acknowledging the importance of the observations of parents and therapists. I have heard the story so many times, that parents are so often reticent to call us. So a week, two weeks, a month, goes by before we put the picture together. We should start our counseling by saying to parents, "Please contact us anytime you observe a change." I think this is essential. Our recognition that parents are the expert on the observation of their children is so critical.

Dr. Seewald: Absolutely. Fortunately, the mom was an assertive mom and made that call and said, "I want a second opinion on this." How important that was ultimately for the child and her performance!

Question: Why do you think the aided thresholds didn't change?

Dr. Seewald: Well, I wasn't sitting next to the audiologist—so there are some unknown factors! There are a couple of possibilities, I think. One is that when we say that the aided thresholds did not change, it assumes that the aided thresholds that were obtained on the day of the initial fitting were valid. The question is, are the aided thresholds that were obtained on the day of the fitting valid, or in fact, was there more real-ear gain there that was simply not being measured? As you recall, I mentioned that the audiologist said the results were only fair. Sometimes we look at our data and it looks tight, but you forget about the "fuzz" that was in there when you were making the measurement, and the struggle you might have had in getting it!

Another hypothesis that I have, and have seen in my own career, is that audiologists sit there doing the measurement and have the previous test result open in front of them! We might call it experimental bias—regardless, I think this is a dangerous activity to engage in, and sometimes we do end up with a good match because that is what we want! I think audiologists tend to be a little bit compulsive in nature and try to keep things tight.

If you go back and look at the aided and unaided audiogram, at some of the frequencies, the unaided results were a little bit better, and the aided thresholds were a little bit poorer at most of the frequencies. Not so surprising, when you look at behavioral measurements that were obtained using five decibel steps to pick out these changes, versus electroacoustic measurements, using a system that is reasonably well calibrated and does not change over time. The real-ear-to-coupler difference measurement, of course, is made with an electroacoustic measurement system and not an "audiometric system" with behavioral data. We were certainly puzzled initially, but we seemed to find where the problem was.

Question: How frequently would you recommend monitoring the real-ear output?

Dr. Seewald: Certainly, any time that there is a change in the earmold, then we remeasure things, because we know that the earmold is going to change the acoustical conditions and, ultimately, the electroacoustics that are delivered into the ear canal. For children of this age, unless there are some strange circumstances, at least through the first three years of life, we see them every six months. Now, in Ontario, we have the advantage that these services are covered by our health plan, and so it doesn't interfere with our getting them back. But definitely, every six months and any time there is a change in the earmold, then these measurements are made.

Do we see a difference between the personal earmold and the standard coupling that comes with the insert earmold? The answer is yes. Sometimes if we don't have a personal earmold available, then we will use the standard coupling as a first approximation. But with children, it is important that the earmold be integrated into the measurement, and there certainly can be a fairly substantial difference between the real-ear-to-coupler difference measurement with just standard coupling versus the personal earmold.

CASE 2

Jackson Roush, Ph.D.

A chronic hearing loss is a particular problem for children with Down syndrome. Several studies have described the hearing loss associated with the condition. Marion Downs (1980), based on an evaluation of over 100 children with Down syndrome, found that over 75% had hearing loss in one or both ears; of that group, 78% had conductive hearing loss. A sensory component to the hearing loss is frequently overlooked with this population. In Downs' survey, one-fourth of the children had a sensory component or a mixed hearing loss; a few also presented with a pure sensory loss. Most children with Down syndrome, however, experience chronic conductive hearing loss.

The usual approach to longstanding conductive loss is the insertion of PE (pressure equalizing) tubes. However, there is a particular problem with PE tubes in this population, and I will briefly share with you a recent study conducted by Selikowitz (1993), which involved a matched group of 24 children with Down syndrome and another group of 24 typically developing children. Both groups had chronic serous otitis media and were candidates for PE tube placement. Hearing was evaluated before and after surgery. Interestingly, these authors found that at the six-week post-op evaluation, 40% of the children with Down syndrome still had hearing loss, compared to only 9% of the children without Down syndrome. Clearly, the usual management strategy, and one that generally works well for most children with chronic serous otitis media, does not necessarily yield the same outcome with this particular group.

The subject of this case study is 5 years old. She has been enrolled in a comprehensive developmental preschool program with speech-language and early intervention services. In many ways this is an optimal situation for a child with Down syndrome. The child has been under the care of a competent ENT physician but one who is not convinced of the need for much audiologic support. This child has had multiple tube placements, but there has been minimal pre- and post-op audiologic assessment and little concern regarding the developmental implications of the conductive hearing loss. In fact, the parents independently sought additional audiologic assessment.

The first audiogram obtained following the fourth tube placement indicated that one of the tubes was patent and the other was closed. A better-ear response obtained by sound field audiometry indicated normal or near-normal hearing in at least one ear. Although high functioning, the child was difficult to test. She wanted nothing on, in, or near her ears, making audiologic assessment a real challenge.

She returned for follow-up with ENT, but no further audiologic assessment was done until eight months later when there was growing concern about her hearing status. Hearing had decreased considerably and probably had been reduced for quite some time. At that time both tubes were nonfunctional, and the child was tubed again for a fifth time. The parents reported a temporary improvement in hearing, followed soon after by concerns regarding hearing sensitivity. Amplification was recommended by the audiologist, but the physician was reluctant to go forward, desiring instead to pursue further traditional medical management.

At the next evaluation three months later, hearing had declined even further. Agreement between the SRT (obtained by identification of body-parts) and the pure tone average was not good. As a result, the physician did not particularly trust the behavioral measures; however, a comparison of air- and bone-conducted SRTs revealed a significant conductive component.

There was such a lack of progress regarding functional hearing up to this point that the parents, in consultation with the audiologist, decided to pursue auditory brainstem response assessment. Air-conduction responses were elevated bilaterally. Bone-conduction ABR supported an air-bone difference; however, there was also evidence that this child, as with many children with Down syndrome, had a slight sensory component as well. On the basis of these findings, the decision was finally made to move forward with the selection and fitting of amplification.

For a period of time, the child was fitted with a loaner ear-level FM system. Almost immediately, impressive results were noted based on the observations of her parents, teachers, and the early intervention specialists who worked with her. There was a problem with retention of the device, however, because of her small ears and her activity level. Presently, she is fitted on a loaner basis, with mini BTEs. Retention is actually very good with these instruments. She has been fitted with Lucite earmolds because she likes to chew on anything rubbery, including earmolds! Other features on the hearing aid were also considered such as restricting battery access with a tamper-proof door.

The reports of parents and professionals regarding her hearing status have been enthusiastic about the benefits of amplification. My experience in other cases where we fitted amplification to children with Down syndrome has been similar. While the limitations of functional gain measures have been discussed by many contributors at this conference, I think they still have a useful, practical application. In this case, we were able to demonstrate to the physician and educational personnel the relative improvement obtained through hearing aid use. This child's unaided air-conduction responses tend to be consistently around 50-60 dB HL, and there seems to be a slight sensory component as well. With hearing aids, her response levels are markedly improved.

We tend to think of most children with Down syndrome as having fluctuating hearing loss. In this case, and I believe this is true of many others as well, hearing was consistently poor. Hearing improved for a few weeks after tube placement and then deteriorated soon after.

This case study would appear to have a happy ending, but all is not well. The parents prefer a mainstream educational setting, and she is now in a public school classroom with 24 other children. This, of course, presents a challenging situation. She is still on a loaner arrangement with BTE amplification until we decide where to go from here. Compared to the small developmental preschool program she attended previously, the challenge of maintaining an appropriate signal-to-noise listening environment in the mainstream setting has arisen. Perhaps our panel members could offer some suggestions.

REFERENCES

Downs, Marion P. 1980. The hearing of Down's individuals. *Seminars in Speech, Language and Hearing*, vol. 1, no. 1.

Selikowitz, Mark. 1993. Short-term efficacy of tympanostomy tubes for secretory otitis media in children with Down syndrome. *Developmental Medicine and Child Neurology* 35:511-515.

Jackson Roush, Ph.D., Discussant
Panel and Participant Exchange

Dr. Flexer: At this point you haven't yet fit her with an FM system or looked at sound field. Where are you with that?

Dr. Roush: We have not attempted sound field FM with her. Her BTEs are, however, capable of direct audio input. Having everything contained at ear level (out of sight, out of mind) is best, as it is not tampered with as much. That is where we are now—without FM at this point.

Dr. Flexer: Is she in a regular kindergarten class?

Dr. Roush: Yes, it is a regular kindergarten class.

Dr. Flexer: It seems to me that there are a lot of other issues, but what might be really helpful for her, and this avoids putting on additional technology, is to amplify the whole classroom, which would help everyone in the class, as well as her, with the BTE hearing aids. A first order issue is to improve the signal-to-noise ratio.

Dr. Roush: With or without wearable amplification?

Dr. Flexer: Yes.

Dr. Tharpe: As I mentioned yesterday, I don't know much about the new 3D-Loop system that is available, but that would result in a lack of additional hardware. As long as she has a good T-coil on her mini BTEs, that may be an option for the classroom.

Dr. Roush: That is a good suggestion. We have gone full circle on that one. Yesterday, Dr. Matkin mentioned looping classrooms back in the sixties, and now we have a more current, advanced technique for applying that.

Ms. Edwards: I found that with some kids with this history, their own speech is very poor because they haven't heard it very well. One of the things we have tried is using the personal FM system but miking it: putting the microphone and the transmitter on the student during speech-production training. When I put an FM system on a student like that, I was just amazed at the fastest change in articulation that I have ever seen! In the space of five minutes, just by bringing the microphone up to their mouth! If that is not possible, you can go to sound field or loop system within the classroom, but I would suggest some specific training with the student—miking her with the personal FM.

Dr. Roush: That's a great suggestion.

Dr. Gravel: I liked Dr. Flexer's suggestion about the sound field FM. She can retain her hearing aids but would benefit from an improved signal-to-noise ratio. So you would get the best of both worlds while having her wear her own amplification. She can hear her peers but also have a better signal-to-noise ratio as well. That should also help her monitor herself, although Carolyn's suggestion is a great one.

Dr. Gravel: Do we have any comments from the audience?

Question: Why not a bone vibrator?

Dr. Roush: My own experience with bone vibrators has been the problem with keeping them in place, even using the Huggie headband or similar arrangement. But I haven't worked much with the ones that are self-contained at the head. With any kind of a body-worn device, we have had some problems. Certainly, her bone line is good enough that a bone-conduction hearing aid can be considered. The biggest problem I have had with these is keeping them on an active child. Did you want to make a follow-up comment?

Comment: I have a 4-year-old who is very happy with them. We started him with just wearing headphones with the FM during storytelling, and over a couple of weeks he enjoyed hearing things better. He had a moderate loss of 40-50 dB. After about a month we then tried his own vibrator with the FM for a limited period. He enjoyed that and was self-motivated and continued to wear it. Now he has his own bone vibrator hearing aid that he uses at home and uses the FM system in school. He is 4½ or 5 now.

Dr. Roush: That's a good suggestion, one I think would be particularly applicable in a case where the child has actively draining ears despite good medical management. Draining ears would preclude some of the other options we've discussed.

Ms. Edwards: What about support services, and how she is doing in the classroom?

Dr. Roush: Yes. Unfortunately, this is in a district with minimal school-based audiologic support, which I guess is not unusual. The feedback we have gotten is that she has done so much better when she has the hearing aids on. It has been a real struggle, however, for this child to adapt to a regular classroom. We talk about the benefits of a family-centered approach, but sometimes families make decisions that are not the ones that we would choose and we then have to try to figure out how to support those as well. I think it is going to be a real challenge to make that big classroom a decent listening environment. We are working on the support systems, and I think they're coming along.

CASE 3

Anne Marie Tharpe, Ph.D.

The case that I would like to present is one that can give us real management problems—at least this was true for me! This little girl had negative pre- and postnatal histories, but a possible family history of hearing loss: an uncle had a hearing loss, but the parents were not sure of etiology. This child had recurrent otitis media from an early age, and was experiencing some academic and social difficulties. When first seen at age 5 years, she had a rather substantial conductive component, although her bone-conduction thresholds were also slightly below normal. She had myringotomy tubes inserted, and the resulting thresholds demonstrated a closed air-bone gap, but bone-conduction responses were still down.

We know that about 90% of children in the United States will have at least one bout of otitis media prior to 6 years of age. Approximately 30% of children have abnormal middle ear function on any given day and will have somewhere between a 20 to 30 dB reduction in hearing sensitivity in the speech frequencies. This, then, is not an uncommon hearing loss to see, although the added slight reduction in bone-conduction thresholds in this case made things a bit more difficult. Our assessment of this child included serial audiologic tests that revealed her hearing thresholds fluctuated periodically when she had clogged or draining myringotomy tubes. We obtained a speech-language assessment that placed her skills grossly within normal limits. We also conducted a Family Needs Survey that I discussed previously (see chapter 17). The Family Needs Survey revealed more discussion with the teacher was necessary. The parents felt that the teacher really didn't believe that there was a hearing loss. I am sure many of you have encountered this situation when the hearing loss is very mild. The teacher thinks the child doesn't pay attention and doesn't really believe that it is a hearing problem. The Family Needs Survey revealed that we needed to go in and have a more in-depth discussion with the teacher regarding that.

In addition, we also obtained results on the SIFTER (Screening Instrument for Targeting Educational Risk), which has been discussed by several of today's speakers, that indicated some academic concerns which were addressed in our discussion with the teacher.

We received a parental report of the classroom acoustics. I always try to include, in the IEPs or IFSPs, an acoustic evaluation of the classroom setting, in case it's needed. I don't always go to make noise measurements in the classroom if it is just obvious, by report, that there is a bad acoustic environment. In this case, the parents reported that there were 20 children in the classroom, there were hard floors, hard ceilings, that sort of thing. We knew it was bad. Had we gotten any resistance from the school system when we went to make acoustic modifications, then I would have made the measurements to prove it. But fortunately, there was not any resistance so that was not a problem.

Amplification options have been discussed in detail throughout this conference. The options include a personal FM system with Walkman-type earphones, or a classroom free-field FM system. The 3D-Loop classroom system is also available with a hearing aid telecoil or a free-field option. So there were several possibilities. We recommended acoustic modification of the classroom, and had carpeting put down, preferential seating and regular audiologic monitoring.

I am sure all of you may be thinking, "Okay, this is not a terribly interesting case, and why did you bring this up as a case study?" What I think is particularly interesting about this case is the question: Should school systems provide special services for children with fluctuating hearing losses secondary to otitis media? Many school systems, knowing that the hearing loss is mild, are not going to provide any special services for this kind of child. The school feels it is not warranted and that the child doesn't fit the state guidelines for classification as hearing impaired.

There is legislative support for special services for minimal or mild hearing losses. Jack Roush did a very nice job of covering the legislative mandates that require services for children with hearing impairment (see chapter 10). One piece of legislation that we may forget about when thinking of school children is the Americans with Disabilities Act—it applies to children as well as adults. What is particularly interesting about this case is that the child is in private school. Many of us may think private schools are not required by law to provide special education services; so, we dismiss the private schools' responsibility. It is true that private schools don't have to abide by the public laws that cover the public school systems. But they do have to abide by the ADA—because this is an *accessibility* issue. Private schools do need to accommodate the public with disorders or disabilities. Just like they would have to put a ramp in for a child in a wheelchair if there was a flight of stairs getting up to the classroom, they must make the classroom acoustically accessible. In fact, surprisingly, there was no resistance from them: we placed the order, they took it, and we are waiting to have the modifications installed. So I am assuming that it's going to be taken care of!

Anne Marie Tharpe, Ph.D., Discussant
Panel and Participant Exchange

Dr. Gravel: Any comments?
Dr. Flexer: I am assuming this was a private, not a parochial, school?
Dr. Tharpe: Yes.
Dr. Flexer: You know that parochial schools are not required to follow federal laws because of the separation between church and state. But our comment is always: "What? God doesn't want this child to hear?" So working with private schools, you can take another track. Certainly, nonparochial schools are covered by ADA.
Dr. Tharpe: Well, actually that is not always true. Although it is true that parochial schools are generally exempt from compliance with the ADA, there are some exceptions. The law actually states that the school is exempt if controlled by a religious organization. The key determinant is whether or not the church or other religious organization actually operates the school.
Ms. Edwards: I think that kids who have had such limited experience with amplification should have opportunities to really explore the sound field FM, using the transmitter with the student in small groups, and then large groups. One of the things that I see with such children is poor discourse tracking—their inability to sustain attention for long periods of time. Having the teacher actually observing change over time in the child's ability to stay on task would also be useful in measuring progress.
Audience Comment (regarding being in private practice, and getting services provided in a private school): In private school, it has been my experience that there are fewer children that have special needs. I think because it is a little unusual, they don't realize they might be opening Pandora's box. Public schools try to keep a tight rein on things. I had one teacher (in a private school) offer to make curtains to put across the windows. (I gave them handouts on classroom modification.) She said, "I have a sewing machine at home and I can do this." I think that is wonderful!

CASE 4

Carol Flexer, Ph.D.

I want to begin with several assumptions. One is that in a mainstream classroom, hearing is a first-order event—so hearing is the first thing we have to manage relative to receiving classroom instruction. Second assumption: a hearing aid alone, no matter how good the hearing aid, is never enough for a child with a hearing problem in a mainstream classroom. In order to hear teacher instruction and improve the speech-to-noise ratio, we have to have some form of remote microphone. Typically, it's FM technology: a well-fit, appropriate personal FM or, for other populations, a classroom or sound field amplification system.

I am not minimizing how tricky it is to fit a personal FM; also, I am not minimizing the in-service required for the classroom teacher and also for kids. The children realize that this is a neat device that this child is wearing! When you pass around the FM receiver and let other children listen through earphones, I'll tell you, almost half of the class wants one. It demystifies the unit, and most of the time makes it desirable; not an object of ridicule.

A point made previously is that for children with minimal hearing losses, rather than fitting the hearing aid first (which is our typical protocol for most severe hearing losses), think about fitting FM technology first. Then, perhaps later, for other settings, add the hearing aid—but start with the FM! With minimal hearing loss, if you start with the hearing aid, it is often difficult to get the FM system (which is what they really need) into a classroom. So, go for what is the most important thing, which is enhancing the speech-to-noise ratio in a classroom setting and hit that first.

The child that I am going to talk about is a child with a unilateral hearing loss. Audiologically, the child has a profound hearing loss in the left ear and essentially normal hearing in the right ear. That part is easy. The important part is what this hearing loss did to this child! Now, we have all been justifiably horrified when we found children with severe-to-profound hearing loss who had been relegated into institutions because people thought they were severely retarded. They got tucked away, and it comes out years later that they had a hearing loss. We just ruined this person by not identifying the problem! Well, we are still doing that.

This is a child who was born with a unilateral hearing loss, left ear, and was identified because he was having other difficulties. He wasn't developing language very well, and he also had otitis media. When you have repeated otitis media on top of unilateral hearing loss, you really are going to have some problems—almost always.

At 1 year of age, the unilateral loss was identified and was deemed minimal. The otitis media was thought not to count because "everyone gets otitis media" and the loss is minimal. Well by 2½ years of age he was in speech-language therapy, and the hearing was still not being managed; it was being *assessed*. It was being monitored, but nothing was being done to access that hearing. Finally, the parents held him back, not starting kindergarten until he was close to 6. About halfway through kindergarten, this child didn't know "up" from "down." He didn't have access to incidental learning from "overhearing," and thus, there was a tremendous deficit in his language and in his knowledge base.

Remember that acoustic filter effect: the invisible impact of the hearing loss that negatively impacts spoken language, reading, and academics, etc.? Halfway through kindergarten, the psychologist tested this child and found an IQ of approximately 70. The school told the parents that they wanted to put this child into a classroom for children with developmental disabilities. They classified this child as retarded. The mother said, "I know he seems to be slow; he is really having problems, but he isn't hearing well. Don't you think that is a problem?" "Oh no! It's a minimal hearing loss; it's just this *little* hearing loss. He is retarded. You just have to accept this and get on with it." This didn't seem right. So the parents looked around and found some of the literature on unilateral hearing loss, made an appointment, and we evaluated this child.

All of the previous audiometric testing had been performed using earphones. The speech test to the good ear was conducted under earphones. Using the WIPI, or whatever the speech material this child could handle, the assumption was made that because he got anywhere from 90% to 100% correct in the acoustically perfect environment of a sound room under earphones, his hearing was fine. So everyone ruled out hearing as a factor in this child's performance and in his development.

We tested him in the test suite in quiet; there he did very well. However, a classroom is not like a soundroom in any way. To make conclusions about classroom listening, the soundroom performance doesn't have relevance. So we tested him in different conditions of quiet and then speech noise. At a typical conversational level of 45 dB HL in sound field where the words were directed to the good ear, he did pretty good. But when the words were directed to the poor ear, even with no competing noise, his word discrimination dropped to approximately 74%; and this is in perfect quiet! When you add noise, with speech to the good side, noise to the poor side, he dropped to between 60% and 70%. And when you direct speech to the poor ear and noise to the good ear, he was down to approximately 8%. We'd all be a bit developmentally delayed if we were getting only 8% to 50% of the information presented around us if there wasn't active direct teaching in a very quiet environment or a way to get the sounds into the good ear!

We presented this information to the teachers and the school who felt that the child was "not deaf, just retarded." The parents said we must have aggressive intervention because we have already wasted his critical learning years. So, we started out with a personal FM system; obviously, very mild gain, low output, fit to the good ear. Now, we have had 6½ years of inaccurate, inconsistent, unreliable input, and the teacher, of course, after two days called and said: "You know he still can't answer questions." Well, it is going to take a little more than 48 hours to fix this! The school speech-language pathologist said she was still working on speech-sound correction, but because the child was diagnosed as developmentally delayed, she didn't expect the speech to get much better. The parents said, "We are not fighting with the school; just leave him in the regular classroom, with the FM system." The parents, on their own, obtained private speech-language therapy, three hours per week. The mother is an elementary school teacher. She tutored this child every single day. We, now we have this huge acoustic filter effect, and we didn't know if there was a cognitive deficit. How could you evaluate the "hard drive" when you have had such an inadequate "keyboard" all these years? The point is that no matter what deficit he may or may not have had cognitively, you have to manage hearing because hearing is the first-order event.

So all through the summer they were doing daily tutoring, with three hours per week of speech-language therapy. They used the FM system at home for all of their instructional sessions. He started first grade, regular school, and was doing better. The parents requested nothing of the school. He continued most of the way through first grade and moved up from the low reading group to the middle reading group. In second grade, he seemed to be more "average" in performance. He continued with the FM system; the parents continued with their heroic intervention. Third grade, this year, the child had his IQ retested and he scored 105: from 70 to 105! Now the school said, "It must have been maturation because it couldn't have been hearing. That minimal hearing loss couldn't have caused all of these problems." If it was maturation, it means that you have no developmentally handicapped (DH) classrooms after third grade, because everyone matures out of this issue!

This child still needs speech-language therapy, and he is still getting tutoring. He still needs some support that the parents continue to provide. I talked to the principal not too long ago, and he asked if the child is still going to need the FM system. Not to be too flippant, I asked: "Do you still need your glasses after all these years? You haven't learned to be able to manage without getting better sensory input? You'd think you would have overcome this need!" The point is the school still doesn't understand that this *minimal problem* could have had such intense negative effects on this child! This child was classified "retarded"; if he had been put in a DH classroom with no management of his hearing, no expectations, guess how he would have performed? His whole life would have been very different! But his parents said, "This doesn't seem right."

Don't you wonder how many kids are sitting in classrooms for children with learning disabilities or emotional disorders, whose primary problem is a minimal hearing loss that has not been managed? As audiologists, it is our job to identify, to advocate, and to manage children's hearing and to access the classroom. We don't know what other problems a child could have—and certainly, there could be other problems besides hearing. But hearing is a first-order event, and no matter what other disabilities the child may have, if we are using speech to communicate, or if we are expecting spoken language to develop, or we are putting a child in a situation where learning depends on receiving auditory information, then we must access that auditory environment and maximize that child's opportunity to receive spoken communication.

Carol Flexer, Ph.D., Discussant
Panel and Participant Exchange

Ms. Edwards: I think that when a student has gone through that much deprivation preschool, what I really encourage the school staff to do is start telling the student *why* they are having difficulties. With this knowledge, they can start to change their own sense of self, from: "I am not capable" (which they obviously got reinforced at a very early point in school), to saying: "I didn't hear, that is why I couldn't respond," then—just give them lots of opportunities for that.

This story is very dramatic, and schools don't hear your points clearly enough. Again, I think it is so easy to underestimate what hearing loss can do. Part of it is because the effects of hearing loss are so ambiguous and appear to be subtle until we look further.

Dr. Flexer: We, the audiologists in the school system, must not be stopped by the guidelines. Many of the state guidelines, especially through special education and IDEA, may not qualify children with minimal hearing loss for services until they have failed so much that we really can't make up for the deficit. Focus on acoustic accessibility and intervene before the child gets so delayed that we can't catch them up.

Author Index

Able-Boone, H., 137, 142
Abraham, S., 33, 50
Abrahamson, J., 276-77, 282
Abrams, S., 383, 386, 397
Ahlstrom, J., 203, 212
Ahmad, N. N., 345, 359
Aittomaki, K., 345, 364
Alencewicz, C. M., 55, 73
Alford, B. R., 383, 386, 397
Alford, C. A., 346, 363, 364-65
Allan, J., 148, 159
Allen, A. A., 353, 359
Allen, L., 236, 240, 241-42, 247, 250
Allen, P., 152, 158
Allum-Mecklenburg, D. J., 305-6
Alpiner, J., 52
Alter, C. A., 345, 359
Ambrose, C. M., 344, 365
American Academy of Pediatrics, 350-51, 359
American National Standards Institute, 33, 45, 47, 48, 50, 80, 81, 102, 194, 197, 202, 210
American Speech-Language-Hearing Association, 112, 120, 127, 142, 245, 247, 277, 279, 281, 316, 319, 402, 412
Amos, C. S., 346, 364-65
Anderson, K. L., 241, 245, 247, 317, 318, 322, 331, 335, 355, 359, 395, 396, 406, 412
Antogenelli, T., 307, 305
Antonelli, A., 83, 102
Anttila, M., 349, 362
Appelbaum, M., 313, 319
Aram, D. M., 313, 319
Arkis, P. N., 148, 158
Arndt, P. L., 305, 307
Aslin, R. N., 30-31, 50
Audiologic-Sarl, 257-61, 271
Auslander, M. C., 151, 159, 350, 352, 359, 403, 414
AVR/Communications Ltd., 256, 260, 271

Bagwell, C., 230, 250
Bailey, D. B., 124, 143, 355, 359
Balkany, T. J., 295, 306, 352, 359, 360

Ball, K., 234, 248
Bamford, J., 232, 247, 426, 429
Bardaji, C., 342, 361
Barker, M. J., 305, 306
Barna, B. P., 348-49, 361
Barr, B., 340, 359
Barta, L., 137, 142
Bateman, R., 236, 247
Battaglia, D., 181, 189, 423
Battaglia, J., 205, 211
Battmer, R., 305-6
Bauer, H., 32, 50, 51
Beauchaine, K. A., 127, 142
Beauchaine, K. L., 152, 155, 158, 159-60, 187, 191, 199, 213, 404, 407, 414
Beck, L. B., 189, 190, 412, 415, 423
Beebe, H. H., 14, 25
Beiter, A. L., 305, 307, 352, 359
Bekassy, A. N., 344, 359
Bell, T. S., 203, 211, 212
Bellman, S., 341, 364
Benafield, N., 236, 240, 247
Bench, J., 232, 247, 426, 429
Bender, R. E., 3, 25
Benitez-Diaz, L., 350, 361
Bennett, D. N., 256, 271
Bennett, F. C., 348, 362
Bennett, R., 200, 213, 230, 250
Benoit, R., 12, 15, 25, 113, 120, 155, 158, 407, 412
Bensen, R. W., 428, 429
Bentler, R., 150-51, 158, 201, 210, 216-18, 226, 229, 249, 403, 404, 405, 412, 413
Bento, L., 342, 361
Beranek, L., 230, 247
Berg, F. S., 230, 236, 241, 244, 246, 247, 249, 311, 319, 322, 324, 325, 331, 332, 335, 389, 396
Berger, K. W., 109, 120, 193, 211
Bergstrom, L., 346, 359
Berlin, C. I., 325, 335, 345, 364
Berliner, K. I., 289, 306
Bernheimer, L. P., 132, 142

455

Bernstein, M. E., 137, 142
Berry, S. W., 288, 298, 307, 371, 382, 406, 414
Bess, F. H., vii, viii, 73, 74, 119, 120, 121, 143, 189, 190, 213, 217, 226, 229-30, 231, 235, 236, 247, 248, 250, 274, 282, 323, 324, 325, 335, 359, 362, 364, 383, 385, 396, 397, 399, 400, 410, 412, 413, 414, 415, 423, 429
Best, C. T., 194, 212
Bilger, R. C., 56, 72, 112, 121
Biscone-Halterman, K., 345, 363
Bisgaard, N., 147, 159
Blair, J. C., 229, 230, 236, 238, 247, 249, 322, 325, 337
Blake, R., 317, 319
Blake-Rahter, P., 236, 240, 250, 313, 315, 320
Blanchard, S., 345, 365
Blood, I., 313, 319
Bluestone, C. D., 351, 361, 365
Bobrow, M., 342, 361
Bocca, E., 83, 102
Bolande, R. P., 344, 359
Bond, L. C., 152, 159
Boney, S., 231, 247, 383, 397
Boothroyd, A., 11, 25, 29, 31, 50, 55, 56, 62, 70, 71, 72-73, 194, 205, 211, 212, 274, 282, 287, 288, 304, 306, 371, 380, 381, 382, 427, 429
Boughman, J. A., 345, 359
Bove, C., 344, 365
Boyer, K. M., 350, 365
Brackett, D., 2, 12, 27, 322, 325, 326, 337, 370, 381, 382, 400, 407, 412
Braida, L. D., 62, 73, 197, 211, 285, 307
Brandsmith, S., 56, 74
Bratt, G., 109, 120, 403, 412
Brey, R. H., 84, 103
Brimacombe, J. A., 305, 307, 352, 359
Brink, B., 147, 159
Brokx, J. P. L., 405, 415
Brook, R. H., 350, 362
Brookhouser, P. E., 340, 345, 350, 352, 359, 363, 410, 412
Brown, D., 87-88, 103
Brown, D. P., 13, 25, 343, 359, 386, 397
Brown, L., 230, 236, 237, 249, 331, 336
Brown, O. E., 342, 360
Brown, S. C., 350, 365
Brown, S. D. M., 345, 365
Brunner, H. G., 345, 360
Buckler, A. J., 344, 365
Buie, C., 236, 241, 249
Bull, D. H., 33, 52

Burkey, J. M., 148, 158
Bustamente, D. K., 62, 73, 197, 211
Butler, K. G., 325, 337
Buyse, M. L., 342, 344, 345, 360
Byers, V. W., 256, 271
Byrne, D., 109, 120, 173-75, 176, 179, 181, 187, 189, 193, 211, 403, 412, 418, 423

Calabrese, L. H., 348-49, 361
Calvert, D. R., 3, 22, 27
Cameron, J. S., 342, 361
Campbell, J. C., 350, 364
Cannoni, M., 347, 365
Cantekin, E. I., 350, 361
Cargill, S., 321, 323, 328, 335
Carhart, R., 15, 25, 78, 79, 81-87, 102, 103, 104, 165, 189, 428, 430
Carney, A. E., 31, 33, 35-40, 45-46, 50-51, 52, 155, 158, 284, 300, 306, 307, 316, 319
Carney, E., 31, 50, 51, 152-54, 159, 160, 284, 306
Carotta, C., 45-46, 50, 51
Carrell, J. A., 15, 21, 27
Cass, S., 340-41, 343-44, 345, 346-47, 363
Cassano, P., 80-81, 103
Cawkwell, S., 288, 306
Cawthon, R., 344, 365
Cervellera, G., 80-81, 103
Chammas, F., 347, 362
Channell, R. W., 84, 103
Chantler, C., 342, 361
Chase, P. A., 119, 120, 399
Chen, A. H., 340, 360
Chen, Q., 71, 72
Cherow, E., 413
Cherow-Skalka, E., 426, 429
Chmiel, R., 148, 159
Chole, R. A., 344, 360
Chute, P. M., 264, 266, 271
Cicci, R., 312, 320
Ciuchi, V., 342, 361
Civitello, B. A., 78, 88, 104
Clark, G. M., 286, 305, 307
Clark, J., 27
Clark, T., 387, 397
Clarke, B. R., 7-8, 25
Clogg, D., 342-43, 361
Cohen, M. M., Jr., 345, 363
Cohen, N. L., 303, 308, 352, 360
Colburn, H. S., 75, 103
Cole, E., 380, 381, 382

Coleman, R. F., 217, 226
Colletti, V., 341, 360
Collier, A., 313, 319
Compton, C., 408, 412
Conde, J., 342, 361
Connolly, C. J., 342-43, 362
Connors, S., 234, 248
Conway, L. C., 326, 335
Cooper, W. A., 181, 190, 196, 212, 404, 413
Coppock, J. S., 345, 363
Cornelisse, L. E., 153, 158, 187, 189, 194, 196, 201, 211, 405, 414
Costello, J. A., 348, 364
Coucke, P., 340, 342, 345, 360
Cox, R. M., 193, 200, 201, 211
Crandell, C. C., 229-30, 231-32, 233, 235, 236, 237, 239, 242, 244, 245-46, 247-48, 274, 282, 312, 319, 320, 329, 335, 383, 385, 389, 397, 407, 412
Crandell, M. A., 91-93, 103
Cremers, C. W., 340, 342-43, 345, 360, 362
Creutz, T., 196, 197, 200, 204, 213
Crowe, S. J., 349, 360
Crowley, J. M., 112, 122, 171, 191
Crum, D., 229, 248
Crum, M. A., 313, 319
Culbertson, J. L., 323, 335
Culpepper, B., 129, 142
Culver, M., 344, 365

Dahle, A. J., 346, 360, 364
Dallos, P., 78, 102
Daly, D. D., 350, 364
Daniel, Z., 56, 74
Daniels, P., 305, 307
Danzer, V., 229, 236, 241, 249
Darby, J. K., 340, 342, 345, 360
Darbyshire, J. O., 137, 143
Davenport, S. L., 343, 345, 360, 363, 365
Davis, H., 9, 25, 336, 428, 429
Davis, H., 350, 360
Davis, J., 216-18, 226, 229, 248, 311, 319, 321, 322, 324, 332, 335, 386, 397
Davis, L. E., 346, 360
Dawson, P., 205, 211
de la Chapelle, A., 345, 364
De La Cruz, A., 347, 361
Deal, A. G., 132, 133, 142, 143
DeGennaro, S., 62, 73, 197, 211
Dehner, L. P., 346, 360
Del Val, M., 346, 362

Dempster, J. H., 151, 158
Dennis, J. M., 346, 360
Derlacki, E. L., 90, 103
DeSouza, C., 352, 360
Dettman, D., 45-46, 51, 305
Devens, J, 229-30, 249
Diefendorf, A. O., 400, 407, 413
Dilka, K., 322, 336
Dillon, H., 109, 120, 174, 181, 189, 193, 196, 205, 211, 213, 403, 412, 418, 423
DiMascio, J., 345, 359
DiRaddo, P., 343, 361
Dirks, D. D., 99, 100, 101, 103, 203, 211, 212, 323, 336
Djoyodiharjo, B., 340, 342, 345, 360
Dobie, R. A., 325, 335
Dodd, B. J., 33, 51
Dodge, P. R., 350, 360
Donaghy, K., 407, 414
Donahue, A., 244, 249
Douville, D. R., 342, 362
Downs, M. P., 29, 52, 250, 320, 321, 322, 324, 335, 336, 337, 443, 445
Doyle, W., 32, 52
Druz, W. S., 255, 271
DuBois, R. W., 350, 362
DuBow, S., 333, 335
Dunn, D., 344, 365
Dunst, C. J., 132, 133, 142, 143
Durieux-Smith, A., 168, 191, 405, 415
Durlach, N. I., 62, 73, 75, 103, 197, 211, 285, 307
Durrant, J. D., 148, 159
Duyao, M.P., 344, 365
Dye, L. L., 289, 306
Dyrlund, O., 147, 158, 159

Early Childhood Curriculum Committee, 384, 397
Eddington, D. K., 305, 308
Edelstein, D. R., 347, 362
Edwards, C., 384, 386, 393, 394, 397, 400, 406, 413, 441, 446, 449, 453
Eichler, J. A., 350, 361
Eilers, R. E., 30, 31, 33, 35-40, 51, 52, 295, 306
Elbert, M., 32, 53
Eldert, E. 428, 429
Eldridge, R., 344, 365
Elfenbein, J., 216-18, 219, 226, 229, 248, 396, 397, 405, 406, 413
Elliott, L., 31, 51, 232, 234, 236, 248, 249, 313,

319, 324, 335, 426, 429
Ellis, M., 383, 397
Elssman, S. F., 312, 319
Emmer, M. B., 148, 159
Engebretson, A. M., 147, 158, 203, 211
Eran, O., 71, 73, 427, 429
Erber, N. P., 55, 56, 73, 171, 175, 179-80, 189, 253-56, 265, 269, 271, 287, 306, 326, 335, 378, 382, 426, 427, 429
Ermocilla, R., 346, 364-65
Escobar, M. W., 400, 407, 413
Evans, P., 217, 226
Everingham, C., 305, 307
Ewing, A. W. G., 13, 20, 25, 26, 27
Ewing, I. R., 13, 20, 25

Fabry, D., 155, 156, 158, 196, 211
Fant, G., 74
Farkashidy, J., 345, 364
Farrior, J. B., 341, 360
Feagans, L., 313, 319
Feagans, L. V., 313, 319
Feigin, J. A., 50, 72, 109, 112, 120, 121, 151, 152, 158, 159-60, 162, 187, 189, 190, 191, 198, 199, 206, 211, 213, 276-77, 280, 282, 403-4, 413, 414, 420, 423, 431, 439, 453
Feigin, R. D., 350, 360
Feldhake, L. J., 107, 120, 122
Ferguson, C. A., 32, 52, 53
Fernandes, M. A., 88, 89-90, 103
Fidell, S., 200, 213, 230, 250
Field, B., 315, 319
Fikret-Pasa, S., 146, 151, 158
Filip, I., 342, 361
Filip, O., 342, 361
Findlay, R. C., 217, 226
Finitzo-Hieber, T., 113, 121, 229-30, 232, 234, 248, 313, 319, 324, 335, 385, 389, 397, 426, 429
Finley, C. C., 305, 308
Fiorino, F. G., 341, 360
Firszt, J., 31, 52-53, 72
Fischer, A., 342, 361
Fischer, E., 217, 226
Fishmann, G., 340, 364
Fitch, W. J., 15, 21, 27
Fletcher, S. G., 311, 319
Flexer, C., 229-30, 231-32, 233, 235, 236, 237, 239, 240, 241, 242, 244-45, 246, 248-49, 315, 319, 320, 321, 323, 324, 327, 328, 329, 331, 335-36, 337, 397, 441, 445-46, 449

Flinter, F. A., 342, 361
Folsom, R. C., 127, 143, 348, 362
Foster, C., 315, 319
Fourcin, A., 229, 249
Foust, K. O., 254-55, 271
Fowler-Brehm, N., 352, 359
Franklin, D., 287, 306
Franklin, L., 263, 271
Frants, R. R., 340, 342, 345, 360
Fraser, F. C., 342-43, 361
Frattali, C., 319
Fravel, R. P., 286, 306
Frederick, L. L., 137, 142
Freeman, B. A., vii, viii, 73, 189, 250, 282
French, N. R., 202, 211
French-St. George, M., 147, 158
Fretz, R. J., 286, 306
Fria, T. J., 350, 361
Frisbie, K. A., 155, 158
Fry, D. B., 13, 28, 29, 51
Fryauf-Bertschy, H., 296, 306
Fukaka, J., 347, 362
Fukushima, K., 340, 360

Gacek, R. R., 343, 361
Gaeth, J. H., 22, 25, 215, 217, 225, 226
Gagné, J. P., 69, 74, 153, 158, 170, 182, 187, 189, 190, 191, 196, 201, 211, 280, 282, 405, 413, 414
Gaines, J., 348, 364
Galambos, R., 125, 142
Gallimore, R., 132, 142
Gananca, M. M., 347, 362
Gantz, B. J., 296, 305, 306, 352, 359
Gardner, W. J., 344, 365
Gatehouse, S., 156, 159, 171-72, 189, 190
Gavin, W., 30, 51
Geer, S., 333, 335
Geers, A., 29, 51
Geffner, D., 33, 51
Gelfand, S. A., 13, 25, 149, 159
Gengel, R., 175, 179, 190, 229, 249, 254-55, 271
George, C. R., 305, 307
Gerber, S. E., 52, 364
Gerlin, I. J., 426, 429
Gerritsen, E. J., 342, 361
Gersell, D. J., 346, 360
Gesteland, R., 344, 365
Giangiacomo, J., 343, 363
Gibson, F., 345, 365
Gilbert, J. H. V., 30, 53

Gilbert, L. E., 323, 335
Gilman, L., 229, 236, 241, 247
Ginsburg, C. M., 342, 360
Giolas, T. G., 51, 56, 74, 229, 250, 311, 320, 323, 336, 429
Glasscock, M. E., III, 341, 361
Glassford, F. E., 230, 236, 240, 250, 316, 320, 331, 336
Gluckman, C., 348, 364
Gluckman, J., 363
Gnadeberg, D., 305-6
Goldstein, D., 76, 104
Goldstein, M., 3-5, 6, 7, 26
Golu, T., 342, 361
Gomolin, R., 303, 308
Gorga, M. P., 109, 120, 127, 142, 151, 152, 158, 162, 189, 198, 206, 211, 386, 397, 403-4, 413, 420, 423, 431, 439
Gorlin, R. J., 340, 341, 347, 362
Graham, J. M., 343, 363
Graser, N. S., 392, 397
Gravel, J. S., 119, 120, 127, 128, 142, 218, 227, 264, 266, 271, 314, 319, 383, 386, 397, 399, 412, 413, 414, 415, 429, 441, 446, 449
Gravel, K. L., 161, 162, 190
Greater Boston Otitis Media Study Group, 314, 320
Green, B. W., 217, 226
Green, H., 238, 249
Green, R. R., 12, 27
Greenberg, D. P., 349-50, 362
Greenwood, J., 217, 226
Griffiths, C., 14, 26
Grimes, A., 112, 121
Griscelli, C., 342, 361
Grissom, T. J., 345, 363
Grose, J. H., 75-76, 83, 90-91, 93-99, 103
Grundfast, K. M., 351, 361
Guilford, P., 345, 365
Guiscafre, H., 350, 361
Gusella, J. F., 344, 365
Gutierrez, C., 342, 361
Guyot, J. P., 343, 361

Haase, V. H., 344, 365
Hack, Z. C., 56, 73
Hagberg, E. N., 109, 120, 193, 211
Haines, J. L., 344, 365
Halal, F., 343, 361
Hall, B. D., 343, 361
Hall, J. W., 75-76, 88, 89-91, 93-99, 103, 143, 362
Haller, G. L., 12, 19, 26
Halligan, P. L., 181, 190, 196, 212
Hamer, A. W., 132, 143
Hammer, M. A., 324, 335
Hanin, L., 71, 72, 427, 429
Harris, C., 230, 249
Harris, J. P., 348, 361
Harris, K. S., 56, 73
Harris, R. W., 84, 103
Haskell, G. B., 166, 190
Haskins, H., 284, 306, 426, 429
Haspiel, G., 426, 430
Hattori, H., 148, 159
Hawkins, D. B., 20, 26, 109, 112, 116, 119, 121, 148, 150, 159, 168-69, 170, 181, 190, 196, 211, 212, 276, 280, 282, 322, 330, 336, 404, 405, 413, 415
Hawkins, J., 427, 429
Hedgecock, L. D., 15, 21, 27
Hedley-Williams, A., 119, 120, 399, 400, 413
Hefner, M. A., 343, 360, 363, 365
Heidbreder, A., 203, 211
Hejtmancik, J. F., 345, 364
Helfrich, M. H., 342, 361
Henderson, F., 313, 319
Hendricks-Munoz, K. D., 348, 361, 365
Hennessey, A., 194, 213
Henningsen, L. B., 147, 159
Herer, G., 348, 363
Hermans, J., 342, 361
Hicks, B. L., 62, 73
Hirsh, I. J., 75, 103, 112, 121, 428, 429
Hirsh, S. K., 350, 360
Hochberg, I., 72, 189, 423
Hochmair, E. S., 307
Hochmair-Desoyer, I. J., 307
Hodgson, M., 389, 397
Hodgson, W. R., 27
Hoekstra, C. 405, 415
Hoene, J., 119, 121
Hoffman, H. E., 346, 360
Hoffman, R., 303, 308
Hohindra, I., 346, 364-65
Holliday, M. J., 344, 364
Holmes, L. B., 345, 361
Holmes, S. J., 350, 360
Holum-Hardegen, L. L, 112, 122, 171, 191
Hosford-Dunn, H., 346, 361
Hou, Z., 203, 212
House, W. F., 289, 306, 347

Houston, I., 342, 361
Hradek, G. T., 303, 306
Hudgins, C. V., 7-8, 26, 55-56, 73
Hudson, S. P., 69, 74, 170, 182, 189, 190, 196, 211, 280, 282, 405, 413, 414
Hughes, G. B., 348-49, 361
Huizing, E. H., 340, 342, 345, 360
Hull, R., 322, 336
Humes, L. E., 112, 121, 168, 190, 203, 212
Humphrey, K., 30, 53
Hustedde, C., 33, 51
Hwang, J. Y., 194, 213

Israel, S. M., 343, 359

Jackler, R. K., 347, 361
Jacobs, M., 347, 362
Jacobson, J. T., 143, 360
Jamieson, D. G., 174, 181, 187, 189, 191, 194, 211, 219, 227, 266, 271, 280, 282, 403-4, 414, 420, 423, 431, 440
Jenison, R. L, 148, 159
Jensen, H., 33, 52
Jerger, J., 87, 88, 103, 148, 159, 383, 386, 397, 427, 429
Jerger, S., 383, 386, 397, 427, 429
Jesteadt, W., 127, 142
John, J. E. J., 20, 26
Johnson, B. H., 134, 142
Johnson, C., 383, 397
Johnson, D., 56, 74
Johnson, K., 78, 103
Johnson, L. G., 346, 360
Johnson, S., 346, 361
Joint Committee on Infant Hearing, 124, 142, 162, 190
Jones, J., 230, 236, 249
Joy, D., 229, 249
Jubelirer, D. P., 350, 360
Jusczyk, P. W., 30, 51

Kaariainen, H., 345, 364
Kalilow, D., 232, 249
Kallio, M. J. T., 349, 362
Kaminski, J. R., 127, 142
Kamm, C. A., 203, 212
Kankkunen, A., 350, 364
Kaplan, J., 345, 365
Kaplan, S. L., 350, 360
Karasek, A., 45-46, 51, 112, 121, 196, 197, 200, 204, 213, 276-77, 280, 282, 305

Karchmer, M. A., 22, 26, 410, 413
Karjalainen, S., 345, 364
Katinsky, S. E., 350, 362
Katz, D., 31, 51, 234, 236, 248, 249, 296, 307, 426, 429
Katz, J., 26, 27, 249, 250
Kaufmann, R. K., 142
Kavanagh, J. F., 52, 53
Kawell, M. E., 405, 413
Kayser, H., 315, 319
Keats, B. J., 345, 364
Keith, R. L., 313, 319
Kelley, P. M., 345, 365
Kelly, C., 33, 52
Kelly, W. J., 340, 350, 359, 410, 412
Kelsay, D. M., 296, 306
Kemink, J., 31, 52-53
Kemker, F. J., 217, 226
Kennedy, M., 229, 249
Kent, R. D., 32, 33, 35, 51, 52
Kessler, D. K., 305, 306, 307
Kessler, K., 288, 300, 307
Kessler, K. S., 371, 382
Kille, E., 234, 248
Killion, M. C., 166, 190, 203, 212, 322, 336
Kilpi, T., 349, 362
Kimberling, W. J., 340, 342, 345, 360, 342-43, 345, 362, 363, 364
Kincaid, G. E., 203, 211, 212
King, M. C., 340, 362
Kinney, S. E., 348-49, 361
Kipp, E., 313, 319
Kirkwood, D. H., 146, 147, 159
Kirn, E. U., 112, 121, 168, 190
Kirwin, L. A., 22, 26
Klatt, D., 51
Klein, J. O., 314, 320, 350, 362, 364
Kleinman, L. C., 350, 362
Kley, N., 344, 365
Knight, J., 229, 249
Knowles, S., 229, 249
Knowlton, R. G., 345, 359
Knox, A. W., 16, 26
Knox, E., 229, 249
Knudsen, V., 230, 249
Kodaras, M., 230, 249
Konigsmark, B. W., 340, 341, 342, 345, 347, 362
Konkle, D. F., 122
Kopun, J. G., 109, 120, 151-52, 153-54, 158, 159, 160, 162, 189, 198, 206, 211, 403-4, 405, 413, 420, 423, 431, 439

AUTHOR INDEX • 461

Kosecoff, J., 350, 362
Koszinowski, U. H., 346, 362
Koval, A., 232, 247, 426, 429
Koziel, V., 348, 364
Kozma-Spytek, L., 295, 308
Kramlinger, M., 407, 413
Kraus, N., 350, 363
Kruger, B., 109, 121, 150, 159, 403, 413
Kuhl, P. K., 30, 51-52, 312, 320
Kuk, F. K., 147, 159
Kumar, S., 342-43, 362

Lacerda, F., 30, 52, 312, 320
Lafayette, R., 33, 52
Lalonde, C. E., 30, 53
Larget-Piet, D., 345, 365
LaRossa, D., 345, 359
Larson, V. D., 169-71, 175, 179, 190, 405, 414
Lass, N., 52
Lauter, J., 72
Lawson, D. T., 305, 308
Lazar, L., 348, 362
Leake, P. A., 303, 306
Leavitt, A. M., 348, 362
Leavitt, R., 229, 249, 326, 327, 328, 336
Lenarz, T., 305-6
Lennenberg, E. H., 13, 26, 325, 336
Leon, P. E., 340, 362
Leonard, L. B., 325, 336
Lerman, J. W., 16, 27, 31, 53, 237, 250, 426, 429
Letowski, T., 244, 249
Levenson, M. J., 347, 362
Levi-Acobas, F., 345, 365
Levilliers, J., 345, 365
Levin, S., 234, 248, 344, 364
Levitt, H., 56, 69, 72, 73, 194, 212, 213, 428, 429
Lew, H. L., 148, 159
Lewis, D., 112, 121, 155, 158, 170, 191, 196, 197, 200, 204, 213, 276-77, 280, 282, 404, 405, 407, 408, 413, 414, 415
Lewis, R. A., 345, 364
Lewis, S., 427, 429
Libby, E. R., 27
Licklider, J. C. R., 75, 103
Lieberman, J. M., 349-50, 362
Liebman, E. P., 350, 362
Liff, S., 12, 26
Lightfoot, R., 113, 122
Lindblom, B., 30, 52, 312, 320

Ling, D., 13, 26, 33, 52, 56-57, 69, 73, 255-56, 271, 324, 325, 326-27, 336, 342-43, 361, 377, 378, 379, 382, 426, 429
Linthicum, F. H., 341, 362
Lippmann, R. P., 62, 73
Liston, S. L., 344, 363
Litwin, A., 348, 362
Loeb, G. M., 305, 306
Logan, S. A., 217, 226
Lounsbury, E., 22, 25, 215, 217, 225, 226
Lovrinic, J. H., 350, 362
Lowder, M. W., 305, 306
Lubinski, R., 319
Lund, G., 345, 363
Lundh, P., 109, 121, 147, 158, 181, 190, 403, 414, 422
Luterman, D., 2, 14, 26, 218, 226
Luxon, L. M., 341, 364
Lybarger, S. F., 12, 19, 26
Lynch, E., 340, 362
Lynch, M., 34, 52
Lyregaard, P. E., 109, 121, 181, 190, 193, 212, 403, 413, 414, 416, 422

Mace, A. L., 152, 160, 410, 413
MacCollin, M. M., 344, 365
MacDonald, M. E., 344, 365
Mackenzie, K., 151, 158
Macpherson, B. J., 405, 413
Macrae, J., 112, 121, 166-67, 190, 405, 413
Madell, J. R., 146, 159, 407, 413
Malachowski, N., 346, 361
Mancl, L. R., 127, 143
Mangabeira-Albernaz, P. L., 347, 362
Manusov, E. G., 342, 362
Maretic, H., 255-56, 271
Margolis, R. H., 78, 88, 104, 120, 122
Marietta, J., 340, 360
Mariman, E. C. M., 345, 360
Marincovich, P. J., 203, 213
Markides, A., 230, 249
Marres, H. A., 342-43, 362
Martin, E. S., 56, 74
Martin, F., 27
Martin, F. N., 161-62, 190
Martin-Evans, B., 62, 73
Martinez, M. A., 342, 361
Martinez, M. C., 350, 361
Martuza, R. L., 344, 365
Matin, M., 229, 249
Matkin, N. D., 2, 27, 29, 52, 132, 134, 142, 174,

177, 190, 227, 229, 248, 312, 319, 323, 332, 336, 383, 385, 395, 396, 397, 406, 412, 426, 429, 446
Mattingly, G., 53
Maxon, A. B., 2, 12, 27, 322, 325, 326, 337, 381, 382, 395, 397
Mburu, P., 345, 365
McCabe, B. F., 348-49, 351, 362-63, 364
McCaffrey, H., 276-77, 282
McCandless, G. A., 181, 190, 193, 212, 403, 413, 416, 422
McCarthy, P., 52
McCarty, D. J., 363
McChord, W., 217, 226
McCollister, F. P., 346, 360, 364-65
McConnell, F., 12, 16, 26, 217, 226, 229-30, 247, 274, 282
McCracken, G. H., Jr., 349, 364
McCroskey, F., 229-30, 249
McDermott, H. J., 304-5, 307
McDonald-McGinn, D. M., 345, 359
McDougall, J. K., 362
McGarr, N. S., 33, 52, 56, 73, 74
McGhee, S., 313, 319
McGonigel, M. J., 134, 142
McGowan, K., 353, 359
McKay, C. M., 304, 307
McKusick, V. A., 348, 363
McNeill, D., 13, 26
Meany, M., 223, 226
Medwetsky, L., 11, 25
Melancon, L., 389, 397
Menapace, C. M., 305, 307
Mencher, G. T., 52, 364
Menn, L., 52
Menon, A.G., 344, 365
Merlob, P., 348, 362
Meskan, M. E., 350, 352, 359
Meyerhoff, W. L., 340-41, 342, 343-44, 345, 346-47, 349, 360, 363
Micallef, M., 392, 397
Miller, G. A., 26
Miller, J. D., 193, 213
Miller, R. W., 84, 103
Millin, J., 230, 236, 237, 249, 331, 336
Mills, D., 221, 226
Mills, M., 242, 249
Mitchell, D. P., 345, 364
Mitchell, J. A., 343, 360, 363, 365
Mitchell, P. R., 35, 52
Mitchell, T. V., 296, 307

Miyamoto, R. T., 31, 51, 52-53, 265, 271, 284, 288, 296, 298, 300, 303, 306, 307, 371, 382, 427, 429
Moeller, M. P., 31, 52, 155, 158, 316, 319, 407, 414
Moller, C. G., 345, 363, 364
Moncur, J. P., 99, 100, 103, 323, 336
Monsen, R. B., 33, 42, 45, 52, 55, 73
Montgomery, A. A., 56, 74, 112, 121, 168-69, 191, 196, 211
Moodie, K. S., 151, 152, 159-60, 174, 181-82, 183, 185, 187, 190, 191, 198-99, 212, 213, 266, 271, 276-77, 280, 282, 403-4, 405, 414, 420, 423, 431, 432-33, 439, 440
Moog, J., 29, 51, 72
Moore, B. C., 197, 213
Moore, J. M., 127, 143
Moore, J. N., 200, 201, 211
Morley, R., 203, 211
Morris, L. J., 161, 190
Morrison, T. M., 181, 190, 196, 212
Morrongiello, B. A., 194, 212
Morrow, J., 340, 362
Mort, J., 229, 249
Moshang, T., Jr., 345, 359
Moss, K. A., 107, 120, 122
Most, T., 70, 73
Mueller, H. G., 112, 116, 121, 203, 212, 282, 322, 336
Mulvihill, J. J., 359, 363
Munnich, A., 345, 365
Munoz, O., 350, 361
Munroe, D., 344, 365
Murrell, J.R., 344, 365
Myers, G. J., 346, 363
Myklebust, H. R., 312, 320
Myres, W. A., 288, 300, 305, 307, 371, 382
Myrup, C., 236, 238, 247

Nabalek, A., 20, 26, 113, 121, 232, 234, 244, 249, 313, 320
Nabelek, I., 20, 26, 232, 249
Nadol, J. B., 352, 359
Nalepa, N. J., 348, 361
Nation, J. E., 313, 319
National Technical Institute for the Deaf, 23, 26
Naulty, C. M., 348, 363
Neely, J. G., 346, 360
Nehlig, A., 348, 364
Nelson Barlow, N. L., 151, 159, 403, 414

Netsell, R., 33, 51
Neuman, A. C., 194, 212
Neuss, D., 236, 238, 249
Newall, P., 181, 189, 403, 412, 423
Newby, H. A., 15, 26
Newton, V. E., 340, 346, 363
Ni, L., 340, 360
Nicholls, S., 81-83, 104
Nickerson, R. S., 56, 73
Nicollas, R., 347, 365
Niebuhr, D., 216-18, 226
Niemoeller, A., 203, 211, 229-30, 250
Nittrouer, S., 194, 212
Noffsinger, D., 77, 83-87, 103
Nogrady, B., 342-43, 361
Northern, J. L., 29, 52, 121, 217, 226, 282, 321, 336, 360
Novak, M., 31, 52-53
Novelli-Olmstead, T., 377, 378, 382
Nozza, R. J., 91-93, 103, 152, 159
Numbers, F. C., 56, 73
Nuutila, A., 345, 363

O'Connell, M. P., 147, 158
O'Connell, P., 344, 365
O'Connor, C. D., 9, 19, 26
O'Neill, M., 340, 360
Odkvist, L. M., 345, 363
Oller, D. K., 31-32, 33, 34-35, 36, 37-40, 51, 52, 295, 306
Olsen, B. R., 345, 360
Olsen, W. O., 77, 83-87, 103, 113, 121, 229-30, 250, 274, 282, 322, 336
Oostra, B. A., 340, 342, 345, 360
Osberger, M. J., 31, 33, 51, 52-53, 56, 72, 74, 265, 271, 284, 288, 296, 298, 300, 303, 306, 307, 371, 382, 427, 429
Otis, W., 56, 74
Otomo, K., 33, 53
Oyler, A. L., 323, 336, 383, 385, 397
Oyler, R. F., 323, 336, 383, 385, 397
Ozdamar, O., 350, 363
Ozdamar, S., 303, 308

Padberg, G. W., 340, 342, 345, 360
Page, L. V., 342, 362
Pagon, R. A., 343, 363
Pakarinen, L., 345, 364
Pantke, O. A., 345, 363
Paparella, M. M., 349, 352, 360, 363
Paradise, J. L., 322, 336, 400, 412

Parisier, S. C., 347, 362
Parkinson, A., 181, 189, 403, 412, 423
Parry, D. M., 344, 365
Parving, A., 340, 363
Paryani, S., 346, 361
Pascoe, D. P., 175, 179, 190, 193, 213
Pashley, N. T., 360
Pass, R. F., 346, 363
Patrick, J. F., 286, 307
Patton, D., 236, 241, 247
Paul, R., 230, 250
Pavlovic, C. V., 194, 201, 203, 210, 212, 213, 404, 412
Pearsons, K., 200, 213, 230, 250
Pelias, M. Z., 345, 364
Peltola, H., 349, 362
Pembrey, M., 341, 364
Penton, J., 229, 249
Perez, B. A., 351, 365
Perez-Abalo, M., 127, 143
Perkell, J., 51
Peters, R. W., 83, 103
Peters-Johnson, C., 141, 143
Peterson, M. E., 229, 247
Peterson, P. M., 62, 73
Petit, C., 345, 365
Phelps, P., 341, 364
Phillips, J. W., 15, 21, 27
Picheny, M., 285, 307
Pickens, J. M., 343, 363
Pickett, J., 113, 121
Pickett, J. M., 56, 74
Pickles, A. M., 12, 26
Picton, T. W., 127, 143
Pijl, S., 305, 307
Pikus, A. T., 344, 363
Pillsbury, H. C., 75, 97-98, 103
Plant, G., 263, 271, 429
Platt, F., 315, 319
Pollack, D., 14, 26, 326, 336
Pollack, M. C., 27, 190, 213, 271, 414
Poole, D., 229, 249
Pope, M. L., 31, 53, 265, 271, 284, 288, 296, 307, 371, 382, 427, 429
Popelka, G. R., 193, 203, 211, 213
Popp, A. L., 264, 266, 270, 271
Porter, T. A., 217, 226
Poth, E. A., 83, 103
Potts, P. L., 217, 226
Powell, C., 229, 249
Prabhu, P. U., 346, 365

Priluck, I., 345, 363
Prockop, D. J., 345, 359
Propst, S., 132, 143
Prosek, R. A., 112, 121, 168-69, 190, 196, 211
Pulaski, K., 344, 365
Punch, J. L., 148, 159
Pyeritz, R., 345, 363

Quaranta, A., 80-81, 103, 104
Quittner, A. L., 296, 307

Rabinowitz, W. M., 62, 73, 305, 308
Raffin, M. J. M., 148, 160, 171, 191
Rai, A., 345, 363
Ramji, K. V., 174, 181, 190, 219, 227, 266, 271, 280, 282, 403-4, 414, 420, 423, 431, 440
Ramsdell, D. A., 326, 336
Rane, R., 109, 120, 193, 211
Rankovic, C. M., 203, 213
Raventos, H., 340, 362
Ray, H., 230, 236, 240, 250, 316, 320, 331, 336
Read, D., 127, 143
Reardon, W., 341, 364
Rebscher, S. J., 303, 306
Reddehase, M. J., 346, 362
Redmond, B., 236, 240, 250
Reed, C. M., 62, 73
Reitz, P. S., 400, 407, 413
Remington, J. S., 364
Renshaw, J. J., 31, 51, 53, 265, 271, 284, 296, 306, 307, 406, 414, 427, 429
Resnick, S. B., 428, 429
Revit, L. J., 146, 151, 158, 404, 405, 414
Reynolds, D. W., 346, 360, 364-65
Reynolds, E. G., 428, 429
Riccardi, V. M., 359
Richards, C., 236, 241, 249
Riedner, E. D., 344, 364
Riggs, D., 274, 282
Rines, D., 151, 159, 403, 414
Ringden, O., 344, 359
Rintelmann, W. F., 122
Risberg, A., 55-56, 74
Robbins, A. M., 31, 51, 53, 265, 271, 284, 288, 296, 298, 300, 303, 306, 307, 371, 382, 406, 414, 427, 429
Robertson, M., 344, 365
Robinson, D. O., 216-17, 226
Robinson, P. K., 234, 249, 313, 320
Robson, R. C., 194, 212
Roeser, R. J., 249, 250, 320, 322, 335, 336, 337, 350, 364
Roger, C., 348, 364
Ronis, M. L., 350, 362
Ropers, H., 345, 360
Rose, D. E., 22, 26
Rosenberg, G., 236, 240, 250, 313, 315, 320
Rosenhall, U., 350, 364
Rosner, B. A., 314, 320
Ross, C., 32, 52
Ross, M., 2, 3, 12, 13, 16, 18-22, 24, 27, 31, 51, 53, 56, 74, 107, 113, 121, 146, 159, 170, 175, 179, 181, 190, 191, 193, 213, 220, 226, 229-30, 237, 248, 250, 266, 271, 273, 274, 282, 311, 320, 321, 322, 325, 326, 335, 337, 406, 412, 413, 414, 423, 426, 429
Rossman, R. N., 152, 159, 203, 211
Roush, J., 2, 27, 218, 227, 441, 443, 445-46, 448
Rowson, V. J., 340, 346, 363
Ruben, R. J., 109, 121, 150, 159, 340, 364, 403, 413
Rubin, J. A., 56, 74
Rubin, M., 21, 27
Rubin-Spitz, J. A., 194, 212
Rushmer, N., 132, 137, 143
Rutter, J.L., 344, 365

Sabo, M. P., 312, 319
Saez-Llorens, X., 349, 364
Sandall, S. R., 137, 142
Sanders, D., 230, 250
Sandlin, R. E., 211
Sanger, D., 393, 397
Sankila, E. M., 345, 364
Sanyal, M., 313, 319
Sarff, L., 230, 236, 240, 250, 316, 320, 323, 331, 336, 337
Savage, H., 315, 319
Scavera, N., 342, 361
Schachern, P., 352, 360
Scheld, W. M., 362, 364
Schell, V., 217, 227
Schilder, A., 386, 398
Schildroth, A. N., 346, 364
Schindler, R. A., 305, 307
Schmael, O., 8, 27
Schoeny, Z., 79, 86, 104
Scholl, M. E., 324, 335
Schuknecht, H. F., 346, 364
Schulte, L., 153, 154, 159
Schum, D., 248, 276, 282
Schum, R., 229, 248, 405, 413

Schuyler, V., 132, 137, 143
Schwaber, M. K., 340-41, 343-44, 345, 346-47, 363
Schwartz, D. M., 109, 112, 121, 122, 169-71, 175, 179, 181, 190, 191, 348, 364, 403, 405, 414, 422
Sculerati, N., 340-41, 343-44, 345, 346-47, 363
Seewald, R. C., 69, 74, 109, 119, 120, 121, 151, 152, 153, 158, 159-60, 163, 170, 174, 175, 181, 182, 183, 185, 187, 189, 190, 191 193-94, 196, 198-99, 201, 210, 211, 212, 213, 219, 227, 266, 271, 276-77, 280, 282, 399, 403-4, 405, 406, 413, 414, 415, 420, 423, 431, 432-33, 439, 440, 441-42
Segel, P. A., 352, 359
Seizinger, B. R., 344, 365
Seligman, P. M., 305, 307
Selikowitz, M., 443, 445
Sell, E., 348, 364
Seltzer, S., 351, 364
Sexton, J., 223, 227
Shallop, J. K., 305, 307
Shapiro, W. H., 303, 308
Sharp, P. A., 348, 361
Shaver, K. A., 345, 359
Shaw, E. A. G., 151, 159, 418, 423
Shea, D., 349, 363
Shea, J. J., Jr., 341, 364
Shemen, L. J., 345, 364
Shepard, N., 386, 397
Sherbecoe, R. L., 194, 203, 213
Shipp, D. B., 305, 307
Shore, I., 112, 121, 175, 179, 190
Short, M. P., 344, 365
Shulman, J., 62, 73
Shumrick, D., 363
Siegenthaler, B., 426, 430
Silman, S., 13, 25, 148, 159
Silverman, C. A., 148, 159
Silverman, S. R., 336, 428, 429
Simeonsson, R. J., 355, 359
Simon, C. S., 324, 325, 337
Simonton, K. M., 348, 364
Sinclair, J. S., vii, viii, 73, 189, 250, 274, 282
Sinclair, S. T., 151, 152, 159-60, 174, 181-82, 183, 185, 187, 190, 191, 198-99, 212, 213, 266, 271, 403-4, 405, 414, 420, 423, 431, 432-33, 439, 440
Singh, R. S., 353, 359
Sinopoli, T. A., 352, 359
Sistonen, P., 345, 364

Skinner, M. W., 146, 153, 160, 171, 174, 191, 193, 213, 303-4, 305, 307, 403, 414
Skinner, P. D., 27
Slattery, W. H., III, 340-41, 343-44, 346-47, 363
Smaldino, J., 119, 121, 229-30, 231-32, 233, 235, 237, 239, 242, 244, 245-46, 248, 320, 329, 335, 397
Smith, A., 127, 143
Smith, C. R., 42, 53, 56, 74, 298, 308
Smith, F., 26
Smith, J., 353, 359
Smith, L., 62, 73
Smith, L. B., 30-31, 50, 296, 307
Smith, R. J., 340, 345, 360, 364
Smith, S., 87-88, 103
Smith, S. D., 340, 342, 345, 360
Snik, A. F. M., 386, 398, 404, 405, 414, 415
Snyder, R. L., 303, 306
Spens, C. E., 429
Sperry, J. L., 84, 104
Spiro, M. K., 175, 179, 191, 423
Springer, N., 62, 73
Sproule, J. R., 343, 361
Stagno, S., 346, 360, 363, 364-65
Staller, S. J., 305, 307
Stanley, S., 386, 398
Stapells, D. R., 127, 143
Stark, R. E., 31, 53, 56, 74
Starling, S. P., 346, 365
Stechenberg, B. W., 350, 360
Steel, K. P., 345, 365
Steffens, M., 34, 52
Stein, D. M., 323, 337
Stein, L., 350, 363
Stein, L. K., 350, 365, 400, 415
Stein, R., 383, 397
Steinberg, J. C., 202, 211
Stelmachowicz, P. G., 50, 72, 109, 112, 119, 120, 121, 151-52, 153-54, 155, 158, 159-60, 162, 170, 181, 187, 189, 190, 191, 196, 197, 198, 199, 200, 204, 206, 211, 213, 276-77, 280, 282, 386, 397, 399, 403-4, 407, 410, 413, 414, 415, 420, 423, 431, 439
Stenstrom, R., 168, 191, 405, 415
Sterling, G. R., 216-17, 226
Stevens, J., 344, 365
Stevens, K. N., 30, 52, 232, 249, 312, 320
Stewart, B. J., 346, 365
Stoel-Gammon, C., 32, 33, 52, 53
Stollman, M. H. P. 404, 414
Stone, M. A., 197, 213

Stoppenbach, D. T., 107, 120, 122
Straatman, H., 386, 398
Strauss, K. P., 333, 335
Streng, A., 15, 21, 27
Stroer, B. S., 31, 52-53, 300, 307
Struthers, G. R., 345, 363
Stuart, A., 168, 191, 405, 415
Stubblefield, J., 76, 104
Studdert-Kennedy, M., 53, 194, 212
Studebaker, G. A., 73, 189, 190, 194, 203, 212, 213, 412, 415, 423
Subtelny, J. D., 55, 74
Sullivan, J. A., 194, 212, 213
Sullivan, R., 280, 282

Tabor, M., 236, 238, 250
Teele, D. W., 314, 320
Tees, R. C., 30, 53
Ternier, F., 347, 365
Tervoort, B., 13, 27
Teter, D., 113, 122
Tharpe, A. M., 119, 120, 229, 247, 323, 335, 399, 400, 407, 410, 412, 413, 414, 415, 429, 441, 445, 447, 449
Thelin, J. W., 343, 360, 363, 365
Thibodeau, L. M., 276-77, 282
Thomas, H., 20, 26
Thompson, C. L., 75, 103
Thompson, D. J., 404, 413
Thompson, G., 127, 129, 142, 143
Thompson, M., 127, 132, 143
Thordardottir, E. T., 107, 120, 122
Thornton, A. R., 148, 160, 171, 191, 203, 212
Tillman, T., 78, 81-83, 102, 103, 104, 113, 121, 229-30, 232, 234, 248, 313, 319, 324, 335, 385, 389, 397, 428, 430
Tinley, S., 342-43, 362
Todd, S. L., 298, 300, 303, 307
Tolan, T., 8-11, 28
Tolk, J., 20, 27
Tonisson, W., 176, 189, 418, 423
Tonokawa, L. L., 289, 306
Tranebjaerg, L., 345, 364
Triglia, J. M., 347, 365
Trivedi, D. V., 342, 362
Trivette, C. M., 132, 133, 142, 143
Trofatter, J. A., 344, 365
Truchon-Gagnon, C., 389, 397
Tucker, B., 23, 27, 28
Tye-Murray, N., 190, 296, 306
Tyler, R. S., 55, 74, 88, 89-90, 103, 248, 296, 305, 306, 308, 382

Updike, C. D., 328, 337

Vaillancourt, M. M., 419, 423
Valente, M., 414, 422
van Beersum, S. E., 345, 360
Van Camp, G. V., 340, 342, 345, 360
Van de Heyning, P. H., 340, 342, 345, 360
van den Borne, S., 405, 415
van den Broek, P., 386, 398
Vandali, A. E., 304, 307
van Loo, I. H., 342, 361
Van Tasell, D. J., 322, 336
Varela, A., 345, 365
Vaughn, G., 113, 122
Vergara, K., 295, 306
Vernon, M., 345, 359
Vert, P., 348, 364
Viehweg, S., 229, 230, 236, 238, 247, 249, 335
Vihman, M., 32, 53
Viskochil, D., 344, 365
Vossen, J. M., 342, 361

Wagenaar, M., 345, 365
Wagner, E. F., 91-93, 103
Walden, B. E., 56, 74, 112, 121, 122, 168-69, 171, 190, 191, 196, 211
Walker, G., 196, 213
Wallace, I. F., 314, 319, 386, 397
Wallace, K. L., 410, 413
Wallach, G. P., 325, 337
Walsh, J., 345, 365
Walton, J. P., 348, 361, 365
Waltzman, S. B., 303, 308, 352, 360
Wang, M. D., 56, 72
Ward, J. I., 349-50, 362
Wark, D. J., 323, 336
Warman, M. L., 345, 360
Watchko, J. F., 348, 362
Watkins, S., 387, 397
Watson, L. A., 8-11, 28
Watson, N. A., 6, 9, 19, 28
Watson, R. B., 6, 9, 19, 28
Watson, T., 229, 249
Watson, T. J., 13, 19-20, 28
Weber, P. C., 351, 365
Wedenberg, E., 3, 28, 340, 359
Weil, D., 345, 365
Weisenberger, J. M., 295, 308
Weisner, T. S., 132, 142

Weiss, I. P., 348, 363
Weiss, R., 344, 365
Weissman, J. L., 351, 365
Werker, J. F., 30, 53
Werner, L. A., 127, 143
Wertz, P., 315, 319
Weston, M. D., 345, 365
Whan, M. A., 410, 413
Whetnall, E., 13, 28
White, R., 344, 365
White, V., 345, 363
Whiteside, S., 182, 187, 191
Whitford, L. A., 305, 307
Wieman, L. A., 32, 52
Wightman, F., 152, 158
Wiley, T. L, 107, 120, 122
Willems, P., 340, 360
Willems, P. J., 340, 342, 345, 360
Williams, D. L, 112, 122, 171, 191
Williams, D. M., 137, 143
Williams, E., 348, 364
Williams, K. A., 30, 52, 312, 320
Willis, D., 56, 74
Wilson, B. S., 287, 305, 308
Wilson, M., 125, 142
Wilson, R. H., 78, 84, 88, 100, 101, 103, 104, 120, 122
Wilson, W. R., 30, 51, 129, 142, 143
Wilson-Vlotman, A., 322, 335, 337
Winchester, R., 217, 226
Winton, P. J., 124, 143
Wispelwey, B., 362, 364
Wolff, A. B., 350, 365
Wolford, R. D., 305, 308
Woodworth, G. G., 296, 305, 306
Wordsworth, P., 345, 363
Worthington, D. W., 340, 350, 359, 410, 412
Wynne, M. K., 400, 407, 413

Xu, G., 344, 365

Yacullo, W. S., 20, 26, 148, 150, 159
Yeni-Komshian, G. H., 52, 53
Yeung, E., 71, 72
Yong, S. L., 343, 363
Yoon, T. H., 352, 360
Yost, W. A., 100, 104
Young, D. F., 344, 365
Younger, A., 346, 361

Zabel, H., 236, 238, 250

Zackai, E. H., 345, 359
Zaphiropoulos, G. C., 345, 363
Zara, C., 370, 382
Zelisko, D. L., 69, 74, 170, 182, 187, 189, 190, 191, 196, 211, 219, 227, 280, 282, 405, 413, 414
Zigmond, N. K., 312, 320
Zimmerman-Phillips, S., 31, 52-53, 300, 307
Zink, G. D., 217, 227
Zizz, C. A., 84, 104
Zonana, J., 343, 363
Zwingle, E., 157, 160

Subject Index

Academic performance, 410
    impact of hearing loss, 311-12, 321-26, 334, 386, 447, 450-52
    monitoring, 331-32, 334, 355, 358, 393-94, 447-48
    reading, 321, 323, 325, 326, 451-52
    with classroom amplification, 230, 236, 238, 240-41, 245-46, 315, 316, 318, 331
Academy of Dispensing Audiologists, vii, viii, 399
Acclimatization, 156, 174, 255, 269
    and speech perception, 56, 171-72
    to cochlear implant, 294-97, 298, 300-1, 302
Acoustic accessibility, 333, 334, 370, 376, 448-49, 453
Acoustic feedback, 146, 147, 153, 219, 246, 402, 409
Acoustic filter effect, 324-25, 326, 451-52
Acoustics, educational setting, 6-7, 19, 22, 229-30, 232-46, 280, 358
    impact on speech perception, 19-20, 112, 202-3, 208, 231-32
    modification, 220, 243, 389, 394, 448-49
    monitoring, 220, 385, 391, 407
    room, 13, 19, 99, 169, 329, 383, 388-90, 395, 396, 448-49
    (See also Distance; Noise; Reverberation)
Adolescents, 66-67, 116-17
Adults, 263-65, 277, 279, 302, 305, 313, 428
Age, 81-83
    at detection of hearing loss, 12, 34, 411
    at onset of hearing loss, 298, 300-1, 302, 303, 305, 340-41, 346
    candidacy criteria, 303, 408-9
    cosmetic concerns, 116-19, 276
    monitoring of hearing loss, 339, 358
    monitoring of amplification, 216, 218, 219, 225, 403
    preselection of device, 146, 150, 332, 356-57, 402, 403, 409
    selection of electroacoustics, 109-10, 146, 175-76
    signal-to-noise ratio, 152, 234-35, 244

    verification of performance, 187, 405, 432
Age differences in,
    academic improvement, 240-41, 316
    assessment techniques, 125, 127-28, 145, 164, 168-69, 178, 187, 401, 403
    auditory skills, 152, 303, 312-14, 372-73, 379-80, 388, 392, 396
    external ear, 109, 145, 150-51, 403-4, 409, 420
    masked level differences, 82-83, 91-97
    real-ear-to-coupler difference, 151-52, 403-4, 420, 421, 432-33, 436-37, 442
    speech perception, 152, 194, 285, 295-97, 298, 300, 302, 305, 313, 332
    speech production, 60, 66-67, 69, 70-71
Aided Audibility Index (AAI), 202, 204, 209, 210
Albers-Schonberg disease, 341-42
Alport's syndrome, 342
American Academy of Pediatrics, 350-51
American Speech-Language-Hearing Association, 1, 108, 279, 316
Americans with Disabilities Act, 448-49
Amplitude, 62, 69, 304
Articulation index, 202-4
Assessment, 322, 408, 432, 436
    in fitting procedure, 15-16, 125-31, 161, 163-64, 172-73, 175, 187, 266, 400, 401-2, 411, 447 (see also Audiometry)
    problems, 23, 172-73, 441-42, 443, 451
Assistive device, 408, 410, 411
Attention, 313, 323, 339, 449
    in educational setting, 314, 328, 331, 384, 393, 394
    with classroom amplification, 241, 313, 315
Attention deficit, 232, 313, 314, 325
Audiologist, 322, 355, 392
    part of multidisciplinary team, 124, 133-34, 135-36, 140, 142, 219, 221, 224, 225, 318, 339, 405-6, 410
    responsibility, 13, 123-24, 131-36, 141, 142, 188-89, 218, 220, 221, 223, 224-25, 279, 281, 318, 333-34, 339, 358, 380-

470 • SUBJECT INDEX

81, 386, 399, 400, 407, 411, 452-53
Audiology, 7, 9, 11, 13, 14, 16, 120, 400, 410
   clinical practice, 14-19, 107-20, 148-50, 161-63, 171-73, 175-76, 178-86, 187, 188, 236, 243, 264-65, 266-69, 279-80, 323, 329, 334, 339, 379-81, 396, 400, 403-7, 442
   goal, 2, 5, 17-18, 21, 24-25, 135, 253, 270, 400
Audiometry, 16, 136, 161, 164, 176-79, 196, 267, 328, 334, 401, 404, 407
   auditory brainstem response, 15-16, 30, 125-26, 156-57, 161-62, 350, 354, 401-2, 408, 410, 444
   behavioral, 16, 91, 125, 127-31, 166, 172-73, 178, 187, 266, 332-33, 350, 355, 401, 410, 442
   changes, 339, 350, 353-58, 447
   play, 15, 91, 129, 357
   transformation to SPL, 176, 178-79, 183-84, 196, 401
   visual reinforcement, 16, 91, 127-31, 355
Auditory sensory deprivation, 13-14, 148, 303
Auditory skills, 29, 152, 312-15, 323, 388, 396, 411
   and academic achievement, 312, 314, 324
   listening, 324, 328, 331, 383-87, 390-96
   measurement, 59-68, 70-71, 303, 313, 318
   monitoring, 406, 407
   training, 5, 7, 13, 15-16, 19, 56, 188, 270, 369-82, 383, 387-88, 390-96
      group, 7, 380, 390-92
      with transposition devices, 255, 263-65
Autoimmune inner ear disease, 348-49, 351

Babbling, 33, 34-40, 44-45
Behavior, 331, 407
   impact of hearing loss, 321, 323, 325, 334
   with classroom amplification, 238, 240-41, 315, 316, 331
Behind-the-ear (BTE) devices, 19, 116, 145-46, 147, 156, 275, 277, 281, 356, 402
   FM systems, 20, 21, 444
Berger method, 109-10
Bilirubin, 347-48
Bill Wilkerson Center (Nashville, Tenn.), vii, 399
Binaural auditory processing, 93-97, 99-102, 148
   impact of hearing loss, 75, 101-2

   localization, 75-76, 78, 90, 93, 102
   masking level difference, 75-76, 78-99
   temporal cues, 75-76, 78, 81-82, 83, 88-90, 93-97
Body-worn device, 9, 11-12, 15, 145, 409
   candidacy criteria, 402-3, 446
   FM unit, 19, 274, 276, 281
   preselection, 146-47, 157-58
   transposition device, 253, 259-60, 262
Bone conduction, 9, 409, 419, 444, 447
Brain lesions, 83-87
Branchio-oto-renal (BOR) syndrome, 342-43, 409

Candidacy criteria, 188, 328, 401-2, 408-9
   classroom amplification, 231-32, 314-15
   cochlear implants, 188, 263-64, 302, 303, 304
   FM systems, 244-45, 276, 328
   transposition devices, 253, 257, 259-60, 262-63, 269
Case studies, 33-49, 148-50, 156-57, 204-9, 353-58, 432-39, 441-53
Central auditory processing disorders, 232, 275, 314
Central nervous system, disorders of, 80-81, 83-86
Child-to-child communication, 4, 8, 20, 273
Classroom (see Educational setting)
Closed captioning, 408
Cochlear implants, 9, 23-24, 256-57, 264-65, 270, 303-5
   candidacy criteria, 147, 188, 262-65, 303-4
   comparison studies, 257, 262-65, 270, 283-303
   meningitis, 352-53, 358
   multichannel, 286, 288-89, 290-97, 298-303, 304-5, 371
   single-channel, 283, 284, 286, 288-89, 301-2
   speech perception, 49, 57, 369-72, 374, 377, 380
Communication mode, 50, 56, 204, 300, 352, 381-82
   auditory/verbal, 60, 69-70, 71, 388
   effect on speech production, 60-61, 64-65, 69-70, 71
   total communication, 45, 60, 69-70, 208
   visual, 369, 373, 374
Compliance, in use of device, 18, 22-23, 289, 317, 356-57, 380, 387

SUBJECT INDEX • 471

Compression ratio, 178, 196, 197, 203-4, 205, 210
Consonant
  discrimination, 371, 372
  perception, 254, 256, 259-62, 263, 264-65, 266, 284, 289, 291-92, 293-94, 296-97, 298, 299, 303, 304
  place, 56, 59, 67-68, 284, 296-97, 298, 299, 301, 371, 372
  voicing, 56, 58, 67, 284, 286, 287, 296-97, 299, 372, 376, 379
Cosmetic concerns, 116-17, 276, 281, 402 (see also Stigma)
Cost, 156, 231, 409
  effectiveness, 240, 242, 243-44, 245, 316, 317, 351
Counseling, 15, 17, 112, 124, 131-42, 154-55, 321, 351-52, 355, 357-58, 400, 410
  content, 124, 136-40, 279, 406, 409
Cytomegalovirus, 346, 409

Day care setting, 312, 314, 315
Deaf, schools for the, 3, 5-9, 22
Deaf community, identity, 23-24
Desired sensation level (DSL) method, 182, 266, 419-21, 431
Developmental delay, 232, 237-38, 241, 312, 314, 410
  language development, delayed, 33-50, 357, 450
Direct audio input, 146, 276, 356, 445
Disabilities,
  developmental, 312, 331, 349, 451-52
  learning, 232, 244, 314, 315, 325, 349
  multiple, 16, 135, 276, 401, 409, 410, 452-53
Distance, 208, 220, 371
  and FM systems, 231, 274, 277, 328, 408
  and speech signal, 152, 193, 204-8, 273, 322
  impact on speech perception, 234-37, 239, 243-44, 266, 322, 324, 326-27, 334
  in educational setting, 280, 332
  (see also Seating)
Distortion, 16, 276, 277
  compression circuitry, 202, 204, 205, 210
  in classroom amplification, 22, 243, 246
  peak clipping, 158, 196-97, 201-2, 204-5, 208, 209, 210
Down syndrome, 443-47
Duffy, John, 17

Early intervention, 133-34, 135, 142, 162, 188-89, 220, 224, 225, 303, 318, 355, 387, 443
  developmental concerns, 12-14, 29, 273, 312, 451
  language development, 30, 326, 373, 379-80
  role of parents, 15, 29, 131-33, 379
  selection, 193, 281, 400, 411
Earmold, 147, 403
  change, 434, 442
  coupling, 164, 168, 328-29, 402, 432, 436
  real-ear-to-coupler differences, 407, 432
  retention, 153-55, 409
Earphones, 311, 329, 331
  insert, 125, 130
  with personal FM system, 317, 448
Earshot (see Distance)
Education of All Handicapped Children Act (P.L. 94-142), 133-34, 311-12, 333 (see also Laws and regulations)
Educational setting, vii, 3-9, 14, 21-22, 23, 230-46, 273, 311-12, 314-18, 321, 323-24, 327, 331-34, 381, 383, 386-96, 445-53
EMILY signal processor, 257-59
English as second language, 233-34, 239, 315
Evaluation of aided hearing performance (see Validation)
External ear, 108-9, 145, 146, 150-51, 403-4, 409, 420, 439

Family, 124, 220, 380
  role in management, 131-35, 218-19, 224, 381, 406, 407, 447
  training, 218-19, 225, 407 (see also Parents)
Family needs questionnaire, 137-39, 447
Family-centered services, 131-33
Fitting, configuration,
  binaural vs. monaural, 9-10, 13, 19, 22, 118, 119, 148-50, 206-8, 215, 402
Fitting procedure, 10-12, 107-20, 123-24, 279, 380, 399-400, 410-11
  goal, 124, 145, 405-6
  prescriptive, 109, 172-87, 193-94, 266-70, 400, 402, 403
  problems, 109, 112, 116, 409
  subjective, 194, 264-66 (see also Assessment; Preselection; Selection; Validation; Verification)
Food and Drug Administration (FDA), 257-58, 304, 369
Freeman E. McConnell Memorial Lecture, 1-

SUBJECT INDEX

28
Frequency, 153, 178, 203, 327, 342, 372, 418
   and speech perception, 194, 204-6, 208, 253-54, 256-57, 259, 260-61, 262, 263
   compression, 259-61
   dynamic range, 269, 304
   high, 172, 196, 260-61, 262, 263, 268-69, 274, 275, 276, 287, 301, 303-4, 342, 344, 371, 374
   low, 349, 381
Frequency modulation (FM) system, 157-58, 164, 220, 256, 261-62, 274, 328-29, 402, 407, 408
   antenna, 274, 275, 277-79, 281
   behind-the-ear (BTE), 113, 114, 146, 156, 262, 273-81, 407, 444
   compared to hearing aid, 329, 334
   cost, 243-44, 317
   coupling, 274, 277, 328-29
   in educational setting, 45, 113, 116, 205-6, 230-46, 327-34, 354, 356-57, 395, 396, 448, 450
   in nonacademic settings, 113, 116, 156
   monitoring, 220, 223-24, 225
   personal, 113, 116, 238, 279, 316, 317, 330, 331, 354, 380, 389, 396, 445-46, 448, 451
   recommended use of, 19, 20, 113, 116, 117, 119, 117, 168
   signal-to-noise ratio, 155-56, 244-45
   sound field, 113, 114, 116, 244-45, 246, 329-31, 333, 354, 358, 389, 391, 445-46, 449
   training, 155, 273, 328
   verification of, 112, 276-77, 279-80
   wireless, 274, 280, 311, 329
   with hearing aid, 274, 275, 277, 278-80, 356-57
Frequency response, 116, 194, 195, 202, 260-61, 276, 356
   target, 178, 182, 217, 269, 279, 280, 405, 410, 416, 419

Gain, 170, 209, 217, 245, 277, 356, 432
   and acoustic feedback, 147, 246
   adjustment, 116, 274-75
   coupler, 182, 184, 421, 424, 437-39
   functional, 17, 112, 280, 444
   high frequencies, 147, 172
   insertion, 174, 267, 416, 417, 418, 424
   target, 174, 178, 186, 267, 279, 403-4
      DSL method, 182, 266, 419-21, 431
      NAL method, 418-19
      POGO method, 181, 416-17
      RECD method, 151
   mild, 313, 316, 317, 328, 354
   muting circuit, 20
   nonlinear, 193-94, 196-97
   real ear, 197-198, 201-2
      measurement, 112, 167, 210, 280, 405
   reserve, 417, 418, 421
Gain curve, 195, 196-97, 201, 202, 210
Gallaudet College, 255
Gallaudet, E. M., 3
Goldstein, Max, 3, 6, 7

Hearing, normal, 30, 78-87, 89-99, 101-2, 130, 153-54, 231-34, 235-38, 239, 240, 241, 242-43, 244, 245, 311-18, 322, 324, 326, 331, 344, 379, 381, 385, 386, 389-92, 395, 408 (see also Hearing loss, degree, minimal)
Hearing aid, 8-12, 14-15, 141, 147, 223, 328, 334, 371, 380, 402, 409, 410
   behind-the-ear (BTE), 145-46, 147, 356, 402, 432
   burden of, 15, 18, 19, 23
   candidacy criteria, 328
   circuitry, 147
      compression, 115, 116, 196-97, 202-5, 208-10, 424-25
      linear, 115, 116, 179, 196-97, 202, 204, 206, 208, 209, 210, 424
      nonlinear, 193-94, 204, 210
   compared with cochlear implants, 283, 286, 287-88, 290-95, 298, 302, 303-4
   cost, 223-24
   direct audio input, 274, 402
   electroacoustics, 166, 173-76, 178-88
      output limiting, 162-63, 166, 178, 179, 182, 186
      verification, 174-75, 177, 182, 187, 204-8, 215-17, 221, 222
   evaluation, 164-72
   in educational setting, 273-74, 334, 449-50
   in the ear, 145, 146, 176, 403
   monitoring, 216-17, 221, 225
   orientation, 218, 225, 406
   personal, 273-74, 280, 383, 387
   programmable, 115-16, 146, 156, 395, 410

SUBJECT INDEX • 473

with FM system, 238, 273, 276-77, 280, 395
Hearing loss, 340-45, 380, 384, 386, 387-89,
  391, 392, 395, 399
  acquired, 263, 298, 300, 302, 305, 346-51
  conductive, 9, 11, 80-81, 83-85, 87-88, 91,
    312, 314, 341, 343, 344, 346, 350, 409,
    417, 419, 421, 443-44, 447
  configuration, 156, 269, 311, 401-2, 409, 412
    asymmetrical, 75, 85-86, 87-88, 91, 97,
      130, 148, 208-9, 312, 343, 402
    unilateral, 232, 312, 323, 324, 326,
      328, 332-33, 334, 345, 346, 348,
      349, 350, 353-54, 383, 385, 386,
      400-1, 410, 412, 450-51
  congenital, 11, 12, 145, 298, 300, 302, 341,
    346
  degree, 56, 130, 164, 269, 273, 275, 281, 322,
    326, 328, 333, 334, 340, 342, 343, 344,
    345, 346, 347, 348, 350, 369, 371, 379,
    386, 400-2, 408, 409, 418, 431
    mild, 9, 33, 113, 115, 116, 117, 119,
      154, 166-67, 238, 241, 311, 322-23,
      324, 326, 328-29, 332, 333, 383,
      385-90, 392, 396, 405, 407, 447-48
    minimal, 119, 154, 232-33, 236-37,
      238-39, 240, 312, 316, 321-22, 324-
      27, 328-29, 331-33, 334, 358, 383,
      385-87, 391, 405, 410, 412, 448,
      450-53
    moderate, 23, 33, 37, 38-40, 42, 43, 45,
      113, 115, 116, 117, 119, 148, 198,
      206, 238, 245, 255, 258, 311, 349,
      357-58, 385, 386, 391, 407
    profound, 11, 15, 33, 39, 40, 44, 45-49,
      59-69, 70, 71, 113, 115, 117, 119,
      146-47, 148, 157, 162, 171, 181,
      195, 205, 253, 254-56, 258, 262,
      263, 283-305, 311, 341, 343, 345,
      347, 352, 353, 355, 369-71, 376-77,
      379-82, 383, 387, 396, 402, 405,
      407, 408, 416, 418, 450
    severe, 11, 15, 23, 33, 38, 40, 42, 43,
      44-45, 59-69, 71, 113, 115, 117, 119,
      146, 147, 148, 151, 162, 171, 181,
      195, 198, 206, 245, 253, 255, 256,
      258, 262, 311, 341, 342, 352, 355,
      369-71, 376-77, 379-82, 383, 387,
      396, 405, 407, 408, 416, 418, 432-
      33, 450
  fluctuating, 148-50, 156, 232, 314, 322, 324,
    326, 328-29, 332, 334, 339-41, 346-49,

350-51, 353-58, 383, 400, 406, 409-10,
  444, 447, 448
frequencies, 79, 130, 146, 147, 208, 312,
  401, 410
incidence, 312, 314, 321, 323, 340, 342-45,
  346, 348, 349, 350, 443
noise-induced, 83-86, 316, 404, 409
progressive, 148-50, 339-41, 342-47, 348-49,
  351-54, 358, 406-7, 409-10, 443-44
sensorineural, 11, 79, 80-81, 83-85, 87-88,
  89-91, 100-2, 164, 177, 203, 231-33,
  234-35, 236-37, 238-39, 240, 244-45,
  273, 311, 340-41, 342-45, 346, 347,
  348, 349, 351, 352, 353, 355, 357-58,
  383, 387, 409, 410, 431, 432, 443-44
Hyperbilirubinemia, 347-48

Individualized Education Plan (IEP), 133, 141,
  220, 223, 225, 333, 448
Individualized Family Service Plan (IFSP), 133-
  34, 135, 141, 220, 224, 225, 448
Individuals with Disabilities Education Act
  (IDEA), 134, 141, 220-25, 312, 318, 333,
  334, 453 (see also Laws and regulations)
Infant and Toddler Program (Part H), 134, 224
Inner ear disorder, 347, 348-49, 351, 352-53
Intensity, signal, 17, 152, 270, 288, 313, 315,
  327, 370, 371, 389
International Phonetic Alphabet, 41, 46-49

Jaundice, 347-48
Joint Committee on Infant Hearing, 162

Knowles Electronics Mannequin for Acoustic
  Research (KEMAR), 235, 236, 239

Language development, 8, 11, 30-32, 253, 333-
  34, 370-71, 379-80, 410
  age, 12-14, 32
  with classroom amplification, 7-8, 316, 331
  impact of hearing loss, 311-12, 321, 323-25,
    400-1, 450
  (see also Auditory skills; Speech perception;
  Speech production)
Laws and regulations, 21, 133-34, 135, 136, 141-
  42, 220-25, 228, 311-12, 333, 334, 448-49,
  453

Least restrictive environment, principle of, 133, 312
Ling, Dan, 13
Listening, incidental, 323, 324, 326-27, 333-34, 408, 450
Listening level,
    comfort, 59, 266, 400, 403, 406, 416, 418
    discomfort, 18, 179-80, 181, 193, 194, 209, 266, 403, 404, 405, 406
Localization, 127, 323
    with binaural hearing, 75-76, 78, 90, 93, 102, 148
Loop system, 274, 276, 277, 281, 311, 445-46, 448
Loudspeaker, 243, 246, 317, 329, 332
Lybarger, Sam, 12

Mainstreaming, 311-12, 383, 445, 452
Maintenance, of device, 141, 155, 224, 243, 245, 246, 380, 387, 406
Malfunction of device, 22, 215-18, 219, 223, 225, 245, 246, 317
    (see also Maintenance; Monitoring)
Masking level difference, 75-102
    in adults, 79-91
    in Ménière's disease, 79-80, 83-85
    postsurgery, 90-91, 97-99
    with asymmetric hearing loss, 83, 85-86, 87-88, 91
Maternal and Child Health Bureau, viii
Ménière's disease, 79-81, 83-86, 349, 351
Meningitis, 300, 302, 349-50, 352-53, 355-56, 358
Mental retardation, 450-51
Microphone, 20, 34, 147, 152, 153, 262, 267
    directional, 118, 119, 150, 156, 374, 395
    in educational setting, 327, 328, 330, 334, 450
    omnidirectional, 118, 150
    placement, 277-79, 281, 424
    probe-tube, 17, 196
        alternatives, 151, 166, 185, 432
        in verification, 32, 109-12, 152, 176-77, 180-81, 182, 204-5, 279-80, 357, 403-4, 405, 432
        real-ear-to-coupler difference, 198-99
        test-retest reliability, 168
    remote, 155, 327, 328, 330, 334, 409, 450
    voice-activated, 155, 156
    with FM system, 155, 230, 231, 274-75, 277-81, 317, 395
Middle ear disorder, 9, 148-49, 314, 340, 342, 343, 348, 350-51, 410
    (see also Otitis media)
Minimal Pairs Test, 284-85, 289, 291-92, 293-94, 296-97, 298, 299, 301
Mobility, 273, 311, 317
Mondini's dysplasia, 347, 353
Monitoring, of device or system performance, 215-26, 407, 434-35, 439
    daily, 219, 220, 221-23, 225, 279, 371
    educational setting, 221-23
    equipment for, 219, 225
    FM system, 279-80, 281, 317, 334
    guidelines, 220, 221-25, 279-80
Monitoring, of hearing loss, 151, 316, 339, 351, 352-53, 354, 356, 357, 358, 409, 410, 436
Monitoring, of hearing performance, 357, 379, 403, 406-7, 442, 448, 450
Mucopolysaccharidoses syndrome, 343-44
Multiband, 20
Multidisciplinary team, 124, 133, 134-36, 140, 142, 219, 220, 224, 225, 352, 358, 406, 410-11
Multiple sclerosis, 83-87

National Acoustic Laboratories method, 109-10, 181, 187, 418-19
National Technical Institute for the Deaf, 23-24
Noise, 19, 75, 220, 273-74, 371, 406
    and binaural processing, 76-102
    and speech perception, 19-20, 109-12, 203, 208, 231-32, 274, 313-14, 378
    effect on language development, 19, 315
    in assessment, 6, 17, 167, 266-67
    in educational setting, 229-30, 231, 232-35, 243, 245, 246, 280, 311-12, 314, 315, 324, 332-33, 334, 358, 387-92, 393-94
    internal to hearing aid, 17, 167, 275
    masking, 76-102, 231-32, 233
    with transposition devices, 254, 256, 266-67, 269-70 (see also Signal-to-noise ratio)

Osteogenesis imperfecta (Van der Hoeve's syndrome), 344
Otitis media, 147, 322, 350-51, 353, 357-58, 409, 450
    and Down syndrome, 443-46

and masked level differences in children, 91, 97-99
  impact of hearing loss, 13, 312, 313, 314, 323, 385
  service delivery, 383, 447-48
Otosclerosis, 90-91, 99, 341
Output, maximum, 162-63, 179-80, 193, 197, 202, 206, 280, 403-4, 410, 417, 424-25, 432, 437
Output limiting, 166, 178, 179-80, 182, 186, 279, 316, 317, 329, 356, 403-5, 416-17, 431, 432, 439
  compression, 202, 205, 209, 424-25
  peak clipping, 202, 205, 209

Parents, 18, 124, 276, 317, 339, 380
  education of, 279, 316, 339, 357, 379, 386, 409
  role in intervention, 14-15, 24, 188, 381, 402, 411, 443, 451-52
  role in maintaining device, 216, 218-19, 224, 225
  role in monitoring hearing loss, 351, 355, 356, 358, 410, 441, 444
  role in monitoring hearing performance, 127, 156-57, 405-6, 434, 436, 439
  training with FM systems, 19, 155 (see also Family)
Perilymphatic fistula, 148, 351, 410
Persistent pulmonary hypertension of the newborn, 348
Phoneme recognition, 284-85, 300, 370, 376, 385
Position statement,
  on amplification for infants and children with hearing loss, 119, 120, 399-415
  on early intervention, 162
Presbycusis, 80-81, 83-85
Prescription of Gain and Output (POGO) method, 109-10, 181, 187, 416-17
Preselection (of device), 16-19, 113-17, 119, 145-47, 153-56, 354, 402, 411, 432
  behind-the-ear hearing aid, 146, 147, 402-3
  classroom amplification, 316-17, 328, 329-31
  cochlear implant, 147, 301-2
  FM systems, 19, 113, 116, 155-56, 231-32, 244-45, 274-79, 281, 316-17, 328, 329
  transposition hearing aid, 147, 263
  vibrotactile device, 147, 287

Real-ear-to-coupler difference (RECD), 17, 181-83, 185, 198, 206, 266, 401, 404, 405, 407, 424-25, 431-33, 436-37, 439, 442
  age, 151-52, 181, 404, 420, 424-25, 431, 437, 439
  method, 151-52, 198-99, 209, 279-80
  variability, 403, 436-37
Reduced aspect feature transcription (RAFT), 40-49
Refsum syndrome, 345
Rehabilitation Act (Section 504), 333, 334 (see also Laws and regulations)
Repetition, 57-68, 70, 71, 386, 393, 394
Research, future directions,
  acclimatization, 156, 171-72
  auditory skills, 49, 69-71, 318, 411-12
  evaluating technology, 263-64, 269-70, 281
  profound hearing loss, 281-305
  selection methods, 187-88, 209-10, 411-12
  sound field amplification, 238, 243, 244, 328
  speech perception, 56-57, 171-72, 411-12
  test development, 318, 411-12
Retention of device, 153, 154-55, 402, 409, 444, 446
Reverberation, 200, 208, 220, 231, 327, 371, 408
  in educational settings, 229-30, 231, 234-35, 236, 242-43, 245, 246, 311, 324, 333, 384, 385, 389
  and speech perception, 274, 313
Rubella, congenital, 346

Safety, 146, 154, 316, 400, 402, 408, 410, 412, 444
Scheibe dysplasia, 347
School district, responsibility, 223-24, 352, 448-49
  (see also Laws and regulations)
School personnel, 331, 339, 407, 410, 411
  attitudes toward amplification, 241-42, 245-46,
  monitoring of device, 216, 219, 220, 221-23, 405-6
  training of, 141, 221, 241-42, 246, 279, 316, 317, 357, 386, 389, 406, 447-48, 450, 451-52
Screening, universal, 188-89
Screening Instrument for Targeting Educational Risk (SIFTER), 241, 317, 318, 331-32, 334, 355, 357, 358, 395, 406, 447-48
  pre-school, 395, 406

Seating, 235, 327
  preferential, 235-37, 328, 333, 394, 448
  (see also Acoustics; Distance)
Selection (of electroacoustic characteristics),
  109-10, 172-76, 178-89, 193-95, 266, 279,
  328, 400, 403-5, 416-22, 424-25
  computer-assisted, 181, 185, 195-210, 266-
    70, 403, 420, 431-32, 437, 439
  methods,
    Berger, 109-10
    DSL, 18, 109-10, 181-86, 187, 219,
      419-22, 424-25, 431-32, 437,
      439
      for transposition device, 266-
        70
    NAL, 109-10, 181, 187, 418-19
    POGO, 109-10, 181, 187, 416-17
    SHARP, 194-210
  (see also Frequency response; Gain; Output
    limiting)
Self-monitoring of speech, 4, 8, 22, 371, 372,
  384, 405, 446
  speech spectrum, 152-53, 200-1, 202, 204-8
  with FM system, 147, 155, 273, 279, 328-29
Self-perception, 390, 386, 396, 453
Sign language, 7, 32, 45
Signal detection, 152, 370, 387, 388 (see also
  Speech perception)
Signal processing, 187, 209, 257-59, 405
  in cochlear implant, 286-87, 300-1, 302-3,
    304-5
Signal-to-noise ratio, 148, 152, 313, 314, 317,
  411
  in educational setting, 229-30, 232-35, 236,
    238, 242-43, 273-74, 314, 324, 326,
    327, 328, 329, 330-31, 334, 358, 384,
    385, 445-46, 450
  with FM system, 19, 20, 116, 155, 231, 244-
    45, 274, 317, 391, 407, 408, 450
Situational hearing aid response profile
  (SHARP), 194-210
Social development, 230, 236, 326-27, 395, 407
  risk of problems, 245, 311, 323, 334, 386,
    447
Sound fidelity, 242-43, 317, 409
Sound field testing, 99-102, 219, 263, 266, 332,
  334, 355, 406
  and speech perception, 169-72, 173
  test-retest variability, 168-69, 196
Sound pressure level, 170, 176, 178-79, 195-96,
  409

  real-ear, 180, 182, 401, 403
  saturation, 152, 162, 184, 195-96, 267, 277,
    404, 425, 433, 437-39
  target, 217, 421-22, 425
Special education, 311, 312, 318, 333, 334, 392,
  448-49, 453
  impact of amplification, 23, 240, 243-44,
    316, 331
Speech discrimination, 152, 322, 323, 325, 334
Speech perception, 8-9, 29-32, 49, 179, 327,
  328, 357, 371-73, 380, 401-2, 405
  across settings, 193, 195, 276
  and frequency, 203, 253-54, 255-57, 261,
    262, 263
  and speech production, 55-71, 376-78
  impact of hearing loss, 32-33, 59-69, 324-25
  in educational settings, 229-46
  in noise, 155, 245, 322-23, 332-33, 385, 386,
    389
  in validation of hearing performance, 164,
    165, 171-72, 173
  temporal cues, 203, 288
  test, 283-86, 288-89, 299, 300, 301, 318, 370,
    377, 406
    with visual cues, 285, 289, 292-93, 295,
      296-97, 298, 299, 374-75
  visual, 56, 68 (see also Speechreading)
  with cochlear implants, 283-302, 304-5
  with FM system, 274, 277, 358
  with transposition devices, 253-55, 256, 263,
    264, 266
  with vibrotactile device, 289-95, 302
Speech production, 31-32, 33-48, 55, 57, 370,
  385, 446
  and speech perception, 56, 57, 62-66, 68-69,
    284, 325, 376-78
  benefits of amplification, 34, 45, 57, 69, 70,
    240-41, 256, 263
  impact of hearing loss, 32, 33-48, 57, 60-69,
    70, 71, 152, 381, 451
  role of auditory capacity, 29, 32, 49-50
  learning opportunity, 57, 69, 70, 377-79
Speech recognition, 233, 244, 279, 289, 304-5,
  313-14, 315, 374-75, 385, 402
  test, 111-12, 238-39, 264, 280, 284-85, 426-
    28
    in noise, 111-12, 231-36, 451
    open-set, 288-89, 292, 294-96, 298,
      299, 300, 302, 303, 305
    with sound field amplification, 236-39,
      242-43

with visual cues, 255, 263, 285, 292-93, 294-95, 296-97, 298, 299, 302
(see also Speech perception; Word recognition)
Speech spectrum, 169, 179, 184, 187, 200-2, 370, 400, 404
across settings, 152-53, 193, 194-95, 202-3, 204-8
audible, 194-210, 202-4, 268-69, 315, 381, 382, 400, 402, 406
feature extraction, 286-87, 299, 300-1, 304-5
long-term average (LTASS), 179, 194, 200-2, 205, 206, 207, 209, 421, 424, 431
target, 433, 439
transposed, 254, 255, 256, 259-60, 263
Speech-language pathologist, 357, 405-9, 411
Speech-language therapy, 357, 392, 450, 451-52
Speech-to-noise ratio (see Signal-to-noise ratio)
Speechreading, 7, 56, 59, 70, 292-93, 294-95, 296
and cochlear implants, 295, 296
and vibrotactile aid, 295, 302
blocking, 285, 288, 289, 373-75
Stickler syndrome, 345, 409
Stigma, 15, 18-19, 243, 245, 276, 317, 358, 450
Syphilis, 346-47, 351

Teacher evaluation,
of amplification, 241-42, 246
for at-risk behaviors, 241, 331-32, 355, 393-95
Teacher performance, 229, 240, 246
Telephone use, 408
Test-retest reliability, 173, 178, 199, 405
of sound field testing, 168-69, 196
of speech recognition tests, 171-72, 285-86
Threshold, 17, 69, 79-80, 130, 139, 178, 181, 195-96, 203, 322, 331, 400-2, 404, 419, 433, 436, 447
and selection of electroacoustics, 404, 418, 420, 421-22, 424
candidacy criteria, 303-4
masked, 17, 78, 167
measurement, 130-31, 441-42
pure tone, 56, 69, 238, 287-88, 298
shift, 340, 350
sound field, 111-12, 130-31, 164, 165-70, 174, 175, 176-78, 182-84, 219, 267, 333, 334, 405, 434-36
comparative, 168-69, 178

limitations, 98-99, 112, 166-69, 170-71, 172-73, 176-77, 196, 266, 280, 401
speech detection, 264, 266
Tone,
control, 8, 17, 168, 274, 275, 395
pure, 197, 209-10, 404, 405, 416
warble, 17, 127, 404
Transposition, device, 253-70, 287, 302, 380
compared with cochlear implant, 263-65

Usher syndrome, 344-45

Validation (of aided performance), 32-33, 161, 215, 331, 370, 404, 405
comparative, 164-66, 168-71, 209, 242-43, 244-45, 283, 288-95, 297, 298-305, 328
with sound field thresholds, 112, 164, 165-71, 176-77, 405
with transposition device, 254-56, 263
(see also Speech recognition tests)
Verification (of electroacoustic characteristics), 17, 32, 109-13, 173-75, 187, 215, 400, 403-5, 432
for FM system, 112, 276-77, 279-80
real-ear-to-coupler difference method, 151-52, 197-99, 209, 279-80
Vibrotactile device, 147, 157, 256, 283, 284, 286, 288, 380, 446
dual-channel, 286, 287, 289-90, 291, 302
multichannel, 286, 287, 289-95, 302
Volume control, 155, 266, 274, 276, 410, 425
Vowel
discrimination, 371, 372
height, 41-48, 56, 58, 67, 284, 296-97, 298, 299, 301
neutralization, 42, 44-48
perception, 254, 256, 260-61, 264-65, 266, 284, 289, 291-92, 293, 296-97, 298, 299, 301, 304
place, 56, 58, 67-68, 284, 296-97, 298, 299, 371, 376
production, 40-48

Waardenburg's syndrome, 345
West, Robert, 1-2
Word recognition, 148-49, 260, 288, 322, 323, 324, 334, 385

test, 31, 33, 165, 171, 255-56, 263, 289, 302, 370
   closed-set, 264, 375
   in noise, 234-35, 313, 332-33, 334
   limitations, 171-73
   open-set, 264, 303
   with sound field amplification, 237-39, 242-43

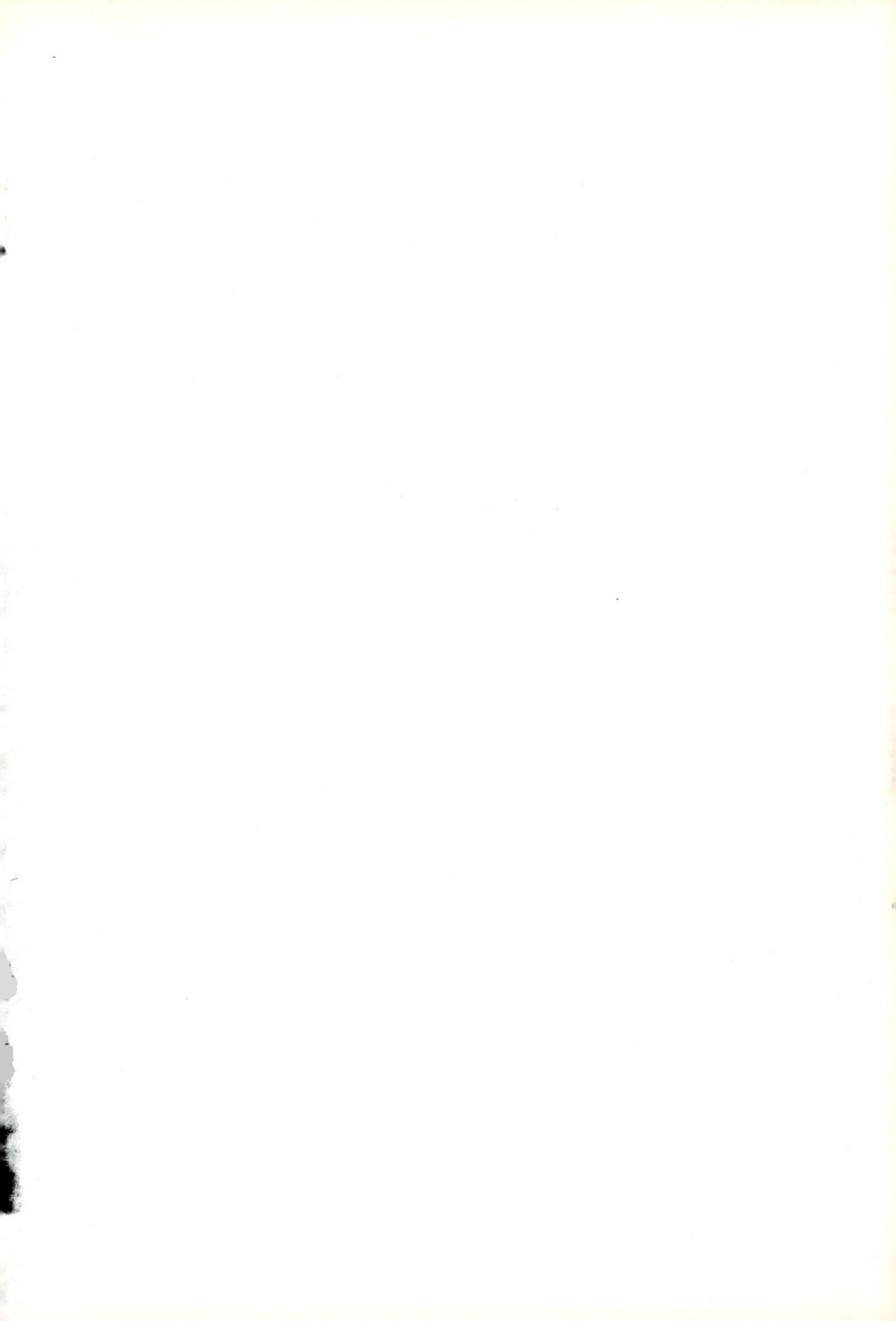